Cardiology
1984

Cardiology: 1984

Printed in the United States of America

First Edition

International Standard Book Number: 0-914316-42-7

International Standard Serial Number: 0275-0066

Cardiology
1984

WILLIAM C. ROBERTS, MD, Editor
Chief, Pathology Branch
National Heart, Lung, and Blood Institute
National Institutes of Health, Bethesda, Maryland, and
Clinical Professor of Pathology and Medicine (Cardiology)
Georgetown University, Washington, D.C.
Editor-in-Chief, The American Journal of Cardiology

CHARLES E. RACKLEY, MD
Chairman, Department of Medicine
Anton and Margaret Fuisz
Professor of Medicine
Georgetown University Medical Center
Washington, D.C.

DEAN T. MASON, MD
Physician-in-Chief
Western Heart Institute
St. Mary's Hospital and Medical Center
San Francisco, California
Editor-in-Chief, American Heart Journal

JAMES T. WILLERSON, MD
Professor of Medicine
Chief, Division of Cardiology
Department of Medicine
University of Texas Health Science Center
Dallas, Texas

THOMAS P. GRAHAM, JR, MD
Professor of Pediatrics
Chief, Division of Pediatric Cardiology
Department of Pediatrics
Vanderbilt University
Nashville, Tennessee

ALBERT D. PACIFICO, MD
Professor of Surgery
Department of Surgery
University of Alabama Medical Center
Birmingham, Alabama

ROBERT B. KARP, MD
Chief, Cardiac Surgery Section
Department of Surgery
University of Chicago Medical Center
Chicago, Illinois

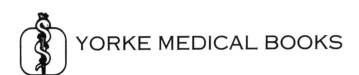

YORKE MEDICAL BOOKS

Contents

5. Valvular Heart Disease

Preface

Cardiology 1984 is the fourth book to be published in this series. Each year the book has gotten bigger. *Cardiology 1981* summarized 446 articles; *Cardiology 1982*, 665 articles; *Cardiology 1983*, 721 articles; and *Cardiology 1984*, 809 articles. Two major reasons account for the 12% increase in the number of articles summarized in the 1984 Edition compared to the 1983 edition. 1) An additional major cardiology journal, namely *The Journal of The American College of Cardiology*, began in January 1983 and 337 articles were published in it during its first year. Of them, 69 were summarized in CARDIOLOGY 1984. 2) The number of articles published in the regular issues of *The American Journal of Cardiology* in 1983 increased by 40% over the number published in this *Journal* in 1982 (from 389 to 643) and therefore the number of articles summarized from this Journal increased accordingly.

The number of articles summarized by each of the 7 authors is tabulated below. Rackley's submissions were from *Circulation*; Mason's, from *The American Heart Journal*; Willerson's, from *The Journal of The American College of Cardiology*. Roberts' contributions were from *The American Journal of Cardiology, The American Journal of Medicine, Annals of Internal Medicine, Archives of Internal Medicine, British Heart Journal, Journal of the American Medical Association, Lancet*, and the *New England Journal of Medicine*. Karp's, Pacifico's and Graham's contributions also were from several journals. The summaries from each contributor were submitted to me, edited and organized into the 9 chapters.

CARDIOLOGY 1984

AUTHOR	CHAPTER NUMBER									TOTALS	
	1	2	3	4	5	6	7	8	9		
WCR	88	71	82	47	63	26	3	21	30	431	(53.28%)
CER	42	18	7	10	10	10	0	9	5	111	(13.72%)
DTM	29	13	13	8	6	4	5	6	2	86	(10.63%)
JTW	25	6	16	0	7	1	0	8	6	69	(8.53%)
TPG Jr	0	0	4	0	0	0	35	0	0	39	(4.82%)
ADP	0	0	0	0	0	0	37	0	0	37	(4.57%)
RBK	19	3	0	0	13	1	0	0	0	36	(4.45%)
TOTALS	203	111	122	65	99	42	80	44	43	809	(100%)

A book of this type is made possible because of unselfish contributions from several individuals, none of whom are rewarded by authorship. I am especially indebted to Margorie Hadsell who typed superbly all 431 summaries contributed by me. Margaret M. M. Moore and Rebecca Fanning organized the figures and tables for photography. Mary McMahon typed the large table of contents. Tamsin Wolff, Leslie Silvernail, Barbara Hassler, Belinda Lambert, Evelyn Woods, and Sue Long also typed numerous summaries. Ann K. Bradley managed to carry the 25 pound package of summaries, references, figures and tables from Bethesda to New York. Gay C. Morgulas, Director of Yorke Medical Books, again coordinated publication with her usual finesse and expertise.

WILLIAM C. ROBERTS, MD
EDITOR

1

Coronary Heart Disease

DETECTION
(HISTORY, PHYSICAL EXAMINATION, ELECTROCARDIOGRAM, VITAL
CAPACITY, COLD PRESSOR TEST, ECHOCARDIOGRAM)

---

*Frequency of utilization of cardiologic tests and of
recommending aortocoronary bypass grafting by various
groups of physicians*

Hlatky and associates[1] from San Francisco, California, and Durham,
North Carolina, provided 91 physicians (26 either full time or clinical
members of the cardiology division of a university hospital, 11 cardiologists
in a prepaid group practice (HMO), and 54 unassociated with either
organization but practicing in the community) with case summaries of the
same patients in a management simulation setting. Using summaries of
actual patients complaining of chest pain and suspected of having CAD, the
physicians rated the need for 2 diagnostic tests, exercise thallium scintigraphy and coronary angiography. Since both tests are relatively expensive
(roughly $600 for thallium scintigraphy and $3,000 for coronary angiography), prescribing these tests obviously can make a significant difference in
terms of dollars. Each cardiologist was first asked to define the groups of
patients in whom he/she would recommend CABG even if the patients'
symptoms could be controlled with medication. Consecutive patients with
chest pain who had undergone both exercise thallium scintigraphy and
coronary angiography were studied. After review of the summaries, the

cardiologists rated the need for the exercise thallium scintiscan and for a coronary angiogram in each case. Community cardiologists had the broadest indications for CABG. The HMO cardiologists chose thallium scintigraphy significantly less often than did the other 2 groups of cardiologists. The HMO and university cardiologists both rated the need for coronary angiography significantly lower than did community cardiologists. Thus, physicians in different practice settings recommend costly diagnostic and therapeutic methods differently, even for identical patients.

Estimating the likelihood of CAD

Pryor and associates[2] from Durham, North Carolina, determined which characteristics obtained by the physician during his initial assessment were important for estimating the likelihood of significant CAD and whether the estimates using these characteristics were valid over time when applied to different patient populations. Among the 23 clinical characteristics examined in 3,627 consecutive, symptomatic patients referred for cardiac catheterization between 1969 and 1979, 9 were found to be important for estimating the likelihood that a patient had significant CAD. These included chest pain, previous AMI, sex, age, smoking history, hyperlipidemia, ST-T wave changes, diabetes mellitus, and the interactions of age with sex, smoking, and hyperlipidemia. A model using these characteristics accurately estimated the likelihood of CAD when applied prospectively to 1,811 patients referred after 1979 and when used to estimate prevalence of CAD in subgroups reported in medical journals.

Noninvasive assessment of CAD

DePace and associates[3] from Philadelphia, Pennsylvania, performed a study to determine whether a mathematical model can be used to assess noninvasively the extent of CAD. The model was based on stepwise multivariate discriminant analysis of data obtained in 99 patients from clinical and nonhemodynamic exercise variables, or from RNA determination of LV function at rest or during exercise, or both. The extent of CAD was assessed by a scoring system and by the number of diseased arteries. The variables selected by this method (Q-wave AMI, exercise LV EF, change in systolic BP from rest to exercise, sex, and diabetes mellitus) yielded a predictive accuracy of 82% for the identification of patients with extensive CAD (score ≥35). Slightly better results were achieved by a subgroup of 77 patients who had adequate exercise end points (exercise heart rate ≥120 beats/min, or angina or ST depression during exercise). In these patients, the predictive accuracy was 84%. The model also identified patients with "light" CAD (score ≤10) with a predictive accuracy of 82%. Thus, noninvasive assessment of the extent of CAD is possible with a stepwise multivariate discriminant analysis of clinical, ECG, and LV function assessed by RNA at rest and during exercise. The scoring system was superior to the conventional method of classifying patients according to the number of significantly narrowed coronary arteries.

Vital capacity as a predictor of CAD

The relation of forced vital capacity (FVC) to the development of the major atherosclerotic cardiovascular diseases (CAD, intermittent claudication, stroke), CHF, and cardiovascular mortality was investigated by Kannel and associates[4] from Boston, Massachusetts, based on 20 years of biennial follow-up of 5,209 subjects in the Framingham study. There was a substantial inverse relation of cardiovascular morbidity and deaths to antecedent FVC (incidence of symptoms and mortality were greater with lesser FVC values) adjusting for age and in nonsmokers and in smokers even excluding subjects with pulmonary disease, chest deformity, and CHF. The association was stronger in women than in men and persisted even when other cardiovascular risk factors were taken into account. The association with the development of CHF was striking, but this did not explain the association with excess cardiovascular morbidity and mortality. The FVC ranked high as a predictor in comparison with the major cardiovascular risk factors, particularly in women. Although the pathogenic mechanism relating FVC to cardiovascular disease is unknown, FVC correlated with handgrip strength, suggesting that FVC may be a measure of general health. It was concluded that FVC is a practical office procedure for predicting cardiovascular morbidity and mortality by selecting asymptomatic adult candidates at high risk for future cardiovascular events.

Usefulness of cold pressor test

Wasserman and coworkers[5] from Washington, D.C., compared cold pressor stimulation (CPS) with supine bicycle exercise during RNA as a procedure for diagnosing CAD in 30 patients. In the 18 patients with angiographically proved CAD, LV EF decreased a mean of 5 EF units in response to CPS. Two patients developed a new wall motion abnormality. In response to maximal supine exercise, the CAD group showed a mean decrease in LV EF from rest of 2%. Nine patients developed an exercise-induced wall motion abnormality. In the 12 patients with angiographically proved normal coronary arteries, LV EF decreased a mean of 6 units in response to CPS and increased a mean of 9% in response to exercise. Thus, the LV EF response to CPS was not significantly different in CAD and in normal groups (5 -vs- 6). These same patients demonstrated the expected difference in LV EF response to exercise. Thus, CPS is not useful in diagnosing CAD.

Mitral E point septal separation

The diagnostic value of E point septal separation (EPSS) was assessed in 108 patients with CAD who underwent coronary angiography and M-mode echo within a 2-year period by Ahmadpour and associates[6] from Los Angeles, California. In patients with remote anterior AMI, EPSS correlated well with EF determined angiography (specificity, 85%; sensitivity, 82%). In remote inferior AMI, a 21% frequency of falsely elevated EPSS values were encountered (sensitivity, 100%; specificity, 67%). In combined remote anterior and inferior AMI, EPSS accurately estimated abnormal EF with a sensitivity and specificity of 100%. An abnormal EPSS (>7 mm) was found to be more sensitive (87%) and specific (75%) in detecting individuals with angiographically determined reduced EF (<50%) compared with other echo indices of pump function. Also, EPSS was effective in estimating LV function in the presence of left BBB, paradoxical septal motion, and angiographic septal, posterior, and anterior wall motion abnormalities.

Exercise (non-RNA) stress testing

Famularo and associates[7] from Long Beach, California, studied septal Q-wave amplitudes in lead CM_5 to evaluate its utility in predicting segmental CAD. Q-wave amplitudes were measured in 41 patients with CAD before and immediately after treadmill exercise. All patients studied had either significant 1-vessel CAD (>70% diameter reduction) or normal coronary anatomy, 13 had LAD CAD, 8 had right coronary occlusions, 8 had LC CAD, and 12 had angiographically determined normal coronary arteries. Septal Q-wave amplitude measurements at rest and during peak exercise were recorded in 0.5 mm increments and classified as increasing in 20 patients, decreasing in 8, and no change in 13 with exercise. All 13 patients with isolated LAD narrowing had either no change (5 patients) or a decrease (8 patients) in the septal Q wave with exercise (Fig. 1-1). Statistical analysis revealed 62% sensitivity and 100% specificity for single LAD narrowing if a decreasing Q wave was noted with exercise. Patients with isolated right or LC CAD or normal coronary anatomy had mixed septal Q-wave responses to exercise. Only patients with LAD narrowing had reductions in Q-wave amplitude with treadmill exercise. This finding suggests that low Q-wave voltage and its failure to increase after exercise imply abnormal septal activation, reflecting loss of contraction associated with ischemia from LAD narrowing.

To determine the frequency and significance of transient intraventricular conduction abnormalities occurring in association with myocardial ischemia during exercise testing, Boran and associates[8] from Lackland Air Force Base, Texas, reviewed the recordings of 2,200 consecutive exercise tests. Ten patients (0.45%) had both ischemia and intraventricular conduction abnormalities that developed transiently during the exercise test. In all 10 patients both typical angina and ECG evidence of ischemia developed during exercise. Among the 10 patients, left anterior hemiblock developed in 4, left posterior hemiblock in 2, right BBB in 2, right BBB with left axis deviation in 1, and left anterior hemiblock progressing to complete left BBB in 1. All 10 patients had cardiac catheterization showing significant obstruction of the LAD coronary artery at or before the origin of the first septal branch. Eight patients were treated surgically and 2 medically, all with relief of ischemic symptoms. Nine of the 10 had repeat exercise stress testing without angina or ECG evidence of ischemia and without recurrence of the transient intraventricular conduction disturbance. Thus, development of transient intraventricular conduction abnormalities associated with myocardial ischemia during exercise testing is uncommon (0.45%). When such conduction disturbances do develop, the existence of significant disease in the proximal portion of the LAD coronary artery is strongly suggested. With control of myocardial ischemia, the transient conduction disturbances during exercise are ameliorated.

Colby and associates[9] from Philadelphia, Pennsylvania, evaluated the results of treadmill exercise ECGs in 179 patients with significant CAD involving ≥1 vessel to determine the prognostic significance of the magnitude of ST-segment depression during exercise. Exercise ECGs were strongly positive in 51 patients, mildly positive (1–1.9 mm ST-segment depression) in 28 patients, falsely negative in 23 patients, and uninterpretable in 77 patients. The degree of exercise-induced ST-segment depression did not

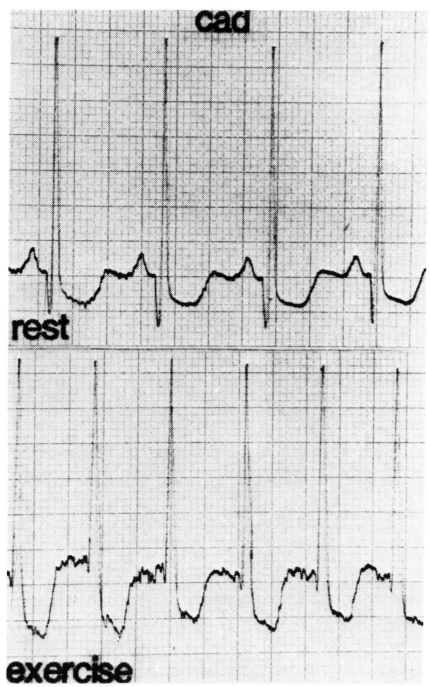

Fig. 1-1. Q–wave response to exercise in patient with 1–vessel LAD coronary artery disease (CAD).

correlate with LV function, extent of CAD, exercise heart rates, and rate-pressure product, or the extent of exercise-induced thallium-201 perfusion abnormality. However, marked ST-segment depression at heart rates of ≥140 beats/minute or an advanced stage of exercise in the Bruce protocol was predictive of less extensive CAD and perfusion abnormalities. Thus, the data obtained in this study demonstrate that the magnitude of ST-segment depression during exercise is not predictive of the extent of CAD, even in patients with ≥3 mm ST-segment depression. However, a strongly positive exercise ECG in the first 2 stages of the Bruce protocol or at a heart rate of >140 beats/minute is related to the extent of CAD and impaired myocardial perfusion.

Currie and associates[10] from Melbourne, Australia, compared exercise-induced ECG ST depression during supine and erect graded bicycle exercise in 43 patients with chest pain but no prior AMI. All had ≥1 mm of ST depression during either erect or supine exercise, 16 had multivessel, 24 had 1-vessel, and 3 had no CAD. Supine exercise used 4 minutes/stage, and erect exercise used either 4 or 3 minutes/stage with identical graded work loads for both postures. Chest pain occurred in 31 patients during erect and in 29 patients during supine exercise. ST depression was ≥1 mm in 28 patients during erect exercise and in all 43 patients during supine exercise ($p <$ 0.001); mean maximal ST depression was 1.3 ± 0.2 mm during erect and 2.6 ± 0.2 mm during supine exercise ($p < 0.001$). Maximal work load was higher during erect than supine exercise (745 ± 32 -vs- 678 ± 32 kpm/min; $p < 0.001$). The accentuation of ST depression by supine posture was not attributable to the changes in heart rate, rate-pressure product, or mean BP during supine -vs- erect exercise. In the 10 patients who had 2 erect bicycle tests using work load durations of 3 and 4 minutes, the maximal ST depression was not significantly different (erect 3 minutes, 1.3 ± 0.5 mm; erect 4 minutes, 1.4 ± 0.4 mm). In 7 patients who also had a maximal treadmill exercise test, the maximal ST depression was significantly greater during supine exercise (2.3 ± 0.4 mm) than during either an erect bicycle test (0.6 ± 0.4 mm) or treadmill exercise (0.7 ± 0.4 mm) ($p < 0.05$). Supine posture should be considered as an important potentiator of exercise-induced myocardial ischemia when comparing indicators such as ECG, RNA, and thallium-201 myocardial perfusion imaging during exercise.

Califf and associates[11] from Durham, North Carolina, evaluated the prognostic information obtained from exercise testing by following patients in whom ventricular arrhythmias developed with treadmill exercise testing. Of 1,293 consecutive nonsurgically treated patients undergoing an exercise test within 6 weeks of cardiac catheterization, 236 patients developed simple ventricular arrhythmias with exercise. These patients had a higher prevalence of significant CAD (57% -vs- 44%), 3-vessel CAD (31 -vs- 17%), and abnormal LV function (43 -vs- 24%) than did patients without ventricular arrhythmias. In patients with complex ventricular ectopic activity, including paired VPC or VT, there was an even higher prevalence of significant CAD (75%), 3-vessel CAD (39%), and abnormal LV function (54%). Those patients with significant CAD and paired VPC or VT had a lower 3-year survival rate (75%) than did patients with simple ventricular arrhythmias (83%) and those with no ventricular arrhythmias (90%). Therefore these data suggest that ventricular arrhythmias developing with treadmill exercise testing have prognostic importance, but they make no independent contribution to prognostic insight once the location and extent of CAD are known. In patients without significant CAD, no relation between ventricular arrhythmias and survival was found.

Radionuclide angiography without exercise

Newman and associates[12] from Sydney, Australia, correlated thalium defects in the LV inferior and lateral walls with right and LC CAD in 405 patients who underwent coronary arteriography. In the 102 patients with either single right or LC CAD, inferior segment defects (anterior view) were associated with right CAD, and both lateral segment defects (40° left anterior oblique [LAO] view) and posteroinferior defects (60° LAO view) were associated with LC CAD. In all 405 patients, inferior segment defects had a sensitivity of 65%, a specificity of 92%, and a predictive accuracy of 89% for right CAD, and lateral segment defects had a sensitivity of 52%, a specificity of 96%, and a predictive accuracy of 90% for LC CAD. Posteroinferior defects had a low predictive accuracy for narrowing in either artery. The presence or absence of concomitant anterior defects did not alter these results. Narrowing in both right and LC coronary arteries was best identified by a combination of inferior and lateral segment defects (sensitivity, 30%; specificity, 96%; predictive accuracy, 72%). Narrowing in only 1 of these 2 arteries was best identified by a combination of inferior segment without lateral segment defects for right CAD (sensitivity, 63%; specificity, 86%; predictive accuracy, 55%) and lateral segment without inferior segment defects for LC CAD (sensitivity, 45%; specificity, 92%; predictive accuracy, 57%). Thallium scanning identifies significant narrowing in the right and LC coronary arteries, and these may be separated by the pattern of defects.

Okada and associates[13] from Boston, Massachusetts, evaluated 30 patients with a new technique for thallium-201 imaging, "split dose thallium-201 administration," with dipyridamole infusion. With the patient supine at rest, 1.0 mC thallium was injected intravenously and imaging performed in the anterior and 50° LAO projections for a preset time. Immediately after acquisition of the rest images, an infusion of dipyridamole at 0.15 mg/kg/minute for 4 minutes was initiated. Two minutes after discontinuing the dipyridamole, 1.0 mC thallium-201 was injected intravenously and the LAO and anterior projection images were acquired once again. Two and a half to 3 hours after the dipyridamole infusion, myocardial imaging was repeated. Images utilizing the same projections were realigned using a computer image registration approach. The rest image was subtracted from the realigned dipyridamole image to produce an image representing perfusion during dipyridamole-induced hyperemia. The subtraction images were of adequate quality for interpretation in 29 of 30 patients. Of 45 stenosed coronary arteries, 84% demonstrated thallium-201 defects in appropriate segments, whereas of 42 normal coronary arteries, 98% demonstrated normal thallium-201 activity in the corresponding segments. The overall sensitivity and specificity of the subtraction versus rest thallium image technique for detecting anatomically important CAD were 91 and 100%, respectively. Thus, this study describes a new method for obtaining thallium-201 evaluation of the patient with chest pain and suggests that this methodology will be an alternative to exercise thallium-201 scintigraphy for purposes of detecting physiologically important CAD.

Radionuclide angiography with exercise

Although exercise radionuclide ventriculography (RVG) was initially reported to be a highly specific test for CAD, later studies reported a high false positive test. To verify this turnabout, Rozanski and associates[14] from Los Angeles, California, analyzed the responses in 77 angiographically normal patients; 32 were studied from 1978–1979 (the early period), and 45 from 1980–1982 (the recent period). Most patients studied in the early period had normal responses (94% for EF and 84% for wall motion). In contrast, normal responses were less frequent in patients studied in the recent period (49% for EF and 36% for wall motion; p < 0.001). The probability of CAD before testing was higher in these patients (38 -vs- 7%; p < 0.001). More patients studied in the recent period underwent RVG before angiography (78 -vs- 22%; p < 0.001), and more of these prior studies had abnormal results than those performed after angiography (55 -vs- 6%; p < 0.0001). Thus, 2 factors are responsible for the temporal decline in specificity: a change in the population being tested (pretest referral bias) and a preferential selection of patients with a positive test response for coronary angiography (post-test referral bias).

Bodenheimer and associates[15] from Philadelphia, Pennsylvania, studied 48 patients to determine relative advantages and disadvantages of isotonic and isometric stress with RVG in the noninvasive detection of CAD. All patients had first-pass RNA using a multicrystal camera at rest, during handgrip exercise, and maximal bicycle exercise; 28 had CAD and 20 had normal coronary arteries. Bicycle exercise caused a significantly higher rate-pressure product. Alterations in LV EF during handgrip exercise did not distinguish patients with or without CAD. However, 82% of the patients with CAD considered significant angiographically demonstrated an increase of <5 units in LV EF during bicycle exercise. Assessment of regional ventricular EF during bicycle exercise indicated a sensitivity of 75% and a specificity of 65% for CAD. The specificity for the global LV EF measurement during bicycle exercise was relatively low regarding specific detection of CAD. Thus, these data suggest that upright bicycle exercise combined with RVG and analysis of regional EF provides a more optimal assessment of the presence or absence of CAD than does isotonic handgrip exercise.

Brown and associates[16] from Boston, Massachusetts, studied 47 patients undergoing angiography for the evaluation of chest pain utilizing exercise-induced changes in hepatic blood volume compared with alterations in RV and LV EF at exercise. Hepatic blood activity was measured on separate 20-second anterior static liver images at rest and peak exercise during supine stress. Average hepatic counts per picture element at exercise compared with rest were used to determine an exercise/rest hepatic blood volume ratio. In patients with normal coronary arteries and those with CAD limited to the left coronary artery, a significant decrease in hepatic counts with exercise occurred. Patients with proximal right CAD had no change in hepatic counts with exercise. Mean hepatic blood volume ratio was greatest among patients demonstrating a decrease in RV EF during exercise (p < 0.01). Thus, alterations in hepatic blood volume in response to exercise can be utilized to predict the presence of proximal right CAD and RV functional alterations during stress.

DePace and associates[17] from Philadelphia, Pennsylvania, evaluated 65 patients to determine the relation between LV function during exercise and the extent of CAD. Among these patients, 26 had CAD (≥70% luminal diameter narrowing) of 1 vessel, 21 had multivessel CAD, and 18 had no significant CAD. Exercise LV EF was significantly higher in patients with no CAD (p < 0.001), but there was considerable overlap among the 3 groups. A fair correlation was found between the extent of CAD and the exercise LV EF (r = −0.70; p < 0.001). In patients whose exercise heart rate was ≥130 beats/minute and who were ≤50 years of age, the correlation between these variables was r = −0.73 and −0.82, respectively. Thus, these data suggest that the exercise EF may be used to estimate the extent of CAD and that the predictive ability of this variable is greatest in patients of younger age who achieve higher heart rates during exercise.

A study by Gewirtz and associates[18] from Providence, Rhode Island, was done to test the hypothesis that recognition of delayed washout of thallium from myocardial scan zones with apparently normal thallium uptake is useful for identifying patients with 3-vessel CAD. Exercise thallium stress tests were performed in 21 patients with angiographically proved 3-vessel CAD (≥50% diameter reduction of all 3 major vessels). Anterior and left anterior oblique thallium images were obtained 5–10 minutes after stress and 2 hours later. Background corrected scans (bilinear interpolative method) were analyzed by computer (radial analysis program) for the presence of initial uptake defects as well as delayed thallium washout. Twenty-five patients with 1- or 2-vessel CAD and 14 patients with normal coronary arteries also were studied to obtain specificity data regarding the diagnosis of 3-vessel CAD. In patients with 3-vessel CAD, 50 (79%) of 63 narrowed vessels were detected by combined use of uptake and washout criteria. However, only 8 (13%) of 63 narrowed arteries were detected by washout criteria alone. Nevertheless, use of washout criteria did increase the number of patients correctly identified as having 3-vessel CAD from 7 (identified on the basis of uptake defects alone) to 10. Accordingly, sensitivity using both uptake and washout criteria was 48% (10 of 21 patients). Specificity for the diagnosis of 3-vessel CAD using combined uptake and washout criteria was 76% for patients with 1- or 2-vessel CAD and 95% for normal patients. This was little different from values obtained based on uptake criteria alone (80 and 100%, respectively). Thus, even though relatively few stenosed vessels in patients with 3-vessel CAD are associated with isolated thallium washout abnormalities, use of washout criteria does increase the sensitivity of the thallium stress test for the detection of such patients and therefore is a worthwhile addition to routine uptake analysis of thallium images of the myocardium.

In an investigation performed by Gutman and associates[19] from Los Angeles, California, the relation between the severity of CAD and the time to completed redistribution of ^{201}Tl defects following maximal exercise was investigated in 59 patients undergoing stress redistribution ^{201}Tl scintigraphy, coronary angiography, and contrast ventriculography. Multiple view ^{201}Tl scintigrams were obtained, beginning 6 minutes (immediately after stress), <1 hour (early), 3–5 hours (average), and 18–24 hours (late) following intravenous ^{201}Tl injection at peak exercise. Angiographic lesions were grouped into 5 levels of severity by percent stenosis. In the 107 defects that were seen on the immediate poststress images, early redistribution was noted in 15 (14%) and late redistribution was found in 23 (21%). In addition, there was a correlation (r = 0.56) between the time to completed redistribution and the severity of the CAD (p = 0.001). In comparison to defects with early and average redistribution, the segments contralateral to those with defects showing late redistribution more often had a critical stenosis supplying that segment. The frequency of healed myocardial infarction on ECG and the number of segments with akinetic and dyskinetic wall motion were less in defects undergoing late rather than no redistribution. Thus, the time to completed ^{201}Tl redistribution following stress appears to be related to the severity of stenosis in the coronary artery supplying the defect. Also, late redistribution is associated with the presence and early redistribution with the absence of a significant stenosis in the coronary artery to the contralateral segment.

Iskandrian and associates[20] from Philadelphia, Pennsylvania, studied 42 symptomatic patients with CAD involving 2 or 3 coronary arteries using exercise ^{201}Tl myocardial scintigraphy. Qualitative analysis of the images predicted multivessel CAD in 75% of the patients with 2-vessel CAD and in 82% of the patients with 3-vessel CAD. Quantitative analysis of the size of the perfusion defect indicated that approximately 40% of the LV perimeter showed abnormal perfusion pattern during stress in these patients, and there was no significant difference in the size of the defect in patients with 2- or 3-vessel CAD (41 ± 17% -vs- 42 ± 14%, respectively, mean ± SD). The exercise heart rate, exercise ECG response, and severity of narrowing did not correlate with the size of the perfusion defect. Patients with anterior infarction had larger defects in the distribution of the LAD than those without infarction. Collaterals offered partial protection during exercise only when they were not jeopardized. This study confirms the value of qualitative analysis of exercise ^{201}Tl imaging in predicting multivessel CAD and describes a simple method of assessing the extent of perfusion abnormalities during stress in patients with multivessel CAD.

LV function was evaluated by Osbakken and associates[21] from Boston, Massachusetts, with rest and supine bicycle exercises multigated blood pool scans in 53 patients who had previously undergone coronary angiography for evaluation of a chest pain syndrome. There were 21 normal patients (<25% stenosis in any coronary artery, LV end-diastolic pressure ≤12 mmHg, and normal left ventriculography) and 32 patients with CAD (>50% narrowing of ≥1 major coronary artery). Thirty-two (60%) were receiving propranolol. The normal patient had a significant increase in mean EF during exercise (+0.08 ± 0.09), but the CAD group had no increase (0 ± 0.11; p < 0.05). Mean ESV decreased significantly in the normal group (-5 ± 8 ml/M^2) but demonstrated no significant change in the CAD group (1 ± 12 ml/M^2; p < 0.05) compared with normal patients. There was no significant change in mean end-diastolic volume in either group. Mean ejection rate, mean peak systolic pressure/ESV ratio, and mean pulmonary blood volume ratio also differed in the normal -vs- CAD patients. Despite mean differences, there was considerable overlap in both groups of individual EF responses: 8 (38%) of 21 of the normal group did not have an increase in EF of 0.05 with exercise, whereas 15 (47%) of 32 of the CAD group did have an increase in EF of 0.05 with exercise. However, the addition of peak systolic pressure/ESV ratio and pulmonary blood volume (exercise/rest) ratio improved the sensitivity for detecting CAD from 53–84% without adversely affecting specificity. Thus, there is a wide spectrum of LV EF responses to supine exercise. EF alone was an insensitive and nonspecific marker of CAD. The addition of other parameters of global LV function that may be generated using RNA helps to distinguish patients with CAD from normal subjects.

Lindsay and colleagues[22] from Washington, D.C., examined the impact of beta adrenergic blocking drugs on the sensitivity and specificity of RNA in 95 patients with angiographically proved CAD and in 22 angiographically normal subjects. Sixty of the former and 7 of the latter were receiving beta adrenergic blocking agents. All had normal regional and global LV function at rest. Exercise-induced asynergy and failure of exercise to increase EF by at least 0.05 were considered abnormal findings. Exercise-induced regional wall motion abnormality was equally frequent (58%) in CAD patients receiving beta blocking drugs and in those who were not. However, the specificity of the criterion, failure to increase EF, was so impaired (87 -vs- 29%) by these agents that the usefulness of that observation for the diagnosis of CAD was negated. Furthermore, an exercise-induced decline in EF of at least 0.05 was observed significantly less frequently in CAD patients receiving beta blockers (30 -vs- 54%; p < 0.025). Therefore the utility of the exercise EF measurement to diagnose CAD is compromised with beta blockers, since that response is often ameliorated by these drugs.

Currie and associates[23] from Melbourne, Australia, assessed the incremental value of clinical assessment, exercise ECG, and biplane RVG in the prediction of CAD in 105 men without AMI in whom coronary angiography had been performed for investigation of chest pain. Graded supine bicycle exercise testing was symptom limited. Right anterior oblique ECG-gated first-pass RVG and left anterior oblique ECG-gated equilibrium RVG were performed at rest and exercise. Regional wall motion abnormalities were defined by agreement of 2 of 3 blinded observers. A combined strongly positive exercise ECG response was defined as ≥2 mm ST depression or 1.0–1.9 mm ST depression with exercise-induced chest pain. A multivariate logistic regression model for the preexercise prediction of CAD was derived from the clinical data and selected 2 variables: chest pain class and cholesterol level. A second model assessed the incremental value of the exercise test in prediction of CAD and found 2 exercise variables that improved prediction: RVG wall motion abnormalities and a combined strongly positive ECG response. Applying the derived predictive models, 37 of the 58 patients (64%) with preexercise probabilities of 10–90% crossed either below the 10% probability threshold or >90% threshold and 28 (48%) also moved across the 5 and 95% thresholds. Supine exercise testing with ECG and biplane RVG together, but neither test alone, effectively adds to clinical prediction of CAD. It is most useful in men with atypical chest pain and when the ECG and RVG results are concordant.

Wackers and associates[24] from New Haven, Connecticut, used sequential first-pass RNA and gold-195m to evaluate 25 patients with known or suspected CAD at the end of each 3-minute stage of exercise and immediately after exercise. The LV EF at rest was assessed with technetium-99m and gold-195m and the results correlated well (r = 0.93). Repeat LV EF at rest with gold-195m correlated closely. Peak LV EF at exercise was abnormal in 20 of 25 patients compared with resting values when gold-195m was used to label the cardiovascular blood pool. These data suggest that multiple, high count rate, first-pass studies of LV function can be performed with accuracy using gold-195m during and after exercise.

Contrast angiography

ANEURYSMAL CAD

Swaye and associates[25] from Miami Beach, Florida, examined the clinical and historic features in the natural history of aneurysmal CAD at 15 participating clinical centers of the multi-institutional Coronary Artery Surgery Study: 978 patients (5% of the total registered population) were identified as having aneurysmal CAD. No significant differences were noted between aneurysmal and nonaneurysmal CAD patients when such features as systemic hypertension, diabetes mellitus, lipid abnormalities, family history, cigarette consumption, incidence of documented AMI, presence and severity of angina, and presence of peripheral vascular disease were examined. No difference in 5-year medical survival was noted between these groups.

CORONARY COLLATERAL VESSELS

The appearance of coronary collateral vessels at coronary angiography generally is believed to provide additional information regarding coronary flow and myocardial oxygen supply beyond that obtained from angiographic assessment of the large coronary arteries. To evaluate the adequacy of this assumption, to determine the relation between angiographic appearance of coronary arteries and of coronary collateral arteries, and to gain additional insight into the mechanisms governing collateral flow in man, Goldberg and associates[26] from New York City examined the coronary angiograms of 121 patients in whom ≥1 coronary artery was narrowed ≥75% in diameter. Collateral vessels were graded absent, poor, or good, based on the size and intensity of filling. Stenosis of the recipient artery significantly affected the angiographic appearance of collateral vessels. No artery with <90% stenosis received angiographically detectable collateral vessels; 118 of the 193 vessels with ≥90% stenosis received collateral vessels: 79 (84%) of 94 totally occluded arteries -vs- 39 (39%) of 99 with ≥90% but <100% stenosis (p < 0.001). Good collateral vessels went to 70 (89%) of the 79 totally occluded arteries, but only 17 (49%) of 39 subtotally occluded arteries (p < 0.001). Of the 87 good collateral vessels, only 16 (18%) were supplied by single arteries manifesting ≥75% stenosis; of 31 poor collateral vessels, 20 (65%) were supplied by arteries with ≥75% stenosis (p < 0.001). When the patency of all the arteries that could supply collateral vessels to the 94 totally occluded was semiquantitated, the extent of obstruction of the potential suppliers was significantly greater in those arteries with none or poor collateral vessels (p < 0.001 for both groups of arteries with good collateral vessels). It was concluded that the angiographic appearance of the recipient and supplying coronary arteries is a major predictive factor in the angiographic appearance of coronary collateral vessels.

DUAL LAD CORONARY ARTERY

An anatomic variant of the LAD coronary artery in 23 of 2140 coronary angiograms is delineated by Spindola-Franco and associates[27] from New York City. This variant, termed dual LAD, consists of 2 branches that supply the usual distribution of the LAD. One branch (short LAD) terminates in the proximal aspect of the anterior interventricular sulcus. A second, longer branch has a variable course outside the anterior interventricular sulcus and returns to this area distally. The long LAD arose from the LAD proper in 21 patients and from the right coronary artery in 2 patients. The initial course of the long LAD was on the epicardial surface of the left ventricle (17 patients), right ventricle (3 patients), or within the ventricular septum (3 patients). Recognition of these dual LAD variants is important for correct surgical identification of the short and long LADs in the performance of CABG.

EXERCISE-INDUCED ISCHEMIA

Carroll and colleagues[28] from Zurich, Switzerland, studied LV pressure decay and early diastolic pressures at rest and during exercise in 3 groups of patients. Patients in the ischemia group had CAD and developed new regional wall motion abnormalities documented by biplane cineangiography during exercise. Patients in the control group had a normal exercise response. Patients in the scar group had prior AMI, akinetic scars, and no ischemia with exercise. Isovolumic pressure data were used to compute the time constant (T) of LV pressure decay from the linear relation of LV pressure and negative dP/dt and an extrapolated baseline pressure (P_B) at dP/dt=0. During exercise in the ischemia group, minimal LV diastolic pressure (P_L) increased from 9–21 mmHg, end-systolic volume increased from 38–55 ml/M^2 and P_B rose from -10–11 mm; T decreased from 55–37 ms compared with the decrease in the control group from 49–22 ms. Relaxation at P_L during exercise was incomplete in the ischemia group and complete in the control group. The time course of LV pressure fall was extrapolated from the isovolumic period into the passive LV filling phase. The extrapolated pressure at the time P_L occurred rose from 0–20 mmHg with ischemia. Thus, the characteristics of LV pressure decay can account for the elevated early diastolic pressure ischemia. In contrast, the scar group maintained a low P_L during exercise even though T decreased inadequately, because P_B did not shift upward. Ischemia-related pressure elevations involve both delayed relaxation and a pressure baseline shift. During exercise, LV pressure decay is normally adjusted to maintain low diastolic pressures; with exercise-induced ischemia, LV pressure decay is abnormal and early diastolic pressures are severely elevated.

RELATION BETWEEN SEVERITY OF CORONARY STENOSES AND MEAN DIASTOLIC PRESSURE GRADIENT

Bateman and colleagues[29] from Los Angeles, California, studied the relation between angiographic severity of CAD and the mean diastolic pressure gradient measured directly at CABG. The pressure measurements were made after the placement of saphenous vein grafts distal to the stenosis. Correlation between mean diastolic gradient and percent stenosis was good (r = 0.78; p = 0.001). Narrowings >90% had a wide range of gradients, whereas narrowings <90% tended to have more predictable gradients (Fig. 1-2). Collaterals invariably identified narrowings causing major pressure gradients. Length of narrowings was not an important influence on gradient. The authors point out that when narrowings are well visualized by standard

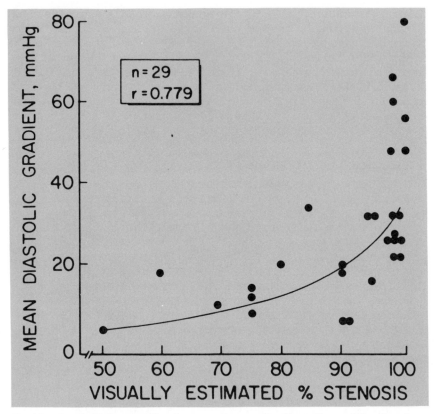

Fig. 1-2. Correlation between directly measured mean diastolic gradient and visually estimated percent stenosis as determined angiographically. Reproduced with permission from Bateman et al.[29]

angiographic techniques, there does appear to be a good correlation between anatomic appearance and the hemodynamic impact of the stenosis. Narrowings of the 51–75% tended to be associated with invariable pressure gradients, but these are generally small. Lesions of 91–100% may produce marked diastolic gradients but also may lead to gradients that are quite mild. Thus, there is overlap between mild, moderate, and severe anatomic stenoses and their associated diastolic pressure gradients. In general, the correlation was good, particularly with visually estimated stenoses as opposed to drawn or traced estimates of the angiographic lesion.

LV FILLING

Left ventricular filling dynamics were examined by Carroll and coworkers[30] from Zurich, Switzerland, at rest and during supine bicycle exercise in 33 patients at cardiac catheterization. Twenty-three had CAD, (ischemia group), 5 with prior AMI had an akinetic area at rest (scar group), and 5 had minimal cardiovascular disease (control). Peak filling rate and mean filling rate during each half of diastole were assessed by biplane angiography. Simultaneous micromanometer pressures were used to compute the time constant of isovolumic pressure decay (T). Peak filling rate and mean filling rate during the first half of diastole increased with exercise in all groups. However, T was greater (reduced rate of pressure decay) with exercise in the ischemia group. Changes in the atrial driving pressure for filling appeared to counterbalance the difference in T. Mean filling rate during the second half of diastole increased with exercise in controls and in the scar group and only modestly in the ischemia group. The reduction in late diastolic filling during exercise-induced ischemia was associated with increased filling in early diastole, with a mid-diastolic volume increase from 160–186 ml and an upward shift in the diastolic pressure-volume relation. Thus LV filling was not impaired at rest in patients with CAD who had a normal EF. Furthermore, the augmentation of early filling induced by exercise was not blunted but was maintained during ischemia, apparently at the expense of elevated LA pressure. However, late filling was restricted with ischemia by an increase in impedance.

LM NARROWING

Reliability of angiographic assessment of the LM coronary artery segment was evaluated by Cameron and colleagues[31] from New York City by review of 106 coronary cineangiograms from the Coronary Artery Surgery Study. The films were interpreted by 3 groups of angiographers: those at a clinical site, those at a quality control site, and those on a study census panel. Among the readings of these 3 groups, there was 41–59% agreement on the severity of the narrowing, with 80% agreement on whether the narrowing was < or >50%. The severity of the narrowing, its location, or presence of ectasia or calcium did not affect the discrepancy rate, whereas segments that were unusually short, diffusely diseased, or obscured by overlapping vessels were especially difficult to interpret.

FOLLOW-UP (7 YEARS) OF APPARENTLY HEALTHY MEN

Erikssen and coworkers[32] from Oslo, Norway, suspected latent CAD in 105 of 2,014 apparently healthy middle-aged men after a baseline cardiovascular survey. Of them, 105 underwent angiography and 36 were found to have normal coronary arteries (group 1). A 7-year follow-up survey revealed that: 1) 3 had died suddenly; 2) 4 had received a diagnosis of cardiomyopathy; 3) 1 had developed aortic dilation and AR since the baseline survey; 4) all had a significantly more rapid decline in their physical performance and maximal heart rate levels from the time of the baseline survey to follow-up than did randomly selected normal controls (group 2); and 5) thallium study results were normal in both groups but technetium ventriculography revealed a subnormal increase in EF during exercise of <5% units in 14 of 27 group 1 subjects and 4 of 26 group 2 subjects. Thus, incipient heart disease may be present in patients in whom coronary angiographic examination has removed a previous suspicion of CAD.

SUBTLE LV ASYNERGY WITH COMPLETE CORONARY OBSTRUCTION

Leighton and associates[33] from Toledo, Ohio, investigated the phenomenon of apparently normal angiographic LV wall motion in the presence of 1 completely obstructed coronary artery in 16 patients with CAD by quantitative phasic biplane cineangiography. Angiographic contours were digitized at quarterly intervals throughout ejection and 9 areas of motion were measured in both right and left anterior oblique planes. Normal values were derived from 18 other patients who had normal coronary arteries and normal LV function. Areas of asynergy undetected when quantitative analysis was applied only at end systole in the right anterior oblique plane were found in 12 of the 16 patients with CAD: in 2 patients by end-systolic analysis in the left anterior oblique plane and in 10 patients by phasic analysis of both planes. Of 19 asynergic areas, 18 corresponded to sites of high grade CAD. All patients had angina pectoris, but only 5 had clinical or ECG evidence of prior AMI.

LOCALIZATION OF CORONARY NARROWINGS

The location of coronary arterial narrowings in CAD is of considerable importance in assessing the mass of myocardium at risk and patient prognosis. Halon and associates[34] from Jerusalem, Israel, mapped the detailed distribution of coronary arterial lesions in 302 patients with CAD who had coronary angiography for chest pain. All identifiable coronary narrowings were measured manually and the site and degree of narrowing were stored in a computer-based multisegmental model of the coronary tree. A high prevalence of CAD was found in proximal vessels, especially at, or adjacent to, proximal points of branching. In the LAD coronary artery, the narrowings were most prevalent immediately after the first diagonal branch and at the origin of this branch. In the right coronary artery, there was a high prevalence of narrowing between the infundibular and acute marginal branches and specifically around the origin of the RV branch. In the LC coronary artery, there was a predilection for narrowing in and around the origin of the first marginal branch. When a ramus intermedius was present, its origin was frequently the site of narrowing.

Pressure gradients across coronary narrowings

Fluid-filled catheter transducer systems have been developed for assessment of phasic pressure gradients across arterial stenoses. In a study reported by Ganz and associates[35] from Boston, Massachusetts, 2 such catheters were employed (3 French and 2 French in diameter). After the catheters were flushed with carbon dioxide and filled with degassed saline solution to remove microbubbles of air, the catheters were attached to a low volume displacement transducer. The frequency response of both catheter transducer systems was adequate to record phasic arterial pressures. The catheters were very flexible and radiopaque, and the ability to monitor phasic pressure continuously at the tip during passage across a stenosis enhanced safety of their use. The catheters were employed successfully to measure phasic pressure gradients across 36 coronary and 5 renal artery stenoses. Maximal pressure gradients were observed in early diastole for coronary stenoses and in systole for renal artery stenoses, consistent with known differences in phasic flow patterns in these vascular beds. The pressure gradients in patients with CAD could be markedly increased by injection of contrast medium (Renografin 76). Since unsatisfactory correlation was observed between the resting pressure gradients and the angiographically defined degree of CAD, this method for measurement of pressure gradients appears to have clinical utility in selected patients.

Digital angiography

Using digital subtraction angiography, Tobis and associates[36] from Irvine, California, obtained left ventriculograms with 10 ml of iodinated contrast material in 21 patients both at rest and during atrial pacing. In 15 patients with significant CAD (>50% diameter narrowing in at least 1 major artery), EF decreased during atrial pacing from a mean of 62 ± 14%–51 ± 15% (p < 0.001). In 14 (93%) of 15 patients, EF decreased or was unchanged during pacing. In 6 patients with chest pain but normal coronary arteries, EF increased from a mean of 66 ± 9% at rest to 72 ± 6% during atrial pacing (p < 0.01). The EF increased by ≥5% during pacing in 5 of 6 patients with normal coronary arteries. Patients with CAD also had an abnormal response in end-systolic volume during atrial pacing (50 ± 31 ml at rest -vs- 47 ± 24 ml during pacing) compared with patients with normal coronary arteries (46 ± 16 ml at rest -vs- 26 ± 9 ml during pacing; p < 0.01). The digital ventriculograms demonstrated new or increased wall motion abnormalities during atrial pacing in 4 of 5 patients with CAD who had wall motion abnormalities at rest and in 8 of 10 patients with CAD who had normal wall motion at rest. Moreover, these wall motion abnormalities occurred in myocardial wall segments that were supplied by coronary arteries with significant lesions. Thus, because digital subtraction angiography allows multiple left ventriculograms to be obtained during routine cardiac catheterization, intervention studies such as atrial pacing can be used to obtain a functional assessment of the severity of coronary arterial lesions.

Johnson and associates[37] from Washington, D.C., evaluated 61 patients to determine whether digital subtraction left ventriculography using intravenous contrast media may be used as a means to detect CAD. Rest studies and an evaluation of LV function during atrial pacing were obtained. Thirty-five ml of contrast media were injected into a central vein (usually the inferior vena cava). Regional wall motion abnormalities were detected equally well by digital subtraction angiography and direct left ventriculography in 40 patients having both tests. Atrial pacing to a maximal heart rate of 150 beats/minute was utilized in those patients with a normal resting digital ventriculogram. Of the 61 patients, 44 had significant CAD and 10 of these had a wall motion abnormality at rest by digital subtraction evaluation. With atrial pacing, 28 of the 34 remaining patients developed a new wall motion abnormality. Thus, these data suggest intravenous injection of contrast media with subsequent digital left ventriculography will be a means of detecting the presence of significant CAD when both rest and stress (atrial pacing) studies are obtained.

Twenty-one patients with CAD were evaluated by Goldberg and associates[38] from New York City at rest and exercise to determine whether exercise left ventriculography accomplished with an intravenous injection and digital angiography could be used to detect abnormal global functional responses. In these patients, EF was 58% at rest and 45% with exercise (p < 0.001 compared with rest values). In 7 patients with no CAD, EF was 65% at rest and 69% with exercise. Sixteen patients had both rest and exercise radionuclide cineangiography and digital subtraction angiography. In these individuals, there was a strong correlation between the 2 techniques for EF at rest (r = 0.78), EF with exercise (r = 0.83), and change in EF from rest to exercise (r = 0.88). Thus, these data suggest that exercise ventriculography utilizing intravenous digital subtraction angiography will provide information comparable to that obtained from radionuclide ventriculography.

PROGNOSIS

Improvement with medical therapy

Several reports have described a decrease in mortality from CAD in the USA in recent years. From 1968–1976, unadjusted mortality rates for CAD decreased 12% and the age-adjusted mortality rate decreased 21%. The decrease represents a potential annual saving of 192,500 lives nationally. The cause of the decrease is not clear. It does not appear to be secondary to artifact or to changes in the coding of death certificates. Fewer persons may be developing CAD, which would represent a decrease in incidence. Alternatively, patients with CAD may be living longer. Pryor and associates[39] from Durham, North Carolina, examined the decrease that occurred over time in cardiovascular mortality and morbidity rates in a consecutive population of patients referred for coronary angiography, and they presented evidence that the prognosis has improved for medically treated patients with angiographically documented CAD. The mortality rate and the total number of cardiovascular events both decreased during the 10 years in 1,911 medically treated patients with significant CAD. The decrease could not be explained by less sick patients being referred for evaluation. Their study suggests that at least part of the decrease in CAD mortality observed nationally is occurring in patients with established CAD.

Fifteen-year survival

Proudfit and associates[40] from Cleveland, Ohio, determined survival rates in 598 patients in whom severe CAD was demonstrated by arteriography; initially they were treated medically and were followed for 15 years. Deaths due to noncoronary causes were uncommon (5% of total) in the first 5-year period but were frequent (36%) in the third period. Survival rates were 48, 28, 18, and 9% for patients with 1-, 2-, and 3-vessel and LM narrowing, respectively. Abnormalities documented by ventriculography were related to survival. In 386 patients who would have been candidates for bypass surgery, survival rates were 58, 35, 26, and 11% for those with 1-, 2-, 3-vessel and LM coronary narrowing, respectively. Cardiac survival curves for 1-, 2-, 3-vessel CAD in candidates for surgery and curves constructed on the basis of 3% mortality per artery per year corresponded fairly closely. When an abnormal ECG was considered as a single variable in multivariate analysis, 5-year survival rates of candidates for surgery were influenced by the following in order of importance: abnormal ECG, symptoms ≥5 years, 3-vessel CAD, 2-artery disease, and arteriosclerosis obliterans. A simple prognostic stratification was devised that used only ECGs and duration of symptoms for each subset based on the number of arteries affected.

By exercise testing

To assess whether exercise testing could help predict cardiac mortality, Weiner and colleagues[41] from Boston, Massachusetts, analyzed 14 exercise and 10 clinical variables in 292 patients treated medically who underwent treadmill exercise testing and cardiac catheterization and were followed annually for a mean of 2.5 years. None of the individual variables could accurately predict subsequent cardiac mortality, with predictive values ranging from 6–44%. Combinations of variables were then analyzed in the subset of 113 patients with multivessel CAD. A high risk subgroup (n, 59) consisting of patients with either severe exercise ischemia ($\geqslant$2 mm ST depression lasting $\geqslant$5 minutes involving $\geqslant$3 leads) or LV dysfunction (treadmill time $\leqslant$3 minutes, S_3 gallop, or cardiac enlargement) had a mortality of 20% at mean follow-up of 26 months; this was significantly greater (p < 0.01) than a low risk subgroup (n, 54) with neither severe exercise ischemia nor LV dysfunction whose mortality was 2%. It was concluded that combining clinical and exercise variables to distinguish high and low risk subgroups of patients with similar coronary pathoanatomy is useful in predicting cardiac mortality.

Gohlke and coworkers[42] from Bad Krozingen, West Germany, examined whether exercise testing with measurement of cardiac output during maximal exercise can provide additional prognostic information for medically treated patients in whom LV function and extent of CAD are known. The investigators followed 1,034 patients with normal or mildly impaired LV function: 410 of these patients (group 1) had 1-vessel CAD, 316 had 2-vessel CAD (group 2), and 308 had 3-vessel CAD (group 3). In addition, 204 patients with 2- or 3-vessel CAD and moderately impaired LV function (group 4) were followed. Mean follow-up in these 1,238 patients was 4.5 years. End point of follow-up was death. Groups 1, 2, and 3 were divided into terciles according to the maximally achieved values of the following exercise variables: exercise tolerance, angina-free exercise tolerance, maximal heart rate, and cardiac output during maximal exercise. Group 4 was divided into halves accordingly. Survival curves for group 2 showed a 15% difference in 5-year survival rate between the highest and lowest terciles by use of the noninvasive variables exercise tolerance, angina-free exercise tolerance, and maximal heart rate. The separation into terciles according to cardiac output during maximal exercise resulted in a significant difference in survival rates between the highest and the lowest terciles in all groups of patients. The differences in 5-year survival rates were 9, 16, 19, and 22% for groups 1, 2, 3, and 4, respectively. The investigators conclude that noninvasive exercise parameters can separate high and low risk subgroups of patients with 2-vessel disease and good LV function. Determination of maximal cardiac output allowed identification of low and high risk subgroups in all 4 angiographically defined groups.

By exertional hypotension

The prognostic and predictive value of exertional hypotension was assessed by Hammermeister and associates[43] from Seattle, Washington, in 1,241 patients having treadmill maximal exercise testing, coronary arteriography, and follow-up averaging 5.4 years. Medically treated patients with CAD with exertional hypotension had poorer survival than did those without such hypotension. Maximal systolic pressure, however, during exercise was a more powerful predictor of survival. Patients with exertional hypotension had more extensive CAD and more LV dysfunction than did patients who had an increase in BP with exertion; these findings probably account for the impaired survival. However, exertional hypotension, was an insensitive indicator of significant LM CAD, 3-vessel CAD, or severe resting LV dysfunction.

With 1-vessel narrowing

The clinical outcome in 688 patients with isolated stenosis of 1 major coronary artery were analyzed by Califf and colleagues[44] from Durham, North Carolina. Survival rate among patients with disease of the right coronary artery was higher than that among patients with LAD or LC CAD. The survival rate among patients in all 3 anatomic groups was >90% at 5 years. The presence of a narrowing proximal to the first septal perforator of the LAD was associated with decreased survival compared with the presence of a more distal narrowing. For the entire group of 1-vessel CAD patients, total ischemic events (death and nonfatal infarction) occurred at similar rates regardless of the anatomic location of the lesion. The LV EF was the baseline descriptor most strongly associated with survival, and the characteristics of the angina had the strongest relation with nonfatal AMI. No differences were found in survival or total cardiac events with surgical or nonsurgical therapy. The relief of angina, however, was superior with surgical therapy, although most nonsurgically treated patients had significant relief of angina. Thus, the investigators concluded that the survival rate of patients with 1-vessel CAD was excellent, and the risk of nonfatal AMI was low.

To permit comparison of PTCA with conventional therapy, Hlatky and associates[45] from Durham, North Carolina, established the clinical outcome in patients who would have been suitable candidates for PTCA had the technique been available. Coronary angiograms were reviewed of patients who met the following criteria: 1-vessel disease with proximal subtotal coronary stenosis, chest pain of at least class II, and cardiac catheterization before 1981. Angiograms were evaluated according to estabished criteria for PTCA by an experienced angiographer. One hundred ten patients (2.1% of the patient population) were judged suitable for PTCA. Clinical and catheterization findings closely resembled those of patients in the national PTCA registry. Five years after catheterization, 97% of PTCA candidates treated medically were alive and 85% had not had AMI. Forty-six patients had CABG within 6 months of catheterization and 10 other patients had subsequent surgery. Five years after surgery, 91% were alive and 87% had not had AMI. At 6 months of follow-up, 78% of all patients had improved at least 1 functional class, and 86% of all patients working before catheterization were still employed. Functional capacity was well maintained during long-term follow-up (median, 6.5 years; range, 1.4–12.2). These data indicate that PTCA candidates have an excellent prognosis for survival, a low risk of AMI, and well-maintained functional capacity when revascularization is reserved for those with inadequate control of symptoms by medical therapy.

With combined proximal LAD and LC narrowings

Combined proximal LAD and proximal LC artery stenosis >70% have been referred to as "LM equivalent" lesions. Chaitman and participants[46] in the Coronary Artery Surgery Study from St. Louis, Missouri, compared the survival rates of medically treated patients who have this type of coronary anatomic characteristics with the survival rates of patients who have LM coronary narrowing >70% by use of a stratified life table approach and a Cox regression model. Comparison of the patients with LM CAD with those who have LM equivalent lesions by use of life table analysis and 3 different calculations of patient exposure time revealed a poorer prognosis for the patients who had LM CAD. The stepwise Cox analysis also determined that patients who had LM CAD had a significantly poorer prognosis than patients who had LM equivalent CAD, even after consideration of important baseline variables known to affect survival rates. The investigators then compared the patients who had combined proximal LAD and proximal LC CAD with patients who had combined stenoses >70% in the nonproximal LAD and proximal circumflex coronary arteries to determine if location of the LAD stenosis influenced survival rates. The 5-year survival rate was not as high for the patients who had proximal LAD CAD (55 -vs- 70%). In conclusion, combined proximal LAD and proximal LC CAD identified a high risk patient subset. It was not prognostically equivalent to LM CAD.

PROGRESSION OF CORONARY NARROWING

In an investigation carried out by Kramer and associates[47] from Cleveland, Ohio, serial coronary angiograms were examined retrospectively in 148 patients with progressive CAD. This evaluation included 2,899 coronary arterial segments that were categorized and compared at first and second study. Progression was defined as a 2-category increase in severity or a new occlusion at second study. Progression was found most frequently in the proximal third of the right coronary artery, and in the middle third of the LAD and right. Progression occurred most often in segments diseased at first study ($p < 0.0001$). The probability of finding a new occlusion at second study was related to the severity of the initial obstruction ($p < 0.0001$) and did not depend directly on time ($p = 0.64$). The CAD progression, excluding occlusion, occurred in relation to both time and the severity of the initial narrowing ($p < 0.0001$).

LIPIDS

Usefulness in predicting CAD

The relations of total cholesterol and the portion of cholesterol in individual lipoprotein classes to CAD are complex. To help simplify these relations, cholesterol values are often combined into a summary estimate to form a single risk factor with a relation to disease that is more easily described. Although summary estimates result in convenient expressions relating cholesterol to CAD, there remains the potential for sacrificing information by ignoring the joint configuration of cholesterols that make up these estimates. Castelli and coworkers[48] from Bethesda, Maryland, investigated the extent of this possibility for the ratio of total to HDL cholesterol and the ratio of LDL to HDL cholesterol. The findings suggest that the summary estimates are useful expressions of combining information and are strong predictors of CAD. Clinicians who choose to use a summary estimate for screening purposes should recognize that a single ratio estimate is not always as informative as a joint configuration of the cholesterols that make up the estimate. This possibility is most clearly exhibited for the ratio of LDL cholesterol to HDL cholesterol, and it may become more apparent in future studies as the capabilities of exploring lipoprotein cholesterol relations improve.

Apolipoprotein A-I for predicting CAD

Maciejko and associates[49] from Rochester, Minnesota, designed a study to determine whether the plasma level of apolipoprotein A-I is a better discriminator of angiographically documented CAD than the level of HDL cholesterol in men. The level of plasma apolipoprotein A-I in 83 patients with CAD was 97 ± 4 mg/dl (mean $\pm$ SEM), which was significantly lower (p < 0.0001) than the level in 25 patients without CAD (147 ± 2 mg/dl) (Fig. 1-3). The levels of HDL cholesterol also were lower (p < 0.0001) in patients with CAD (32 ± 1 mg/dl) than in those without CAD (46 ± 2 mg/dl). A stepwise discriminant analysis, however, indicated the superiority of apolipoprotein A-I over HDL cholesterol in detecting CAD. Furthermore, a linear discriminant analysis suggested that, although HDL cholesterol by itself was a discriminator of CAD, it did not provide a substantial increase in discriminatory value over that provided by apolipoprotein A-I; in contrast, apolipoprotein A-I levels added discriminatory value to the information obtained by measuring HDL cholesterol alone. The authors concluded that apolipoprotein A-I by itself was more useful than HDL cholesterol for identifying patients with CAD.

Levels in British men aged 40–59 years

Thelle and associates[50] from Birmingham, England, measured the concentrations of serum total cholesterol (TC), HDL cholesterol, and triglycerides in 7,735 men aged 40–59 years from 24 towns in England, Wales, and Scotland. The distribution of these blood lipids, their interrelations, and their association with age, social class, body mass index, cigarette smoking, alcohol intake, and physical activity at work have been examined. Body mass index emerges as the factor most strongly associated with these 3 blood lipids. Serum TC increased with increasing body mass index until about 28 kg/M^2 but thereafter showed no further rise. The relation between body mass index and HDL cholesterol was negative and linear; that between body mass index and triglycerides was positive and linear. The inverse relation between HDL cholesterol and triglycerides was independent of the fact that both were related to body mass index. Alcohol intake was associated with increased

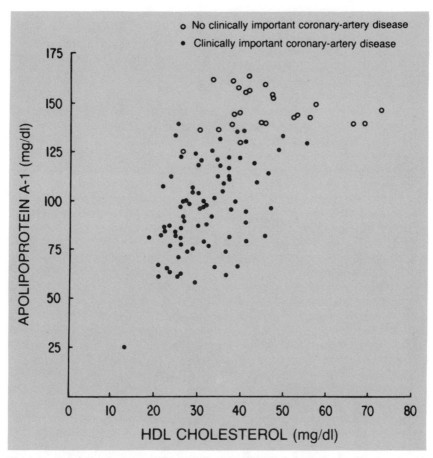

Fig. 1-3. Correlation between apolipoprotein A-1 and HDL cholesterol concentrations in 108 patients studied by angiography. Despite overall correlation between HDL cholesterol and apolipoprotein A-1 (r = 0.60, p < 0.001), at given level of apolipoprotein A-1 there was a wide range of corresponding HDL cholesterol levels. Reproduced with permission from Maciejko et al.[49]

HDL cholesterol concentrations and cigarette smoking with lowered HDL concentrations; the association with alcohol appeared to be dominant. No significant trends with age were observed for the 3 blood lipids. In this population, body mass index was closely associated with the concentration of blood lipids but its effects are probably indirect and mediated by a complex of dietary and other factors.

HDL cholesterol levels from quadriplegics to marathon runners

Studies of physical activity, HDL cholesterol, and CAD suggest that increased activity is associated with high HDL cholesterol levels and a reduced risk of CAD. LaPorte and associates[51] from Pittsburgh, Pennsylvania,

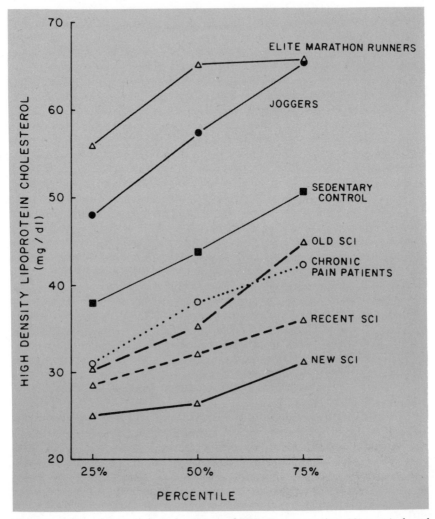

Fig. 1-4. Relation between physical activity and HDL–C concentration. SCI = spinal cord injury. Reproduced with permission from LaPorte et al.[51]

measured HDL cholesterol levels in 56 spinal injury patients (25 quadriple-gics, 31 paraplegics), 11 patients disabled with chronic pain (usually back pain), 197 normal control subjects, 16 joggers, and 7 marathon runners. All were men aged 18–60 years. The joggers averaged 2–40 miles/week and the marathon runners, 80 miles/week. There was a clear gradient in HDL cholesterol, ranging from a mean of 27 mg/dl in the new spinal cord injured patients to 61 mg/dl for the marathon runners (Fig. 1-4). The levels in the disabled were consistently below those in the nondisabled. All new spinal cord injured cases were below the fifth percentile of the normal population. If risk estimates for various HDL cholesterol levels were applied to the values, these authors found that spinal cord injured patients would be at a 90% greater risk of heart attack than the controls and at a 350% greater likelihood of a heart attack than the runners. These findings provide a pattern of diverse causes of impaired activity associated with low levels of HDL cholesterol and increased CAD risk. This pattern suggests that at least part of the increased CAD risk in the disabled is associated with inactivity. More than 15% of the population of western countries are disabled. For older persons, the figure exceeds 30%. The disabled therefore represent a large population who may be at very high risk for cardiovascular disease. Perhaps increasing the activity of disabled persons makes more public health sense than trying to turn sedentary workers into marathon runners.

Familial aggregation

Widespread screening of adults and children for the presence of elevated blood lipids is an expensive and inefficient process. As far back as 1910, Osler observed that CAD tended to cluster in families (Osler W: Lumleian lectures on angina pectoris. *Lancet* 1:697–702 and 2:839–844, 1910). Investigators in 1974 and 1976 (Glueck CJ, Fallat RW, Tsang R, et al: Hyperlipidemia in progeny of parents with myocardial infarction before age 50. *Am J Dis Child* 127:70–75, 1974; Hennekens CH, Jesse MJ, Klein BE, et al: Cholesterol among children of men with myocardial infarction. *Pediatrics* 58:211–217, 1976) studied offspring of parents with premature AMI and found higher mean total cholesterol levels than in control children, and the prevalence of familial dyslipoproteinemia in children whose parents had sustained early AMI also was much higher than expected. This hyperlipidemic proband-generated sampling strategy is more attractive epidemilogically than sampling strategies based on family history of premature CAD for the following reasons: 1) although the offspring of parents with premature CAD ($\leqslant 50$ years) have significantly elevated total cholesterol and LDL cholesterol levels, and a greatly increased proportion of them have familial hypercholesterolemia, premature CAD is itself relatively rare and, thus, identifies few children in the population who probably will be at risk for CAD; and 2) waiting until the parent or sibling has CAD before identifying other persons at risk may lose the opportunity for early identification and conservative intervention. Accordingly, Morrison and associates[52] from Cincinnati, Ohio, and Chapel Hill, North Carolina, studied 841 offspring and 1,236 siblings of normocholesterolemic probands, 833 offspring and 1,194 siblings of hypercholesterolemic probands, 806 offspring and 1,099 siblings of normotriglyceridemic probands, and 877 offspring and 1,108 siblings of hypertriglyceridemic probands in the Lipid Research Clinics Collaborative Family Study Program. These authors documented the fact that identification of subjects at high risk for CAD because of dyslipoproteinemia can be facilitated by using the phenomenon of family aggregation of lipoprotein risk factors for CAD. Comparing offspring and siblings of probands having persistent and severe hypercholesterolemia with offspring and siblings of normal probands, the frequency of top decile total cholesterol levels was increased 2-fold to 3-fold for offspring and 2-fold to 4-fold for siblings; the frequency of top decile LDL cholesterol levels was increased 2-fold to 3-fold for offspring and 2-fold to 5-fold for siblings. In addition, there was almost a 2-fold increase in the frequency of top decile triglyceride levels in siblings of high total cholesterol probands, reflecting the expression of combined hyperlipidemia and the phenotypic expression of elevated triglyceride levels, which would be more common in adult siblings than in pediatric offspring of probands. These authors concluded that lipid and lipoprotein measurements, along with determination of BP in late adolescence and early adulthood, may be more predictive of CAD than measurements taken later in life. This may explain why total cholesterol and LDL cholesterol values have less predictive power for future CAD in men >50 years compared with men <50 years. The authors recommended for patients with elevated values of total cholesterol that 2 repeat determinations be obtained to verify persistent elevation of total cholesterol levels and to document whether LDL or HDL cholesterol levels predominately accounted for the hypercholesterolemia. Probands with sporadic hypercholesterolemia (only 1 of 3 values ≥ the 90th percentile) in their study were much less likely than those with 2 or 3 elevated values to have hypercholesterolemic siblings and offspring. Patients found to have persistent elevations of total cholesterol and LDL cholesterol levels should be advised to have their siblings and offspring tested.

New reference values

The diagnosis of several common varieties of hypolipidemia is based on the use of high reference values, usually the 95th percentile of the distribution of cholesterol, triglyceride, or lipoprotein cholesterol for a given population. Low reference values (usually the 5th percentile of the distribution of cholesterol, LDL, and HDL) used to identify persons with unusually low levels of lipids or lipoproteins also are used to screen for various lipoprotein deficiency disorders. To define a reference value based on a percentile, it is necessary to establish the distribution of the relevant lipid or lipoprotein levels through study of a well-defined population sample. The existing data for lipid distributions in the North American population, from which reference values have been derived, have been limited. The 12 Lipid

TABLE 1-1. *50th and 90th percentiles for plasma lipid concentration.* Reproduced with permission from Rifkind and Segal.*[53]*

	MEN				WOMEN			
	PERCENTILE				PERCENTILE			
AGE, YR	50TH	90TH	50TH	90TH	50TH	90TH	50TH	90TH
	TOTAL CHOLESTEROL, MG/DL		TRIGLYCERIDES, MG/DL		TOTAL CHOLESTEROL, MG/DL		TRIGLYCERIDES, MG/DL	
20–29	172	215	90	182	164	207	65	114
30–39	194	234	109	232	176	219	71	130
40–49	206	254	123	250	195	241	84	163
50–59	211	261	122	242	222	275	111	194
60–69	210	258	116	222	228	280	108	203
70–79	205	249	112	212	228	280	110	200

* From the Lipid Research Clinic data.

TABLE 1-2. *50th and critical percentiles for LDL* and HDL* cholesterol† . Reproduced with permission from Rifkind and Segal.*[53]

	LDL CHOLESTEROL, MG/DL				HDL CHOLESTEROL, MG/DL			
	MEN		WOMEN		MEN		WOMEN	
	PERCENTILE				PERCENTILE			
AGE, YR	50TH	90TH	50TH	90TH	50TH	10TH	50TH	10TH
20–29	108	147	100	138	45	32	52	38
30–39	128	171	113	151	44	32	54	39
40–49	138	180	124	168	44	32	56	39
50–59	144	188	144	196	45	31	58	40

* LDL indicates low-density lipoprotein; HDL, high-density lipoprotein.
† From the Lipid Research Clinic data.

Research Clinics in North America, started in 1973, provide detailed information on the distribution of levels of plasma lipids and lipoproteins in a random sample of a variety of well-defined North American populations. Rifkind and Segal[53] from Bethesda, Maryland, analyzed plasma cholesterol and triglyceride distributions for 60,502 participants in a survey of 10 separate Lipid Research Clinics. Lipoprotein cholesterol levels were measured in a random sample of 7,055 white participants. From these data, new age- and sex-specific reference values were selected for the diagnosis of hyperlipidemia and hypolipidemia (Tables 1-1 to 1-8). The use of these new reference values for population screening would result in the conditions of more young subjects being diagnosed as hypercholesterolemic and a very significant decrease in the proportion of the adult population being diagnosed as having hypertriglyceridemia.

TABLE 1-3. *Selected reference values for plasma high–density lipoprotein cholesterol (mg/dL) in white male subjects. Reproduced with permission for Rifkind and Segal.*[80]

| | | | PERCENTILES | | |
AGE, YR	NO.	MEAN	5	10	95
5–14	438	55	35	40	75
15–19	299	45	30	35	65
20–24	118	45	30	30	65
25–29	253	45	30	30	65
30–34	403	45	30	30	65
35–39	371	45	30	30	60
40–44	383	45	25	30	65
45–69	1,162	50	30	30	70
70+	119	50	30	35	75

TABLE 1-4. *Selected reference values for plasma total cholesterol (mg/dL) in white female subjects. Reproduced with permission from Rifkind and Segal.*[53]

AGE, YR	NO.	MEAN	PERCENTILES			
			5	75	90	95
0–19	5,470	160	120	175	190	200
20–24	1,566	170	125	190	215	230
25–34	4,340	175	130	195	220	235
35–39	2,012	185	140	205	230	245
40–44	2,050	195	145	215	235	255
45–49	2,149	205	150	225	250	270
50–54	1,992	220	165	240	265	285
55+	4,478	230	170	250	275	295

Dietary and pharmacologic therapy

The Council of Scientific Affairs report[54] by a select AMA committee made the following recommendations: 1) Initial search for the presence of hyperlipidemia ideally should be done at or before age 20 years. 2) Before initiating treatment, fasting levels of plasma cholesterol and triglyceride should be measured at least twice to determine a baseline value. Full lipoprotein profiles are not ordinarily necessary before initiation of therapy. 3) Underlying disorders (e.g., alcoholism, diabetes mellitus, or hypothyroidism) known to cause elevation of plasma lipoprotein levels should be identified and treated directly when present. 4) Vigorous dietary therapy should be initiated in patients who have mean serum cholesterol levels >90th percentile for age and sex. Patients <60 years of age who continue to have plasma lipid elevations unresponsive to dietary therapy deserve a trial of long-term drug therapy. 5) Patients with plasma lipid levels in the range of

TABLE 1-5. *Selected reference values for plasma low–density lipoprotein cholesterol (mg/dL) in white female subjects. Reproduced with permission from Rifkind and Segal.*[53]

AGE, YR	NO.	MEAN	PERCENTILES			
			5	75	90	95
5–19	652	100	65	110	125	140
20–24	199	105	55	120	140	160
25–34	646	110	70	125	145	160
35–39	299	120	75	140	160	170
40–44	318	125	75	145	165	175
45–49	326	130	80	150	175	185
50–54	256	140	90	160	185	200
55+	668	150	95	170	195	215

TABLE 1-6.   *Selected reference values for plasma high–density lipoprotein cholesterol (mg/dL) in white female subjects. Reproduced with permission from Rifkind and Segal.*[53]

| AGE, YR | NO. | MEAN | PERCENTILES | | |
			5	10	95
5–19	666	55	35	40	70
20–24	199	55	35	35	80
25–34	649	55	35	40	80
35–39	298	55	35	40	80
40–44	318	60	35	40	90
45–49	328	60	35	40	85
50–54	256	60	35	40	90
55+	668	60	35	40	95

the 50th–90th percentile for age and sex also may benefit from diet therapy, because most patients with CAD emerge from this group. Factors such as age, sex, family history, other risk factors, accompanying disease, prognosis, and anticipated compliance may all influence the clinical decision to treat the hyperlipidemia. 6) Diet therapy for hypercholesterolemia and hypertri-glyceridemia should include instruction in attaining and maintaining a desirable body weight. Further measures include a diet that contains no more than 30–35% of calories as fat, <10% of calories from sources of saturated fat, and at least 10% of calories from oils rich in polyunsaturated fatty acids. There should be <300 mg/day of cholesterol with an adequate protein intake. 7) In patients who have not reached an optimal level of plasma cholesterol on the preceding diet, further restriction of fat to <30% of

TABLE 1-7.   *Selected reference values for plasma triglycerides (mg/dL) in white male subjects. Reproduced with permission from Rifkind and Segal.*[53]

| AGE, YR | NO. | MEAN | PERCENTILES | | |
			5	90	95
0–9	1,491	55	30	85	100
10–14	2,278	65	30	100	125
15–19	1,980	80	35	120	150
20–24	882	100	45	165	200
25–29	2,042	115	45	200	250
30–34	2,444	130	50	215	265
35–39	2,320	145	55	250	320
40–54	6,862	150	55	250	320
55–64	2,526	140	60	235	290
65+	1,600	135	55	210	260

TABLE 1-8. *Selected reference values for plasma triglycerides (mg/dL) in white female subjects. Reproduced with permission from Rifkind and Segal.*[53]

| | | | PERCENTILES | | |
AGE, YR	NO.	MEAN	5	90	95
0–9	1,304	60	35	95	110
10–19	4,166	75	40	115	130
20–34	5,906	90	40	145	170
35–39	2,012	95	40	160	195
40–44	2,050	105	45	170	210
45–49	2,149	110	45	185	230
50–54	1,992	120	55	190	240
55–64	2,768	125	55	200	250
65+	1,710	130	60	205	240

calories and cholesterol to <250 mg/day may be warranted. 8) If the plasma triglyceride level remains >90th percentile, alcohol should be proscribed and carbohydrate restriction may be necessary. Drug therapy is not usually justified in an isolated hypertriglyceridemia. 9) Because 1 family member with hyperlipidemia suggests that other members may be at risk and because dietary management is a family affair, consideration should be given to extending the dietary recommendations to the patient's entire family. 10) Control of plasma lipid levels is only one facet in cardiovascular risk management. Other factors such as cessation of cigarette smoking, BP control, and the medical management of glucose intolerance must not be ignored.

Treatment of heterozygous hypercholesterolemia

Mabuchi and associates[55] from Kanazawa, Japan, studied the effects of the bile acid sequestrant cholestryamine alone and in combination with the experimental agent compactin (ML-236B), a competitive inhibitor of 3-hydroxy-3 methylglutaryl coenzyme A reductase, on serum levels of lipoproteins in 10 heterozygous patients with familial hypercholesterolemia. After cholestyramine treatment alone for 2–16 months, serum total and LDL cholesterol decreased by 20 and 28%, respectively. With the addition of compactin for 12 weeks, there was a 39% total decrease in serum cholesterol from the control value (356 ± 14–217 ± 10 mg/dl; p < 0.001) and a 53% decrease in LDL cholesterol (263 ± 13–125 ± 10 mg/dl) (Fig. 1-5). HDL cholesterol, which had increased during cholestyramine treatment, remained at its higher level. No adverse effects were observed. If long-term safety can be demonstrated, the compactin-cholestyramine regimen may prove useful in heterozygous familial hypercholesterolemia.

Homozygous hypercholesterolemia

The lesions of the aortic root that are supravalvular AS and coronary ostial stenosis in familial hypercholesterolemia were studied by Beppu and

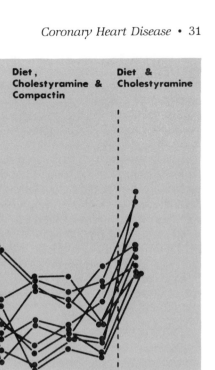

Fig. 1-5. Cholesterol levels during the treatment sequence. To convert cholesterol values to millimoles per liter, multiply by 0.026. "F" denotes final determination made in that treatment period. † denotes values obtained before "F" values. Reproduced with permission from Mabuchi et al.[55]

associates[56] from Osaka, Japan, using 2-D echo. The subjects were 25 heterozygotes, 6 homozygotes, and 30 control subjects. The internal diameters of the aortic ring, the sinus of Valsalva, and the supravalvular aortic ring were measured. Measurement variation due to body size was avoided by normalizing the latter 2 values by the diameter of the aortic ring. Four heterozygotes and all homozygotes were judged to have stenosis of the supravalvular aortic ring, none of the heterozygotes and 4 homozygotes had stenosis of the sinus of Valsalva. In 3 of the 4 patients with stenosis of both the supravalvular aortic ring and the sinus of Valsalva, a pressure gradient was demonstrated. The degree of supravalvular AS correlated with the serum cholesterol level but not with the patient's age. All homozygotes, even the very young, had a severe aortic root lesion. In the short axis view of the aortic root, a lump or raised mass on the aortic wall indicating atheromatous plaquing was demonstrated in 5 heterozygotes and all homozygotes. Coronary ostial stenosis was shown in 3 of the 4 patients whose plaquing echoes were adjacent to the coronary orifice. The authors concluded that 2-D echo was useful in diagnosing lesions of the aortic root in patients with hypercholesterolemia.

Patients with homozygous familial hypercholesterolemia have premature atherosclerosis that preferentially involves the ascending aorta and coronary arteries. The aortic valve cusps and wall of ascending aorta may be thickened by actual atherosclerotic plaque. Aortography in these patients has shown characteristic aortic root "funnelling." Ribeiro and associates[57] from London, England, utilized cross-sectional echo to identify aortic root lesions and coronary ostial stenosis in 35 patients with familial type IIa and IIb hyperlipoproteinemia, including 3 homozygotes and 32 heterozygotes. Two homozygotes showed abnormal bright echoes encircling the proximal aortic root, and they interfered with full excursion of the aortic valve cusps. One homozygote had typical echo features of supravalvular AS at the superior border of the sinus of Valsalva with normal aortic cusps. Catheterization disclosed peak systolic pressure gradients of 15 and 30 mmHg in 2 homozygotes and a supravalvular gradient of 40 mmHg in the third. Left coronary ostial stenosis was identified by echo in all 3 homozygotes.

CIGARETTE SMOKING

Lipid values of smokers

Cigarette smoking is an important risk factor for CAD. Its mechanisms of action, however, remain unclear. Brischetto and associates[58] from Portland, Oregon, tested the hypothesis that a mechanism by which cigarette smoking enhances CAD might be through its effects on plasma lipids. They measured the plasma lipids and lipoproteins in cigarette smokers, exsmokers, and nonsmokers from 233 randomly selected American families. Cigarette smokers (men and women) had significantly lower HDL levels and higher VLDL cholesterol and plasma triglyceride levels than the exsmokers and nonsmokers. The plasma levels of lipids and lipoproteins were related to the number of cigarettes smoked a day. Heavier cigarette smokers (>25 cigarettes/day) had significantly lower HDL levels and significantly higher VLDL cholesterol, total cholesterol, and plasma triglyceride levels than those who smoked <25 cigarettes/day, nonsmokers, and exsmokers. The lipid and lipoprotein values of those who smoked <15 cigarettes/day were similar to those of exsmokers and nonsmokers. Inasmuch as exsmokers had levels of plasma lipids and lipoproteins similar to those of nonsmokers, these findings add another health-enhancing benefit to the cessation of cigarette smoking.

Willett and associates[59] from Boston, Massachusetts, examined the relations of cigarette smoking with fasting triglycerides, total cholesterol, and HDL cholesterol levels among a group of 191 white women aged 20–40 years. The mean triglyceride level among current smokers was 100 mg/100 ml, and among nonsmokers it was 68 mg/dl (p $<$ 0.005). Mean total cholesterol values among current smokers and nonsmokers were 197 and 189 mg/dl (p $<$ 0.1), respectively. Mean HDL levels were 45 mg/dl among smokers and 52 mg/dl among nonsmokers (p $<$ 0.005). Simultaneous adjustments for the effects of age, weight, height, blood glucose, resting pulse, and oral contraceptive use did not materially alter these relations.

Therefore at least a modest portion of the effect of cigarette smoking on risk of CAD may be explained by an adverse effect of cigarette smoking on blood lipids.

Relation to body weight and mortality

Cigarette smoking is a potential confounder of the relation between obesity and mortality, and statistical control for this factor needs careful consideration. Garrison and associates[60] from Framingham, Massachusetts, reported results of studies in the Framingham Heart Study subjects who were weighed, their stature measured, and their cigarette smoking histories obtained at the first biennial examination beginning in 1949. Of men under desirable weight (Metropolitan relative weight [MRW], <100%), >80% were smokers, but only about 55% of the extremely overweight men were cigarette smokers. When age-, smoking-, and MRW-specific mortalities for 26 years of follow-up were calculated in these men, it was found that smokers had higher mortality than nonsmokers, but that in both smokers and nonsmokers minimum mortalities occurred for subjects who were initially in the "desirable weight" group (MRW, 100–109%). Among cigarette smokers, lean men (MRW, <100%) experienced considerably elevated mortality, often higher than that in all but the most overweight cigarette smokers. These findings suggest that elevated mortality in low weight American men results from the mortality risks associated with cigarette smoking and demonstrates the need for controlling for cigarette smoking when considering the relation between relative weight and mortality. Furthermore, the concept of "desirable weight" developed by the Metropolitan Life Insurance Company in 1959 and subsequently distributed in tabular form is validated by this long-term study. Thus, even those men who were near the average weight (about 20% above "desirable weight") showed appreciably elevated mortality. This finding is contrary to the widely held view that moderate overweight carries no increased risk.

Relation to survival after onset of angina pectoris or acute myocardial infarction

Hickey and associates[61] from Dublin, Ireland, followed 634 men <60 years of age, who survived a first attack of angina pectoris or AMI. The patients were followed for 4 years, and details of initial and follow-up smoking habits were examined. Patients who continued to smoke cigarettes or cigars had an excess mortality compared with nonsmokers, those who stopped smoking, and cigarette smokers who changed to pipe smoking. Pipe smokers who continued smoking the pipe had an observed mortality that was greater than that of the nonsmokers, but the numbers were small and the results were not statistically significant. The effect of smoking on mortality was not influenced by 2 other determinants of prognosis: age and severity of initial attack. These results confirm that the long-term prognosis of patients after unstable angina or AMI may be significantly influenced by smoking habits. They are consistent with the hypothesis that cigar and pipe smoking may have an adverse effect after AMI, but further studies are needed to corroborate the association between cigar and pipe smoking and prognosis of CAD.

Relation of acute myocardial infarction to nicotine and carbon monoxide content

To evaluate whether the nicotine and carbon monoxide content of cigarette smoke is related to the risk of nonfatal first AMI in young men, Kaufman and associates[62] from Boston, Massachusetts, compared 502 cases with 835 hospital controls, all between the ages of 30 and 54 years. The estimated risk of AMI increased with the number of cigarettes smoked. Overall, the relative-risk estimate for current smokers was 2.8 (95% confidence interval). The risk did not appear to vary according to the amount of nicotine or carbon monoxide in the cigarette, and the mean amounts of both substances per cigarette were similar for the cases and controls. The results suggest that men who smoke the newer cigarettes with reduced amounts of nicotine and carbon monoxide do not have a lower risk of AMI than those who smoke cigarettes containing larger amounts of these substances.

Effects on coronary circulation

Klein and associates[63] from New York City evaluated the effects of smoking on the coronary circulation in 12 chronic smokers and 10 nonsmokers. Coronary vascular reserve was measured by analyzing the hyperemic response to selective coronary injection of contrast media. There was no statistically significant difference between the patients of the 2 groups with regard to age, ECG, or response to treadmill or thallium-201 exercise tests. However, mean coronary reserve was reduced in the smokers compared with the nonsmokers ($p < 0.02$). In patients who smoked ≤ 1 pack a day and in those who smoked >1 pack a day, the mean coronary reserve was 90 and 65%, respectively. These data suggest that coronary vascular reserve is significantly less in chronic smokers than in nonsmokers and that this decrease is more pronounced in heavy smokers.

BODY WEIGHT

Obesity as a risk factor

The relation between the degree of obesity and the incidence of cardiovascular disease (CVD) was reexamined by Hubert and colleagues[64] from Framingham, Massachusetts, in the 5,209 men and women of the original Framingham cohort. Recent observations of disease over 26 years indicate that obesity, measured by Metropolitan relative weight, was a significant independent predictor of CVD, particularly among women. Multiple logistic regression analyses showed that Metropolitan relative weight, or percentage of desirable weight, on initial examination predicted 26-year incidence of CAD (both angina and CAD other than angina), coronary death, and CHF in men independent of age, cholesterol, systolic BP, cigarettes, LV hypertrophy, and glucose intolerance. Relative weight in women also was positively and independently associated with CAD, stroke, CHF, and CAD and CVD death. These data further show that weight gain after the young adult years conveyed an increased risk of CVD in both sexes that could not be attributed either to the initial weight or the levels of the risk factors that may have resulted from weight gain. Thus, this long-range epidemiologic study suggests that intervention in obesity in addition to the well-established risk factors appears to be an advisable goal in the primary prevention of CVD.

To assess associations between current weight, weight at age 18 years, and weight change from age 18 to ages 30–55 years with current levels of plasma cholesterol, HDL and LDL cholesterol, triglycerides (TG), and systolic and diastolic BP, Khoury and associates[65] from Cincinnati, Ohio, calculated weight change from self-reported weight at age 18 years and measured weight at ages 30–55 years in 308 white and 69 black subjects in a random recall group and in 244 whites and 66 blacks in a hyperlipidemic recall group in the Princeton School Study. In random recall group whites, mean weight gain over time was greater in men than in women; black women had greater weight gain than black men, and nearly twice the weight gain of white women. Current weight and/or weight gain from age 18 years to ages 30–55 years in whites were inversely associated with HDL cholesterol level and positively associated with TG level and systolic and diastolic BP. Similar, but less consistent and significant, trends were observed for blacks. Although weight at age 18 years had no consistent independent explanatory relation to cholesterol, TG, HDL cholesterol, and LDL cholesterol values, random recall group of white men who were in the lowest quartile for weight at age 18 years had current levels of cholesterol, TG, and systolic and diastolic BP that were all lower than those observed in white men who had been in the upper quartile of weight at age 18 years.

In westernized countries cross-sectional and longitudinal studies have shown a progressive increase in weight and relative ponderosity from young adulthood to ages 55–65 years. Similarly, from late adolescence through the sixth decade of life in westernized countries, there are gradual, progressive increments in total serum cholesterol, TG, LDL cholesterol, and BP values. Conversely, when largely rural subjects in Third World countries ingest their habitual "native" diets, there is no progressive increase in weight gain over time, nor are the age-related patterns of increase in total cholesterol, TG, and LDL cholesterol levels as noticeable as in the USA. The current study supports cross-sectional and longitudinal evidence that atherogenic increments in TG level, systolic and diastolic BP from age 18 to 30–55 years are a function, in part, of current weight and weight gain during these years.

PHYSICAL ACTIVITY

Relation to blood lipids

Gordon and coworkers[66] from Bethesda, Maryland, in the Lipid Research Clinics Coronary Primary Prevention Trial, examined the association of habitual physical activity with plasma HDL cholesterol and total triglyceride (TG) in 7,106 asymptomatic 35–59-year-old white men with primary type II hyperlipoproteinemia. Subjects were rated by usual level of physical activity at work and outside of work and the frequency of strenuous physical labor or exercise. By each of these 3 criteria, physical activity was monotonically related to HDL cholesterol and TG: the most physically active men with the highest HDL cholesterol and the lowest TG level. With respect to physical activity outside of work, mean HDL cholesterol and TG were 46 and 152 mg/dl, respectively, in the most active group and 41 and 187 mg/dl in the most sedentary group. Physical activity remains significantly predictive of HDL cholesterol and TG when other known correlates of these plasma constituents—age, Quetelet index, plasma total cholesterol, cigarette smoking, alcohol intake, and clinic—were controlled individually by 2-way analysis of variance or jointly by analysis of covariance. The association of physical activity with very low density lipoprotein cholesterol was parallel to but weaker than its association with TG. Low density lipoprotein and total cholesterol were not significantly related to physical activity.

In a study carried out by Heath and associates[67] from St. Louis, Missouri, the effects of endurance exercise training on plasma lipoprotein lipids were determined in 10 men, aged 46–62 years, with CAD. Patients maintained body weight, health-related behaviors, and stable diets throughout the program. Training was at 50–85% of maximal oxygen consumption $\dot{V}O_2$ max) for 40–60 minutes, 3–5 days/week for 29 ± 7 weeks. Training increased $\dot{V}O_2$ max (31 ± 19%; $p < 0.001$), reduced plasma cholesterol (C) ($-8 ± 4\%$; $p < 0.01$), LDL cholesterol ($-9 ± 9\%$; $p < 0.01$), and triglyceride ($-13 ± 32\%$; $p < 0.05$) concentrations, and increased HDL cholesterol levels (11 ± 13%; $p < 0.05$) and HDL cholesterol/LDL cholesterol ratios (25 ± 20%; $p < 0.01$). Changes in LDL cholesterol and $\dot{V}O_2$ max were correlated ($r = -0.73$; $p ± 0.01$), whereas the changes in LDL cholesterol and HDL cholesterol each correlated inversely with pretraining lipoprotein levels (LDL cholesterol = -0.77; $p < 0.01$; HDL cholesterol = -0.68; $p < 0.05$). Thus potentially antiatherogenic benefits of exercise appear to be due to a training effect, since they correlate best with changes in $\dot{V}O_2$ max and are maximal in patients with initially low $\dot{V}O_2$ max, high LDL cholesterol, and low HDL cholesterol levels.

Risk factors related to physical fitness

Gibbons and colleagues[68] from Dallas, Texas, examined associations between physical fitness and risk factors for CAD in healthy women aged 18–65 years. Physical fitness was objectively determined by the duration of a maximal treadmill exercise test. Six physical fitness categories (very poor to superior) specific within 10-year increments were established. Mean risk factor levels varied across categories, but so did potential confounders, such as age and weight. Multiple linear regression modeling was used to control for the effects of age, weight, and year of examination on coronary risk factors. After adjustment, physical fitness was independently associated with triglycerides, HDL cholesterol, total cholesterol, BP, and cigarette smoking.

Peters and associates[69] from Los Angeles, California, assessed physical work capacity (PWC), a measure of physical fitness, by bicycle ergometry in 2,779 healthy men <55 years of age who were subsequently followed an average of 4.8 years. Thirty-six developed AMI. The relative risk of AMI for below median PWC, adjusted for conventional risk factors for heart disease, was 2.2 (95% confidence limits, 1.1 and 4.7). This increased risk appeared to be limited to men with certain other risk factors present simultaneously:

above median cholesterol level, smoking, above median systolic BP, or a combination of these. Among men with at least 2 of these factors, the adjusted relative risk for below median PWC was 6.6 (95% confidence limits, 2.3 and 27.8). Poor physical fitness may be an important risk factor for heart disease, especially when conventional risk factors are also present.

COFFEE

Thelle and associates[70] from Asgard sykehus, Norway, examined the relation between coffee consumption and levels of serum total cholesterol, HDL cholesterol, and triglycerides among 7,213 women and 7,368 men aged 20–54 years. Coffee consumption was positively associated with levels of total cholesterol and triglycerides in both sexes and was inversely associated with levels of HDL cholesterol in women. The coffee-cholesterol relation remained strong and statistically significant ($p < 0.0001$ in a covariance analysis) after adjustment for age, logarithm of body-mass index, physical activity in leisure time, cigarette smoking, and alcohol consumption. After adjustment for all covariates, the total cholesterol level was 5.56 ± 0.05 mmol/liter (mean ± SE) in men drinking <1 cup of coffee a day compared with 6.23 ± 0.03 mmol/liter in those consuming >9 cups a day. The corresponding figures for women were 5.32 ± 0.05 and 5.92 ± 0.04 mmol/liter. None of the other variables considered could explain this relation. Thus, coffee consumption is a major contributor to the variation of total cholesterol levels.

VASECTOMY

Goldacre and associates[71] from New Haven, Connecticut, performed 2 epidemiologic studies using routine abstracts of medical records to test the hypothesis that vasectomy may predispose men to cardiovascular disease. In a case control study 1,512 men who were <55 years of age and had a history of AMI, stroke, or systemic hypertension were matched with 3,024 controls with other conditions; 2.4% of the cases and 2.7% of the controls were identified as having undergone vasectomy (risk ratio, 0.9; 95% confidence limits, 0.6–1.3). In a cohort study data covering a mean period of 6.5 years after surgery were available on 1,764 men who had had a vasectomy and on 3 comparison cohorts of men who had had other minor surgical procedures. There was no evidence of an increased risk of cardiovascular disease associated with vasectomy. There is no consistent evidence from the studies to support the hypothesis that in the short term vasectomy predisposes young men to cardiovascular disease.

BLOOD HEMATOCRIT

Carter and associates[72] from Honolulu, Hawaii, describe the relation between baseline hematocrit (HCT) level and morbidity and mortality in 10 years in a cohort of 8,006 Japanese-American men. Significantly higher baseline HCT levels were found in the men who subsequently died of CAD compared with the total population. Elevated HCT levels were not found to be significantly associated with any other major cause of death studied. In bivariate analyses, the relation between elevated HCT and the incidence of CAD was found to be significant for nonfatal myocardial infarctions and deaths due to CAD, but not significant for angina pectoris. Using a multiple logistic function, however, the relation of HCT to CAD risk disappeared after adjustment for the correlated risk variables, the most influential being diastolic BP, serum cholesterol, and smoking. These findings indicate that, although there is a significant relation between HCT and CAD mortality and the incidence of some manifestations of CAD morbidity, these relations are not independent of the stronger influences of diastolic BP and serum cholesterol on disease outcome.

ALCOHOL INTAKE

The relation of alcohol intake to development of cardiovascular disease is receiving renewed attention. Alcohol drinking has been incriminated as a cause of dilated cardiomyopathy and of sudden death. It has been reported to be related to the development of systemic hypertension and of stroke. A protective influence against CAD, however, has been noted in some studies. Much of the evidence for these conclusions has come from investigations of alcohol abuse and not from studies of general populations. Gordon and Kannel[73] from Framingham, Massachusetts, observed drinking habits and other characteristics for 20 years in a cohort of 5,209 men and women. During this period, the average amount of alcohol consumed rose 63%. The percent increase was greater for women than men and greater for younger persons than older persons. Serum uric acid and phospholipid concentrations were higher at higher levels of alcohol consumption. Lipoprotein levels of 0–12 and 100–400 Svedberg units were positively associated with alcohol consumption in men but negatively associated with alcohol consumption in women. The BP was higher in nondrinkers than light drinkers, but among drinkers BPs were higher at higher consumption levels. Although cigarette smokers had lower BPs than nonsmokers, this seemed to be due to their lower weight. Persons who increased their alcohol consumption during follow-up had a small mean increase in serum phospholipid and uric acid levels, BP, and weight relative to the average changes for these variables.

Hartung and associates[74] from Houston, Texas, measured plasma HDL cholesterol levels before and after alcohol abstinence and after resumption of a controlled alcohol dose in 16 marathon runners, 15 joggers, and in 13 inactive men. A 3-week period of abstinence resulted in a significant decrease in HDL concentration in the inactive men (50–42 mg/dl). Three weeks of alcohol consumption (1,065 ml/day of beer) produced a significant increase in HDL cholesterol level to 51 mg/dl. No change in HDL cholesterol level was found for the marathon group or the joggers during abstinence or 3 weeks of alcohol intake. The consumption of alcohol in moderation therefore seems to be associated with increased HDL concentration levels in inactive men but not in men who engage in regular running or jogging.

In a prospective study of cardiovascular disease involving 5,209 men and women from Framingham, Massachusetts, alcohol consumption was determined on 4 occasions during the first 24 years of follow-up. Based on this information, it was found by Gordon and Kannel[75] from Boston, Massachusetts, that the incidence of cardiovascular disease in general, and of CAD and intermittent claudication in particular, was inversely related to the amount of alcohol regularly consumed. These relations were weak but statistically significant. In men, the inverse relation to CAD was equally strong for all manifestations of the disease, except sudden death. There was a suggestion that sudden death was more commonly unexpected among men drinking >90 ounces of ethanol a month than among other men. In women, the strongest inverse relation was with angina pectoris. No relation could be demonstrated for either sex between the amount of alcohol consumed and the incidence of CHF, hemorrhagic stroke, or atherothrombotic stroke.

Thornton and associates[76] from Bristol, England, measured the effect of alcohol on plasma HDL cholesterol and on bile cholesterol saturation in 12 healthy volunteers with a very low initial alcohol intake. The subjects drank 39 g of alcohol daily for 6 weeks, and then abstained from alcohol for 6 weeks. The HDL cholesterol rose significantly from 1.07 ± 0.05–1.25 ± 0.08 mmol/liter (41.4 ± 1.9–48.3 ± 3.1 mg/dl) when alcohol was being consumed and fell to 1.04 ± 0.06 mmol/liter (40.2 ± 2.3 mg/dl) during abstention. Bile cholesterol saturation index fell from 1.31 ± 0.06–1.08 ± 0.06 during the period of alcohol consumption and rose to 1.27 ± 0.09 during absention. There was a significant inverse correlation between bile saturation index and HDL cholesterol ($r = -0.56$). These data provide further evidence of a biochemical link between cardiovascular disease and cholesterol gallstones and suggest that moderate alcohol intake has some protective effect against both diseases.

EXERCISE ECG RESPONSE

Giagnoni and associates[77] from Milan, Italy, studied 135 asymptomatic normotensive subjects with exercise-induced ST ischemic depression of $\geqslant 1$ mm and compared them with 379 controls. At least 2 controls with negative responses on the exercise ECG test were selected for each case and were matched for age, sex, work, community, and coronary-risk factors index. The end points considered were the following coronary events: angina pectoris, AMI, and sudden death. After a median follow-up period of 6.0 years for the cases and 6.4 years for the controls, the relative risk was 5.55 (95% confidence limits, 2.75–11.22). Coronary events occurred significantly earlier in the cases than in the controls (Fig. 1-6). The data also suggest that the exercise ECG response is a particularly good prognostic indicator for AMI. In addition, the analysis has confirmed the predictive roles of age, smoking, BP, and the index of coronary risk factors and suggests that the exercise ECG response is an additional independent risk indicator for coronary events.

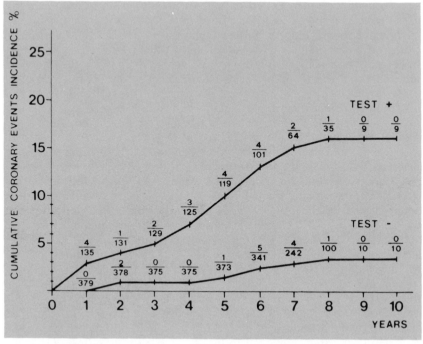

Fig. 1-6. Cumulative curves for incidence of coronary events in cases (test +) and controls (test −). For each year of follow–up the number of coronary events observed (numerator) and number of subjects exposed to risk (denominator) are indicated. Relative risk as determined by Cox's regression model is 5.55 (95% confidence limits, 2.75–11.22); as determined by logistic matched set analysis, 5.03 (95% confidence limits, 2.41–10.49). Reproduced with permission from Giagnoni et al.[77]

MISCELLANEOUS TOPICS

Heart disease prevention projects (Belgian and UK)

The UK Heart Disease Prevention Project and the Goteborg trial were the first randomized population-based trials set up to study how much health education can change the major CAD risk factors in a population and how such changes affect the mortality and incidence of CAD. Subsequently, the US Multiple Risk Factor Intervention Trial and the Oslo Heart Study were set up to evaluate prevention in selected high risk groups. To increase its power and to test the consistency of the findings in various populations, the UK study was later extended to 4 other European countries to form the WHO European Collaborative Trial in the Multifactorial Prevention of CAD with a total of 60,881 participants. From the outset, the 5 centers were recognized as autonomous; a common protocol was adopted to permit both pooling of combined results and analysis of contrast between national findings. Rose and associates[78] from London and Dundee, England, reported results of the UK center and Kornitzer and associates[79] from Brussels and Gent, Belgium, reported results from the Belgian Heart Disease prevention project, both of which were part of the WHO European Collaborative Trial in the Multifactorial Prevention of Coronary Heart Disease. In the UK center trials, 18,210 men took part, aged 40–59 years. They were employed in 24 factories, which formed the allocation units for randomized control trial lasting 5–6 years. Intervention comprised advice on cholesterol lowering diet, smoking cessation, weight control, exercise, and treatment of systemic hypertension. Advice was given mainly through factory medical departments. There was an overall average net reduction of 4% CAD risk but there was no clear effect on CAD end points (coronary deaths and AMI) or on all-causes mortality. There was, however, a 36% reduction in the rate at which intervention subjects reported ill with other CAD (principally angina pectoris) during the study, and fewer intervention men gave positive responses to a self-administered questionnaire on angina and chest pain.

In the Belgian Heart Disease Prevention Project, 19,409 men aged 40–59 years took part. They were employed in 30 factories that formed the allocation units for randomized control trial lasting 5–6 years. The intervention package was similar to the UK study. The coronary risk profile was reduced in the intervention group compared with that in the control group, especially during the first 4 years by effects on serum cholesterol, number of cigarettes smoked daily, and arterial BP. Total mortality was 18% lower in the intervention group than in the control group. Coronary mortality was reduced by a nonsignificant 21%, whereas CAD incidence (nonfatal AMI plus fatal AMI plus sudden death) was reduced by 25%. Nonfatal AMI (not a major end point) was similarly reduced by 26%.

Secular trends

Kimm and coworkers[80] in Durham, North Carolina, compared secular trends in CAD mortality in North Carolina, Georgia, South Carolina, and Virginia with those in California, New York, and Utah. Mortality data were obtained from US Vital Statistics and population informaton from the US Census Bureau. Age-adjusted CAD mortality increased until 1968 in the Southeastern states and then declined, and declines were greatest in nonwhite women. In contrast, CAD mortality in all groups in California and in women in New York and Utah began to decline in the early 1950s, with accelerated declines since 1968. In all states, the decline in rates in nonwhites have been greatest in the younger age groups. This has not been true in the white populations. Declining CAD mortality correlated moderately well with the decline in death from all cardiovascular disease and from all causes, but not with the declining cerebrovascular disease mortality. Respiratory cancer mortality increased in similar proportions in California and South Carolina, 2 states with dissimilar CAD trends. These findings suggest that improved control of systemic hypertension and changing patterns of cigarette smoking may not be responsible for the recent decline in CAD mortality.

ANGINA PECTORIS

Effects on ECG, LV function, and prognosis

Complete occlusion of the LM coronary artery is rare and, prior to this report, only 64 patients had been reported. Ward and associates[81] from London, England, described 5 patients aged 24–62 years, each with angina pectoris for a long time with complete occlusion of the LM coronary artery. In 1 of the 5 the right coronary artery also was completely occluded. All patients had a dominant right coronary circulation and the right coronary was significantly narrowed in only 1 patient. Ventricular function was severely impaired in only 1 patient. Only 1 of the 5 patients had a history of AMI.

In 18 consecutive patients without a history of AMI, prolonged angina pectoris with persistent T waves in the precordial leads was associated in a study by Figueras and associates[82] from Barcelona, Spain, with a high frequency of in-hospital spontaneous angina (14 of 18, 78%), usually accompanied by ST-segment elevation, and occasionally in-hospital AMI (4 of 18, 22%). Angina and AMI always involved the ECG leads with negative T waves. Coronary arteriography, performed in 16 patients, revealed ≥90% proximal diameter reduction of the LAD coronary artery in 14 patients. No patient had severe narrowing of all 3 major coronary arteries, but the 3 who had 100% LAD occlusion lacked collateral circulation. The EF was ≥50% in 13 patients. Atrial pacing performed in 11 patients at an average rate of 142 beats/minute produced a 1.0 mm ST-segment change in only 5 patients (45%), 3 of whom had an associated lactate production. Arterial systemic hypertension induced by methoxamine in 14 patients caused reversal of negative T waves without significant ST-segment shifts or chest pain and failed to elicit lactate extraction abnormalities in each of the 5 patients in whom it was determined. Thus, prolonged angina with persistent negative T waves in the precordial leads is almost invariably associated with a critical and proximal LAD obstruction, severe narrowing of 1 or 2 coronary arteries, and poor or absent collateral vessels. The relatively preserved coronary reserve in 55% of patients suggests that negative T waves do not represent active myocardial ischemia. The study also suggests that transient "positivization" of the negative T waves may not necessarily relate to myocardial ischemia when associated with acute systemic hypertension.

Deanfield and associates[83] from London, England, in 30 patients with stable angina pectoris and positive exercise tests used ambulatory ST segment monitoring to record episodes of transient myocardial ischemia during daily life. All patients had 4 consecutive days of monitoring and in 20 patients long-term variability was assessed by repeated 48-hour monitoring and exercise testing over 18 months. There were 1,934 episodes of rectilinear or downsloping ST depression (911, 1 mm; 638, 2 mm; 385, > 3 mm) in 446 days of recording, of which only 470 (24%) were accompanied by angina. Positron emission tomography showed evidence of regional myocardial ischemia during both symptomatic and asymptomatic ST depression. On average, heart rate at the onset of both symptomatic and asymptomatic ST episodes was significantly lower than the rate at the onset of ST depression during exercise testing (98 ± 21 -vs- 124 ± 17 beats/min). Heart rate rose by more than 10 beats in the minute preceding ST depression in only 23% of episodes. Over 18 months, 8 (40%) patients exhibited marked variability in the number of daily ST episodes. Variability of ST depression was consistently underestimated by symptoms and not reflected by exercise testing. Thus, patients with stable angina showed frequent, variable, and often asymptomatic ECG evidence of ischemia. Heart rate increase was not common before myocardial ischemia, suggesting that, in such patients, transient impairment in coronary supply may be at least as important as excessive increase in demand in the genesis of ischemia during daily life.

Simultaneous and accurate recording of the systemic arterial BP and ST segment changes is fraught with technical difficulties. Davies and associates[84] from Harrow, England, developed a new system to enable accurate reproduction of the ECG and intraarterial BP, using a transducer/-perfusion unit conventionally used to study hypertensive subjects, linked to a frequency modulated tape recorder. Detailed methods of digital analysis have been developed to process the data. This system has been used to study 22 patients with arteriographically proved severe obstructive CAD who had frequent attacks of angina. Control data from quantified dynamic exercise in the laboratory were used for comparison with the effects of normal daily activities outside the hospital and to test the hypothesis that double product (heart rate times systolic BP) is relevant to the onset of angina in such patients. The most important finding was that both angina and asymptomatic episodes of ST-segment depression were invariably accompanied by an increase in heart rate, whereas there was considerable variation in BP changes, ranging from an increase to a substantial fall. This suggests that heart rate changes are more important in determining ischemic episodes than BP. Furthermore, the double product was not reproducible during repeated episodes of angina and asymptomatic ischemia and did not appear to have an important role in the pathogenesis of intermittent myocardial ischemia in this group of patients.

Haines and associates[85] from Burlington, Vermont, studied the significance of the development of new T-wave inversion in 118 consecutive patients with unstable angina pectoris. The ECGs during hospitalization in the coronary care unit were analyzed for occurrence of new T-wave inversion ≥2 mm and correlated with findings at coronary angiography (73 patients) and at follow-up (112 patients). Twenty-nine patients had anterior T-wave inversion. Of these, 25 patients (86%) had ≥70% diameter reduction of the LAD artery, compared with 11 (26%) of 42 patients without anterior T-wave inversion (p < 0.001). The sensitivity of T-wave inversion for significant LAD stenosis was 69%, specificity was 89%, and positive predictive value was 86%. Two patients had T-wave inversion in the inferior leads. Both patients had significant right CAD, compared with 18 of 55 patients without inferior T-wave inversion (p, NS). Seventy-one patients who were treated medically had 16 ± 9 months of follow-up. Of 26 patients who had T-wave inversion, 10 (38%) had cardiac events, compared with 7 (16%) of the remaining 45 patients without T-wave inversion (p < 0.05). Forty-one patients who had undergone CABG had 19 ± 9 months of follow-up. Of 22 patients with T-wave inversion, 4 (18%) had cardiac events, compared with 2 (11%) of the remaining 19 patients without T-wave inversion (p, NS). Thus, development of new T-wave inversion ≥2 mm in patients with unstable angina is predictive of significant CAD, and identifies a subgroup with poor prognosis when treated medically.

M-mode echo has been used during exercise to evaluate changes in LV size and performance in response to various types of exercise and cardiac drugs. Crawford and associates[86] from San Antonio, Texas, utilized 2-D echo for quantitating LV size and performance in 25 patients with angina pectoris from CAD and in 10 normal subjects. In 18 (72%) of the 25 patients, suitable biapical 2-D echoes for quantitative analysis were recorded during upright bicycle exercise. The LV volume, EF, and wall motion score were measured at rest and at peak exercise, 30 minutes later at rest, after nitroglycerin at rest, and at peak exercise. The EF increased during control exercise in the normal subjects from 57 ± 16–71 ± 22%, but was unchanged in the patients during exercise before nitroglycerin. In 7 patients (39%) marked increases in EF during exercise occurred after nitroglycerin. The wall motion score increased significantly in the patients during control exercise but was less at maximum exercise after nitroglycerin. Thus, quantitation of LV performance during exercise by biapical 2-D echo can be accomplished in a large proportion of patients with angina pectoris from CAD and can be used to assess the effects of therapeutic interventions.

Boden and associates[87] from Providence, Rhode Island, evaluated 15 patients with episodic angina at rest, recurrent ST-segment elevation, and nontransmural AMI who continued to have rest angina despite intensive nitrate and beta adrenergic antagonist therapy. Eleven patients required intraaortic balloon counterpulsation for refractory angina and 13 underwent cardiac catheterization. High grade (≥90%) diameter reduction of the proximal LAD coronary artery was demonstrated in 11 of the 13 patients and coronary arterial spasm without significant fixed occlusive disease in 2. Urgent coronary arterial revascularization was performed in 7 patients, with 1 late death after a later reoperation. Eight patients not requiring surgery initially were followed on medical therapy, but 5 of these subsequently developed large transmural anterior infarcts and 3 died from pump failure. Thus, repetitive episodes of rest angina with marked ST-segment elevation across the precordial leads and mild creatine kinase elevations may define a subset of patients at major risk for massive transmural AMI.

Moise and associates[88] from Montreal, Canada, studied the progression of atherosclerotic narrowings in 38 patients who had previously undergone coronary angiography and were later hospitalized for an episode of unstable angina pectoris, and 38 matched patients with stable angina who had also undergone prior catheterization. Patients with unstable angina and those with stable angina were similar in terms of age (mean, 49 and 50 years, respectively), number of risk factors (1.5/patient in both groups), interval between studies (mean ± SD, 44 ± 31 and 35 ± 31 months, respectively), number of diseased vessels on the first angiogram (1.52 in both groups), and initial EF (65 and 63%, respectively). Progression of coronary narrowing was demonstrated in 29 of the 38 patients with unstable angina, compared with 12 of the 38 with stable angina (p < 0.0005). Progression to ≥70% stenosis was recorded in 21 patients with unstable angina but in only 5 with stable angina (p < 0.0005). Also, more frequent in the patients with unstable angina were multifocal progression (11 -vs- 2; p < 0.01) or progression of the LM or preseptal LAD artery or both (9 -vs- 1; p < 0.01). Thus, unstable angina is associated with progression in the extent and severity of CAD.

Progression of CAD was assessed prospectively by Frick and associates[89] from Helsinki, Finland, in a randomized series of 36 medically treated and 42 surgically treated patients with angina pectoris. The medical patients were reexamined after 5 years and the surgical patients at 3 weeks, 1 year, and 5 years after operation. Sixty-seven percent of the medical patients and 69% of the surgical patients had progression. The frequency of new lesions in initially normal segments after 5 years in the medical group was 7% -vs- 4% in ungrafted normal segments in the surgical group (p = 0.05, and p < 0.01). The frequency of progression in abnormal arteries was 24% in the medical group -vs- 23% in the ungrafted arteries of the surgical group (p = 0.90, and p < 0.95). The rate of progression of obstructed segments proximal to the graft over 5 years was 43 -vs- 27% of the corresponding segments in the medical group (p < 0.01). Progression took place in 12% of normal segments proximal to the graft -vs- 2% of the corresponding segments in the medical group (p < 0.05); 69% of progression occurring in segments proximal to the graft had reached total occlusion -vs- 38% of the corresponding segments in the medical group (p < 0.01). Progression developed in 4% of segments distal to the graft -vs- 3% of the corresponding segments in the medical group. Progression takes place at identical rates in medically treated patients and in ungrafted arteries and segments distal to the graft in surgical patients. Proximal to the graft, the rates differ and total occlusions appear as early as 3 weeks after operation.

Treatment with nitrates and/or comparison with nitroprusside

Kimchi and associates[90] from Sacramento, California, evaluated the prophylactic antianginal efficacy of nitroglycerin (NTG) oral spray in 20 patients with angiographically documented CAD and stable angina pectoris. The evaluation was performed by a randomized crossover trial involving treadmill exercise testing. On study day 1, a control treadmill exercise test was performed, followed 30 minutes later by a second exercise test 2 minutes after administration of either placebo (group A, 10 patients) or NTG 0.8 mg (group B, 10 patients). One week later, on study day 2, the patients again underwent control treadmill exercise testing followed by a second exercise test after either NTG spray (group A) or placebo (group B). NTG spray delayed the onset of anginal pain during exercise by a mean of 100 ± 64 seconds in 13 patients and prevented pain entirely in 7 individuals. Placebo did not significantly delay the appearance of angina and prevented chest pain in only 1 patient. NTG spray increased treadmill exercise duration by 31% before the onset of angina, but placebo did not significantly alter the duration of exercise. NTG spray abolished in 6 patients and delayed in 14 patients the onset of exercise-induced ST-segment depression of 1 mm. Patients achieved a higher heart rate at peak exercise with NTG spray, and yet the maximal exercise-induced ST-segment depression of 2.1 ± 1 mm during the control study declined to 1.3 ± 0.9 mm with the spray. The placebo had no effect on exercise ST-segment depression. These investigators concluded that oral NTG spray is an effective prophylactic for exercise-induced angina.

In 10 men with documented CAD and stable exertional angina pectoris Degré and associates[91] from Brussels, Belgium, examined the benefit and duration of action on their symptom-limited exercise capacity in a double-blind crossover study of 2 doses (2.5 and 6.5 mg) of sustained release NTG. A multistage bicycle test was performed in the sitting position by steps of 30 watts each 3 minutes until the onset of typical angina pectoris. It was performed 24 hours before the start of the study; 1 and 5 hours after administration of placebo, and repeated after 2.5 and 6.5 mg of NTG administered in a double-blind crossover study according to a 4-successive-days protocol. No differences appeared between administration of placebo (1 and 5 hours) and the results obtained at the first exercise test. The dose of 2.5 mg of NTG was effective on the symptom-limited working capacity but only at 1 hour (+9%; $p < 0.01$). The dose of 6.5 mg was more effective both at 1 hour (+25%; $p < 0.001$) and at 5 hours (+27%; $p < 0.001$). All patients had angina at a higher heart rate (+5–8%; p, NS and $p < 0.01$), whereas systolic BP and double product tended to be slightly but insignificantly increased. ST depression at the onset of angina was insignificantly changed with placebo and 2.5 and 6.5 mg of NTG. It is concluded that 6.5 mg of orally administered sustained release NTG was effective during at least 5 hours, and that the magnitude of the benefit and its duration are dose related.

A prospective randomized trial of intravenous NTG in the management of repetitive spontaneous angina was undertaken by Curfman and colleagues[92] from Buffalo, New York, in 40 consecutive patients. The clinical effectiveness of intravenous NTG (group A) was compared with that of oral isosorbide dinitrate (ISDN) and topical 2% NTG ointment in combination (group B) during a 72-hour treatment period. The doses of both nitrate regimens were adjusted so that the mean arterial pressure in the 2 groups was reduced by 15% of control values to the same level (77 mmHg). The intravenous NTG dose of 10–200 mg/minute produced arterial plasma levels of 1.2–65.3 ng/ml and estimated plasma clearance of 106 ml/min/kg of body weight. In group B the doses were 20–60 mg of oral ISDN and 0.5–2 inches NTG ointment every 6 hours. Intravenous NTG reduced the number of spontaneous ischemic episodes from 3.3/24 hours during the control period to 1/24 hours during the treatment period, whereas the oral and topical ISDN/oral NTG combination reduced the number of episodes from 3–1.4. Overall, the magnitude of the therapeutic effect of the intravenous NTG was statistically indistinguishable from that of ISDN/oral NTG combination, although the intravenous NTG did have somewhat greater clinical benefit on day 2 of the 3-day treatment period. Although both regimens markedly reduced the frequency of spontaneous ischemic episodes, only 36% of patients in group A and 17% in group B experienced no ischemic episodes during the study period. In group A 43% of patients and in group B 61% of patients required early CABG to control recurrent ischemic episodes refractory to medical therapy. The investigators concluded that intravenous NTG and ISDN/oral NTG when administered in doses adjusted to produce similar effects on systemic arterial pressure have nearly equivalent clinical effects in the management of recurrent episodes of spontaneous angina pectoris. The recurrence rate of spontaneous ischemic episodes during medical therapy remained high with both regimens, and early CABG may be required for long-term management.

Kaplan and associates[93] from Chicago, Illinois, treated 35 patients with angina at rest that was unresponsive to oral or topical nitrates and beta blocking drugs with a continuous infusion of intravenous NTG. The infusion was started at 10 μg/minute and increased by 10 μg/minute increments every 5 minutes until an infusion rate of 50 μg/minute was reached. After each episode of rest angina, the infusion was increased by 50 μg/minute in the same stepwise manner. Data from a 24-hour baseline control period were compared with those from a 24-hour intravenous NTG end point period at which time the highest intravenous NTG infusion rate was administered. The average intravenous NTG infusion rate was 140 ± 15 μg/minute. With intravenous NTG therapy, the number of episodes of angina at rest decreased from 3.5 ± 0.4–0.3 ± 0.1, sublingual NTG decreased from 1.9 ± 0.3–0.4 ± 0.1 mg/day, and morphine sulfate administration decreased from 5.5 ± 1.3–0.4 ± 0.2 mg/day (all p < 0.001). When each patient's response on the end point day was analyzed, 25 were defined as complete (no rest angina), 8 as partial (>50% decrease in the number of episodes/day from control values), and 2 as nonresponders. No significant drug-induced adverse effects occurred. Intravenous NTG appears to be effective therapy for angina at rest refractory to standard oral and topical medications.

Dalal and associates[94] from Kingston, Canada, evaluated 10 patients in a randomized, double-blind crossover study to determine acute and sustained effects of oral ISDN. Circulatory changes in exercise performance were evaluated before and 2 and 6 hours after medication. Sublingual NTG was administered 30 minutes after the 2- and 6-hour exercise tests and the exercise test was repeated after another 5 minutes. Systolic blood pressure at rest 2 hours after ISDN decreased by 25% during the acute phase, but by only 11% during the sustained phase and was not decreased further by NTG during acute therapy but was decreased during sustained therapy. Six hours after ISDN, systolic BP remained below control values during sustained therapy. Exercise time to moderate angina was prolonged 2 hours after ISDN during both acute and sustained phases. However, during the sustained phase, there was no difference from control values after 6 hours. The NTG did not increase walking time 2 hours after ISDN during either acute or chronic therapy, but at 6 hours NTG increased walking time during sustained therapy. Thus, these data demonstrate that 1) tolerance to the hemodynamic and antianginal effects of ISDN develops; 2) NTG does not further prolong exercise duration 2 hours after ISDN, but it does prolong exercise duration 6 hours after this agent is administered; and 3) there is possible cross-tolerance between ISDN and NTG.

Parker and coworkers[95] from Ontario, Canada, determined the circulatory response and plasma concentrations of ISDN in 10 patients with chronic stable angina administration of 5 mg sublingual ISDN during the control stage, after 48 hours of therapy 15 mg ISDN orally every 6 hours, and subsequently after a 48-hour period when ISDN was substituted by placebo 4 times daily. Initially, sublingual ISDN induced major reductions in both supine and standing systolic and diastolic BP, but after 45 hours of therapy with oral ISDN, there was a significantly diminished vasodepressor response in both positions. Subsequently, when placebo was substituted for ISDN, the circulatory response initially seen was restored within 21 hours. Plasma ISDN concentrations after the test sublingual dose were slightly higher after 48 hours of oral ISDN dosing than at the start of the study. This suggests that tolerance is unlikely to be caused by reduced bioavailability or accelerated elimination of ISDN. It is possible that tolerance is related to accumulation of ISDN metabolites. The attenuation of the circulatory response to ISDN may be related to the altered antianginal efficacy commonly seen during sustained therapy with ISDN.

Feldman and associates[96] from Gainesville, Florida, compared the coronary hemodynamic effects of an infusion of nitroprusside and of sublingual NTG in the same patients. The coronary hemodynamic responses of the anterior LV region to both drugs were studied in 9 patients in whom the LAD was filled by collaterals. Before and during administration of each drug (given in doses designed to produce similar changes in LV diastolic pressure), heart rate, LV and aortic pressure, and anterior regional flow, oxygen delivery, and lactate metabolism were measured. Given in this manner, as expected, both drugs decreased the double product of heart rate and systolic BP. Concomitant with these changes, anterior regional blood flow increased or decreased modest amounts or did not change with either drug. Similar directional flow changes or no change occurred in 6 patients and directionally different changes in the other 3 patients. The ratio of mean aortic pressure or of the double product to anterior regional flow consistently decreased during the administration of both drugs. Additionally, anterior regional myocardial oxygen uptake remained similar during both drug periods compared with control values. Anterior region lactate extraction was abnormal (<10%) in 4 of the 9 patients during the initial control period. Lactate extraction was usually normal during both the nitroprusside and the NTG periods. In general, coronary hemodynamic values were remarkably similar during both of these periods. Thus, although relative differences in systemic arterial and venous dilation were obtained with nitroprusside and NTG, similar and beneficial coronary hemodynamic changes generally occurred.

Treatment with propranolol

To determine whether propranolol can be administered twice daily without any loss of antianginal effect, Bassan and Weiler-Ravell[97] from Jerusalem, Israel, studied 9 men receiving long-term propranolol therapy for stable angina pectoris. Each patient performed bicycle exercise to the point of angina on 2 consecutive mornings. By means of double-blind placebo and propranolol administration before the test, the study created a situation whereby on 1 day the exercise took place 12 hours after the last dose of propranolol, and on the other day, 1.5 hours after a dose. Despite markedly lower blood levels of propranolol on the day that exercise was performed 12 hours after the last dose, exercise time to angina was nearly identical on the 2 days. It was concluded that long-term therapy with propranolol for angina pectoris can be administered on a twice daily basis with no loss of effectiveness.

Morris and associates[98] from Durham, North Carolina, compared the effects of medium dose (160 mg/day) and high dose (480 mg/day) oral propranolol in 22 patients with typical angina pectoris and objective evidence of myocardial ischemia during exercise. The LV EF and wall motion score (WMS) (an index of regional LV dysfunction) were assessed by RNA both at rest and during exercise to the pretreatment maximum work load. Functional class improved in 11 of the 22 patients during medium dose propranolol therapy. Medium dose propranolol reduced mean resting heart rate from 71–55 beats/minute, exercise heart rate from 122–93 beats/minute, and exercise systolic BP from 183–162 mmHg (p < 0.001 for each). The frequencies of exercise-induced chest pain and ST-segment depression were reduced from 19–9 patients (p < 0.001), and from 20–10 patients (p = 0.002), respectively. Medium dose propranolol had no effect on mean EF or WMS at rest, but improved function in ischemic regions during exercise; WMS decreased (p = 0.001), and mean exercise EF increased from 0.51–0.56 (p = 0.025). Compared with the medium dose, high dose propranolol improved functional class in 3 additional patients, and further reduced mean resting heart rate (from 55–52 beats/min; p = 0.001) and mean exercise heart rate (from 93–86 beats/min; p = 0.001). Exercise-induced chest pain and ST-segment depression were abolished in another 7 and 6 patients, respectively. Exercise EF and WMS improved further in several patients, but the changes were not statistically significant for the group (p = 0.095 and 0.082, respectively). Thus, in patients with CAD and exercise-induced ischemia, propranolol reduced heart rate and BP and the incidence of exercise-induced chest pain, ECG changes, and ischemic LV dysfunction. Although most of these effects were seen with medium dose propranolol, higher doses provided additional relief of chest pain and ST-segment depression, and further improved global and regional LV function in several patients.

Although beta adrenergic blocking agents reduce myocardial oxygen consumption and symptoms of myocardial ischemia in patients with CAD, propranolol has been reported to exacerbate coronary artery spasm in some patients with variant angina. To determine whether increased coronary vasomotor tone can be induced by beta adrenergic blockade, Kern and colleagues[99] from Boston, Massachusetts, measured the changes in coronary vascular resistance (CVR) during cold pressor testing (CPT) in 15 patients, 9 with severe CAD and 6 with normal left coronary anatomy before and after intravenous propranolol. Coronary blood flow was measured by coronary sinus thermodilution. The CVR was calculated as mean arterial pressure divided by coronary sinus blood flow. Heart rate was maintained constant at a paced subanginal rate of 95 beats/minute. Before propranolol, CPT induced significant increases in CVR in patients with CAD but no increase in CVR in normal patients. After propranolol, the CVR change during CPT was augmented for patients with CAD, 29%, and for the normal population, 9%. The potentiated increase in CVR occurred without significant changes in resting CVR or in the magnitude of the hypertensive response to CPT. These investigators conclude that beta adrenergic blockade for propranolol can potentiate coronary artery vasoconstriction in some patients with CAD, possibly mediated by unopposed alpha adrenergic vasomotor tone. These changes may be important in patients in whom intense adrenergic stimulation may increase coronary artery tone and adversely influence the balance between myocardial oxygen supply and demand.

Comparison of propranolol and pindolol

Parker[100] from Kingston, Canada, assessed 22 patients with chronic, stable, exercise-induced angina pectoris during periods of therapy with propranolol, standard formulation pindolol, and a slow release preparation of pindolol. Patients maintained diaries of the frequency of angina pectoris and nitroglycerin consumption and underwent treadmill exercise testing at 2 weekly intervals. No significant differences were observed in nitroglycerin consumption or anginal frequency during these 3 treatment programs.

Resting heart rates were higher with pindolol than with propranolol, but no differences were noted between periods on standard and slow release pindolol. Systolic and diastolic BP was similar during therapy with these 3 treatment programs. Treadmill walking time to the development of moderate angina and systolic and diastolic BP was similar during treatment with propranolol, standard formulation pindolol, and slow release pindolol. Exercise heart rates were slightly higher during therapy with slow release pindolol than during standard formulation pindolol. Thus, propranolol, pindolol, and slow release pindolol are equally effective in the management of patients with chronic, stable, exercise-induced angina.

A similar study also was reported by Manyari and associates[101] from London, Canada.

Effects of dobutamine

Pacold and colleagues[102] from Hines, Illinois, studied 14 patients with CAD and normal or near normal LV function at rest and during atrial pacing until the occurrence of angina (12 patients) before and during infusion of dobutamine (3.80 µg/kg/min). At rest, during the infusion, 3 patients developed chest pain, mean ST-segment depression increased from 0.02–0.08 mV, and myocardial lactate extraction fell from 18––1.4%. These ischemic changes were associated with significant increases in arterial systolic pressure (134–149 mmHg), heart rate (79–91 beats/min), coronary sinus flow (89–113 ml/min), and myocardial oxygen consumption (11–14 ml/min). In contrast, during atrial pacing, dobutamine did not reduce the pacing threshold or further increase myocardial oxygen consumption or ST-segment changes; however, arterial mean and diastolic pressures were significantly lower with pacing during dobutamine infusion compared with control pacing. In the absence of heart failure, dobutamine in low doses can cause myocardial ischemia in patients with CAD. The absence of increased ischemia from dobutamine during pacing may reflect reversal of pacing-induced ventricular dysfunction.

Treatment with calcium channel blockers alone and/or comparison to other agents

The clinical outcome after the initial year of therapy with either diltiazem (D), nifedipine (N), or verapamil (V) was examined in 45 patients with rest angina in an investigation reported by Pepine and associates[103] from Gainesville, Florida. Age, frequency of angina, duration of symptoms, and EF were similar in all 3 treatment groups. CAD was present in 60% of patients (5 of 13 given D, 8 of 16 given N, and 14 of 16 given V). Coronary spasm was suspected (ST elevation with angina) or documented (angiographically) in 35 (78%) patients. Twenty-nine (64%) patients had >50% decrease in angina without a coronary event (9 taking D, 11 taking N, and 9 taking V). Coronary events (sudden death, AMI, and hospitalization for unacceptable angina control or CABG) occurred in 13 (29%) patients (2 taking D, 4 taking N, and 7 taking V). To achieve these responses, 20 (44%) patients required additional antianginal drugs (long-acting nitrates, beta blockers, or other calcium channel blockers). Four of these 20 patients were taking D, 9 were taking N, and 7 were taking V. Seventeen (38%) patients experienced a side effect (6 taking N, and 11 taking V). Although rest angina can be controlled in most patients during the initial year of treatment with calcium channel blockers, additional therapy is often required. Furthermore, the clinical course of patients presenting with rest angina remains unpredictable, even during calcium channel blocker treatment. Morbid events continue to occur, related in part to the extent of CAD.

Subramanian and associates[104] from Harrow, England, evaluated 21 patients with chronic stable angina pectoris to determine the ideal dose of diltiazem in effectively treating their symptoms. Dose titration studies utilized 180, 270, and 360 mg/day, and a blinded, objective protocol was used to determine which dose was most effective. Improvement in exercise tolerance was found at all dose levels, but the most effective dosage for reduction of angina and nitroglycerin consumption and improving exercise capacity was 360 mg/day. Only 1 patient was withdrawn from the study while receiving 360 mg of diltiazem, and this was necessitated by pedal edema. Thus, diltiazem is an effective antianginal medication in dosages ranging from 180–360 mg/day, but the most effective dosage in the treatment of angina pectoris appears to be 360 mg/day.

The effects of oral diltiazem (360 mg/day) on exercise tolerance, LV performance, and plasma lactate and catecholamine levels were studied by Petru and coworkers[105] from San Antonio, Texas, in 13 patients with atherosclerotic CAD in a placebo-controlled, randomized, double-blind protocol. Exercise duration to the onset of ischemic ST-segment depression, time to angina pectoris, and time to peak exercise improved by 120, 174, and 144 seconds, respectively. The LV EF, as determined by RNA, increased in patients at rest from 52% during placebo therapy to 58% during diltiazem therapy; at peak exercise EF increased from 44% during placebo therapy to 52% during diltiazem. The mean plasma norepinephrine level in patients at rest increased from 498 pg/ml during placebo treatment to 667 pg/ml during diltiazem therapy. Resting standing BP and supine and standing diastolic BP decreased significantly with diltiazem. In all 10 patients followed over a long term, oral diltiazem caused persistent improvement in exercise performance at 12–20 weeks, without evidence of placebo effects. Thus, diltiazem is highly effective in divided doses of 360 mg/day for the therapy of chronic angina pectoris.

Lindenberg and associates[106] from Boston, Massachusetts, gave 20 patients with moderate to severe exertional angina incremental doses of diltiazem. Diltiazem produced a dose-related improvement in anginal frequency and exercise capacity, so that weekly anginal attacks were reduced to 7.5, 5.6, and 4.9 with diltiazem dosages of 120, 240, and 360 mg/day, respectively, compared with 11.9 episodes on placebo. Treadmill exercise time was also increased by high dose diltiazem and time to ischemic ST-segment depression was reduced. These beneficial effects of diltiazem were sustained during a follow-up period of 6 months without major side effects from diltiazem. Thus, these data indicate that diltiazem reduces the frequency of symptoms and provides protection for patients with stable angina.

Klein and associates[107] from Kfar-Saba, Israel, examined the acute hemodynamic effects of an intravenous bolus of verapamil (0.1 mg/kg or 0.06–0.075 mg/kg) by serial RNA in 46 patients with CAD. In 20 patients with EF >35% (group 1A) verapamil (0.1 mg/kg) administered over 1–1.5

minutes had a biphasic effect: first, a transient decrease in EF accompanied by increased LV volumes and cardiac output equivalents, then an overshoot of EF to values above control accompanied by a decrease in peripheral vascular resistance and a drastic decrease in LV volumes, whereas cardiac output equivalent remained slightly elevated. In 8 patients with an EF <35% (group 1B), only the first effect on EF was noted. In 10 patients with an EF >35% (group 2) verapamil (0.06–0.075 mg/kg) exerted quantitatively similar but milder effects on hemodynamic function. Finally, verapamil (0.1 mg/kg) given more slowly over 2–2.5 minutes produced no significant changes in EF or LV volumes in another 8 patients (group 3). Thus, the acute effects of verapamil are both time related and dose dependent. These effects also are related to the baseline functional LV reserve. These observations demonstrate that verapamil exerts a depressant effect on LV function, but the transient nature of this depression and the quick recovery to normal or above normal values indicate that verapamil in the doses employed in this study is safe to use intravenously in patients with CAD.

Chew and associates[108] from Los Angeles, California, studied the effect of intravenous verapamil on systemic and coronary hemodynamic function at cardiac catheterization in 12 patients with CAD. Verapamil was administered as a 2-minute bolus (0.145 mg/kg) followed by an infusion (0.005 mg/kg/min). Cardiac output and coronary sinus blood flow were measured by thermodilution techniques. Caliber of the large coronary arteries and of diseased segments was determined from the coronary angiogram using a computer-assisted method. Verapamil reduced mean arterial pressure by 14% (p < 0.001), systemic vascular resistance by 21% (p < 0.01), and stroke work index by 16% (p < 0.001). Coronary vascular resistance decreased 24% (p < 0.01), with a small increase in coronary sinus blood flow (+13%, difference not significant). Myocardial oxygen consumption determined in 5 patients showed no significant change with verapamil. Luminal area in 39 coronary lesions was measured in the "normal" portion of the diseased segment and at its maximal constriction, and an estimate of flow resistance in the stenosis was computed. Overall, 50% of "normal" and of diseased coronary segments dilated significantly with verapamil. Stenosis dilation resulted in an average 14% reduction (p < 0.01) in estimated flow resistance. In 8 patients, the luminal changes (n, 27) induced by sublingual nitroglycerin were compared with those induced by verapamil. Nitroglycerin induced a significantly greater increase in coronary caliber in both normal and diseased segments; estimated stenosis flow resistance decreased 28% with nitroglycerin compared with 14% with verapamil (p < 0.01). Thus, verapamil moderately dilates the systemic and coronary small vessel resistance bed without apparently increasing myocardial metabolic demand. Furthermore, verapamil mildly dilates large coronary conductance vessels in both "normal" and diseased segments, although significantly less than does nitroglycerin.

Weiner and associates[109] from Boston, Massachusetts, assessed the long-term efficacy and safety of high dose verapamil (480 mg/day) in 26 patients with chronic stable angina pectoris during a 3-phase protocol: phase 1, an initial 6-week placebo-controlled, double-blind crossover assessment; phase 2, an open label, 1-year follow-up; and phase 3, a final drug withdrawal and rechallenge 10-week study. Three patients withdrew during phase 2 (1 had hepatitis and 2 underwent coronary bypass surgery). Adverse effects during phase 2 were mild, consisting of constipation (6 patients) and prolongation of the P-R interval (5 patients); however, no patient required alteration of the 480 mg/day dosage. At the end of phase 2, 10 patients underwent the phase 3 study, commencing with a 2-week period in which verapamil was either tapered gradually or abruptly discontinued. This was followed by an 8-week double-blind, placebo-controlled crossover rechallenge study with verapamil. The clinical and exercise responses to verapamil compared with placebo were similar during the phase 3 protocol and the initial phase 1 study (treadmill time increased by 55% and anginal attacks/week decreased by 63% during phase 3, compared with a 28% increase and a 42% decrease, respectively, during phase 1; p, NS). Withdrawal of verapamil produced a similar return of anginal symptoms whether the drug was abruptly discontinued or its administration tapered. No patient had unstable angina pectoris or AMI. These investigations demonstrate that verapamil is safe and effective when evaluated after 1 year of continuous therapy using a dosage of 480 mg/day. There is no evidence of drug tachyphylaxis, nor does verapamil appear to cause an abrupt withdrawal syndrome in patients with chronic stable angina pectoris.

In an investigation carried out by Mauritson and colleagues[110] from Dallas, Texas, to assess the efficacy of verapamil in individuals with unstable angina at rest, 11 patients (5 men and 6 women; average age, 55 years) with recurrent chest pain at rest and transient ST-segment deviation (elevation or depression ≥ 0.1 mV) on continuous ECG monitoring were enrolled in a 3-day double-blind, randomized study. The day before randomization (day 1), all received single-blind placebo. On day 2, they were randomized to placebo (n, 6) or verapamil 320 mg/day (n, 5). On placebo, the number of chest pains (day 1, 2.8 ± 2.1; day 2, 2.2 ± 2.5; p, NS), nitroglycerin used (day 1, 2.7 ± 4.4 tablets; day 2, 2.2 ± 3.5 tablets; p, NS) and ST-segment deviations (day 1, 8.5 ± 5.9; day 2, 5.3 ± 7.1; p, NS) did not change. On verapamil, the number of chest pains (day 1, 5.4 ± 2.2; day 2, 1.6 ± 2.1; p < 0.1), nitroglycerin used (day 1, 5.0 ± 4.5 tablets; day 2, 1.6 ± 2.6 tablets; p = 0.057), and ST-segment deviations (day 1, 12.6 ± 4.7; day 2, 6.2 ± 6.2; p < 0.05) fell. Since 5 of 6 patients on placebo had frequent chest pain and ST-segment deviations on day 2, they were changed blindly to verapamil 320 mg/day. Of the 5 verapamil patients, 3 had no chest pain or ST-segment deviations on day 2, but 2 had continued chest pain and ST-segment deviations and were increased blindly to verapamil 480 mg/day. Of the 8 patients given verapamil (320 mg/day) on day 3, 5 had chest pain or ST-segment deviations and were increased blindly to verapamil 480 mg/day on day 4. Of the 7 who received verapamil 480 mg/day on day 4, 3 had chest pain and ST-segment deviations similar in frequency to that occurring on day 1. Thus, in patients with unstable angina at rest, verapamil exerts an initial beneficial effect, but in some individuals this salutary influence is not sustained.

Therapy of patients with rest angina is a difficult clinical problem. Mehta and associates[111] from Gainesville, Florida, demonstrated clinical efficacy of oral verapamil in the short-term therapy of 15 patients with rest angina in a double-blind placebo-controlled trial. Twelve patients responsive to oral verapamil were then maintained on verapamil (240–640 mg daily) and followed for up to 21 months. Two patients died within 1 week of discharge from the hospital, 2 had myocardial infarction at 2 weeks and 12 months of follow-up, another patient underwent elective CABG at 6 months of follow-up, and 1 patient had intolerable side effects. Until the episode of myocardial infarction, most patients had marked decrease in chest pain frequency and nitroglycerin consumption. Long-term outcome with verapamil therapy could not be predicted from clinical findings or initial response to treatment. Most frequent side effects observed were constipation and prolongation of ECG P-R interval. This study shows that long-term therapy with verapamil in patients with rest angina is associated with relief of chest pain, but myocardial infarction and sudden death do occur in some patients.

To evaluate the influence of oral verapamil (80 and 120 mg) on angina threshold, coronary blood flow, myocardial oxygen consumption, and LV function, Rouleau and associates[112] from San Francisco, California, subjected 13 patients with effort angina and fixed obstructive CAD to atrial pacing and progressively higher heart rates. After administration of 120 mg of verapamil, the time to onset of angina and the heart rate at the onset of ST-segment depression increased by 18 and 10%, respectively, without any change in the angina threshold (rate-pressure product at the onset of angina). The rate-pressure product, coronary blood flow, and myocardial oxygen consumption were lower at rest than at preangina heart rates, but not when the angina threshold was released. The beneficial effect of verapamil seemed to be due to decreased myocardial oxygen demand rather than to increased coronary blood flow. The decreased demand resulted from a lower arterial pressure at each pacing rate and in these patients without heart failure LV mechanical function did not deteriorate. The response to 80 mg oral verapamil was less beneficial than the 120 mg dose. The authors concluded that oral verapamil has a potential role in the management of patients with effort angina due to fixed obstructive CAD.

Sherman and Liang[113] from Boston, Massachusetts, studied in a double-blind prospective placebo-controlled crossover trial 30 patients with chronic stable angina pectoris to assess the efficacy of nifedipine (30–60 mg/day orally) in controlling symptoms and objective signs of myocardial ischemia using a symptom-limited treadmill exercise test. Adverse effects that occurred during both nifedipine and placebo treatment were minor and generally well tolerated. Twenty-three patients were analyzed from the crossover phase of the study. Nifedipine significantly reduced the frequency of angina by 55% and nitroglycerin consumption by 59% and increased exercise time by 34%. These changes were significantly greater than those in the placebo group. Hemodynamic evaluation during exercise revealed a significant reduction in systolic and diastolic BP in the nifedipine group at the onset of angina and at maximal exercise without significant differences in heart rate responses in the nifedipine and placebo groups. The pressure-rate product during submaximal exercise was significantly smaller in the nifedipine group than in the placebo group, but it did not differ significantly in the 2 groups at the onset of angina or on maximal exericse. Furthermore, ST-segment depressions that occurred during exercise at the same pressure-rate products were smaller in the nifedipine period than in the placebo period. Thus, it appears that the antianginal effects of nifedipine are caused by a reduced myocardial oxygen demand for a specific work load and possibly by an increased blood supply to ischemic myocardium.

Sellers and associates[114] from Charlottesville, Virginia, studied 77 patients hospitalized for unstable angina in whom oral, dermal, or intravenous nitrates and/or beta blockade had failed. Of these, 81% with negligible or 1-

vessel CAD and of the 55% with 2- or 3-vessel CAD showed significant response to nifedipine. Patients with either ST elevation or no change during pain responded better (31 of 45) than those with any ST depression (16 of 32; $p < 0.05$). Patients with negligible or 1-vessel CAD had a higher prevalence of ST elevation (13 of 16) than patients with 2- or 3-vessel CAD (15 of 31; $p = 0.004$). ST motion did not predict response in patients with 2- or 3-vessel CAD, but did predict response in patients with negligible or 1-vessel disease. On follow-up study at 9 ± 8 (range, 1–33) months, 39 of 42 who had shown response were free from pain. Three died from AMI without unstable angina. Five who showed response had elective CABG. The addition of nifedipine abolished or reduced pain episodes by more than 50% in 61% of patients with refractory unstable angina pectoris. Patients with negligible or 1-vessel CAD with ST elevation benefited most. In patients with 2- or 3-vessel CAD, the type of ST motion did not predict response. Follow-up of all those with response indicated sustained amelioration by nifedipine therapy. Failure of nifedipine therapy should not be accepted until a dose of 120 mg/day has been achieved or until intolerable side effects appear.

To elucidate the mechanisms of action of nifedipine in angina pectoris, 14 patients were studied by Emanuelsson and Holmberg[115] from Goteborg, Sweden, before and after sublingual administration of 10 mg nifedipine. Systemic and coronary hemodynamic and myocardial metabolic measurements were taken at rest and during pacing. At the pacing rate that induced pain in the control situation, no patient experienced angina after nifedipine administration. Lactate production during control turned into extraction after nifedipine administration and the double product was reduced. Systemic and coronary vascular resistance were reduced by 26 and 19%, respectively. Systolic BP fell from 160–127 mmHg and diastolic from 100–79 mmHg. Pulmonary artery diastolic BP fell from 14–10 mmHg. When the pacing rate was further increased after nifedipine administration until pain developed, the double product and the degree of lactate production were the same as during pain before nifedipine was administered. The pacing rate was 131 compared with 119 during control. Both the systolic and diastolic BP were still significantly reduced compared with control pacing values. These data demonstrate that the antianginal efficiency can be partly explained by afterload reduction, which decreases myocardial oxygen consumption. The data also suggest additional mechanisms, possibly an increase in collateral flow, direct dilation of the stenotic parts of epicardial arteries, or a decrease in myocardial back pressure secondary to reduced LV filling pressure.

Nifedipine is an effective antianginal agent, but its efficacy in patients with angina refractory to maximally tolerated conventional therapy has not been well studied. Stone and colleagues[116] from Boston, Massachusetts, report their experience using nifedipine in an unblinded manner in 716 patients with refractory angina, all of whom underwent cardiac catheterization. Patients were treated with nifedipine when maximally tolerated conventional therapy (nitrates, beta blockers) was inadequate to control angina. Patients were divided into 3 mutually exclusive clinical groups based on the apparent pathophysiologic mechanism responsible for angina. Group I consisted of 389 patients with Prinzmetal's angina and coronary vasospasm documented by the observation of spontaneous angina with ST-segment elevation and/or vasospasm observed during coronary angiography. Group II was composed of 292 patients with mixed angina, defined as those patients who exhibited evidence of both classic exertional angina and possible superimposed coronary vasospasm. No patient had documented coronary vasospasm or ST-segment elevation with angina. Group II included 35 patients with classic stable exertional angina, without rest pain or ST-segment elevation associated with episodes of ischemia. Angina frequency and nitroglycerin use were compared on conventional therapy before and after the addition of nifedipine. Mean duration of nifedipine therapy was 6.5 months. The addition of nifedipine (median dosage, 60 mg/day; range 10–200 mg) significantly decreased the mean frequency of angina attacks a week in group I from 14–3 (p < 0.001), in group II from 20–6 (p < 0.001), and in group III from 11–7 (p < 0.03). Complete prevention of angina was most frequent in patients with documented vasospasm (42% of group I patients), intermediate in those clinically suspected of, but not proved, having vasospasm (20% of group II patients), and least frequent in patients with classic exertional angina alone (3% of group III patients) (p < 0.001). In 78% of the 716 patients the weekly angina rate decreased by ⩾50% of baseline values obtained during maximally tolerated conventional therapy, but the degree of improvement was significantly better in patients with either suspected or documented vasospasm. Treatment with nifedipine was associated with an increase of angina frequency in 13–29% of the 716 patients; this increase was most frequently observed in those with no evidence of vasospasm (group III). Nifedipine efficacy did not vary on the basis of the presence or absence of fixed obstructive CAD. These results suggest that nifedipine is efficacious for patients with angina refractory to maximally tolerated conventional therapy and that efficacy is greatest when coronary vasospasm also is present.

Blaustein and associates[117] from Boston, Massachusetts, reported the results of adding nifedipine to aggressive therapy with nitrates and beta blocking drugs in 47 hospitalized patients with unstable angina pectoris. The patients were followed up for an average of 12 months. Twenty-two (47%) improved sufficiently to be discharged; despite this symptomatic improvement, 8 had cardiac events within 4 months. Eighteen patients had no symptomatic improvement and 7 of them had cardiac events in 4 months. In 7 others, relief was insufficient to permit discharge, and 1 of these patients had AMI. In all, 31 patients were treated with medical therapy only. Twenty-one of these patients had a favorable short-term response to nefedipine; 13 died or had an AMI in <4 months. Two of 16 patients who underwent CABG had cardiac events. The presence of ECG changes with pain did not identify either a group at higher risk or a group with a better outcome with nifedipine. Thus, in a high risk subset of patients with unstable angina pectoris nifedipine does not reduce morbidity or mortality or the need for CABG, but it relieves symptoms in many patients. An early symptomatic response to nifedipine did not predict a reduced frequency of subsequent cardiac events.

To investigate the mechanism by which nifedipine improves exercise tolerance in patients with CAD, Specchia and coworkers[118] from Pavia, Italy, studied 14 patients with stable exertional angina and LAD CAD by measuring great cardiac vein flow (GCVF) and calculating anterior regional coronary resistance (CR) during exercise before and after sublingual administration of 20 mg of nifedipine. After nifedipine, 7 patients (group 1) had no increase in exercise capacity and showed a similar magnitude of ST-segment depression at peak exercise, and another 7 patients (group II) had prolonged exercise duration with less ST-segment depression at peak exercise. Such effects were achieved despite a significant increase in double product, an indirect index of myocardial oxygen consumption. In group I patients no significant change was induced by nifedipine in GCVF or in CR either at rest or at peak exercise. In contrast, in group II patients nifedipine significantly increased GCVF at rest and at peak exercise. Moreover, resting CR was decreased and remained significantly lower at peak exercise compared with the prenifedipine values. These data show that nifedipine may increase GCVF and decrease CR at rest and at peak exercise in patients with LAD CAD. Such increase in myocardial oxygen supply seems the most likely mechanism by which nifedipine may improve exercise capacity in patients with stable exertional angina.

Platelet function was studied by Dale and colleagues[119] from Oslo, Norway, before and 1 hour after ingestion of 20 mg nifedipine in 20 patients with CAD. Platelet counts remained unchanged. Platelet adhesiveness, measured as retention in glass bead columns with Hellem's method for native blood, did not drop significantly either when 0.9 or 3.6 ml of blood was used. Platelet aggregation, which is dependent on extracellular calcium, was induced in citrated platelet-rich plasma. The mean maximal rate of primary aggregation, initiated with 3 different concentrations of adenosine diphosphate, was reduced by 20–26%. The rate of irreversible collagen-induced aggregation was on average 23% lower after nifedipine. The mean bleeding time was 36 seconds (12%) longer after ingestion of the drug. The moderate but significant reduction of platelet aggregation and prolongation of the bleeding time by nifedipine may be mediated through inhibition of calcium transport across the platelet membrane.

Detry and associates[120] from Brussels, Belgium, examined the antianginal effects of felodipine, a new calcium channel blocking agent, in 8 patients with CAD and exertional angina pectoris. Hemodynamic measurements were made at rest, during submaximal exercise, and during angina-limited exercise before and 30 minutes after oral administration of 0.1 mg/kg of felodipine. Angina pectoris was always prevented after the drug was given and the exercise intensity was increased until recurrence of angina (5 patients) or exhaustion (3 patients). Hemodynamic data were also recorded at this higher exercise capacity. At rest and during submaximal exercise, felodipine increased heart rate and decreased arterial BP and systemic vascular resistance. The prevention of angina pectoris was accompanied by lower mean PA wedge pressure, systemic vascular resistance, and ST-segment depression; the pressure-rate product was unchanged. The 20% greater exercise capacity after felodipine was attended by a 20% increase in maximal cardiac output, a 17% increase in maximal heart rate, and a 13% increase in maximal pressure-rate product; the maximal arterial BP and ST-segment abnormalities were unchanged and the systemic vascular resistance was lower. The relation between ST-segment depression and the pressure-rate product during exercise was favorably influenced by felodipine. Thus, felodipine is an active antianginal drug; its major mechanism of action is to lower the systemic vascular resistance. The data also suggest that it improves coronary blood flow during exercise.

Hung and colleagues[121] from Stanford, California, compared the effects of oral diltiazem and propranolol alone and in combination with those of placebo in 12 patients with stable effort angina. Patients performed symptom-limited, multistage, upright bicycle ergometric exercise while undergoing equilibrium-gated RNA examination after 2-week periods of 90 mg diltiazem 4 times daily, 60 mg propranolol 4 times daily, a combination 90 mg diltiazem and 60 mg propranolol 4 times daily, and placebo. All drugs were given double blind and in randomized order. Diltiazem, propranolol, and the combination significantly increased exercise duration compared with placebo; the drugs also increased time to onset of angina pectoris and ischemic ST-segment depression. Compared with placebo, heart rate-pressure product at a fixed submaximal workload were decreased after diltiazem but were unchanged at peak effort. Heart rate and rate-pressure product at both submaximal and peak effort were decreased by propranolol and were decreased further by the combination of diltiazem and propranolol. Diltiazem and the combination of diltiazem and propranolol decreased maximal exercise ST-segment depression. The mean exercise LV EF was higher in patients on diltiazem than in those on placebo, propranolol, or the combination of diltiazem and propranolol. Adverse side effects severe enough to require dosage reduction (severe sinus bradycardia or orthostatic hypotension) occurred in 4 patients on combination therapy. High dose diltiazem alone appears to be as effective as or more effective than moderate dose propranolol or the combination of diltiazem and propranolol in improving exercise tolerance, myocardial ischemia, and LV function in patients with stable effort angina.

Winniford and associates[122] from Dallas, Texas, evaluated 13 men with severe, limiting angina of effort to determine whether propranolol alone or propranolol combined with verapamil best relieved symptoms and improved exercise performance. A stable dose of propranolol was maintained throughout the study (295 ± 83 mg/day, mean ± SD) and in addition to propranolol therapy each patient was given 2 weeks of up-titration of open label verapamil at 2-week periods of randomized, double-blind therapy, 1 of placebo and the other of verapamil (431 ± 77 mg/day). Propranolol and verapamil together resulted in a decline in anginal episodes (7.3 ± 6.9/week during propranolol-placebo to 4.7 ± 5.0/week during propranolol-verapamil, p = 0.03) and the number of nitroglycerin tablets used in a week (7.6 ± 6.6/week during placebo and propranolol to 4.4 ± 4.2/week during propranolol-verapamil, p = 0.008). With propranolol and placebo, all 13 patients had angina after 4.6 ± 2.1 minutes of supine bicycle exercise, but with propranolol-verapamil, 5 had no angina with exercise even though the duration of exercise increased; in the remaining 8 patients, time to angina increased from 4.0 ± 1.5 minutes with propranolol-placebo to 5.3 ± 1.6 minutes with propranolol-verapamil, p = 0.01. A propranolol-verapamil combination caused no change in rest or peak exercise LV volumes or EF as assessed by equilibrium gated blood pool scintigraphy compared with values obtained with propranolol alone. However, propranolol and verapamil together caused P-R interval prolongation in 4 patients and 2 patients developed increased fatigue and dyspnea. Two additional patients had marked sinus bradycardia with junctional escape rhythm that required a reduction in verapamil dosage. No patient developed CHF or high grade AV block. Thus, these data suggest that combined verapamil and propranolol are superior to propranolol alone in reducing the frequency of angina and improving exercise tolerance in patients with severe, limiting angina. However, the combination of verapamil and propranolol together must be used with caution because of potentially serious side effects.

With the use of equilibrium RNA, Johnston and coinvestigators[123] from London, Canada, compared the effects on LV function of 160 mg oral propranolol daily and 360 mg verapamil daily alone and in combination in 18 patients with chronic exertional angina. A randomized, double-blind, placebo-controlled, crossover protocol was used. The reduction in exercise rate-pressure product induced by the combination was significantly greater than that by propranolol or verapamil alone. In patients at rest, neither single nor combined therapy altered global or regional LV EF. Verapamil, but not propranolol, increased cardiac volumes of resting subjects; used in combination, no further increase in LV volume occurred. With placebo, exercise global EF did not decrease from the level at rest and therefore no drug effect could be demonstrated for this parameter of LV function. By an evaluation of normalized regional EF measurements, the combination was shown to reduce exercise-induced hypokinesis. No significant improvement was noted with propranolol or verapamil alone; only the combination prevented a significant increase in end-systolic and end-diastolic volumes during exercise. Thus, propranolol and verapamil used alone and in moderate doses exert no beneficial effect on exercise LV function as measured by EF and volume changes, and resting function deteriorates slightly with verapamil. Combined with single-drug therapy, the combination causes no further change in LV function of resting subjects and improves exercise function. This improvement was most likely due to a reduction in myocardial oxygen demand.

In a study by Bowles and associates[124] from Harrow, England, propranolol (240 mg daily) and verapamil (360 mg daily) were objectively compared for their respective efficacy in the treatment of chronic stable angina pectoris. Twenty-two patients were studied in a randomized placebo-controlled, double-blind crossover trial with 4 weeks on each active drug treatment. Multistage treadmill exercise with computer-assisted ECG analysis was performed after 2 weeks on placebo and at the end of each 4-week active drug treatment. The mean exercise time to produce angina was 5.5 minutes (SEM ± 0.4 min) on placebo and this increased to 7.8 (±0.5) minutes on propranolol and 9.1 (±0.5) minutes on verapamil. The improvement in exercise time of verapamil over propranolol was statistically significant ($p < 0.01$). Ten patients became free of angina with verapamil and 4 with propranolol. Resting and maximal exercise heart rates were significantly reduced by propranolol; verapamil did not reduce the maximal heart rate but reduced the resting heart rate slightly. However, the heart rate increase per minute of exercise was significantly diminished ($p < 0.001$). ST-segment changes showed improvement with both drugs despite marked differences in heart rate profile. The overall efficacy of verapamil compares favorably with that of propranolol, thus providing a new perspective in the management of angina pectoris. These 2 classes of drugs seem to act by different mechanisms, and it is suggested that if patients are resistant or intolerant to 1 of these drugs, the other can be used to yield a beneficial response.

Schanzenbacher and associates[125] from Bonn, West Germany, studied the effect of intravenous and intracoronary nifedipine on coronary sinus blood flow, coronary vascular resistance, and myocardial oxygen consumption on 20 patients with CAD. An intravenous infusion of 1.0 mg nifedipine resulted in a decrease in mean aortic pressure, an increase in heart rate and coronary blood flow, and no significant change in myocardial oxygen consumption. In contrast, the intracoronary injection of 0.1 mg nifedipine led to a moderate reduction in mean aortic pressure, no change in heart rate, an increase in coronary blood flow, and a significant reduction in myocardial oxygen consumption. During rapid atrial pacing before and approximately 6 minutes after the intracoronary nifedipine injection, coronary blood flow and myocardial oxygen consumption reached identical levels. Thus, only intracoronary injection of nifedipine increases coronary flow in the presence of reduced myocardial oxygen consumption. After intravenous administration, reflex tachycardia counteracts the direct myocardial effect of nifedipine and the potential oxygen-saving effect of afterload reduction. There is no evidence of prolonged oxygen-sparing effect after cessation of the immediate effects.

In 10 men with stable angina not fully relieved by optimal doses of propranolol, Bassan and colleagues[126] in Jerusalem, Israel, administered on each of 4 mornings a single dose of 10 mg nifedipine, 120 mg verapamil, isosorbide dinitrate (5–30 mg), or placebo in double-blind fashion. Bicycle exercise to angina was performed hourly for 8 hours thereafter. All three vasodilators increased exercise time by at least 50% by the first hour, with a gradually diminishing effect persisting for 6–8 hours. Although for the group there were no differences in magnitude and duration of effect among the 3 drugs, in 5 individual patients there were important differences in response favoring 1 or another vasodilator. The investigators conclude that nifedipine, verapamil, and isosorbide dinitrate are equally effective and reasonably long-acting antianginal supplements to propranolol, although some patients may benefit more from 1 than the other 2.

Treatment with aspirin

Lewis and associates[127] from Washington, D.C., conducted a multicenter (Veterans Administrative Cooperative Group) double-blind, placebo-controlled randomized trial of aspirin treatment (324 mg in buffered solution daily) for 12 weeks in 1,266 men with unstable angina (625 taking aspirin and 641, placebo). The principal end points were death and AMI diagnosed by the presence of creatine kinase MB or pathologic Q-wave changes on ECG. The incidence of death or AMI was 51% lower in the aspirin group than in the placebo group: 31 patients (5%) compared with 65 (10.1%); $p = 0.0005$. Nonfatal AMI was 51% lower in the aspirin group: 21 patients (3.4%) compared with 44 (6.9%); $p = 0.005$. The reduction in mortality in the aspirin group was also 51%—10 patients (1.6%) compared with 21 (3.3%)—although it was not statistically significant; $p = 0.054$. There was no difference in gastrointestinal symptoms or evidence of blood loss between the treatment and control groups. These data show that aspirin has a protective effect against AMI in men with unstable angina, and they suggest a similar effect on mortality.

Treatment with intraaortic balloon counterpulsation

Intraaortic balloon counterpulsation (IABC) is capable of reducing afterload in patients with unstable angina. Whether it is also capable of augmenting coronary blood flow to poststenotic myocardium is controversial. Fuchs and associates[128] from Baltimore, Maryland, studied 7 patients receiving maximal drug therapy and requiring IABC for unstable angina. All

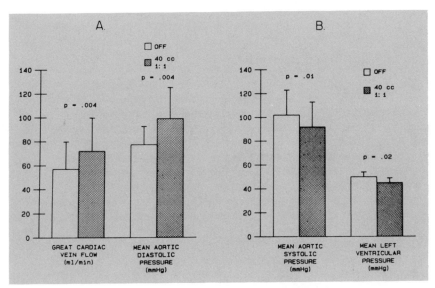

Fig. 1-7. Effect of maximal augmentation by balloon pumping on great cardiac vein flow, mean aortic diastolic pressure, mean aortic systolic pressure, and mean LV pressure. Brackets indicate standard deviations. Reproduced with permission from Fuchs et al.[128]

patients had >90% diameter stenosis of the proximal LAD coronary artery. With maximal augmentation (40 ml balloon volume, 1/1 assist ratio) great cardiac vein flow representing the efflux from the LAD coronary artery bed rose from a baseline of 52 ± 20–67 ± 25 ml/minute (p = 0.004) (Fig. 1-7). Increased cardiac vein flow correlated with increased mean aortic diastolic pressure across changes in balloon volumes and changes in assist ratio. However, the intermediate balloon volumes produced great cardiac vein flows at an intermediate level between full assist and no assist (p < 0.5), whereas the intermediate assist ratios did not augment flow. Ischemic pain was relieved. The authors could not state whether the increase in coronary flow or the decrease in mean LV pressure (thus demand) was of greater importance. The study suggests that graded reduction in balloon volume rather than graded reduction in assist ratio would be more appropriate for weaning from IABC support. They demonstrated that there was increased flow to beds distal to critical stenoses and that this increased flow correlated with increased aortic diastolic pressure, indicating probable loss of autoregulatory ability in the area of the stenosis.

Exercise training

Hagberg and coworkers[129] from St. Louis, Missouri, studied 11 men to determine whether 12 months of intense endurance exercise training can induce an increase in LV stroke volume and in stroke work during exercise in patients with CAD. With training, mean maximal oxygen uptake (VO_2 max) increased 39%, from 1.85–2.57 liters/minute. Stroke volume during upright exercise that required 35–65% of VO_2 max was 18% higher after training. At the same percentage of VO_2 max, mean BP was the same before and after training; as a result, LV stroke work (mean BP times stroke volume) increased 18%. These findings suggest that in patients with CAD prolonged intense training induces an increase in stroke volume, and this is a result of cardiac rather than peripheral adaptations.

Stress management

To evaluate the short-term effects of an intervention consisting of stress management training and dietary changes in patients with CAD, Ornish and associates[130] from Houston, Texas, compared the cardiovascular status of 23 patients who received this intervention with a randomized control group of 23 patients who did not. After 24 days, patients in the experimental group demonstrated a 44% mean increase in duration of exercise, a 55% mean increase in total work performed, somewhat improved LV regional wall motion during peak exercise, and a net change in the LV EF from rest to maximum exercise of +6%. Also, the authors measured a 21% mean decrease in plasma cholesterol levels and a 91% mean reduction in frequency of anginal episodes. In this selected sample short-term improvements in cardiovascular status seemed to result from these adjuncts to conventional treatments of CAD.

VARIANT ANGINA AND/OR CORONARY SPASM

Reduced vasodilator reserve of the small arteries

Cannon and associates[131] from Bethesda, Maryland, evaluated 22 patients to determine the mechanism of chest pain in patients with insignificant large vessel coronary arterial stenoses. In this evaluation, great cardiac vein flow and coronary resistance were measured and lactate content determined at rest and during coronary sinus pacing. Nine patients developing chest pain with pacing demonstrated significantly less increase in flow from baseline values, less decrease from baseline in coronary vascular resistance, and less lactate consumption compared with 13 patients without pacing-induced chest pain. Pacing performed during cold pressor testing elicited similar abnormalities in those patients experiencing chest pain compared with those who did not; 4 of 8 patients developing chest pain demonstrated a lower or new anginal threshold compared with that during the control study. Coronary arteriography during the cold pressor test revealed no significant change in epicardial coronary arterial dimension. Ergonovine administration, 0.15 mg intravenous, caused 2 of 20 patients to have chest pain associated with a marked decrease in coronary flow and increase in coronary vascular resistance. Pacing performed during ergonovine administration resulted in chest pain in 10 of the remaining 18 patients, including 5 who had not had pain during the control pacing study. No patient had significant epicardial CAD on arteriography, but their coronary flow increased less, their coronary vascular resistance decreased less, and less lactate consumption occurred than in patients not experiencing chest pain. These data suggest that some patients with chest pain but without significant narrowing of epicardial coronary arteries may have inappropriate arteriolar or small vessel coronary arterial constriction with abnormal vasodilator reserve in response to increases in oxygen demand.

Diurnal distribution of ST-segment elevation and related arrhythmias

Araki and coworkers[132] from Fukuoka, Japan, performed 24-hour ambulatory ECG recording in 26 patients with variant angina to evaluate the diurnal distribution of ST-segment elevation in relation to chest pain and the incidence of arrhythmias during the episodes. During a recording period of 52 days, 364 ST-segment elevations of 1 mm or greater were observed and 79% were asymptomatic. ST-segment elevation frequently occurred between 0:00 and 9:00 hours and most frequently between 5:00 and 6:00 hours on a 24-hour schedule. Only a few episodes occurred between 10:00 and 18:00 hours. Premature atrial contractions, VPC, VT, and complete AV block occurred in 12% of the episodes and were more common during painful than during painless episodes. However, VT and severe forms of VPC (couplets and bigeminy) appeared 8 times during painless and 9 times during painful episodes. Arrhythmias occurred more frequently when the elevated ST segment started to return or was returning to the control level than when it was rising. The frequency of arrhythmias was lower when the daily frequency of ischemic episodes was high. This study demonstrates that episodes of asymptomatic coronary artery spasm predominately occur early in the morning as symptomatic episodes; complex arrhythmias occur during asymptomatic episodes; arrhythmias occur predominately during the reperfusion period, and more arrhythmias accompany infrequent daily episodes of ischemia than frequent ones.

Ventricular tachyarrhythmias and relation to ST segment elevation

Previtali and associates[133] from Pavia, Italy, studied 46 patients with Prinzmetal's variant angina to determine the frequency and clinical significance of ventricular tachyarrhythmias and to correlate the arrhythmias with the degree and time course of ST-segment changes during ischemic attacks. Twenty-nine patients (group I) had no ventricular arrhythmias in any of the 1,083 recorded episodes, but 27 patients (group II) developed arrhythmias in 18% of the attacks. No significant differences in clinical, ECG, angiographic, or hemodynamic findings were found between the 2 groups. In 23 of the 27 group II patients, ventricular arrhythmias developed during maximal ST segment elevation (occlusion arrhythmias), but in 10 they occurred during resolution of ST-segment changes (reperfusion arrhythmias); 6 of the latter patients also had occlusion arrhythmias. Eight of 23 patients with occlusion arrhythmias and 6 of 10 with reperfusion arrhythmias had VF or VT. Maximal ST-segment elevation was significantly greater ($p < 0.001$) in patients with occlusion arrhythmias than in those without arrhythmias. The episodes with reperfusion arrhythmias were significantly longer ($p < 0.001$) and showed a significantly greater ST-segment elevation ($p < 0.001$) than those without arrhythmias in group I patients. This study shows that significant ventricular tachyarrhythmias develop during ischemic attacks in about 50% of patients with active variant angina; clinical and angiographic features are not useful in distinguishing patients with arrhythmias from the others. Their findings suggest that in variant angina ventricular arrhythmias may be due to the effects of both coronary artery occlusion and reperfusion; both types of arrhythmias correlated with the severity of ischemia, as measured by the degree of ST-segment elevation. Reperfusion arrhythmias also appear to correlate with the duration of ischemia.

Mechanism of arrhythmias

In a study by Kerin and associates[134] from Detroit, Michigan, 36 patients with variant angina pectoris were analyzed to investigate whether the mechanism underlying arrhythmia was related to coronary occlusion or reperfusion. Fifteen (42%) of the 36 patients had arrhythmias. Twelve (80%) of 15 patients experienced arrhythmias before the peak ST-segment elevation (occlusive arrhythmia), and those of the tachyarrhythmia type were characterized by the presence of VPC initially isolated, increasing in frequency, and preceding the more malignant forms of arrhythmias, such as VT or VF. The occlusive arrhythmias included ventricular arrhythmia (VPC, VT, slow VT, VF) in 8 patients and conduction abnormalities (second- and third-degree AV block, left posterior fascicular block) in 4 patients. Thirteen episodes at variant angina were fully recorded by ECG. The average time to onset of arrhythmia, after the beginning of ST-segment elevation, was 4.9 minutes ±1.5. The duration of the episodes without arrhythmias was 0.86 minute ±0.53. The reperfusion arrhythmia occurred in 3 patients (20%) and was characterized by the appearance of isolated couplets of VPC, VT, or VF without prodromal ectopic activity. The arrhythmia occurred in 1 patient during the resolution of ST-segment elevation and in 2 patients within seconds of ST-segment normalization. It was concluded that the occlusive-related arrhythmias are the most important mechanism in variant angina and that they are dependent on the duration of the ischemic episode.

Comparative sensitivity of exercise, cold pressor, and ergonovine testing in provoking attacks

Exercise, ergonovine, and the cold pressor test have been employed to provoke variant angina attacks. Waters and colleagues[135] from Montreal, Canada, compared the sensitivity of these 3 tests in 34 hospitalized patients with well-documented active variant angina who had recently undergone coronary arteriography. The 3 tests were performed on 3 consecutive days and 28 of the 34 had the 3 tests within 1 week. Angina was provoked by ergonovine in all 34 patients, by exercise in 17, and by the cold pressor test in only 5. ST-segment elevation developed during the ergonovine test in 32 (94%), during exercise in 10 (29%), and during the cold pressor test in only 3 (9%). With ergonovine administration, 1 patient had only ST-segment depression and 1 had no ECG changes. During the cold pressor test, 2 patients had pseudonormalization of abnormally negative T waves and 29 had no ECG changes. Exercise induced T-wave pseudonormalization in 4 patients, ST depression in 9 others, and no ECG changes in 11. ST-segment elevation was more frequent with ergonovine than with either of the other tests. The investigators concluded that the sensitivity of the ergonovine test is high in patients with variant angina and that exercise will provoke angina with ST-segment elevation in about 30% of these individuals. In contrast, the sensitivity of the cold pressor test is too low to be of much clinical value in the diagnosis of variant angina.

ECG changes

In a study by Feldman and associates[136] from Gainesville, Florida, the presence or absence of important ECG changes (ST elevation or depression ≥1 mm) was evaluated in 79 consecutive patients with coronary artery spasm. In 8 patients, ECG changes usually did not accompany episodes of rest angina. Evaluation before, during, and after cardiac catheterization included multiple ECGs and ambulatory monitoring during angina. These observations suggest that the ECG may not always be a sensitive indicator of coronary spasm. Thus, the diagnosis of transient myocardial ischemia secondary to coronary spasm should not necessarily be excluded because of a lack of ECG changes during rest angina.

Coronary arteriography and left ventriculography during ST-segment elevation

Matsuda and colleagues[137] from Yamaguchi, Japan, carried out an angiographic demonstration of coronary artery spasm during both spontaneous and exercise-induced angina in 3 patients with variant angina. In each patient, clinical, ECG, coronary angiographic, and left ventriculographic observations were made at rest, during spontaneous angina, and during exercise-induced angina. The character of chest pain was similar during spontaneous and exercise-induced episodes. ST-segment elevation was present in the anterior ECG leads during both episodes. The LAD coronary artery became partially or totally obstructed during both types of attacks. When coronary spasm was demonstrated during both types of attacks, left ventriculography disclosed akinetic or dyskinetic wall motion in the area supplied by the involved artery. In those patients with reproducible exercise-induced ST-segment elevation and chest pain, thallium-201 scintigraphy showed areas of reversible anteroseptal hypoperfusion. Thus, in selected patients with variant angina, exercise-induced attacks of angina were similar to spontaneous episodes.

Catheter-induced spasm

During a 4-year period, 33 patients with angiographic coronary artery spasm in the absence of significant fixed CAD were evaluated by Mautner and colleagues[138] from New Orleans, Louisiana. Sixteen patients had typical variant angina and 17 had catheter-induced spasm. All patients had ≥1 episode of rest angina. Left ventriculography demonstrated MVP in 14 patients (42%) and end-systolic cavity obliteration in 6 (18%). Spasm was demonstrated to occur in the right coronary artery in 26 patients and in the left coronary artery in 7. Two patients had multivessel spasm. Comparing patients with variant angina and catheter-induced spasm demonstrated no significant difference in clinical, ECG, or angiographic parameters. Two patients with catheter-induced spasm had healed myocardial infarcts and both developed spontaneous noncatheter-induced spasm in the infarct-related artery. Most patients responded to long-acting nitrate therapy, although those with catheter-induced spasm tended to have more recurrent chest pain. Six patients were placed on calcium channel blocker drugs, with marked symptomatic improvement in 5. This study suggests that patients with catheter-induced spasm are similar to those with variant angina and its angiographic documentation may be a marker for the identification of patients with vasospastic angina.

Variability in coronary hemodynamics in response to ergonovine

Schwartz and associates[139] from San Francisco, California, evaluated 15 patients without angina and with normal coronary arteries to determine their responsiveness to ergonovine (0.05, 0.10, and 0.20 mg intravenous). Heart rate-BP product increased significantly (p < 0.001) without any change in coronary sinus flow, coronary vascular resistance, myocardial oxygen extraction, arterial-coronary sinus oxygen difference, and lactate extraction. However, in 7 of the 15 patients, coronary vascular resistance did increase (mean increase, 39%), and coronary sinus flow decreased (14%; p < 0.001), despite an increase in heart rate-BP product. No ECG, metabolic, or thallium-201 scintigraphic abnormalities occurred. These data suggest that increases in coronary vascular resistance do occur in response to ergonovine in some patients with normal coronary arteries and atypical chest pain.

Natural history

Bott-Silverman and Heupler[140] from Cleveland, Ohio, evaluated 59 patients with variant angina and fixed important CAD. There were 32 women and 27 men, and they were followed an average of 5.9 years. Angina at rest was the main symptom (93%) and AMI occurred in 19%. With spontaneous anginal attacks, 64% of the patients had ST-segment elevation and 17%, ST-segment depression, whereas 15% had no ECG changes. Major arrhythmias occurred during angina in 24%, and permanent pacemakers were required in 10%. Long-acting nitrate therapy controlled symptoms in only 31% of patients, whereas calcium channel blockers controlled symptoms in 83% of those who were unresponsive to nitrates. Spontaneous remission of angina for ⩾1 month while receiving no medical therapy occurred in 39% of patients; 15% had an indefinite remission with no recurrence of symptoms for ⩾2 years. There were no cardiac deaths. Thus, this evaluation of the natural history of coronary arterial spasm in patients with variant angina demonstrated frequent spontaneous remission, a relatively poor response to long-acting nitrate therapy, a good response to calcium channel blockers, and a low frequency of cardiac mortality.

Spontaneous remission

Waters and associates[141] from Montreal, Canada, evaluated 100 patients with variant angina pectoris to determine the prevalence of spontaneous remission during a follow-up of ⩾1 year. Remission in anginal activity was found in 45 of 100 patients who had received no treatment for >3 months (mean, 18.3). The remaining 55 patients were receiving medical therapy; 37

had been angina-free for $\geqslant$6 months (mean, 22.5), but angina persisted in 18 patients. In those patients with continuing angina pectoris despite medical therapy, there was a lower prevalence of important CAD and a longer history of angina at rest before treatment. These data indicate that patients with variant angina frequently have remission of their symptoms, and this should be kept in mind when patients are treated medically.

Factors influencing prognosis

To determine the prognosis of variant angina and the factors influencing it, 169 consecutive patients hospitalized in a coronary care unit were followed by Waters and colleagues[142] from Montreal, Canada, for a mean of 15 months (range, 1–68). Survival at 1, 2, and 3 years was 95, 90, and 87% respectively. Survival without AMI was 80, 78, and 75%. Twenty of the 22 AMI and 8 of the 14 deaths occurred within the first 3 months. Mantel-Haenszel log-rank analysis demonstrated that CAD, LV function, and the degree of disease activity were significantly independent variables that influenced both survival and survival without AMI. At 1, 2, and 3 years, survival for patients with multivessel CAD was 81, 76, and 66%; for patients with 1-vessel CAD, it was 97, 92, and 92%; and for patients without stenosis >70%, it was 98% at each year. Survival without AMI at 1 year was 88% in patients with no stenosis >70% and 82% in patients with 1-vessel CAD; it did not change thereafter in either group, but was 62, 58, and 50% at 1, 2, and 3 years in patients with multivessel CAD. Treatment did not influence survival in any subgroup or survival without AMI in patients with multivessel CAD. However, in patients without multivessel CAD treatment with nifedipine, diltiazem, and verapamil improved survival without AMI compared with treatment with perhexiline maleate or long-acting nitrates alone. Thus, in addition to preventing angina, nifedipine, diltiazem, and verapamil appear to reduce complications in patients with variant angina without multivessel CAD.

Ergonovine provocation to assess efficacy of calcium channel blocking therapy

In the patient with Prinzmetal's variant angina, the response to therapy with calcium channel blocking agents may be assessed symptomatically, by ambulatory ECG monitoring, or by response to ergonovine provocation. Although some studies have suggested a good relation between anginal frequency and ergonovine responsiveness, none has compared ambulatory ECG activity with the results of ergonovine provocation during the long-term administration of calcium channel blocking agents. Winniford and associates[143] from Dallas, Texas, compared ergonovine responsivenes with both clinical and ambulatory ECG activity in 27 patients with Prinzmetal's variant angina during long-term therapy with placebo, verapamil, and nifedipine. The patients received placebo and verapamil for 2 months each, after which 23 of the 27 also received nifedipine for 2 months. All patients kept a diary of chest pains, and all had weekly 24-hour 2-channel ambulatory ECG (Holter) monitoring from which episodes of transient ST-segment deviation were quantitated. During the final week of therapy with each agent, ergonovine was administered, beginning at 0.025 mg and incrementally increasing to

0.20 mg. It was discontinued when the patient had chest pain with ST-segment elevation ≥0.1 mV or received a total dose of 0.50 mg. Of the 74 tests, 59 were negative; 6 of the negative tests occurred during a treatment period in which the patient had >10 chest pains a week and >25 episodes of ST segment deviation a week. Of the 15 positive tests, 8 became positive during administraiton of <0.20 mg ergonovine; 5 of the positive tests occurred during a treatment period in which the patient had no chest pain or ST-segment deviation. Thus, in patients with variant angina, disease activity cannot be monitored reliably by ergonovine provocation because some patients have negative ergonovine tests at a time of marked clinical and ECG activity, whereas others have positive tests at a time of little (or no) disease activity.

Diltiazem therapy

Schroeder and associates[144] from Stanford, California, evaluated the efficacy of 43 patients with variant angina (starting dosage, 60 mg orally every 6 hours, increasing to 90 mg every 6 hours if tolerated) followed for 20 months (range, 6–29 months). AMI, sudden death, and hospitalization for prolonged angina were decreased significantly (p < 0.01) during the initial 6 months and for the mean period of therapy. There were 22 events during follow-up before therapy and 2 events during an equal time period on therapy. No patient died. Anginal frequency was decreased by 94% in the patients receiving diltiazem. Diltiazem was well tolerated by all patients and no patient had to discontinue therapy because of side effects. Thus, these data suggest that long-term diltiazem therapy is beneficial in patients with variant angina pectoris.

Propranolol therapy

Tilmant and associates[145] from Lille, France, determined with quantitative variables if propranolol was detrimental in patients with documented coronary arterial spasm and if this drug can be used in combination with calcium channel blocking agents. Eleven patients with documented coronary spasm were entered prospectively in a study with 4 phases of 2 days each: 1) control; 2) diltiazem or propranolol (mean, 225 ± 75 mg/day); 3) propranolol or diltiazem (360 mg/day); 4) propranolol and diltiazem. The effects of the drugs were assessed by the detection of ischemic ECG episodes (24-hour ECG monitoring) and provocative tests with ergonovine. During the period of treatment with propranolol, the number and the duration of attacks increased and provocative tests had positive results in all patients. Diltiazem completely abolished spontaneous episodes, but 6 of 11 patients remained sensitive to the administration of ergonovine. The association of the 2 drugs led to a disappearance of ischemic episodes. In conclusion, propranolol is ineffective in patients with coronary artery spasm. It can be used in combination with diltiazem, but without any advantage over diltiazem alone.

Nifedipine therapy

Hill and associates[146] from Gainesville, Florida, compared nifedipine with isosorbide dinitrate in a randomized crossover trial of 26 patients with angina and coronary spasm: 18 had a short-term beneficial response to nifedipine and 14 of them were followed for an average period of 9.4 months. During follow-up, nifedipine was the primary therapy in these 14 patients, but other drugs were added when clinically necessary to control angina. There was an overall 86% beneficial response rate (>50% decrease in angina frequency). However, 2 patients had a large increase (>10 times) and 4 patients had a slight increase (transient) in angina frequency in long-term compared with short-term response. The other 8 patients had a similar angina frequency compared with short-term response. Of the 12 patients with a good response (transient slight increase or no change), 8 (67%) required additional drug therapy to control angina. Nifedipine was discontinued in 2, and the dose was decreased in 3 of the 14 patients because of adverse effects. Three patients had a marked increase in angina at 9, 14, and 3 months, requiring hospitalization; 1 patient had coronary bypass for symptom control. Thus, patients with coronary spasm selected because of a favorable short-term response to nifedipine were effectively treated over the long term with nifedipine; however, additional therapy was often needed to control symptoms. Adverse effects were common, but simple reduction of nifedipine dose usually diminished the unwanted effects of the drug.

Alpha-adrenergic blockade (prazosin) therapy

Robertson and associates[147] from Nashville, Tennessee, evaluated 6 patients with variant angina to determine the efficacy of alpha$_1$ adrenergic antagonism with prazosin in a double-blind, randomized, placebo-controlled evaluation. Despite plasma prazosin levels adequate to produce a 6-fold shift in the response to phenylephrine, there was no significant difference in the number of ischemic episodes while taking prazosin compared with placebo. Similarly, there was no difference in the length of the ischemic episodes. Chest pain and nitroglycerin usage were not different during treatment periods with prazosin and placebo. Thus, these data suggest that alpha$_1$ adrenergic antagonism with prazosin does not reduce the frequency of anginal attacks in patients with coronary arterial spasm.

In an investigation carried out by Tzivoni and colleagues[148] from Jerusalem, Israel, prazosin was used to abolish Prinzmetal's variant angina in 6 patients during a follow-up period of 4–6 months. All had a recent transmural AMI, after which the anginal attacks with transient ST-segment elevation developed, and 3 of them had already had variant angina prior to the infarction. Therapeutic trials with high doses of nifedipine, verapamil, nitrates, beta blockers, and (in 1 case) phenoxybenzamine were ineffective in all 6 patients. Prazosin 8–30 mg/day combined with low dose nitrates of nifedipine completely abolished the attacks in 4 patients, markedly reduced their frequency and intensity in 1 patient, and had to be stopped in the sixth because of hypotension and dizziness. Except for this last patient, the drug was well tolerated, and no changes in BP were observed. In 4 patients discontinuation or reduction of prazosin resulted in exacerbation of symptoms, and its renewal was followed by disappearance of the attacks. Thus, postsynaptic alpha$_1$ blockade without norepinephrine elevation effected by prazosin provides potent coronary vasodilation that may be superior to conventional agents, and chronic application of prazosin constitutes a new therapeutic approach in selected patients with refractory variant angina.

Winniford and coworkers[149] from Dallas, Texas, assessed the efficacy of prazosin in 6 men (mean age, 49 years) with variant angina. Prazosin, 14 mg/day in 3 equal doses, was compared with placebo in a double-blind, randomized, double-crossover trial lasting 4.5 months: 2 weeks of open label prazosin followed by 4 1-month periods of blinded alternating therapy. No other vasoactive medications were administered during the period. Prazosin reduced sitting systolic arterial BP from 145–127 mmHg, but exerted no effect on diastolic arterial pressure or heart rate. Prazosin did not change the weekly number of episodes of chest pain (2.5 with placebo -vs- 3.1 with prazosin), nitroglycerin tablets used (3.9 with placebo -vs- 4.6 with prazosin), or transient ST-segment deviations (by calibrated 2-channel Holter monitoring for 24 h/week throughout the study) (6.5 with placebo -vs- 11.8 with prazosin). During prazosin therapy, 3 patients had orthostatic dizziness and 1 patient had headache. Thus, in this long-term randomized double-blind trial, prazosin exerted no obvious beneficial effect in patients with variant angina.

Aspirin therapy

Recent studies suggest that large doses of aspirin or indomethacin can contract coronary arteries and thereby may induce coronary spasm in patients with variant angina. To evaluate this phenomenon, Miwa and colleagues[150] from Kyoto, Japan, administered aspirin (4.0 g/day) orally to 4 patients with Prinzmetal's variant angina to examine the effect of this drug on anginal attacks. The administration of aspirin increased the frequency of resting anginal attacks markedly, and the attacks that occurred only during the night or early morning during the control period occurred also in the daytime when the 4 patients were receiving aspirin. Exercise stress testing done in the afternoon was repeatedly negative during the control period and became positive with ST elevation during the aspirin administration period in the 3 patients who were able to perform the test. Thus, a large amount of aspirin can aggravate coronary arterial spasm in some patients with Prinzmetal's variant angina. It was postulated that large amounts of aspirin may act on the endothelium of coronary vessels and inhibit the protective effect against vasoconstriction by blocking prostacyclin synthesis through inactivation of cyclooxygenase.

Partial sympathetic denervation plus CABG

Poor results of CABG in the treatment of variant angina have been ascribed to recurrent vasospastic activity due to autonomic imbalance. Cardiac sympathetic denervation (plexectomy) may represent a rational approach in the prevention of vasospasm. To test the value of plexectomy in the treatment of variant angina, Betriu and associates[151] from Montreal, Canada, studied 31 patients, 17 of whom (group 1) underwent conventional CABG and the remaining 14 (group 2) underwent cardiac sympathetic denervation also. The 2 groups were similar with respect to age (54 ± 8 -vs- 50 ± 7 years), sex distribution (male/female ratio 12/5 -vs- 9/5), prevalence of coexisting effort angina (10 -vs- 12 patients), previous AMI (7 -vs- 4 patients), and duration of variant angina (3.3 ± 5.4 -vs- 2.4 ± 2.7 months). The LV EF was comparable in both groups (60 ± 11 -vs- 60 ± 4%) as were LV and end-diastolic pressure (15 ± 4 -vs- 5 mmHg) and extent of CAD (65 -vs- 71% prevalence of multivessel disease). The average duration of follow-

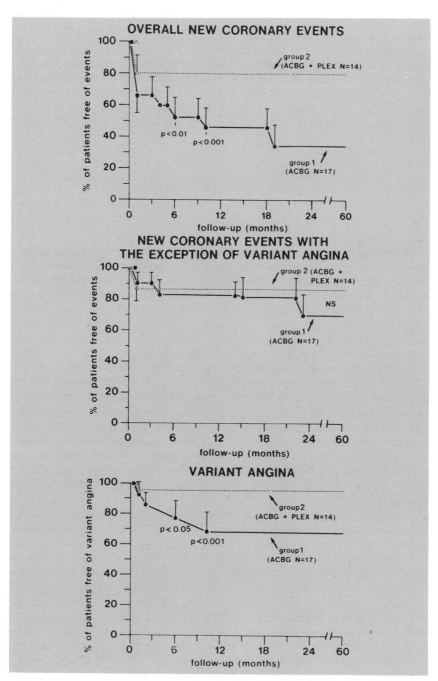

Fig. 1-8. Actuarial curves with standard error of mean showing the cumulative probability of overall new coronary events (top), new coronary events with exception of variant angina (middle), variant angina (bottom). Note that when only myocardial infarction and death were selected as endpoints, actuarial analysis failed to show differences in the 2 groups. The differences reach significance at 6- and 10-month points (arrow). ACBG = aortocoronary bypass graft; PLEX = plexectomy.

up was 23 ± 15 months in group 1 and 22 ± 18 months in group 2 (p, NS). There were no operative deaths. Four patients, 2 in each group, had a perioperative AMI. Seven patients in group 1 and 1 patient in group 2 had recurrent variant angina. There was sudden death and 2 infarcts in group 1. Actuarial curves showed the cumulative probability of recurrent variant angina to be significantly lower (p < 0.05 and p < 0.001 at 6 and 10 months, respectively) in group 2 (Fig. 1-8). This study suggests that cardiac sympathetic denervation may prevent recurrent vasospastic activity in variant angina.

CORONARY ARTERY BYPASS GRAFTING

Results with or without comparison to medical therapy alone

There has been debate during the past decade about how many conduits should be inserted in patients undergoing CABG. Jones and associates[152] from Atlanta, Georgia, analyzed 1,238 patients with 3-vessel CAD ($\geq$50% diameter reduction) who had undergone CABG. The patients were divided into 2 groups, depending on whether complete (773 patients) or incomplete (465 patients) revascularization had been done. Patients with complete revascularization had a higher frequency of a normal preoperative ECG than did patients with incomplete revascularization (23 -vs- 14%). The EF for both completely and incompletely revascularized patients was good (60 and 57%). The mean number of grafts per patient for the 2 groups was 3.8 and 2.6. No significant differences between the 2 groups were observed with regard to postoperative inotropic requirements (8 and 7%), ventricular arrhythmias (1.8 and <1%), necessity for intraoperative balloon pumping (1.6 and 1.5%), hospital mortality (1.2 and 2.8%), or AMI (4.3 and 4.8%). Survival at 5 years was significantly greater in patients with complete (89%) than in those with incomplete revascularization (84%). Reemployment occurred more often in patients with complete (52%) than in those with incomplete revascularization (40%), and more patients were free of angina pectoris after complete (70%) than after incomplete revascularization (58%). Thus, long-term survival appeared to be mediated primarily through improved revascularization rather than through differences in LV function.

Miller and associates[153] from Stanford, California, examined the changing risks of CABG over a 10-year period. Using univariate and multivariate logistic regression analyses, they investigated the effects of 42 variables on the incidence of perioperative AMI and operative mortality for 2 cohorts undergoing CABG (group A 1971–1975 and group B 1977–1979) (Figs. 1-9, 1-10). Group B patients were at higher potential risk than those in group A. The postoperative AMI and operative mortality rates declined from 8.7% ± 0.9–4.6% ± 0.7% (p = 0.005) and from 2.4% ± 0.5–1.2% ± 0.4% (p = 0.07), respectively. Additionally the independent determinants of AMI and mortality for the 2 time intervals were distinctly different. The multivariate determinants for predicting perioperative AMI rate in the group A patients were the presence of LM CAD, age, the presence of a preoperative AMI, and the mode of myocardial protection. In the later group B cohort, gender and coronary thromboendarterectomy were the only significant predictive variables. For prediction of operative mortality rate in the earlier group A patients,

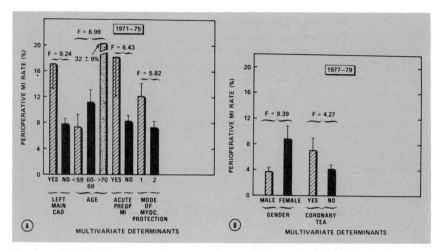

Fig. 1-9. (A) Clinical impact of 4 independent determinants of perioperative myocardial infarction (*PMI*) in group A. The PMI rates are presented with 70% confidence limits. (B) Clinical influence of independent determinants of PMI for group B. Gender and coronary thromboendarterectomy (*TEA*) were the only significant predictive variables. *CAD* = coronary artery disease; *MI* = myocardial infarction; *MYOC* = myocardial. *Mode 1* myocardial protection was continuous VF without ischemic arrest. *Mode 2* was aortic cross clamping using continuous profound topical hypothermia. Reproduced with permission from Miller et al.[153]

the variables were emergency operation, LM CAD, severity of CHF, systemic hypertension, and degree of MR. This was opposed to the later group B in which operative mortality was related only to emergency operation and the presence of CHF. During the last year of the study (1979), the operative

Fig. 1-10. (A) Clinical impact of 5 independent determinants of operative mortality (*OM*) for group A. These OM rates (±70% confidence limits) varied markedly from 1–21% according to patient classification. (B) Clinical impact of independent determinants of OM for group B (1977–1979). Compared to group A only emergency operation and CHF remained significant predictors of OM, and variation in OM rates was less dramatic. *CAD* = coronary artery disease; *CHF* = congestive heart failure; *MR* = mitral regurgitation. Reproduced with permission from Miller et al.[153]

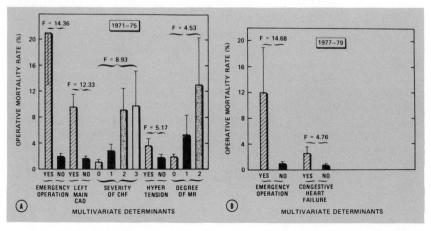

mortality rate for 15 who had emergency operation was 6.7 ± 7% compared with 0.47 ± 0.4% for those who did not (p, NS). Patients with a history of CHF had an operative mortality rate of 1.75% ± 1.3% compared with 0.31% ± 0.3% for those without congestive heart failure (p, NS). Those trends suggested to the authors that even the adverse effects of CHF and emergency operation on operative mortality seen in the later cohort were not present in the last year of the study. The specific factors responsible for those reductions and operative risks remain uncharacterized.

Loop and associates[154] from Cleveland, Ohio, evaluated surgical results in 2,445 consecutive women undergoing isolated CABG and compared them with surgical results in 18,079 consecutive men. The indication for CABG was severe or unstable angina in 60% of women and 45% of men. Women had a higher operative mortality rate (2.9 -vs- 1.3%) despite having less 3-vessel CAD (44 -vs- 56%, p < 0.001) and better LV function (normal LV EF in 60% of women and 53% of men, p < 0.001). When matched for age, severity of angina, and extent of CAD, women still had twice the operative mortality of men. Further analysis revealed that body surface area was the strongest predictor of operative risks. Women also had a lower overall graft patency (76%) than men (82%), and at 5 and 10 years postoperatively, a higher percentage of men were angina-free. However, survival for women and men at 5 and at 10 years postoperatively was similar. Thus, the smaller size of women rather than their sex appears to explain the difference in operative risks.

Salomon and colleagues[155] from Portland, Oregon, addressed the problem of diabetes mellitus associated with CABG. In a retrospective analysis, 412 diabetic patients were compared with 3,295 nondiabetic patients. There were 20 preoperative and 18 intraoperative variables examined. The diabetic group differed from the nondiabetic patients in that there was evidence of greater CAD judged angiographically and a higher incidence of systemic hypertension, LV hypertrophy, and tobacco consumption and a longer duration of angina. The diabetic group had a higher average number of grafts than the nondiabetic group. Postoperative mortality and morbidity was greater in the diabetic group (Table 1-9). Follow-up extending to 10 years revealed that survival was less good in diabetic compared with nondiabetic patients (Fig. 1-11). Surviving patients had a higher incidence of CAD-related events among the diabetic than the nondiabetic groups (p < 0.001). CABG should be done on diabetic patients. These data help to advise patients with diabetes of their prognosis after CABG. Studies of the natural history of diabetics with CAD treated medically are not readily available.

Of 2,144 patients aged ≥65 years entered into the registry of the Coronary Artery Surgery Study (CASS) who had coronary arteriography, Gersh and participants[156] from Seattle, Washington, reviewed 1,086 who underwent isolated CABG. Complications of angiography included death in 4 patients and nonfatal AMI in 17. Eight patients had neurologic complications, which were transient in 5. The perioperative mortality was 5.2% (57 of 1,086), which is significantly greater than the perioperative mortality of 1.9% (151 of 7,827) in patients <65 years entered in CASS. There was a trend toward an increased mortality rate with age: 4.6% in patients aged 65–69 years, 6.6% in those 70–74 years, and 9.5% in those ≥75 years. Also, the duration of hospital stay after operation was significantly longer for patients ≥65 years than for those <65 (13 days -vs- 11 days). Stepwise linear discriminant

TABLE 1-9. *Perioperative mortality and morbidity data. Reproduced with permission from Salomon et al.*[155]

%	NONDIABETIC PATIENTS (N = 3,295)	DIABETIC PATIENTS TREATED (N = 250)	INSULIN-DEPENDENT DIABETIC PATIENTS (N = 162)
Hospital deaths	2.5	5.1*	4.5*
Sternotomy complications	0.5	2.0*	3.0*
Renal failure	0.1	3.1*	3.0*
Neurologic complications	1.0	2.1	3.1
Total hospital days (mean ± S.D.)	10.7 ± 6.4	12.2 ± 9.0*	13.3 ± 11.3*
Perioperative infarction	3.1	4.0	4.2

* p < 0.05 difference from nondiabetic group.

analysis identified 5 variables predictive of perioperative mortality: presence of ≥70% stenosis of the LM coronary artery and a left dominant circulation, LV end-diastolic pressure, a history of current cigarette smoking, pulmonary rales, and presence of ≥1 associated medical disease. A second linear discriminant analysis incorporating 7,658 CASS patients who underwent isolated CABG irrespective of age examined whether age ≥65 years was an independent predictor of perioperative mortality. The variables selected in order of significance were CHF score, LM CAD, and a left dominant circulation, age ≥65 years, LV wall motion score, sex, and history of unstable angina pectoris. These investigators concluded that in patients aged ≥65 years, the mortality from coronary arteriography is low, whereas mortality from CABG is greater than that in CASS patients <65 years of age.

Fig. 1-11. Actuarial survival comparison: A = nondiabetic patients (n = 3,295); B = diabetic patients treated with diet or oral medication (n = 250); C = insulin–dependent diabetic patients (n = 162). Reproduced with permission from Salomon et al.[155]

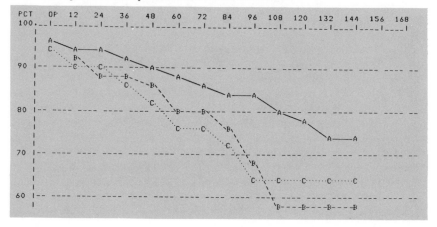

Frick and colleagues[157] from Helsinki, Finland, examined 100 patients with angina pectoris who fulfilled specific entry criteria randomly assigned to either medical therapy or CABG. These groups were subjected to annual exercise testing during a 5-year follow-up period. The degree of revascularization was assessed by graft and native vessel angiography at 3 weeks, 1 year, and 5 years after the operation. The exercise tolerance of the medical group remained largely unchanged in the follow-up period. Eighty-five to 95% of the patients were using beta blocking agents at the successive testing situations. The surgical group had a sustained improvement in exercise tolerance: total work increased by 39–66%, maximal ergometric load by 23–35%, and maximal ST depression decreased by 39–61%. The use of beta blocking agents in the surgical group steadily increased from 44% at 6 months after operation to 63% of patients at 5 years. Division of the surgical group into subsets of complete and incomplete revascularization revealed that the improvement was confined to complete revascularization. Thus, the investigators concluded the improved exercise tolerance after CABG was the result of successful reestablishment of effective coronary perfusion; despite graft attrition (15% in 5 years) and new narrowings in the native arteries, this improvement persisted for 5 years with appropriate medical therapy.

Rahimtoola and associates[158] from Portland, Oregon, assessed the long-term results of CABG performed for unstable angina in 1,282 patients from 1970–1982. The operative mortality was 1.8%; in the first 4 years it was 2.5%, and in the last 8.5 years it was 1.7%. Using actuarial techniques, the 5-year and 10-year survival rates (mean ± SE) were 92 ± 1 and 83 ± 2%, respectively, for the whole group (Fig. 1-12). For patients with normal LV function, they were 92 ± 2 and 86 ± 3%, and for patients with abnormal LV function, 91 ± 2 and 79 ± 4% (p = 0.14) (Fig. 1-13). No significant differences were observed in the long-term survival for any of the 3 clinical subgroups of patients with unstable angina: angina at rest, angina after recovery from AMI, and progressive angina of recent onset (p = 0.49). The

Fig. 1-12. Actuarially determined expected survival for all patients undergoing coronary bypass surgery for unstable angina. Those at risk include all patients who were known to be alive and in whom follow-up was obtained. Reproduced with permission from Rahimtoola et al.[158]

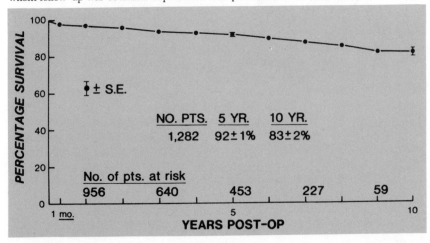

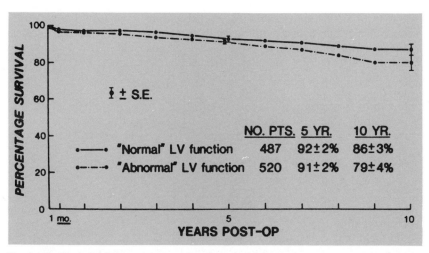

Fig. 1-13. Survival after surgery as predicted on the basis of LV function. Reproduced with permission from Rahimtoola et al.[158]

reoperation rates at 5 and 10 years were 6 ± 1 and 17 ± 3%. Currently, 61% of the survivors had no angina; angina occurred on severe exertion in 20%, on ordinary exertion in 14%, and on mild exertion in 5%. Thus, CABG is an effective form of therapy (for up to 10 years) in patients with unstable angina.

Gibson and associates[159] from Charlottesville, Virginia, determined the value of thallium-201 exercise scintigraphy in predicting responses to CABG in 47 consecutive patients. All patients underwent thallium-201 scintigraphy and coronary angiography 4.3 ± 3.1 weeks (mean ± SD) before and 7.5 ± 1.6 weeks after CABG. Thallium uptake and washout were computer quantified and each of the 6 segments was defined as normal, showing total or partial redistribution or a persistent defect. Persistent defects were further classified according to the percent reduction in regional thallium activity. Of 82 segments with total redistribution before CABG, 76 (93%) had normal thallium uptake and washout postoperatively compared with only 16 (73%) of 22 with partial redistribution (p = 0.01). Preoperative angiography revealed that 95% of the segments with total redistribution had preserved wall motion -vs- only 74% of those with partial redistribution (p = 0.01). Of 42 persistent defects thought to represent AMI before CABG, 19 (45%) demonstrated normal perfusion postoperatively. Of the persistent defects that showed improved thallium perfusion postoperatively, 75% had normal or hypokinetic wall motion before CABG -vs- only 14% of those without improvement (p < 0.001). These data suggest that preoperative quantitative thallium-201 scintigraphy is useful in predicting responses to revascularization surgery, and some persistent defects may revert to normal thallium uptake after surgery.

To assess the benefits of regular participation in a medically supervised cardiac rehabilitation program, Waites and associates[160] from Atlanta, Georgia, studied retrospectively 22 patients who had undergone CABG (2 groups of 11 each). Group I (mean age, 53 years) was currently enrolled in the rehabilitation program. Group II (mean age, 56 years) had begun but had discontinued the program. The stated reasons for discontinuation were not medical. There was no difference in entry exercise tests, and presurgical catheterization data in both groups were comparable. Mean peak oxygen consumption (VO_2) by modified Douglas bag technique, heart rate times systolic BP product, and treadmill duration time were recorded in a single testing period. Results revealed that group I had higher peak VO_2 (30 ml/kg/min) than group II (24 ml/kg/min) (p < 0.005) and greater treadmill time (11 min) than group II (8 min) (p < 0.01). Nine of 11 subjects in group I were fully employed -vs- 4 of 11 in group II (p < 0.01). One of 11 subjects in group I had been rehospitalized -vs- 5 in group II. None in group I but 4 in group II smoked. Thus, based on the sampling and methodology of this study, it was concluded that CABG patients in rehabilitation programs have greater peak VO_2 and treadmill test time, smoke less, are less often rehospitalized, and are more often fully employed than those who are not in such programs.

Pantely and colleagues[161] from Portland, Oregon, in 1981 initiated a prospective randomized study comparing CABG (group 1, 51 patients) to drug therapy (group 2, 49 patients). Supine graded exercise testing (SGXT) was performed initially at 6 months and annually with a bicycle ergometer. The presence or absence of ischemic ST-segment changes (positive or negative SGXT) and chest pain were recorded. Initially, 63% of all patients had positive SGXT. For group 2 the frequency of positive SGXT results did not change significantly at 6 months (58%) or at 5 years (52%). At 6 months the number of patients without chest pain increased in group 1 compared with group 2, but there was no difference in the frequency of positive SGXT results. This occurred because a majority of the group 1 patients with positive SGXT no longer had associated chest pain. This response was associated with incomplete revascularization in 8 of these 11 group 1 patients and may result from silent ischemia. At 5 years, no significant difference existed in the incidence of positive SGXT (group 1 -vs- group 2), but group 1 continued to have a reduction in the number of patients without chest pain. The incidences of death and AMI were not significantly different between groups. Fewer episodes of unstable angina occurred in group 1. Thus, the prognosis of group 1 patients with positive SGXT and no chest pain and incomplete revascularization was not different from that of group 2.

Reoperations for CAD will assuredly be more frequent in the future. Loop and colleagues[162] from Cleveland, Ohio, analyzed the first 1,000 operations for isolated CABG reoperation. They divided the patients into 4 cohorts of 250 patients each in time frames between 1969 and 1982. Operative mortality declined from 5–2% over that period and most other forms of perioperative morbidity declined also. The number of grafts per patient increased from 1.4–2.3 and the incidence of complete revascularization at reoperation increased from 65–76%. After a mean of 29 months, graft patency was 81% in the 154 patients restudied. Patency was similar for grafts to arteries previously involved with graft failure and to arteries not previously grafted. Five-year actuarial survival for patients in the first 3 cohorts was 89%. Survival was affected significantly by extent of CAD and LV performance before reoperation and by completeness of revascularization. Survival was not affected by the reason for reoperation, that is, graft closure, progressive atherosclerosis, or both. Patients who received complete revascularization (all major arteries >1 mm in diameter and narrowed ≥50% in diameter were grafted) had a 5-year survival of 92% after reoperation compared with an 86% survival for those classified as having incomplete revascularization. The authors add that there were 130,000 CABG operations done in 1980. Among survivors of CABG at 10 years, there will be a 10% chance of reoperation, and thus they suggest that in 1985, 7,900 reoperations will be done and in 1990 13,700 reoperations will be done. These data are important and suggest that the reoperative procedure will be of benefit in terms of survival and relief of symptoms.

From the CASS registry Alderman and colleagues[163] from Stanford, California, identified 420 medically treated and 231 surgically treated patients who had severe LV dysfunction manifested by an EF <36% and markedly abnormal wall motion. Compared with medically treated patients, those treated surgically had more severe angina, (57 -vs- 29% class III or class IV; p < 0.001), less CHF as predominant symptoms (11 -vs- 19%; p < 0.03), more severe CAD (67 -vs- 50% 3-vessel CAD; p < 0.001), greater LM CAD (13 -vs- 4%; p < 0.001) and a greater estimated extent of jeopardized myocardium (p < 0.001). Multivariate regression analysis of survival showed that surgical treatment prolonged survival (p < 0.05) (Fig. 1-14). However, it ranked below severity of CHF, age, EF, and LM CAD in determining prognosis. Surgical benefit was more apparent for patients with an EF <26% (43% 5-year survival with medical treatment -vs- 63%). Surgically treated patients had substantial symptomatic benefit compared with medically treated patients if the presenting symptom was predominantly angina (Fig. 1-15). However, there was no relief of symptoms caused primarily by CHF

Fig. 1-14. Life table cumulative survival for all patients. Method B was used for survival analyses. Survival curves are adjusted for all other significant prognostic variables; p values associated with each analysis are shown in bottom left corner. Reproduced with permission from Alderman et al.[163]

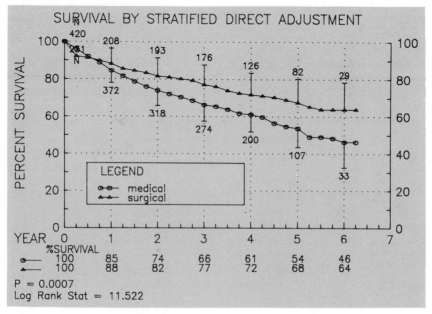

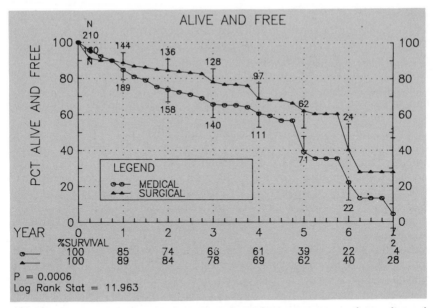

Fig. 1-15. Percentage of patients with angina as the predominant symptom who are alive *and* free of moderate or severe limitation. Reproduced with permission from Alderman et al.[163]

Fig. 1-16. Percentage of patients with heart failure as the predominant symptom who are alive *and* free of moderate or severe limitation. Reproduced with permission from Alderman et al.[163]

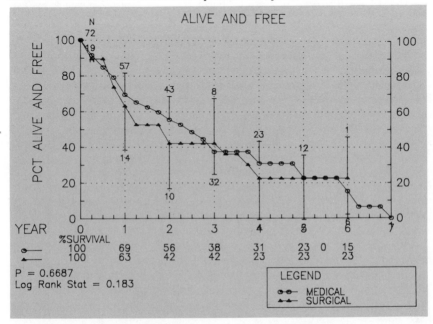

(Fig. 1-16). The authors concluded that patients with angina and a severely depressed EF should not be excluded from CABG.

At the time of 3-year follow-up, 30% of surgically treated and 10% of medically treated patients whose primary presenting symptom was chest pain became free of functional limitation. Thirty-two percent of the medically treated patients had died -vs- 16% of the surgically treated patients. Death within 30 days of operation occurred in 7% of the surgical patients. The superiority for recommending operation in patients presenting with CHF symptoms (as opposed to angina) was not demonstrated. Caution should be exercised in recommending patients with a low EF and CHF symptoms for operation and operative mortality should be ≤7%.

Coronary Artery Surgery Study (CASS) includes a multicenter patient registry and a randomized controlled clinical trial. From August 1975 to May 1979, 780 patients with stable CAD were randomly assigned to receive surgical (n, 390) or nonsurgical (n, 390) treatment and were followed through April 15, 1983.[164] The CASS registry includes a total of 24,959 patients who during the interval from July 1974 to May 31, 1979, underwent coronary arteriographic examination at the 15 participating CASS registry sites. The 780 patients randomized are part of 1,319 patients randomizable who were but a small number of patients (16,626) who were available to the CASS registry at randomizing sites. Patients excluded were those with inoperable arteries, a large group of patients with class II or class IV angina, and patients with LM CAD. Patients additionally excluded were those with prior CABG, CHF, and age >65 years. At 5 years, the average annual mortality rate in patients assigned to surgical treatment was 1.1%, and the mortality rate in those receiving medical therapy was 1.6%. The differences for this comparison and for comparisons by number of arteries narrowed was not statistically significant. Nearly 75% of the patients had an entry EF of ≥50% and minimal or no angina pectoris. The annual rate of CABG in patients who were initially assigned to receive medical treatment (crossover) was 4.7%. The excellent survival rates observed both in CASS patients assigned to receive medical and those assigned to receive surgical therapy and the similarity of survival rates in the 2 groups of patients in this randomized trial lead to a conclusion that patients similar to those enrolled in that trial can safely defer CABG until symptoms worsen to the point that surgical palliation is required. One must also conclude that patients in this category need not have angiography if LV function appears good and symptom status is minimal. The study might be criticized because the number of patients randomized was a small percent of the total patients analyzed in CASS. However, other criticisms are not valid, including those regarding surgical risks (1.4% in the present study), number of grafts performed, or late patency rates.

In a companion paper to the survival statistics from CASS, the principal investigators[165] evaluated the comparative effects of medical or surgical therapy on quality of life in patients with stable CAD. Patients in the surgical group reported significantly less chest pain, fewer activity limitations, and required less therapy with nitrates and beta blockers than did patients in the medical group. Treadmill exercise test documented significantly longer treadmill time, less exercise-induced angina, and less ST-segment depression among the surgical patients. However, employment status and recreational status did not differ significantly between medical and surgical groups. These are corroborative data showing that surgery indeed has a positive and saluatory affect on the quality of life and exercise physiology in CAD patients. Even in these mildly symptomatic patients, there was marked improvement in exercise status and freedom from angina.

Internal mammary artery as conduit

Singh and associates[166] from Pittsburgh, Pennsylvania, Albany, New York, and New Hyde Park, New York, studied 33 patients up to 10 years after CABG in whom each patient had at least 1 saphenous vein conduit and at least 1 internal mammary artery as a conduit. Eleven symptom-free patients studied 1 month to 5 years (mean, 1.9 years) after CABG had intact internal mammary artery and saphenous vein grafts in a good state of preservation. Of the 6 patients developing symptoms within the first year after CABG, 3 had evidence of poor flow in the internal mammary artery graft because of large side branches and the other 3 had stenosis or occlusion of the saphenous vein grafts. Sixteen patients developed symptoms after several years of being symptom-free and were studied 3–10 years (mean, 6) after operation. Of the 23 saphenous vein grafts in this group, 17 (74%) were either occluded or severely narrowed and 6 (26%) were in good condition. One internal mammary artery graft was occluded and the remaining 15 were in good condition. Saphenous vein graft failure was the predominant cause of late development of symptoms in patients with combined revascularization. Long-term performance of the internal mammary artery grafts appears superior to that of the saphenous vein grafts.

Lytle and colleagues[167] from Cleveland, Ohio, studied 76 consecutive patients with multivessel CAD who underwent CABG with bilateral mammary artery grafts during the period from 1971–1980. There were no hospital deaths. Thirty-three free and 119 in situ grafts were used. Postoperative arteriograms obtained 1–108 months (mean, 26) postoperatively revealed that of 55 grafts in 28 patients, 49 were patent (89%). Of the 71 late survivors, 49 patients (69%) were asymptomatic at follow-up. There were 22 patients experiencing angina, but 18 were New York Heart Association class II and only 4 were class III. Comparison of postoperative functional class with preoperative symptom status showed 59 patients (83%) improved by at least 1 functional class. Actuarial survival was 97% at 7 years and 90% at 9 years after operation. The authors believe that bilateral mammary artery grafting yielded excellent graft patency and relief of symptoms. When saphenous vein is unsuitable, bilateral mammary artery grafts can be used before other conduits are considered.

Results of reoperation

Schaff and colleagues[168] from Rochester, Minnesota, analyzed the survival and functional status of 106 consecutive patients after second CABG procedures for CAD. Before reoperation, 95% of the patients were judged to be New York Heart Association class II or IV with angina and 76% had 3-vessel CAD. Angina recurrence was most commonly caused by bypass graft occlusion alone or in combination with further narrowing of the native arteries. Reoperative mortality was 2.8%, each death resulting from AMI.

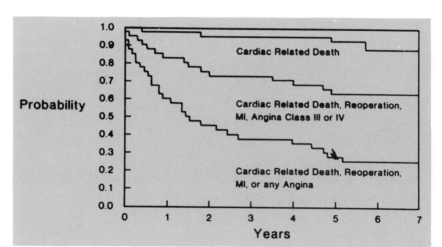

Fig. 1-17. Event–free interval was computed with cardiac–related death *(top curve)* as an end point, in addition to reoperation (third revascularization), myocardial infarction *(MI)*, and recurrence of angina. Probability of remaining free of these cardiac events is 26% at 7 years. However, when mild angina (NYHA Class II) is not included as a serious cardiac event, event–free survival is 73% at 3 years and 63% at 5 and 7 years. Reproduced with permission from Schaff et al.[168]

Actuarial survival of patients dismissed alive was 94% at 5 years and 89% at 7 years, figures similar to that reported by others for patients with 3-vessel CAD having primary operation and similar to other reports of groups of patients having reoperation (Fig. 1-17). However, when recurrence of any angina, need for a third operation, and AMI were included with cardiac-related deaths, event-free survival drops to 28% at 5 years and 26% at 7 years. There was no significant difference in survival or event-free survival according to the cause of recurrent CAD nor did the risk factors of diabetes mellitus, lipid abnormalities, or systemic hypertension adversely affect the late results of reoperation. Whether bypass graft occlusion, additional narrowing in native arteries, or narrowed but not bypassed arteries at initial operation caused reoperation did not influence incrementally late results. Reoperation could be done at low risk but was attendant with increased perioperative morbidity and persistent cardiac-related events in the follow-up period.

Laird-Meeter and associates[169] from Rotterdam, The Netherlands, ana-lyzed 53 patients who underwent a second CABG during a mean follow-up time of 3.5 years. The 53 patients were among 1,041 patients having CABG at their hospital. The operative mortality of the first operation was 1.2% and of the second CABG, 3.8%. The anatomic reason for reoperation was occlusion of the bypass graft in 41 (77%) patients, which in 18 was accompanied by progressive narrowing in the native coronary arteries. Progressive narrowing alone was observed in the native coronary arteries in 7 (13%). When symptoms occurred within 6 months after the first operation, occlusion of the bypass graft was found in 32 of 36 instances. Progressive narrowing in native coronary arteries not bypassed was seen only when symptoms occurred later. Late results in angina pectoris were less favorable in the group undergoing reoperation: 31 (65%) of the 48 operated on twice and 406

(46%) of the 877 operated on once still had angina at late follow-up. Both groups were improved equally by operation (88 -vs- 89%).

Effect on left ventricular function

Austin and associates[170] from Durham, North Carolina, studied 14 patients before, 8 days after, and 3 months after CABG. They used RNA at rest and during exercise to determine LV EF and they calculated end-systolic volume, stroke volume, and cardiac index. An index of contractility was calculated as a peak systolic pressure/end-systolic volume ratio. Resting function was unaltered after operation, although mild increases in heart rate and end-diastolic volume were observed on the eighth postoperative day. In contrast, exercise function was significantly improved at both postoperative time periods. Exercise EF was 0.54 ± 0.10 before operation, 0.73 ± 0.12 at 8 days, and 0.64 ± 0.13 at 3 months ($p = 0.0001$ at 8 days; $p = 0.002$ at 3 months). The contractility index during exercise increased from 2.2 ± 1.0 before operation to 4.5 ± 2.2 ($p = 0.001$) at 8 days and remained elevated at 3.9 ± 1.8 at 3 months ($p = 0.001$ -vs- before operation). Myocardial protection was accomplished with cold potassium cardioplegia. The present study revealed no improvement in resting function with CABG. This group of patients had normal resting EF before CABG. Patients with significant CAD decreased their LV EF with exercise before CABG. The most striking difference in hemodynamics during exercise was the increase in EF. Both heart rate and heart rate-pressure product achieved during exercise were the same as before operation; therefore the increase in EF documented improvement in LV function and probably reflected augmented myocardial contractility. This increase in contractility also was apparent in the ratio of systolic pressure to end-systolic volume. These results were noted up to 3 months after operation and probably are the result of the elimination of ischemia by CABG.

Taylor and associates[171] from Cambridge, England, studied the effect of CABG on global LV EF and regional contraction in 56 consecutive patients with chronic stable angina pectoris by means of multigated ventricular scintigraphy at rest and during dynamic supine exercise before and 6 weeks after CABG. Before operation, exercise induced a significant fall in EF and regional wall motion score. Six weeks after operation, 52 patients were symptomless. Resting EF and regional wall motion score was unchanged, but exercise EF increased significantly and the previous exercise-induced regional wall motion abnormalities were abolished. The 4 patients with persisting angina all showed the same pattern as before operation with a fall in LV EF and regional wall motion score during exercise. Thus, multigated ventricular scintigraphy affords a safe, objective, reproducible, and noninvasive means of assessing serial LV function at rest and during exercise in patients with CAD. The technique confirms that CABG abolishes exercise-induced abnormalities of LV function but has no influence on resting function.

Kronenberg and associates[172] from Nashville, Tennessee, studied global LV performance (EF) and regional LV function by rest-exercise radionuclide ventriculography in 36 patients before and after (23 ± 8 weeks) CABG for stable angina pectoris. The exercise EF was less than the resting EF before but not after CABG. The degree of postoperative improvement correlated with the degree of preoperative dysfunction. Improvement was most likely to occur if exercise-induced dysfunction was present preoperatively, even with healed AMI. Regional dysfunction during preoperative exercise was also likely to improve postoperatively. Protocol design is important in determining the results and their interpretation. Matching postoperative exercise loads to preoperative loads and using regional analysis with 2 imaging projections improved judgment of the results. Regional dysfunction was more common than global dysfunction and was less sensitive to workloads than was EF. This study shows that CABG can improve LV performance on exercise if preoperative tests indicate the presence of ischemia-induced dysfunction.

Preoperative and serial postoperative ECGs in 104 patients undergoing rest and exercise RNA before and 1–12 months after CABG were reviewed by Floyd and associates[173] from Durham, North Carolina. Five patient groups were defined by ECG findings before and after CABG: group I, normal ECG before and no ECG change after CABG; group II, prior AMI by ECG before but no QRS change after CABG; group III, all patients with a minor QRS cahnge (<0.04 s Q wave, loss of R-wave amplitude) after CABG; group IV, all patients with a major QRS change (≥0.04 s Q wave) after CABG; group V, all patients without new Q waves or loss of R-wave amplitude but with a major QRS change (conduction disturbance) after CABG. Mean resting EF changed little after CABG in all groups, although the 0.03 increase in group I was significant ($p < 0.05$). Group IV had the largest decrease in resting EF after CABG (0.04), but this was not statistically significant. Mean exercise EF increased significantly ($p < 0.0001$) in groups I, II, and III but not in groups IV and V. QRS changes do not consistently reflect impairment of LV function after CABG.

Effect on subsequent hospitalization, employment, and medical costs

Reasonable evidence now exists to document the efficacy of CABG in prolonging survival (LM and 3-vessel CAD) and in relieving symptoms of angina pectoris. The efficacy, however, of CABG in reducing other measures of morbidity, such as frequency of hospitalization, was lacking until the study by Hamilton and associates[174] from Seattle, Washington, who compared the rates of hospitalization during follow-up for a matched pair cohort of medically and surgically treated patients from the Angiography Registry of the Seattle Heart Watch. Medically and surgically treated patients were matched according to extent of CAD, LV EF, age, and 3 other survival rate-related characteristics. There was a 26% reduction in cardiovascular hospitalizations in the surgically treated patients (19%/year) compared with medically treated patients (26%/year). This was due to a significant reduction in hospitalization rate for AMI (surgically treated patients, 1.1%/year; medically treated patients, 2.6%/year), and for other cardiovascular reasons (surgically treated patients, 12.5%/year; medically treated patients, 15.7%/year). No significant ($p = 0.146$) reduction occurred in hospitalization rate for chest pain not due to AMI (surgically treated patients, 5.6%/year; medically treated patients, 7.7%/year). When the perioperative AMI is included for the surgical cohort, the overall AMI rate is not significantly different ($p = 0.173$) between the 2 treatment groups (surgically treated patients, 1.9%/year; medically treated patients, 2.6%/year). Acute AMI was an uncommon reason for hospitalization, accounting for only 8% (55 of 685) of all cardiovascular hospitalizations, and was not related to the number of stenotic vessels in medically treated patients.

Stanton and associates[175] from Boston, Massachusetts, studied preoperative predictors of postoperative employment status in 228 patients (aged 25–64 years) who underwent CABG, cardiac valve replacement, or both. Of the 150 patients working in the year before surgery, 73% returned within 6 months. Of those not employed, 18% started working. Patients who expected preoperatively to return to work did so at an 82% rate compared with 39% of the others. This was a strong predictor in the multiple regression analysis. Educational level and family income were stronger predictors than occupation or level of physical exertion required (Table 1-10). Rates of return were higher in patients with less severe angina and less fatigue preoperatively, but they did not differ significantly by sex, surgical procedure, or duration of illness. Seven variables predicted work status correctly for 86% of persons. These results suggest that determinants of return to work are largely present before surgery and that patients' attitudes and expectations play an important role.

Loop and associates[176] from Cleveland, Ohio described results of examining patients with multivessel CAD and stable angina pectoris by outpatient testing and admitted to a staging area with their families on the morning of CABG. This experimental group was not hospitalized before CABG. Their hospital charges were compared to those of cohorts of CABG from 1977–1981 who met the same entrance criteria. Length of stay in the hospital was reduced by 2 days. A 10% savings in hospital charges was realized in the 1981 experimental group compared with the 1981 control group. A comparison of total hospital charges, adjusted for inflation, shows that 1981 experimental group patients paid 35% less for their hospital room, 45% less for their intensive care period, and 17% less in total charges than the 1977 control group. Interviews indicated that these patients with stable cardiac conditions preferred to stay with their families or friends before surgery.

To evaluate the benefits of CABG, Jenkins and associates[177] from Galveston, Texas, interviewed and tested 318 patients <70 years of age before and 6 months after elective CABG. Biomedical, psychoneurologic, physical function, role function, occupational, social, family, sexual, emotional, and attitudinal variables were assessed. Quantitative comparisons showed improvement on many factors. Angina was completely relieved for 69–85% of persons, depending on whether it had been induced by exertion or other events. Disability days were reduced >80%. Seventy-five percent of employed

TABLE 1-10. *Percent of preoperatively employed who return to work postoperatively, by income. Reproduced with permission from Stanton et al.[175]*

INCOME LEVEL	N	% RETURNING TO WORK
<$10,000	9	44.4
$10,000–$19,999	50	56.0
$20,000–$29,999	47	89.4
$30,000+	29	93.1
Total	**135***	...

* Fifteen persons failed to respond to this question. χ^2 = 24.23; 3 df; P = .0001.

persons had returned to work. Anxiety, depression, fatigue, and sleep problems declined. Vigor and well-being scores rose significantly. When losses were expected (e.g., psychoneurologic function, marital adjustment), they generally were not found. For none of the >60 outcome variables was widespread serious worsening found. The findings suggest that most patients are able to resume normal economic and social functioning within 6 months after CABG.

Complications: low cardiac output, supraventricular conduction abnormalities, systemic hypertension, new Q waves and myocardial infarction, diabetes insipidus, aortic dissection and aortic false aneurysm, and graft occlusion

Low cardiac output associated with irreversible myocardial necrosis accounts for a small percentage of patients who have inotropic requirement postoperatively. More commonly transient depression of myocardial function is the indication for inotropic support. The period for postoperative myocardial depression is usually limited to the first 24 hours and is marked by progressive stabilization of hemodynamics and diminished requirements for inotropic agents. Inotropic support is gradually withdrawn using a tapering dosage while several hemodynamic variables are monitored. Van Trigt and associates[178] from Durham, North Carolina, used pressure and dimension analyses in 7 postoperative CABG patients to quantitate the changing cardiac response to dopamine over a 24-hour interval postoperatively. Ultrasonic dimension transducers were utilized to measure the minor axis LV diameter, and matched micromanometers were inserted to measure intracavitary LV

Fig. 1-18. The effect of dopamine on peripheral vascular resistance (PVR) 2–4 hours after early CABG and 18–24 hours after late CABG. Reproduced with permission from Van Trigt et al.[178]

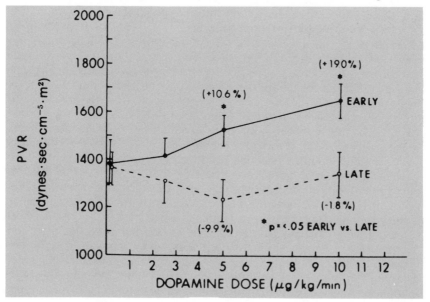

pressure and intrathoracic pressure. Pressure and dimension data were recorded and analyzed by computer during dopamine infusion at 0, 2.5, 5.0, and 10 μg/kg/minute at periods designated as early (2–4 hours after CABG) and late (8–24 hours after CABG). Myocardial contractile responses to dopamine (peak velocity of minor axis shortening, maximal excursion) were similar at each dose in the early and late studies. Overall hydraulic performance, as reflected by cardiac outputs in the areas of the pressure-diameter loops, had augmented late dose responses. Cardiac output increased during the early period from control 3.2 ± 0.7 liters/minute to 3.9 ± 0.7 liters/minute at 10 μg/minute dopamine. Cardiac output during the late period increased from a control of 3.9 ± 0.5 liters/minute to 5.3 ± 0.7 liters/minute at 10 μg/kg/minute ($p < 0.05$) early versus late response at an equal dose of dopamine. Dopamine produced a progressive increase in the maximum velocity of minor axis shortening in both periods; comparison of the augmentation of contractility by similar doses of dopamine in the early and late postoperative periods revealed no significant difference. The response of the pressure-diameter loop, which the authors thought a sensitive and reproducible means of quantitating global mechanical performance, was dramatically influenced by dopamine, and this response also showed a significant difference with respect to time paralleling the response of cardiac output. At the 2 higher doses of dopamine, the increase in the area of the pressure diameter loop was substantially greater in the later period. The differences in the early -vs- late response can be attributed to changes in peripheral vascular resistance. During the early period, infusion of dopamine increased peripheral vascular resistance. During the later period peripheral vascular resistance did not change significantly and thus peripheral vascular resistance at 10 μg/minute dopamine infusion during the late period was significantly different from that during the early period (Fig. 1-18). These data indicate that moderate doses of dopamine affect a more pronounced augmentation of cardiac performance with time following CABG, probably because the lower associated peripheral vascular resistance offers less of an impediment to ventricular ejection later in the postoperative period. This may be a baroreceptor mediated response.

Smith and colleagues[179] from Durham, North Carolina, argue that coincident with the use of longer aortic cross-clamp times with cardioplegic myocardial protection there has developed an increased incidence of postoperative conduction block and supraventricular tachyarrhythmias. In 8 patients undergoing CABG, a marked disparity was noted in the ability to cool the atrial septum compared with ventricular septum (mean temperatures, $26 \pm 1°C$ -vs- $16 \pm 1°C$, respectively; $p < 0.05$) (Fig. 1-19). Moreover, atrial septal temperature returned to the temperature of the systemic perfusate (28°C) within 3 minutes following cessation of cardioplegic infusion, whereas ventricular septal temperature remained at 15–20°C. The effect of intermittent topical ice saline slush on atrial septal temperature was transient. Cardiopulmonary bypass was conducted using a 2-stage single venous cannula. However, similar findings were noted in 10 dogs in which cardiopulmonary bypass and cardioplegic myocardial protection were conducted using 2 venous cannulas with caval tapes. Temperature gradients between the atrial and ventricular septums were due in part to differential delivery of the cardioplegic solution; the atrial septum receiving much less solution per gram of tissue than the ventricular septum. In the clinical setting

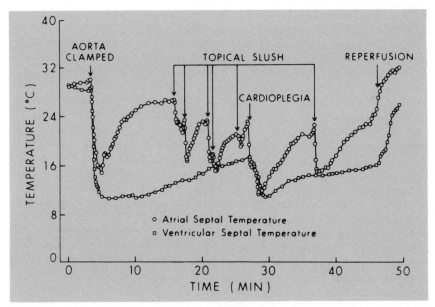

Fig. 1-19. Atrial septal and ventricular septal temperature curves in a patient undergoing quadruple aortacoronary bypass grafting. Systemic perfusion temperature was maintained at 28°C throughout period of cardioplegic arrest. Note the rapid decline in both atrial septal and ventricular septal temperatures during initial infusion of cardioplegic solution coincident with time of aortic cross clamping. Ventricular septal temperature reached 10°C within 30 seconds, atrial septal temperature decreased only to 15°C. Ventricular septal temperature gradually increased during the next 20 minutes to 16°C, when a second infusion of cardioplegic solution was instituted. Within 3–5 minutes following completion of initial cardioplegic infusion, atrial septal temperature increased to 25–26°C and stayed at that level until topical iced saline slush was applied to the heart. Although topical saline slush did not affect gradual rewarming of ventricular septum, it caused an abrupt decrease in atrial septal temperature each time it was applied to the heart. However, the effect of topical slush was transient, with atrial septal rewarming beginning shortly after each application of iced saline slush. Twenty minutes following completion of initial cardioplegic infusion, a second cardioplegic infusion was accomplished and resulted in rapid decrease in both the atrial septal and ventricular septal temperatures. Again, however, the atrial septal rewarmed rapidly. Topical iced saline slush was again applied with rapid cooling of atrial septum but with no demonstrable effect on ventricular septal temperature. Atrial septum again began to rewarm rapidly until time of release of aortic cross clamp and reperfusion of coronary arteries at 28°C. Reproduced with permission from Smith et al.[179]

the use of a single venous cannula may partially explain the rise in atrial tissue temperature during cardioplegic myocardial arrest. There is, however, a difference in the distribution of cardioplegic solution to the atria and ventricles, and thus the temperature gradient can only partially be abolished by core cooling and the use of pericardial iced saline solution. The frequency and morbidity attributable to postoperative atrial arrhythmias is unknown. However, prudence dictates that certain attempts be made to improve protection of all the myocardium during aortic clamping. If this is accomplished, then perhaps it will be reflected in a decreased incidence of supraventricular arrhythmias.

Hypertension occurs during the first 3 hours after CABG in 30–60% of patients. It is often treated with nitroprusside. Although therapy will reduce afterload and preload, coronary perfusion pressure is also reduced and may result in myocardial metabolic derangements. Fremes and colleagues[180] from Toronto, Canada, investigated 31 patients undergoing elective CABG. Each had a hypertensive episode with a mean arterial pressure equal to 119 ± 18 mmHg. Studies were done during nitroprusside therapy at a mean arterial pressure of 97 ± 11 and again at a mean arterial pressure of 80 ± 11 mmHg. Nitroprusside produced a significant (p < 0.05) decrease in LA pressure, LV end-diastolic volume index, stroke index, and stroke-work index. Cardiac lactate extraction and the ratio of lactate extraction to stroke-work index increased (p < 0.05) with the initial nitroprusside therapy, but lactate production resulted when the mean arterial pressure was lowered to 80 mmHg. Volume loading studies were then performed during hypertension in 4 patients and during nitroprusside therapy in 15 patients. Neither performance nor compliance was significantly altered at a mean arterial pressure of 9 mmHg, but compliance decreased at normotension (80 mmHg). Coronary sinus blood flow was not significantly altered with nitroprusside therapy. At mean arterial BP equal to 80, there was a significant decrease in lactate extraction to net lactate production along with a decrease in cardiac index. The authors concluded that hypertension and its treatment can result in inadequate myocardial metabolism. They suggest that nitroprusside should be titrated to maintain mean arterial pressure between 90 and 100 mmHg.

Chaitman and members[181] of participating Coronary Artery Surgery Study (CASS) medical centers followed 1,340 patients who underwent CABG in 1978 at 10 hospitals. The incidence of perioperative Q-wave AMI was 4.6% (range, 0.0–10.3% by hospital). The rate of AMI was higher in patients who had increased LV end-diastolic pressure or cardiomegaly on the preoperative chest radiograph. Patients who receive more grafts or who had longer cardiopulmonary bypass time also were at higher risk of AMI. Long-term survival was adversely affected by the appearance of new postoperative Q waves. The hospital mortality was 10% in the 62 patients who had new postoperative Q waves and 1% in the 1,278 patients who did not (p < 0.001); the 3-year cumulative survival rates were 85 and 95%, respectively (p < 0.001). However, in patients who survived to hospital discharge the presence of new postoperative Q waves did not adversely affect the 3-year survival (94 and 96%, respectively). The survival rates were worse in patients who had a preoperative history of AMI or who had impaired LV function preoperatively. The number of hospital readmissions after CABG among the patients who had transmural perioperative AMI was similar to that among patients who did not. The major impact of new Q waves after CABG on mortality occurred before hospital discharge. Patients who were destined to have perioperative AMI could not be predicted from commonly measured preoperative and angiographic variables.

Val and colleagues[182] from Montreal, Canada, evaluated 112 patients undergoing isolated CABG with total creatine kinase MB, electrocardiogram, and pyrophosphate myocardial scan. Of the 112 patients, 81 had all tests negative. A diagnosis of perioperative AMI was established if 2 of the 3 techniques were positive, and that diagnosis was made in 15 patients. The most important predictive factor for AMI was the duration of myocardial

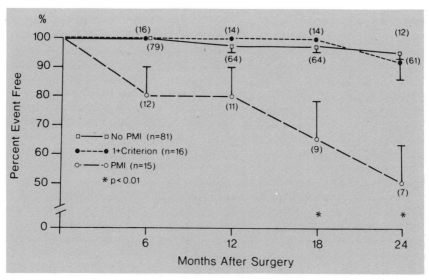

Fig. 1-20. Actuarial probability of remaining free of new coronary events following coronary bypass. Significant difference is presented at 18 and 24 months. Numbers in *parentheses* indicate patients at risk in each group at beginning of intervals. PMI = perioperative myocardial infarction; *vertical bars* indicate standard deviation. Reproduced with permission from Val et al.[182]

ischemia during operation. Patients who had an AMI had more frequent early complications and their prognosis at 2 years showed a 51% probability of remaining free of new cardiac events compared with 96% for the group of patients without an AMI early postoperatively (p < 0.001) (Fig. 1-20). An AMI is not a benign complication of CABG, and its detection appears to be improved by a combination of diagnostic tests. Other factors predictive of perioperative AMI were LM CAD and proximal right CAD, duration of cardiopulmonary bypass, duration of anesthesia, and number of grafts per patient.

Kuan and associates[183] from Long Beach and Irvine, California, described 3 patients with transient central diabetes insipidus after cardiopulmonary bypass. All 3 patients responded promptly to administration of vasopressin and were completely recovered from polyuria 10 days after cardiac surgery. It is postulated that transient diabetes insipidus after cardiac operation occurred in some patients who had preexisting selective osmoreceptor dysfunction when cardiac standstill during extracorporeal circulation alters the LA nonosmotic receptor function, resulting in suppression of antidiuretic hormone release.

Ascending aortic dissection is a rare but often catastrophic complication of cardiac surgical procedures. Murphy and colleagues[184] from Atlanta, Georgia, retrospectively analyzed the hospital records of 24 patients who developed ascending aortic dissection during or following 6,943 cardiac surgical procedures. Fifteen patients had their dissection recognized intraoperatively during CABG. Nine patients, 7 of whom had CABG and 2 of whom had aortic valve replacement, developed dissection 30 minutes to 21 days after cardiac operation. Only 4 patients had poorly controlled systemic hypertension postoperatively. The mortality in the first group was 33% and the overall mortality in the second group was 78%; the major factor in this high mortality, was a delay in diagnosis and surgical treatment. The authors suggest that early diagnosis of the intraoperative or postoperative dissection process is essential to minimize the extent of dissection and prevent delay of definitive surgical therapy. Closed aortic plication of the intimal injury rather than more extensive aortic repair may reduce the morbidity and mortality in selected patients. The authors found that most of the dissections were due to misadventures associated with aortic cannulation and with application of either total occlusion or partial exclusion vascular clamps. Other sites of the dissection occurred less frequently and these included the cardioplegia infusion site and the area of a proximal saphenous vein anastomosis. The authors have raised an important point relating to an operation that is usually associated with a 1% mortality. It has been suggested that prevention of this complication might be appropriately addressed by using less proximal anastomoses and more sequential vein grafts, a single period of aortic clamping for both proximal and distal grafts, and femoral cannulation when the ascending aorta appears diseased.

Saffitz and associates[185] from Bethesda, Maryland, reported 4 patients who had large false aneurysms of the ascending aorta after CABG. The principle illustrated by each of their 4 patients was that an incision into the wall of the ascending aorta for any purpose potentially sets the stage for the aorta to form a medial dissection and/or a false aneurysm at or near the site of initial entrance into the aorta. The incision into the aorta may be an aortotomy or AVR, a cannulation site for cardiopulmonary bypass, or an incision for insertion of a conduit between aorta and coronary artery. These incisions, if not perfectly closed, can allow leakage of blood into the adjacent wall. The resulting dissecting hematoma may progressively enlarge and produce a false aneurysm. The appearance on the chest roentgenogram of a dilated aorta after any open heart operation that includes an incision into the aorta or the insertion of an instrument into the aorta suggests that a dissection or false aneurysm has occurred, and it has the potential to rupture.

Brower and associates[186] from Rotterdam, The Netherlands, studied 221 patients angiographically 1 and 3 years after CABG. The extent of CAD was scored according to the recommendations of the American Heart Association and quantified by the method of Leaman. Patency in 570 grafts at 1 year was 80% and at 3 years, 77%. Of the conduits, 84% had no change from 1–3 years, 11% had more narrowing, and 5% had less narrowing. The authors concluded that most grafts that occlude do so in the first year after CABG. (Of course, however, the authors only studied the patients 1 additional time and that was at 3 years.) The coronary score before CABG was 14 ± 2 and dropped to 5 ± 1 at 1 year when corrected for patent grafts. The coronary score remained >0 because of early graft closure and/or untreated narrowings. By 3 years, the corrected coronary score increased to 7.2 ± 1.1 primarily because of the progression of narrowing in the native coronary arteries. Two subgroups, formed on the basis of angina pectoris at 3 years, showed that progression of disease in the native arteries was identical, but that return of angina was highly correlated with whether or not this narrowing occurred in segments perfused by patent grafts. Those factors known to be risk factors for CAD did not appear to have a bearing on progression or regression of narrowing in the graft, nor did the extent of CAD at the time of CABG correlate with eventual graft patency.

TABLE 1-11. *Serum lipids and graft atherosclerosis.*[A] *Reproduced with permission from Campeau et al.*[187]

	PATIENTS WITHOUT ATHEROSCLEROSIS (N = 26)	PATIENTS WITH ATHEROSCLEROSIS (N = 39)
Total cholesterol	244 ± 37	280 ± 57
HDL[B]	60 ± 19	47 ± 12
LDL[B]	163 ± 37	206 ± 52
LDL-β[B]	108 ± 15	162 ± 28
Triglycerides	157 ± 58	208 ± 125

HDL = high-density lipoprotein; LDL = low-density lipoprotein; LDL-β = low-density β-lipoprotein.
[A] Seventeen patients with late occlusion of grafts without previously documented atherosclerosis were excluded. Methods previously described.
[B] $p < .05$.

It has been generally recognized that saphenous vein graft closure is infrequent after the first year and up to 5–7 years after CABG. Graft closure during the first weeks and also during the first year after operation has been found to be related to poor distal runoff and to inadequate surgical techniques. Average yearly attrition rates between 1 and 5 years vary between 0.4 and 3.2%. Campeau and colleagues[187] from Montreal, Canada, studied 82 unselected patients at 2 weeks, 1 year, 5–7 years, and 10–12 years after CABG. The average yearly attrition rate increased 2.5-fold between 7 and 12 years compared with that of the previous 5 years. The authors attributed that late attrition to the development of atherosclerosis. These late changes in the saphenous vein grafts were not related to classic risk factors except for the presence of LDL and low density beta lipoprotein cholesterol (Table 1-11). The mean yearly attrition rate augmented from 2–5.3%/year. The graft patency was superior in multiple grafts compared with single grafts when analyzed at 10–12 years, but the incidence of atherosclerosis in patent grafts was the same (Table 1-12). Total graft patency in this group of patients was 63% at 10–12 years. This study identifies again inadequacies of surgical technique and poor distal runoff as predominant causes of graft occlusion during the first year. It also identifies the development of atherosclerosis as

TABLE 1-12. *Fate of grafts related to type of distal anastomosis. Reproduced with permission from Campeau et al.*[187]

TYPE OF GRAFTS	PATENT AT 1 YR	UNCHANGED N	UNCHANGED %	OCCLUDED AT 10–12 YR N	OCCLUDED AT 10–12 YR %	ATHEROSCLEROSIS IN PATENT GRAFTS N	ATHEROSCLEROSIS IN PATENT GRAFTS %
Single	70	24	34.3	25	35.7	21	30
Multiple	62	26	39.4	14	21.2	22	33.3
p value		NS		$p < .05$		NS	

the apparent cause of late closure when patients are followed for up to 12 years. The atherosclerosis seems to be related to serum lipids.

To determine the value of nondynamic computed tomography (CT) in assessing CABG patency, Daniel and coinvestigators[188] in Hanover, West Germany, studied 67 patients with 125 grafts by CT and by coronary angiography at close time intervals. The CT scans were performed before and after 1–3 intravenous bolus injections of contrast material. Of 92 grafts patent at angiography, 84 were also visualized by CT; 29 of 33 grafts closed at angiography were considered to be occluded by CT. Of 13 grafts demonstrated 11 had ≥1 severe obstruction at angiography and were considered to be patent by CT. Interobserver disagreement existed in 4 of 125 grafts and interobserver variability was 1.6%. Although nondynamic CT allows a correct assessment of graft patency in many cases, it does not provide sufficient information on graft stenosis and function to replace angiography in patients who are symptomatic after surgery.

PERCUTANEOUS TRANSLUMINAL CORONARY ANGIOPLASTY

In stable and unstable angina pectoris

In an investigation by Meyer and associates[189] from Aachen, West Germany, PTCA was performed in 50 patients with stable and in 50 patients with unstable angina pectoris, each patient showing an isolated stenosis >80% of the luminal diameter of a single coronary artery. The technical success rate was 66% in the stable group (26 of 37 patients, 70%, with LAD; 7 of 12 patients, 58%, with right) and 74% in the unstable group (27 of 34 patients, 79%, with LAD; 10 of 15 patients, 67%, with right). The increase in stenotic area in the unstable group exceeded that in the stable group for LAD stenoses (42 ± 15% -vs- 32 ± 15%; p < 0.03), whereas in right stenoses the results in the stable group were better (45 ± 18% -vs- 33 ± 12%; p, NS). One acute artery occlusion necessitating an emergency CABG occurred in each group (2%). The patient in the stable group died (total mortality rate, 1%). Sixty-three of the successfully treated patients were routinely restudied 6 months later. According to clinical symptoms, 23% of the stable and 36% of the unstable group were in functional classes III and IV. From an anatomic viewpoint, a restenosis (>85%) luminal diameter narrowing was found in 17% of the stable and in 24% of the unstable group. A further spontaneous decrease (>10%) of the artery obstruction was found in 47% of the stable group and in 12% of the unstable group. The results show that PTCA can be carried out with equally low risks and comparable satisfactory early and late results, both in patients with stable and with unstable angina.

Effect of length or eccentricity on results

In 526 patients undergoing a first PTCA of a single native coronary artery, Meier and coworkers[190] from Atlanta, Georgia, studied the influence of length and eccentricity of the lesion on complications and primary success. Stenoses >5 mm did not differ from stenosis <4 mm in terms of overall complications or gain in lumen diameter and distal pressure. Eccentric stenosis showed a lower rate of primary success than concentric stenoses (80 -vs- 89%). Inability to cross the stenosis was the main reason for failure. Stenoses that were long and eccentric had the highest frequency of complication (24%) and stenoses that were short and concentric, the lowest (12%). The average outcome expressed by gain in lumen diameter and distal pressure was equal in both groups and was more dependent on technical factors than on anatomy.

In arteries narrowed <60% in diameter

Ischinger and coinvestigators[191] from Atlanta, Georgia, evaluated all patients receiving PTCA in the past year for mild stenosis (≤60% diameter narrowing in 64 patients, group 1) and compared them with 66 patients with >60% stenosis (group 2) treated during the same year. The degree of CAD before PTCA was 52% in group 1 and 79% in group 2. The primary success rate was 90% in group 1 -vs- 86% in group 2. The frequency of complications requiring CABG after PTCA failed was similar in both groups, but there were 4 occurrences of AMI in group 1 and none in group 2. Recurrence of stenosis was judged on the basis of objective data, 76% of which were angiographic data, in 97% of the patients with primary success. At a mean interval of 5 months, with a mean follow-up period of 7 months, 17 of 58 patients with primary success in group 1 and 24 of 57 patients in group 2 developed restenosis. In group 1, restenosis was markedly more severe than initial stenosis, which was not the case in group 2. In conclusion, PTCA in mild stenosis has favorable primary and long-term results, yet carries the risk of AMI and emergency CABG and may, in some cases, even accelerate the disease process.

Effect on exercise performance

In their first 169 consecutive patients having CABG, Meier and coworkers[192] from Atlanta, Georgia, scheduled serial bicycle ergometric exercise sessions to assess long-term exercise performance. In 160 of these 169 patients an average of 7 ergometric measurements were available during a mean follow-up period of 29 months. One group consisted of 132 patients in whom PTCA was successful and the other group consisted of 28 patients with failure of PTCA who subsequently underwent CABG either on an emergency basis (12 patients) or as an elective procedure (16 patients). Exercise performance was expressed as work capacity in watts according to the highest completed exercise stage. In the successful PTCA group, the actual work capacities increased from 74 before PTCA to 122 watts at the most recent follow-up examination. In patients who underwent emergency or elective CABG the respective figures were 73 and 65 watts before CABG and 120 and 119 watts at the most recent follow-up examination. Successful PTCA and CABG after failed PTCA improved work capacity significantly. Comparison of the PTCA results with surgical studies indicates that a failed attempt at PTCA before CABG does not compromise the functional outcome of the operation, regardless of whether it is done on an emergency or on an elective basis.

Intraaortic balloon counterpulsation

In a study carried out by Alcan and colleagues[193] from New York City over a 3-year period, 14 patients required intraaortic balloon counterpulsation (IABP) in conjunction with PTCA. The indications for IABP in the perform- ance of PTCA were: 1) clinically unstable situations in which PTCA might otherwise be contraindicated (LM narrowing, multivessel CAD, unstable anginal syndromes, and cardiogenic shock); 2) preoperative insertion of IABP for added safety following unsuccessful angioplasty; 3) abrupt artery closure during PTCA in which the patient becomes hemodynamically unstable; and 4) late artery closure following initially successful angioplasty resulting in hemodynamic compromise. Of the 14 cases requiring IABP, 13 survived hospitalization and were alive at the time of the present report. Thus, IABP is a useful adjunct to PTCA in a variety of clinical circumstances.

After previous aortocoronary bypass grafting

Douglas and associates[194] from Atlanta, Georgia, determined the efficacy of PTCA in 116 patients after disabling angina pectoris 27 months after CABG: 88% had marked angiographic improvement (>30% reduction in diameter) in 122 initial procedures and in all 7 repetitions. Mean coronary stenosis was reduced from 78 ± 13% (mean ± SD) to 25 ± 13% and mean pressure gradient from 49 ± 15–11 ± 8 mmHg (p < 0.001). Complications in these patients included: 1) emergency CABG in 3 patients; 2) AMI as evident from Q-wave development in 1 patient and only by enzyme elevations in 4 patients; and 3) nonoccluding coronary dissection in 1 patient. One late death occurred 14 months after an unsuccessful but uncomplicated PTCA. Eight months later, 76% of patients were without angina or in improved condition. Thus, when the coronary anatomy is suitable, PTCA is an alternative to reoperation in symptomatic patients with prior CABG.

Effect on employment and recreation

Holmes and associates[195] from Rochester, Minnesota, Bethesda, Mary- land, Richmond, Virginia, Milwaukee, Wisconsin, and Atlanta, Georgia, analyzed employment and recreational patterns in 279 patients who under- went PTCA for symptomatic CAD. The PTCA was successful in 180 patients (65%). When it was unsuccessful, CABG was usually performed (80%). Return to work rates were high irrespective of the outcome of PTCA. Of patients employed full or part time before treatment, 98.5% of those who had successful PTCA alone and 97% of those whose PTCA was unsuccessful but who underwent uncomplicated CABG maintained or improved their work status. In a subgroup of men who had been employed in occupations requiring physical labor, 85% whose PTCA was successful returned to work, compared with 68% of those whose PTCA was unsuccessful. The interval from attempted PTCA to return to work was significantly shorter in the successfully treated group; in patients with successful PTCA, the median time to return to work was 14 days, compared with 60 days in patients in whom PTCA was unsuccessful (p < 0.001). During follow-up, patients with successful PTCA had less angina and were more active in recreational activities than patients who required alternative treatments.

Complications (NHLBI PTCA Registry)

Complications in the first 1,500 patients enrolled in the National Heart, Lung, and Blood Institute PTCA Registry were analyzed by Dorros and participating investigators[196] from Milwaukee, Wisconsin. Data were contributed from 73 centers between September 1977 and April 1981. PTCA was successful in 63% of attempts: 543 in-hospital complications occurred in 314 patients (21%). The most frequent complications were prolonged angina in 121, AMI in 72, and coronary occlusion in 70; 138 patients (9%) had major complications (AMI, emergency CABG or in-hospital death); 102 patients (7%) required emergency CABG, usually for coronary dissection or coronary occlusion; 16 patients (1%) died in the hospital. The mortality rate was 0.85% in patients with 1-vessel CAD and 1.9% in those with multivessel CAD. Mortality rate was significantly higher in patients who had had CABG. Nonfatal complications were significantly influenced by the presence of unstable angina and initial narrowing >90% in diameter. These results support the relative safety of PTCA.

Spasm after PTCA

Hollman and associates[197] from Atlanta, Georgia, described 5 patients who developed coronary arterial spasm at the site of previous successful PTCA. These patients developed coronary arterial spasm on hemodynamically insignificant (<50% diameter narrowing) intrinsic CAD. Four patients did not respond to therapy with slow channel calcium blockers and nitrates, and subsequently developed recurrent CAD. One patient died 2 months after CABG. Thus, coronary arterial spasm may occur during the healing period after PTCA and recurrent symptoms should be considered as possibly being due to coronary arterial spasm rather than recurrent, fixed obstruction.

Bentivoglio and associates[198] from Philadelphia, Pennsylvania, discovered coronary spasm superimposed on fixed CAD in 14 of 74 candidates for PTCA. In 3 of the 14, spasm developed during PTCA and was presumably catheter induced. Eleven of the 14 with unprovoked spasm were the subject of this study. Three of the 11, in whom the fixed component of the mixed stenosis was subcritical, were treated medically, with good results in 2 but with persistent angina pectoris and eventual AMI in 1. Nitroglycerin administered by the intracoronary route relieved spasm resistant to sublingual nitroglycerin in 1 of the 3. In 8 of the 11 with critical fixed CAD, spasm was discovered either before PTCA (7 patients) or on follow-up (1 patient). Six of the 8 had successful PTCA, with no or mild symptoms on follow-up. Of the 2 failures, 1, uncomplicated, was followed by successful elective CABG, and the other, complicated, led to successful emergency CABG, with disappearance of symptoms in both. The rate of success was similar in patients with documented unprovoked spasm (6 of 8) and patients without (39 of 63, 62%). Thus, 1) coronary spasm, if properly sought for, is probably common in 1-vessel candidates for PTCA; 2) patients considered candidates for PTCA should have intracoronary nitroglycerin administered before PTCA; 3) in patients with critical, fixed CAD, associated spasm does not reduce the chances of successful PTCA; 4) coronary spasm may outlast the relief by PTCA of the fixed component of the mixed stenosis and requires long-term vasodilator therapy; and 5) the lack of adverse effects when PTCA is performed in patients with spasm superimposed on critical fixed 1-vessel CAD appears to justify its use.

Between July 1980 and November 1982, 935 coronary angioplasties were performed by Hollman and coworkers[199] from Atlanta, Georgia. Of these patients, 20 developed acute occlusion, 19 of whom presented within 3 hours of surgery or within 3 hours after stopping a continuous heparin infusion. Five had emergency CABG, but in 15 nitrates, nifedipine, and/or repeat PTCA reopened the artery and the patient could be stabilized on continuous infusions of heparin and nitroglycerin. In only 1 case was an occluding thrombus evident by angiography. The mechanism of acute occlusion remains unknown, but coronary artery spasm may play a role.

In completely occluded artery

In 47 consecutive patients referred for coronary angioplasty, Dervan and coworkers[200] from Boston, Massachusetts, attempted the procedure in 13 patients despite occlusion of the involved artery. This included 4 patients with total occlusion and 9 with "functional" coronary occlusion (faint, late antegrade opacification in the absence of a discernible luminal continuity). All procedures were performed with an angioplasty system in which the leading guide wire could be moved independently of the dilation catheter. Primary success was obtained in 54% of patients with coronary occlusion compared with 85% in the remaining patients with stenoses between 75 and 95%. In patients with coronary occlusion, the mean residual stenosis after angioplasty (41%), the abrupt reclosure rate (8%), and the frequency of angiographically evident dissection (29%) were similar to those seen in 34 patients who underwent angioplasty of conventional stenoses, although restenoses tended to be more common (43 -vs- 23%) in patients with coronary occlusion. No evidence of coronary perforation or distal emboliza- tion was found in either group, and no patient undergoing angioplasty of an occluded vessel required emergency CABG, despite 1 case of abrupt reclo- sure. All patients with coronary occlusion had prominent collateral flow to the occluded artery, which could no longer be visualized after successful PTCA. The collaterals were associated with a higher distal pressure (35 mmHg) in patients with coronary occlusion than that seen in patients with less severe stenoses and no visible collaterals (distal occluded pressure, 20 mmHg). Although the primary success rate was lower than that associated with nontotal lesions, PTCA can be performed safely and successfully in most patients with coronary occlusion.

Aneurysm formation

Little information is available regarding coronary artery remodeling over time as a result of this "controlled" injury. Aneurysms at sites of PTCA have not previously been described until the report by Hill and associates[201] from Gainesville, Florida, who described 5 men who developed coronary arterial aneurysms at sites of PTCA. All patients were in New York Heart Association functional class III or IV at the time of PTCA. In 2 patients AMI was evolving and both had acute coronary occlusion. The other 3 patients had angiograph- ic evidence of intimal disruption or acute coronary reocclusion as a result of PTCA, 1 of whom had undergone emergency CABG. Three patients received intracoronary streptokinase during PTCA. One patient was asymptomatic and 4 were symptomatic when the aneurysms were identified between 11 days and 4 months after PTCA. Other than the complex course and anatomy of the patients before and immediately after PTCA, no other features distinguished them from others undergoing this procedure.

Necropsy findings late

Several studies have described morphologic changes early (<60 days) in coronary arteries in the human and in nonhuman animals after PTCA. Morphologic observations have not been reported in coronary arteries in patients subjected to PTCA >60 days before death. Waller and associates[202] from Bethesda, Maryland, described certain clinical and necropsy cardiac findings in 3 men who had PTCA of the LAD coronary artery 80, 90, and 150 days, respectively, before sudden death. Each patient had a decrease in the mean transstenotic coronary gradient (17, 38, and 43 mmHg) and an angiographic increase in the LAD luminal diameter (55, 60, and 65%). At necropsy, the LAD coronary artery in the area of the PTCA in each patient was narrowed 76–95% in cross-sectional area by atherosclerotic plaques. No cracks in plaques or other lesions that may have resulted from the PTCA procedure were identified histologically in the LAD coronary artery of any patient.

Fig. 1-21. Age–adjusted death rates (per 100,000) for CAD in the population 30–74 years old. Twin Cities denotes the Minneapolis—St. Paul metropolitan area. Rates for the United States for 1979 and 1980 were not available. Disease classified according to ICDA codes 410–413; discontinuity between 1978 and 1979 is due to change from the eighth to the ninth revision of ICDA. Reproduced with permission from Gillum et al.[203]

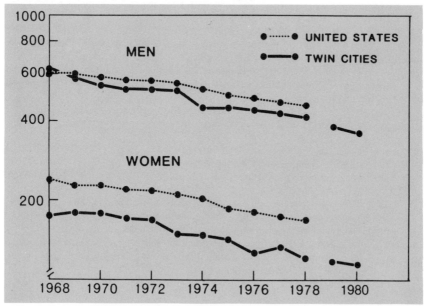

DECLINING CAD DEATH RATES

To determine the causes of the nationwide decline in deaths due to CAD, Gillum and associates[203] from Minneapolis, Minnesota, enumerated cardiac deaths among persons 30–74 years old in Minneapolis-St. Paul. The survey also ascertained rates of hospitalization and case fatality during hospitalization for AMI. For deaths occurring between 1970 and 1978 that were due to CAD, the rates outside the hospital declined by 43% in men and 40% in women, and the rates in hospital emergency rooms increased by 311% in men and 200% in women (Fig. 1–21). In both these years about two-thirds of all such deaths occurred outside hospital wards. Between 1970 and 1980, hospitalization rates for AMI in persons 30–74 years old declined 8% among men and 26% among women, and case fatality in the hospital in persons 45–74 years old declined 29% in men and 27% in women. These changes are probably due to the combined influence of changes in risk factors in the population and improved care of patients with AMI before and during hospitalization.

References

1. HLATKY MA, LEE KL, BOTVINICK EH, BRUNDAGE BH: Diagnostic test use in different practice settings: a controlled comparison. Arch Intern Med 143:1886–1889, Oct 1983.

2. PRYOR DB, HARRELL FE, LEE KL, CALIFF RM, ROSATI RA: Estimating the likelihood of significant coronary artery disease. Am J Med 75:771–780, Nov 1983.

3. DePACE NL, HAKKI A, WEINRICH DJ, ISKANDRIAN AS: Noninvasive assessment of coronary artery disease. Am J Cardiol 52:714–720, Oct 1983.

4. KANNEL WB, HUBERT H, LEW EA: Vital capacity as a predictor of cardiovascular disease: the Framingham Study. Am Heart J 105:311–315, Feb 1983.

5. WASSERMAN AG, REISS L, KATZ RJ, LEIBOFF R, CLEARY P, VARMA VM, REBA RC, ROSS AM: Insensitivity of the cold pressor stimulation test for the diagnosis of coronary artery disease. Circulation 67:1189–1193, June 1983.

6. AHMADPOUR H, SHAH AA, ALLEN JW, EDMISTON WA, KIM SJ, HAYWOOD LJ: Mitral E point septal separation: a reliable index of left ventricular performance in coronary artery disease. Am Heart J 106:21–28, July 1983.

7. FAMULARO MA, PALIWAL Y, REDD R, ELLESTAD MH: Identification of septal ischemia during exercise by Q-wave analysis: correlation with coronary angiography. Am J Cardiol 51:440–443, Feb 1983.

8. BORAN KJ, OLIVEROS RA, BOUCHER CA, BECKMANN CH, SEAWORTH JF: Ischemia–associated intraventricular conduction disturbances during exercise testing as a predictor of proximal left anterior descending coronary artery disease. Am J Cardiol 51:1098–1102, Apr 1983.

9. COLBY J, HAKKI AH, ISKANDRIAN AS, MATTLEMAN S: Hemodynamic, angiographic and scintigraphic correlates of positive exercise electrocardiograms: emphasis on strongly positive exercise electrocardiograms. J Am Coll Cardiol 2:21–29, July 1983.

10. CURRIE PJ, KELLY MJ, PITT A: Comparison of supine and erect bicycle exercise electrocardiography in coronary heart disease: accentuation of exercise-induced ischemic ST depression by supine posture. Am J Cardiol 52:1167–1173, Dec 1983.

11. CALIFF RM, McKINNIS RA, McNEER JF, HARRELL FE, LEE KL, PRYOR DB, WAUGH RA, HARRIS PJ, ROSATI RA, WAGNER GS: Prognostic value of ventricular arrhythmias associated with

treadmill exercise testing in patients with cardiac catheterization for suspected ischemic heart disease. J Am Coll Cardiol 2:1060–1067, Dec 1983.

12. NEWMAN HN, DUNN RF, HARRIS PJ, BAUTOVICH GJ, MCLAUGHLIN AF, KELLY DT: Differentiation between right and circumflex coronary artery disease on thallium myocardial perfusion scanning. Am J Cardiol 51:1052–1056, Apr 1983.

13. OKADA RD, LIM YL, ROTHENDLER J, BOUCHER CA, BLOCK PC, POHOST GM: Split dose thallium–201 dipyridamole imaging: a new technique for obtaining thallium images before and immediately after an intervention. J Am Coll Cardiol 1:1302–1310, May 1983.

14. ROZANSKI A, DIAMOND GA, BERMAN D, FORRESTER JS, MORRIS D, SWAN HJC: The declining specificity of exercise radionuclide ventriculography. N Engl J Med 309:518–522, Sept 1, 1983.

15. BODENHEIMER MM, BANKA VS, AGARWAL JB, WEINTRAUB WS, HELFANT RH: Relative value of isotonic and isometric exercise radionuclide angiography to detect coronary heart disease. J Am Coll Cardiol 1:790–796, March 1983.

16. BROWN KA, OKADA RD, BOUCHER CA, ROTHENDLER JA, STRAUSS HW, POHOST GM: Exercise-induced changes in hepatic blood volume measured during routine cardiac equilibrium cineangiography: relation to coronary anatomy and right ventricular function. J Am Coll Cardiol 2:514–521, Sept 1983.

17. DEPACE NL, ISKANDRIAN AS, HAKKI AH, KANE SA, SEGAL BL: Value of left ventricular ejection fraction during exercise in predicting the extent of coronary artery disease. J Am Coll Cardiol 1:1002–1010, Apr 1983.

18. GEWIRTZ H, PALADINO W, SULLIVAN M, MOST AS: Value and limitations of myocardial thallium washout rate in the noninvasive diagnosis of patients with triple-vessel coronary artery disease. Am Heart J 106:681–686, Oct 1983.

19. GUTMAN J, BERMAN DS, FREEMAN M, ROZANSKI A, MADDAHI J, WAXMAN A, SWAN HJC: Time to completed redistribution of thallium–201 in exercise myocardial scintigraphy: relationship to the degree of coronary artery stenosis. Am Heart J 106:989–995, Nov 1983.

20. ISKANDRIAN AS, HAKKI A-H, SEGAL BL, KANE SA, AMENTA A: Assessment of the myocardial perfusion pattern in patients with multivessel coronary artery disease. Am Heart J 106:1089–1096, Nov 1983.

21. OSBAKKEN MD, BOUCHER CA, OKADA RD, BINGHAM JB, STRAUSS HW, POHOST GM: Spectrum of global left ventricular responses to supine exercise: limitation in the use of ejection fraction in identifying patients with coronary artery disease. Am J Cardiol 51:28–35, Jan 1983.

22. LINDSAY J JR, NOLAN NG, GOLDSTEIN SA, BACOS JM: Effects of beta–adrenergic blocking drugs on sensitivity and specificity of radionuclide ventriculography during exercise in patients with coronary heart disease. Am Heart J 106:271–278, Aug 1983.

23. CURRIE PJ, KELLY MJ, HARPER RW, FEDERMAN J, KALFF V, ANDERSON ST, PITT A: Incremental value of clinical assessment, supine exercise electrocardiography, and biplane exercise radionuclide ventriculography in the prediction of coronary artery disease in men with chest pain. Am J Cardiol 52:927–935, Nov 1983.

24. WACKERS FJ, STEIN R, PYTLIK L, PLANKEY MW, LANGE R, HOFFER PB, SANDS MJ, ZARET BL, BERGER HJ: Gold–195m for serial first pass radionuclide angiocardiography during upright exercise in patients with coronary artery disease. J Am Coll Cardiol 2:497–505, Sept 1983.

25. SWAYE PS, FISHER LD, LITWIN P, VIGNOLA PA, JUDKINS MP, KEMP HG, MUDD JG, GOSSELIN AJ: Aneurysmal coronary artery disease. Circulation 67:134–138, Jan 1983.

26. GOLDBERG HL, GOLDSTEIN J, BORER JS, COLLINS MB, MOSES JW, ELLIS G: Determination of the angiographic appearance of coronary collateral vessels: the importance of supplying and recipient arteries. Am J Cardiol 51:434–439, Feb 1983.

27. SPINDOLA-FRANCO H, GROSE R, SOLOMON N: Dual left anterior descending coronary artery: angiographic description of important variants and surgical implications. Am Heart J 105:445–455, March 1983.

28. CARROLL JD, HESS OM, HIRZEL HO, KRAYENBUEHL HP: Exercised-induced ischemia: the influence of altered relaxation on early diastolic pressures: Circulation 67:521–528, March 1983.

29. BATEMAN TM, GRAY RJ, RAYMOND MJ, MIYAMOTO AT, CHAUX A, KASS RM, LEE ME, STEWART ME,

MATLOFF JM: Coronary artery stenoses: relationship between angiographic severity and impact on mean diastolic pressure gradient. J Thorac Cardiovasc Surg 85:499–507, Apr 1983.

30. CARROLL JD, HESS OM, HIRZEL HO, KRAYENBUEHL HP: Dynamics of left ventricular filling at rest and during exercise. Circulation 68:59–67, July 1983.

31. CAMERON A, KEMP HG JR, FISHER LD, GOSSELIN A, JUDKINS MP, KENNEDY JW, LESPERANCE J, MUDD JG, RYAN TJ, SILVERMAN JF, TRISTANI F, VLIETSTRA RE, WEXLER LF: Left main coronary artery stenosis: angiographic determination. Circulation 68:484–489, Sept 1983.

32. ERIKSSEN J, DALE J, ROOTWELT K, MYHRE E: False suspicion of coronary heart disease: a 7 year follow–up study of 36 apparently healthy middle–aged men. Circulation 68:490–497, Sept 1983.

33. LEIGHTON RF, NELSON AD, BREWSTER P: Subtle left ventricular asynergy with completely obstructed coronary arteries. Am J Cardiol 52:693–697, Oct 1983.

34. HALON DA, SAPOZNIKOV D, LEWIS BS, GOTSMAN MS: Localization of lesions in the coronary circulation. Am J Cardiol 52:921–926, Nov 1983.

35. GANZ P, HARRINGTON DP, GASPAR J, BARRY WH: Phasic pressure gradients across coronary and renal artery stenoses in humans. Am Heart J 106:1399–1406, Dec 1983.

36. TOBIS J, NALCIOGLU O, JOHNSTON WD, SEIBERT A, ISERI LT, ROECK W, HENRY WL: Digital angiography in assessment of ventricular function and wall motion during pacing in patients with coronary artery disease. Am J Cardiol 51:668–675, March 1983.

37. JOHNSON RA, WASSERMAN AG, LEIBOFF RH, KATZ RJ, BREN GB, VARGHESE PJ, ROSS AM: Intravenous digital left ventriculography at rest and with atrial pacing as a screening procedure for coronary artery disease. J Am Coll Cardiol 2:905–910, Nov 1983.

38. GOLDBERG HL, MOSES JW, BORER JS, FISHER J, TAMARI I, SKELLY NT, COHEN B: Exercise left ventriculography utilizing intravenous digital angiography. J Am Coll Cardiol 2:1092–1098, Dec 1983.

39. PRYOR DB, HARRELL FE, LEE KL, CALIFF RM, ROSATI RA: An improving prognosis over time in medically treated patients with coronary artery disease. Am J Cardiol 52:444–448, Sept 1983.

40. PROUDFIT WL, BRUSCHKE AVG, MACMILLAN JP, WILLIAMS GW, SONES FM JR: Fifteen year survival study of patients with coronary artery disease. Circulation 68:986–997, Nov 1983.

41. WEINER DA, MCCABE CH, RYAN TJ: Prognostic assessment of patients with coronary artery disease by exercise testing. Am Heart J 105:749–755, May 1983.

42. GOHLKE H, SAMEK L, BETZ P, ROSKAMM H: Exercise testing provides additional prognostic information in angiographically defined subgroups of patients with coronary artery disease. Circulation 68:979–985, Nov 1983.

43. HAMMERMEISTER KE, DEROUEN TA, DODGE HT, ZIA M: Prognostic and predictive value of exertional hypotension in suspected coronary heart disease. Am J Cardiol 51:1261–1266, May 1983.

44. CALIFF RM, TOMABECHI Y, LEE KL, PHILLIPS H, PRYOR DB, HARRELL FE, HARRIS PJ, PETER RH, BEHAR VS, KONG Y, ROSATI RA: Outcome in 1–vessel coronary artery disease. Circulation 67:283–290, Feb 1983.

45. HLATKY MA, CALIFF RM, KONG Y, HARRELL FE, ROSATI RA: Natural history of patients with single–vessel disease suitable for percutaneous transluminal coronary angioplasty. Am J Cardiol 52:225–229, Aug 1983.

46. CHAITMAN BR, DAVIS K, FISHER LD, BOURASSA MG, MOCK MB, LESPERANCE J, ROGERS WJ, FRAY D, TYRAS DH, JUDKINS MP, RINGQVIST I, KILLIP T, PARTICIPATING CASS HOSPITALS: A life table and Cox regression analysis of patients with combined proximal left anterior descending and proximal left circumflex coronary disease: non-left main equivalent lesions (CASS). Circulation 68:1163–1170, Dec 1983.

47. KRAMER JR, KITAZUME H, PROUDFIT WL, MATSUDA Y, GOORMASTIC M, WILLIAMS GW, SONES FM JR: Segmental analysis of the rate of progression in patients with progressive coronary atherosclerosis. Am Heart J 106:1427–1431, Dec 1983.

48. CASTELLI WP, ABBOTT RD, MCNAMARA PM: Summary estimates of cholesterol used to predict coronary heart disease. Circulation 67:730–734, Apr 1983.

49. Maciejko JJ, Holmes DR, Kottke BA, Zinsmeister AR, Dinh DM, Mao SJT: Apolipoprotein A–I as a marker of angiographically assessed coronary artery disease. N Engl J Med 309:385–389, Aug 18, 1983.

50. Thelle DS, Shaper AG, Whitehead TP, Bullock DG, Ashby D, Patel I: Blood lipids in middle–aged British men. Br Heart J 49:205–13, March 1983.

51. LaPorte RE, Brenes G, Dearwater S, Murphy MA, Cauley JA, Dietrick R, Robertson R: HDL cholesterol across a spectrum of physical activity from quadraplegia to marathon running. Lancet 1:1212–1213, May 28, 1983.

52. Morrison JA, Namboodiri K, Green P, Martin J, Glueck CJ: Familial aggregation of lipids and lipoproteins and early identification of dyslipoproteinemia. JAMA 250:1860–1868, Oct 14, 1983.

53. Rifkind BM, Segal P: Lipid research clinics program reference values for hyperlipidemia and hypolipidemia. JAMA 250:1869–1872, Oct 14, 1983.

54. Council on Scientific Affairs, Division of Scientific Analysis and Technology, American Medical Association: Dietary and pharmacologic therapy for the lipid risk factors. JAMA 250:1873–1879, Oct 14, 1983.

55. Mabuchi H, Sakai T, Sakai Y, Yoshimura A, Watanabe A, Wakasugi T, Koizumi J, Takeda R: Reduction of serum cholesterol in heterozygous patients with familial hypercholesterolemia: additive effects of compactin and cholestyramine. N Engl J Med 308:609–613, March 17, 1983.

56. Beppu S, Minura Y, Sakakibara H, Nagata S, Park YD, Nambu S, Yamamoto A: Supravalvular aortic stenosis and coronary ostial stenosis in familial hypercholesterolemia: 2–dimensional echocardiographic assessment. Circulation 67:878–884, Apr 1983.

57. Ribeiro P, Shapiro LM, Gonzalez A, Thompson GR, Oakley CM: Cross sectional echocardiographic assessment of the aortic root and coronary ostial stenosis in familial hypercholesterolaemia. Br Heart J 50:432–437, Nov 1983.

58. Brischetto CS, Connor WE, Connor SL, Matarazzo JD: Plasma lipid and lipoprotein profiles of cigarette smokers from randomly selected families: enhancement of hyperlipidemia and depression of high–density lipoprotein. Am J Cardiol 52:675–680, Oct 1983.

59. Willett W, Hennekens CH, Castelli W, Rosner B, Evans D, Taylor J, Kass EH: Effects of cigarette smoking on fasting triglyceride, total cholesterol, and HDL cholesterol in women. Am Heart J 105:417–421, March 1983.

60. Garrison RJ, Feinleib M, Castelli WP, McNamara PM: Cigarette smoking as a confounder of the relationship between relative weight and long–term mortality. JAMA 249:2199–2203, Apr 22/29, 1983.

61. Hickey N, Mulcahy R, Daly L, Graham I, O'Donoghue S, Kennedy C: Cigar and pipe smoking related to 4 year survival of coronary patients. Br Heart J 49:423–426, May 1983.

62. Kaufman DW, Helmrich SP, Rosenberg L, Miettinen OS, Shapiro S: Nicotine and carbon monoxide content of cigarette smoke and the risk of myocardial infarction in young men. N Engl J Med 308:409–413, Feb 24, 1983.

63. Klein LW, Pichard AD, Holt J, Smith H, Gorlin R, Teichholz LE: Effects of chronic tobacco smoking on the coronary circulation. J Am Coll Cardiol 1:421–426, Feb 1983.

64. Hubert HB, Feinleib M, McNamara PM, Castelli WP: Obesity as an independent risk factor for cardiovascular disease: a 26 year follow–up of participants in the Framingham heart study. Circulation 67:968–977, May 1983.

65. Khoury P, Morrison JA, Mellies MJ, Glueck CJ: Weight change since age 18 years in 30–55 year old whites and blacks: associations with lipid values, lipoprotein levels, and blood pressure. JAMA 250:3179–3187, Dec 16, 1983.

66. Gordon DJ, Witztum JL, Hunninghake D, Gates S, Glueck CJ: Habitual physical activity and high–density lipoprotein cholesterol in men with primary hypercholesterolemia: the Lipid Research Clinic's coronary primary prevention trial. Circulation 67:512–520, March 1983.

67. Heath GW, Ehsani AA, Hagberg JM, Hinderliter JM, Goldberg AP: Exercise training improves lipoprotein lipid profiles in patients with coronary artery disease. Am Heart J 105:889–895, June 1983.

68. GIBBONS LW, BLAIR SN, COOPER KH, SMITH M: Association between coronary heart disease risk factors and physical fitness in healthy adult women. Circulation 67:977–983, Apr 1983.

69. PETERS RK, CADY LD, BISCHOFF DP, BERNSTEIN L, PIKE MC: Physical fitness and subsequent myocardial infarction in healthy workers. JAMA 249:3052–3056, June 10, 1983.

70. THELLE DS, ARNESEN E, FORDE OH: The tromso heart study: does coffee raise serum cholesterol. N Engl J Med 308:1454–1457, June 16, 1983.

71. GOLDACRE MJ, HOLFORD TR, VESSEY MP: Cardiovascular disease and vasectomy: findings from 2 epidemiologic studies. N Engl J Med 308:805–808, Apr 7, 1983.

72. CARTER C, McGEE D, REED D, YANO K, STEMMERMANN G: Hematocrit and the risk of coronary heart disease: the Honolulu Heart Program. Am Heart J 105:674–679, Apr 1983.

73. GORDON TA, KANNEL WB: Drinking and its relation to smoking, BP, blood lipids, and uric acid. Arch Intern Med 143:1366–1374, July 1983.

74. HARTUNG GH, FOREYT JP, MITCHELL RE, MITCHELL JG, REEVES RS, GOTTO AM: Effect of alcohol intake on high-density lipoprotein cholesterol levels in runners and inactive men. JAMA 249:747–750, Feb 11, 1983.

75. GORDON T, KANNEL WB: Drinking habits and cardiovascular disease: the Framingham study. Am Heart J 105:667–673, Apr 1983.

76. THORNTON J, SYMES C, HEATON K: Moderate alcohol intake reduces bile cholesterol saturation and raises HDL cholesterol. Lancet 2:819–822, Oct 8, 1983.

77. GIAGNONI E, SECCHI MB, WU SC, MORABITO A, OLTRONA L, MANCARELLA S, VOLPIN N, FOSSA L, BETTAZZI L, ARANGIO G, SACHERO A, FOLLI G: Prognostic value of exercise ECG testing in asymptomatic normotensive subjects: a prospective matched study. N Engl J Med 309:1085–1089, Nov 3, 1983.

78. ROSE G, TUNSTALL-PEDOE HD, HELLER RF: UK heart disease prevention project: incidence and mortality results. Lancet 1:1062–1065, May 14, 1983.

79. KORNITZER M, DRAMAIX M, THILLY C, DEBACKER G, KITTEL F, GRAFFAR M, VUYLSTEEK: Belgian heart disease prevention project: incidence and mortality results. Lancet 1:1066–1072, May 14, 1983.

80. KIMM SYS, ORNSTEIN SM, DeLONG ER, GRUFFERMAN S: Secular trends in ischemic heart disease mortality: regional variation. Circulation 68:3–8, July 1983.

81. WARD DE, VALANTINE H, HUI W: Occluded left main stem coronary artery: report of 5 patients and review of published reports. Br Heart J 49:276–279, March 1983.

82. FIGUERAS J, CINCA J, GUTIERREZ L, SEGURA R, RIUS J: Prolonged angina pectoris and persistent negative T waves in the precordial leads: response to atrial pacing and to methoxamine-induced hypertension. Am J Cardiol 51:1599–1607, June 1983.

83. DEANFIELD JE, SELWYN AP, CHIERCHIA S, MASERI A, RIBEIRO P, KRIKLER S, MORGAN M: Myocardial ischaemia during daily life in patients with stable angina: its relation to symptoms and heart rate changes. Lancet 2:753–758, Oct 1, 1983.

84. DAVIES AB, SUBRAMANIAN VG, CASHMAN PMM, RAFTERY EB: Simultaneous recording of continuous arterial pressure, heart rate, and ST segment in ambulant patients with stable angina pectoris. Br Heart J 50:85–91, July 1983.

85. HAINES DE, RAABE DS, GUNDEL WD, WACKERS FJ: Anatomic and prognostic significance of new T wave inversion in unstable angina. Am J Cardiol 52:14–18, July 1983.

86. CRAWFORD MH, AMON KW, VANCE WS: Exercise 2–dimensional echocardiography: quantitation of left ventricular performance in patients with severe angina pectoris. Am J Cardiol 51:1–6, Jan 1983.

87. BODEN WE, BOUGH EW, BENHAM I, SHULMAN RS: Unstable angina with episodic ST segment elevation and minimal creatine kinase release culminating in extensive, recurrent infarction. J Am Coll Cardiol 2:11–20, July 1983.

88. MOISE A, THEROUX P, TAEYMANS Y, DESCOINGS B, LESPERANCE J, WATERS DD, PELLETIER GB, BOURASSA MG: Unstable angina and progression of coronary atherosclerosis. N Engl J Med 309:685–689, Sept 22, 1983.

89. FRICK MH, VALLE M, HARJOLA PT: Progression of coronary artery disease in randomized medical and surgical patients over a 5 year angiographic follow–up. Am J Cardiol 52:681–685, Oct 1983.

90. KIMCHI A, LEE G, AMSTERDAM E, FUJII K, KRIEG P, MASON DT: Increased exercise tolerance after nitroglycerin oral spray: a new and effective therapeutic modality in angina pectoris. Circulation 67:124–127, Jan 1983.

91. DEGRÉ SG, STRAPPART GM, SOBOLSKI JC, BERKENBOOM GM, STOUPEL EE, VANDERMOTEN PP: Effect of oral sustained release nitroglycerin on exercise capacity in angina pectoris: dose response relation and duration of action during double–blind crossover randomized acute therapy. Am J Cardiol 51:1595–1598, June 1983.

92. CURFMAN GD, JEINSIMER JA, LOZNER EC, FUNG HL: Intravenous nitroglycerin in the treatment of spontaneous angina pectoris: a prospective, randomized, trial. Circulation 67:276–282, Feb 1983.

93. KAPLAN K, DAVISON R, PARKER M, PRZYBYLEK J, TEAGARDEN JR, LESCH M: Intravenous nitroglycerin for the treatment of angina at rest unresponsive to standard nitrate therapy. Am J Cardiol 51:694–698, March 1983.

94. DALAL JJ, YAO L, PARKER JO: Nitrate tolerance: influence of isosorbide dinitrate on the hemodynamic and antianginal effects of nitroglycerin. J Am Coll Cardiol 2:115–120, July 1983.

95. PARKER JO, JUNG HL, RUGGIRELLO D, STONE JA: Tolerance to isosorbide dinitrate: rate of development and reversal. Circulation 68:1074–1080, Nov 1983.

96. FELDMAN RL, CONTI CR, PEPINE CJ: Comparison of coronary hemodynamic effects of nitroprusside and sublingual nitroglycerin with anterior descending coronary arterial occlusion. Am J Cardiol 52:915–920, Nov 1983.

97. BASSAN MM, WEILER-RAVELL D: Effect of a 12–hour hiatus in propranolol therapy on exercise tolerance in patients with angina pectoris. Am Heart J 105:234–239, Feb 1983.

98. MORRIS KG, HIGGINBOTHAM MB, COLEMAN RE, SHAND DG, COBB FR: Comparison of high dose and medium dose propranolol in the relief of exercise–induced myocardial ischemia. Am J Cardiol 52:7–13, June 1983.

99. KERN MJ, GANZ P, HOROWITZ JD, GASPAR J, BARRY WH, LORELL BH, GROSSMAN W, MUDGE GH JR: Potentiation of coronary vasoconstriction by beta–adrenergic blockage in patients with coronary artery disease. Circulation 67:1178–1185, June 1983.

100. PARKER JO: Comparison of slow release pindolol, standard pindolol, and propranolol in angina pectoris. Am J Cardiol 51:1062–1066, Apr 1983.

101. MANYARI DE, KOSTUK WJ, CARRUTHERS SG, JOHNSTON DJ, PURVES P: Pindolol and propranolol in patients with angina pectoris and normal or near normal ventricular function: lack of influence of intrinsic sympathomimetic activity on global and segmental left ventricular function assessed by radionuclide ventriculography. Am J Cardiol 51:427–433, Feb 1983.

102. PACOLD I, KLEINMAN B, GUNNAR R, LOEB HS: Effects of low dose dobutamine on coronary hemodynamics, myocardial metabolism, and anginal threshold in patients with coronary artery disease. Circulation 68:1044–1050, Nov 1983.

103. PEPINE CJ, FELDMAN RL, HILL JA, CONTI CR, MEHTA J, HILL C, SCOTT E: Clinical outcome after treatment of rest angina with calcium blockers: comparative experience during the initial year of therapy with diltiazem, nifedipine, and verapamil. Am Heart J 106:1341–1347, Dec 1983.

104. SUBRAMANIAN VB, KHURMI NS, BOWLES MJ, O'HARA M, RAFTERY EB: Objective evaluation of 3 dose levels of diltiazem in patients with chronic stable angina. J Am Coll Cardiol 1:1144–1153, Apr 1983.

105. PETRU MA, CRAWFORD MH, SORENSEN SG, CHAUDHURI TK, LEVINE S, O'ROURKE R: Short– and long–term efficacy of high dose oral diltiazem for angina due to coronary artery disease: a placebo controlled, randomized, double–blind crossover study. Circulation 68:139–147, July 1983.

106. LINDENBERG BS, WEINER DA, MCCABE CH, CUTLER SS, RYAN TJ, KLEIN MD: Efficacy and safety of incremental doses of diltiazem for the treatment of stable angina pectoris. J Am Coll Cardiol 2:1129–1133, Dec 1983.

107. KLEIN HO, NINIO R, OREN V, LANG R, SARELI P, DISEGNI E, DAVID D, GUERRERO J, KAPLINSKY E: The acute hemodynamic effects of intravenous verapamil in coronary artery disease: assessment by equilibrium–gated radionuclide ventriculography. Circulation 67:101–110, Jan 1983.

108. Chew CYC, Brown BG, Singh BN, Wong MM, Pierce C, Petersen R: Effects of verapamil on coronary hemodynamic function and vasomobility relative to its mechanism of antianginal action. Am J Cardiol 51:699–705, March 1983.

109. Weiner DA, McCabe CH, Cutler SS, Creager MA, Ryan TJ, Klein MD: Efficacy and safety of verapamil in patients with angina pectoris after 1 year of continuous, high dose therapy. Am J Cardiol 51:1251–1255, May 1983.

110. Mauritson DR, Johnson SM, Winniford MD, Cary JR, Willerson JT, Hillis LD: Verapamil for unstable angina at rest: a short–term randomized double–blind study. Am Heart J 106:652–658, Oct 1983.

111. Mehta J, Conti CR, Pepine CJ: Long–term oral verapamil therapy in patients with rest angina. Am Heart J 106:1133–1137, Nov 1983.

112. Rouleau JL, Chatterjee K, Ports TA, Doyle MB, Hiramatsu B, Parmley WW: Mechanism of relief of pacing–induced angina with oral verapamil: reduced oxygen demand. Circulation 67:94–100, Jan 1983.

113. Sherman LG, Liang CS: Nifedipine in chronic stable angina: a double-blind placebo controlled crossover trial. Am J Cardiol 51:706–711, March 1983.

114. Sellers TD, Gibson RS, Taylor GJ, Beller GA, Martin RP, McGuire LB, Carabello BA, Gascho JA, Ayers CR, DiMarco JP, Beckwith JR, Burwell LR, Craddock GA, Crampton RS: Relation of therapeutic response to nifedipine to coronary anatomy and motion of ST segment during unstable angina pectoris. Am J Med 75:57–64, July 1983.

115. Emanuelsson H, Holmberg S: Mechanisms of angina relief after nifedipine: a hemodynamic and myocardial metabolic study. Circulation 68:124–130, July 1983.

116. Stone PH, Muller JE, Turi ZG, Geltman E, Jaffe AS, Braunwald E: Efficacy of nifedipine therapy in patients with refractory angina pectoris: significance of the presence of coronary vasospasm. Am Heart J 106:644–652, Oct 1983.

117. Blaustein AS, Heller GV, Kolman BS: Adjunctive nifedipine therapy in high risk, medically refractory, unstable angina pectoris. Am J Cardiol 52:950–954, Nov 1983.

118. Specchia G, de Servi S, Falcone C, Angoli L, Gavazzi A, Bramucci E, Mussini A, Ferrario M, Salerno J, Montemartini C: Effects of nifedipine on coronary hemodynamic findings during exericse in patients with stable exertional angina. Circulation 68:1035–1043, Nov 1983.

119. Dale J, Landmark KH, Myhre E: The effects of nifedipine, a calcium antagonist, on platelet function. Am Heart J 105:103–105, Jan 1983.

120. Detry JMR, Decoster PM, Renkin J: Hemodynamic effects of felodipine at rest and during exercise in exertional angina pectoris. Am J Cardiol 52:453–457, Sept 1983.

121. Hung J, Lamb IH, Connolly SJ, Jutzy KR, Goris ML, Schroeder JS: The effect of diltiazem and propranolol, alone and in combination, on exercise performance and left ventricular function in patients with stable effort angina: a double–blind, randomized and placebo controlled study. Circulation 68:560–567, Sept 1983.

122. Winniford MD, Huxley RL, Hillis LD: Randomized, double–blind comparison of propranolol alone and a propranolol–verapamil combination in patients with severe angina of effort. J Am Coll Cardiol 1:492–498, Feb 1983.

123. Johnston DL, Gebhardt VA, Donald A, Kostuk WJ: Comparative effects of propranolol and verapamil alone and in combination on left ventricular function and volumes in patients with chronic exertional angina: a double–blind, placebo controlled, randomized, crossover study with radionuclide ventriculography. Circulation 68:1280–1289, Dec 1983.

124. Bowles MJ, Subramanian VB, Davies AB, Raftery EB: Double–blind randomized crossover trial of verapamil and propranolol in chronic stable angina. Am Heart J 106:1297–1306, Dec 1983.

125. Schanzenbacher P, Liebau G, Deeg P, Kochsiek K: Effect of intravenous and intracoronary nifedipine on coronary blood flow and myocardial oxygen consumption. Am J Cardiol 51:712–717, March 1983.

126. Bassan MM, Weiler–Ravell D, Shalev O: Comparison of the antianginal effectiveness of nifedipine, verapamil, and isosorbide dinitrate in patients receivng propranolol: a double–blind study. Circulation 68:568–575, Sept 1983.

127. Lewis HD, Davis JW, Archibald DG, Steinke WE, Smitherman TC, Doherty JE, Schnaper HW,

LEWINTER MM, LINARES E, POUGET JM, SABHARWAL SC, CHESLER E, DEMOTS H: Protective effects of aspirin against acute myocardial infarction and death in men with unstable angina: results of a Veterans Administration cooperative study. N Engl J Med 309:396–403, Aug 18, 1983.

128. FUCHS RM, BRIN KP, BRINKER JA, GUZMAN PA, HEUSER RR, YIN FCP: Augmentation of regional coronary blood flow by intraaortic balloon counterpulsation in patients with unstable angina. Circulation 68:117–123, July 1983.

129. HAGBERG JM, EHSANI AA, HOLLOSZY JO: Effect of 12 months of intense exercise training on stroke volume in patients with coronary artery disease. Circulation 67:1194–1199, June 1983.

130. ORNISH D, SCHERWITZ LW, DOODY RS, KESTEN D, McLANAHAN SM, BROWN SE, DEPUEY G, SONNEMAKER R, HAYNES C, LESTER J, McALLISTER GK, HALL RJ, BURDINE JA, GOTTO AM: Effects of stress management training and dietary changes in treating ischemic heart disease. JAMA 249:54–59, Jan 7, 1983.

131. CANNON RO, WATSON RM, ROSING DR, EPSTEIN SE: Angina caused by reduced vasodilator reserve of the small coronary arteries. J Am Coll Cardiol 1:1359–1373, June 1983.

132. ARAKI H, KOIWAYA Y, NAKAGAKI O, NAKAMURA M: Diurnal distribution of ST segment elevation and related arrhythmias in patients with variant angina: a study by ambulatory ECG monitoring. Circulation 67:995–1000, May 1983.

133. PREVITALI M, KLERSY C, SALERNO JA, CHIMIENTI M, PANCIROLI C, MARANGONI E, SPECCHIA G, COMOLLI M, BOBBA P: Ventricular tachyarrhythmias in Prinzmetal's variant angina: clinical significance and relation to the degree and time course of ST segment elevation. Am J Cardiol 52:19–25, July 1983.

134. KERIN NZ, RUBENFIRE M, WILLENS HJ, RAO P, CASCADE PN: The mechanism of dysrhythmias in variant angina pectoris: occlusive versus reperfusion. Am Heart J 106:1332–1340, Dec 1983.

135. WATERS DD, SZLACHCIC J, BONAN R, MILLER DD, DAUWE F, THEROUX P: Comparative sensitivity of exercise, cold pressor and ergonovine testing in provoking attacks of variant angina in patients with active disease. Circulation 67:310–315, Feb 1983.

136. FELDMAN RL, HILL JA, WHITTLE JL, CONTI CR, PEPINE CJ: Electrocardiographic changes with coronary artery spasm. Am Heart J 106:1288–1297, Dec 1983.

137. MATSUDA Y, OZAKI M, OGAWA H, NAITO H, YOSHINO F, KATAYAMA K, FUJII T, MATSUZAKI M, KUSUKAWA R: Coronary arteriography and left ventriculography during spontaneous and exercise-induced ST segment elevation in patients with variant angina. Am Heart J 106:509–515, Sept 1983.

138. MAUTNER RK, COOPER MC, PHILLIPS JH: Catheter induced coronary artery spasm: an angiographic manifestation of vasospastic angina. Am Heart J 106:659–665, Oct 1983.

139. SCHWARTZ AB, DONMICHAEL TA, BOTVINICK EH, ISHIMORI T, PARMLEY WW, CHATTERJEE K: Variability in coronary hemodynamics in response to ergonovine in patients with normal coronary arteries and atypical chest pain. J Am Coll Cardiol 1:797–803, March 1983.

140. BOTT-SILVERMAN C, HEUPLER FA: Natural history of pure coronary artery spasm in patients treated medically. J Am Coll Cardiol 2:200–205, Aug 1983.

141. WATERS DD, BOUCHARD A, THEROUX P: Spontaneous remission is a frequent outcome of variant angina. J Am Coll Cardiol 2:195–199, Aug 1983.

142. WATERS DD, MILLER DD, SZLACHCIC J, BOUCHARD A, METHE M, KREEFT J, THEROUX P: Factors influencing the long–term prognosis of treated patients with variant angina. Circulation 68:258–265, Aug 1983.

143. WINNIFORD MD, JOHNSON SM, MAURITSON DR, HILLIS LD: Ergonovine provocation to assess efficacy of long–term therapy with calcium antagonists in Prinzmetal's variant angina. Am J Cardiol 51:684–688, March 1983.

144. SCHROEDER JS, LAMB IH, BRISTOW MR, GINSBURG R, HUNG J, McAULEY BJ: Prevention of cardiovascular events in variant angina by long–term diltiazem therapy. J Am Coll Cardiol 1:1507–1511, June 1983.

145. TILMANT PY, LABLANCHE JM, THIEULEUX FA, DUPUIS BA, BERTRAND ME: Detrimental effect of propranolol in patients with coronary arterial spasm countered by combination with diltiazem. Am J Cardiol 52:230–233, Aug 1983.

146. HILL JA, FELDMAN RL, CONTI CR, HILL CK, PEPINE CJ: Long–term responses to nifedipine in

patients with coronary spasm who have an initial favorable response. Am J Cardiol 52:26–29, July 1983.

147. ROBERTSON RM, BERNARD YD, CARR RK, ROBERTSON D: Alpha–adrenergic blockade in vasotonic angina: lack of efficacy of specific Alpha₁-Receptor blockade with prazosin. J Am Coll Cardiol 2:1146–1150, Dec 1983.

148. TZIVONI D, KEREN A, BENHORIN J, GOTTLIEB S, ATLAS D, STERN S: Prazosin therapy for refractory variant angina. Am Heart J 105:262–266, Feb 1983.

149. WINNIFORD MD, FILIPCHUK N, HILLIS LD: Alpha–adrenergic blockade for variant angina: a long–term, double–blind, randomized trial. Circulation 67:1185–1188, June 1983.

150. MIWA K, KAMBARA H, KAWAI C: Effect of aspirin in large doses on attacks of variant angina. Am Heart J 105:351–355, Feb 1983.

151. BETRIU A, POMAR JL, BOURASSA MG, GRONDIN CM: Influence of partial sympathetic denervation on the results of myocardial revascularization in variant angina. Am J Cardiol 51:661–667, March 1983.

152. JONES EL, CRAVER JM, GUYTON RA, BONE DK, HATCHER CR, RIECHWALD N: Importance of complete revascularization in performance of the coronary bypass operation. Am J Cardiol 51:7–12, Jan 1983.

153. MILLER DC, STINSON EB, OYER PE, JAMIESON SW, MITCHELL RS, REITZ BA, BAUMGARTNER WA, SHUMWAY NE: Discriminant analysis of the changing risks of coronary artery operations: 1971–1979. J Thorac Cardiovasc Surg 85:197–213, Feb 1983.

154. LOOP FD, GOLDING LR, MACMILLAN JP, COSGROVE DM, LYTLE BW, SHELDON WC: Coronary artery surgery in women compared with men: analyses of risks and long–term results. J Am Coll Cardiovasc 1:383–390, Feb 1983.

155. SALOMON NW, PAGE US, OKIES JE, STEPHENS J, KRAUSE AH, BIGELOW JC: Diabetes mellitus and coronary artery bypass: short–term risk and long–term prognosis. J Thorac Cardiovasc Surg 85:264–271, Feb 1983.

156. GERSH BJ, KRONMAL RA, FRYE RL, SCHAFF HV, RYAN TJ, GOSSELIN AJ, KAISER GC, KILLIP T III: Participants in coronary artery surgery study. Circulation 67:483–491, March 1983.

157. FRICK MH, JARJOLA PT, VALLE M: Persistent improvement after coronary bypass surgery: ergometric and angiographic correlations at 5 years. Circulation 67:491–496, March 1983.

158. RAHIMTOOLA SH, NUNLEY D, GRUNKEMEIER G, TEPLEY J, LAMBERT L, STARR A: Ten–year survival after coronary bypass surgery for unstable angina. N Engl J Med 308:676–681, March 24, 1983.

159. GIBSON RS, WATSON DD, TAYLOR GJ, CROSBY IK, WELLONS HL, HOLT ND, BELLER GA: Prospective assessment of regional myocardial perfusion before and after coronary revascularization surgery by quantitative thallium–201 scintigraphy. J Am Coll Cardiol 1:804–815, March 1983.

160. WAITES TF, WATT EW, FLETCHER GF: Comparative functional and physiologic status of active and dropout coronary bypass patients of a rehabilitation program. Am J Cardiol 51:1087–1090, Apr 1983.

161. PANTELY GA, KLOSTER FE, MORRIS CD: Late exercise test results from a prospective randomized study of bypass surgery for stable angina. Circulation 68:413–419, Aug 1983.

162. LOOP FD, LYTLE BW, GILL CC, GOLDING LAR, COSGROVE DM, TAYLOR PC: Trends in selection and results of coronary artery reoperations. Ann Thorac Surg 36:380–388, Oct 1983.

163. ALDERMAN EL, FISHER LD, LITWIN P, KAISER GC, MYERS WO, MAYNARD E, LEVINE F, SCHLOSS M: Results of coronary artery surgery in patients with poor left ventricular function (CASS). Circulation 68:785–795, Oct 1983.

164. CASS PRINCIPAL INVESTIGATORS AND THEIR ASSOCIATES: CORONARY ARTERY SURGERY STUDY (CASS): A randomized trial of coronary artery bypass surgery: survival data. Circulation 68:939–950, Nov 1983.

165. CASS PRINCIPAL INVESTIGATORS AND THEIR ASSOCIATES: CORONARY ARTERY SURGERY STUDY (CASS): A randomized trial of coronary artery bypass surgery: quality of life in patients randomly assigned to treatment groups. Circulation 68:951–960, Nov 1983.

166. SINGH RN, SOSA JA, GREEN GE: Internal mammary artery versus saphenous vein graft: comparative performance in patients with combined revascularisation. Br Heart J 50:48–58, July 1983.

167. LYTLE BW, COSGROVE DM, SALTUS GL, TAYLOR PC, LOOP FD: Multivessel coronary revascularization without saphenous vein: long–term results of bilateral internal mammary artery grafting. Ann Thorac Surg 36:540–547, Nov 1983.

168. SCHAFF HV, ORSZULAK TA, GERSH BJ, PHIL D, PIEHLER JM, PUGA FJ, DANIELSON GK, PLUTH JR: The morbidity and mortality of reoperation for coronary artery disease and analysis of late results with use of actuarial estimate of event–free interval. J Thorac Cardiovasc Surg 85:508–515, Apr 1983.

169. LAIRD–MEETER K, VANDENBRAND MJBM, SERRUYS PW, PENN OCKM, HAALEBOS MMP, BOS E, HUGENHOLTZ PG: Reoperation after aortocoronary bypass procedure: results in 53 patients in a group of 1041 with consecutive first operations. Br Heart J 50:157–162, Aug 1983.

170. AUSTIN EH, OLDHAM HN, SABISTON DC, JONES RH: Early assessment of rest and exercise left ventricular function following coronary artery surgery. Ann Thorac Surg 32:159–169, Jan 1983.

171. TAYLOR NC, BARBER RW, CROSSLAND P, ENGLISH TAH, WRAIGHT EP, PETCH MC: Effects of coronary artery bypass grafting on left ventricular function assessed by multiple gated ventricular scintigraphy. Br Heart J 50:149–156, Aug 1983.

172. KRONENBERG MW, PEDERSON RW, HARSTON WE, BORN ML, BENDER HW, FRIESINGER GC: Left ventricular performance after coronary artery bypass surgery. Ann Intern Med 99:305–313, Sept 1983.

173. FLOYD RD, WAGNER GS, AUSTIN EH, SABISTON DC, JONES RH: Relation between QRS changes and left ventricular function after coronary artery bypass grafting. Am J Cardiol 52:943–949, Nov 1983.

174. HAMILTON WM, HAMMERMEISTER KE, DEROUEN TA, ZIA MS, DODGE HT: Effect of coronary artery bypass grafting on subsequent hospitalization. Am J Cardiol 51:353–360, Feb 1983.

175. STANTON BA, JENKINS CD, DENLINGER P, SAVAGEAU JA, WEINTRAUB RM, GOLDSTEIN RL: Predictors of employment status after cardiac surgery. JAMA 249:907–911, Feb 18, 1983.

176. LOOP FD, CHRISTIANSEN EK, LESTER JL, COSGROVE DM, FRANCO I, GOLDING LR: A strategy for cost containment in coronary surgery. JAMA 250:63–66, July 1, 1983.

177. JENKINS CD, STANTON BA, SAVAGEAU JA, DENLINGER P, KLEIN MD: Coronary artery bypass surgery: physical, psychological, social, and economic outcomes 6 months later. JAMA 250:782–788, Aug 12, 1983.

178. VAN TRIGT P, SPRAY TL, PASQUE MK, PEYTON RB, PELLOM GL, CHRISTIAN CM, FAGRAEUS L, WECHSLER AS: The influence of time on the response to dopamine after coronary artery bypass grafting: assessment of left ventricular performance and contractility using pressure/dimension analyses. Ann Thorac Surg 32:3–13, Jan 1983.

179. SMITH PK, BUHRMAN WC, LEVETT JM, FERGUSON TB, HOLMAN WL, COX JL: Supraventricular conduction abnormalities following cardiac operations: a complication of inadequate atrial perservation. J Thorac Cardiovasc Surg 85:105–115, Jan 1983.

180. FREMES SE, WEISEL RD, BAIRD RJ, MICKLEBOROUGH LL, BURNS RJ, TEASDALE SJ, IVANOV J, SEAWRIGHT SJ, MADONIK MM, MICKLE DAG, SCULLY HE, GOLDMAN BS, MCLAUGHLIN PR: Effects of postoperative hypertension and its treatment. J Thorac Cardiovasc Surg 86:47–56, July 1983.

181. CHAITMAN BR, ALDERMAN EL, SHEFFIELD LT, TONG T, FISHER L, MOCK MB, WEINS RD, KAISER GC, ROITMAN D, BERGER R, GERSH B, SCHAFF H, BOURASSA MG, KILLIP T, PARTICIPATING CASS MEDICAL CENTERS. Circulation 67:302–309, Feb 1983.

182. VAL PG, PELLETIER LC, HERNANDEZ MG, JAIS JM, CHAITMAN BR, DUPRAS G, SOLYMOSS BC: Diagnostic criteria and prognosis of perioperative myocardial infarction following coronary bypass. J Thorac Cardiovasc Surg 86:878–886, Dec 1983.

183. KUAN P, MESSENGER JC, ELLESTAD MH: Transient central diabetes insipidus after aortocoronary bypass operations. Am J Cardiol 52:1181–1183, Dec 1983.

184. Murphy DA, Craver JM, Jones EL, Bone DK, Guyton RA, Hatcher CR Jr: Recognition and management of ascending aortic dissection complicating cardiac surgical operations. J Thorac Cardiovasc Surg 85:247–256, Feb 1983.

185. Saffitz JE, Ganote CE, Peterson CE, Roberts WC: False aneurysm of ascending aorta after aortocoronary bypass grafting. Am J Cardiol 52:907–909, Oct 1983.

186. Brower RW, Laird–Meeter K, Serruys PW, Meester GT, Hugenholtz PG: Long–term follow-up after coronary artery bypass graft surgery: progression and regression of disease in native coronary circulation and bypass grafts. Br Heart J 50:42–47, July 1983.

187. Campeau L, Enjalbert M, Lesperance J, Vaislic C, Grondon CM, Bourassa MG: Atherosclerosis and late closure of aortocoronary saphenous vein grafts: sequential angiographic studies at 2 weeks, 1 year, 5–7 years, and 10–12 years after surgery. Circulation 68(suppl II):II-1–II-7, Sept 1983.

188. Daniel WG, Dohring W, Stender HS, Lichtlen PR: Value and limitations of computed tomography in assessing aortocoronary bypass graft patency. Circulation 67:983–987, May 1983.

189. Meyer J, Schmitz H–J, Kiesslich T, Erbel R, Krebs W, Schulz W, Bardos P, Minale C, Messmer BJ, Effert S: Percutaneous transluminal coronary angioplasty in patients with stable and unstable angina pectoris: analysis of early and late results. Am Heart J 106:973–980, Nov 1983.

190. Meier B, Gruentzig AR, Hollman J, Ischinger T, Bradford JM: Does length of eccentricity of coronary stenoses influence the outcome of transluminal dilatation. Circulation 67:497–499, March 1983.

191. Ischinger T, Gruentzig AR, Hollman J, King S III, Douglas J, Meier B, Bradford J, Tankersley R: Should coronary arteries with less than 60% diameter stenosis be treated by angioplasty. Circulation 68:148–154, July 1983.

192. Meier B, Gruentzig AR, Siegenthaler WE, Schlumpf M: Long–term exercise performance after percutaneous transluminal coronary angioplasty and coronary artery bypass grafting. Circulation 68:796–802, Oct 1983.

193. Alcan KE, Stertzer SH, Wallsh E, DePasquale NP, Bruno MS: The role of intraaortic balloon counterpulsation in patients undergoing percutaneous transluminal coronary angioplasty. Am Heart J 105:527–530, March 1983.

194. Douglas JS, Gruentig, King SB, Hollman J, Ischinger T, Meier B, Craver JM, Jones EL, Waller JL, Bcne DK, Guyton R: Percutaneous transluminal coronary angioplasty in patients with prior coronary bypass surgery. J Am Coll Cardiol 2:745–754, Oct 1983.

195. Holmes DR, Vlietstra RE, Mock MB, Smith HC, Dorros G, Cowley MJ, Kent KM, Hammes LN, Janke L, Elveback LR, Vetrovec GW: Employment and recreation patterns in patients treated by percutaneous transluminal coronary angioplasty: a multicenter study. Am J Cardiol 52:710–713, Oct 1983.

196. Dorros G, Cowley MJ, Simpson J, Bentivoglio LG, Block PC, Bourassa M, Detre K, Gosselin AJ, Gruntzig A, Kelsey SF, Kent KM, Mock MB, Mullin SM, Myler RK, Passamani ER, Stertzer SH, Williams DO: Percutaneous transluminal coronary angioplasty: report of complications from the national heart, lung, and blood institute PTCA registry. Circulation 67:723–730, Apr 1983.

197. Hollman J, Austin GE, Gruentzig AR, Douglas JS, King SB: Coronary artery spasm at the site of angioplasty in the first 2 months after successful percutaneous transluminal coronary angioplasty. J Am Coll Cardiol 2:1039–1045, Dec 1983.

198. Bentivoglio LG, Leo LR, Wolf NM, Meister SG: Frequency and importance of unprovoked coronary spasm in patients with angina pectoris undergoing percutaneous transluminal coronary angioplasty. Am J Cardiol 52:1067–1071, Apr 1983.

199. Hollman J, Gruentzig AR, Douglas JS, King SB III, Ischinger T, Meier B: Acute occlusion after percutaneous transluminal coronary angioplasty: a new approach. Circulation 68:725–732, Oct 1983.

200. Dervan JP, Baim DS, Cherniles J, Grossman W: Transluminal angioplasty of occluded coronary arteries: use of a movable guide wire system. Circulation 68:776–784, Oct 1983.

201. Hill JA, Margolis JR, Feldman RL, Conti CR, Pepine CJ: Coronary arterial aneurysm formation after balloon angioplasty. Am J Cardiol 52:261–264, Aug 1983.

202. WALLER BF, McMANUS BM, GORFINKEL HJ, KISHEL JC, SCHMIDT ECH, KENT KM, ROBERTS WC: Status of the major epicardial coronary arteries 80–150 days after percutaneous transluminal coronary angioplasty. Am J Cardiol 51:81–84, Jan 1983.

203. GILLUM RF, FOLSOM A, LUEPKER RV, JACOBS DR, KOTTKE TE, GOMEZ–MARIN O, PRINEAS RJ, TAYLOR HL, BLACKBURN H: Sudden death and acute myocardial infarction in a metropolitan area, 1970–1980: the Minnesota heart survey. N Engl J Med 309:1353–1358, Dec 1, 1983.

2

Acute Myocardial Infarction and Its Consequences

DIAGNOSIS OF AMI AND OF THE HIGH RISK PATIENT

Electrocardiographic aids

Over a 35-month period, Rude and associates[1] from Dallas, Texas, St. Louis, Missouri, Boston, Massachusetts, Burlington, Vermont, screened all admissions to 5 university hospital coronary care units for eligibility for the Multicenter Investigation of the Limitation of Infarct Size (MILIS), an ongoing study of the effects of hyaluronidase, propranolol, and placebo on AMI size. Of 3,697 patients with $\geq$30 minutes of discomfort that was thought to reflect myocardial ischemia who were assessed for the presence or absence of certain ECG abnormalities at the time of hospital admission, the ECG was considered predictive of AMI if $\geq$1 of the following abnormalities was present: new or presumably new Q waves ($\geq$30 ms wide and 0.20 mV deep) in at least 2 of the 3 diaphragmatic leads (II, III, aVF), or in at least 2 of the 6 precordial leads (V_1–V_6), or in I and aVL; new or presumably new ST-segment elevation or depression of $\geq$0.10 mV in 1 of the same lead combinations; or complete left BBB. In the screened population, the diagnostic sensitivity of the ECG criteria was 81%, whereas the overall AMI rate in the total population screened was 49%. The diagnostic specificity of these entry criteria was 69% and the predictive value was 72%. Further application of readily ascertainable study exclusion criteria (age >75 years; qualifying symptoms commencing >18 hours before presentation; previous MILIS participation; geographic, physical, or psychologic impediments to follow-up; cardiogenic shock; recent AMI; and other major cardiac or medical problems likely to affect prognosis) resulted in an overall AMI rate of 86% in patients determined to be eligible. This represents the overall value of the criteria in selecting, before serial ECG or serum enzyme data are available, a population with a high prevalence of acute AMI.

Warner and associates[2] from Syracuse, New York, reported a systematic evaluation of a large number of ECG variables that might be useful for diagnosing anterior wall AMI. Previous anterior AMI was shown to be present or absent by cardiac catheterization in 199 patients. The best discriminator between cases and noncases of anterior AMI in most patients is the presence of a Q wave of any magnitude or an initial R wave <20 ms in lead V_2. In patients with ECG evidence of associated LV or type C RV enlargement, the more stringent criterion of a Q wave of any magnitude in lead V_2 yielded the optimal combination of sensitivity and specificity for diagnosing anterior AMI. The diagnostic performance of the proposed criteria for anterior AMI was superior to that of more traditional criteria that use measurements of the absolute and relative amplitudes of precordial R waves.

Warner and associates[3] from Syracuse, New York, proposed new ECG criteria for diagnosing the combination of inferior AMI and left anterior hemiblock. The proposed criteria are based upon the relations between portions of the vectorcardiographic QRS loop in the frontal plane and the corresponding portions of the QRS complexes recorded by the limb leads. The application of the proposed criteria requires that the tracings be obtained with 3-channel ECG machines. The proposed criteria for the diagnosis of inferior AMI and left anterior hemiblock were as follows: 1) leads aVR and aVL both end in R waves, with the peak of the terminal R wave in lead aVR occurring later than in lead aVL, and 2) a Q wave of any magnitude in lead II. The performance of the proposed criteria was superior to that of 10 combinations of traditional ECG criteria for inferior AMI and left anterior hemiblock.

To determine whether morphologic analysis of VPC can aid in the ECG diagnosis of AMI, 12-lead ECGs were evaluated by Dash and Ciotola[4] from Hershey, Pennsylvania, in 760 consecutive patients who underwent cardiac catheterization, and 2-minute multiple lead rhythm strips were evaluated in 515 of the 760 patients. The VPC occurred in 58 patients; 21 had prior AMI diagnosed by regional akinesia of dyskinesia on LV cineangiogram. Standard criteria were used to diagnose prior AMI from the sinus beats of the electrocardiogram. The AMI was diagnosed from the morphology of a VPC when it had a QR or QRS sensitivity (29%) but high specificity (97%) and high predictive value (86%). Sinus beats diagnosed AMI with higher sensitivity (52%, and 69% if patients with left BBB and LV hypertrophy were excluded from analysis) than VPC morphologic analysis ($p < 0.05$),), but with similar specificity (97%) and predictive value (92%). Two patients with angiographic AMI had no AMI according to standard ECG criteria but did have an AMI manifested by VPB morphologic analysis. Despite low sensitivity, analysis of the morphology of VPC may be useful for the diagnosis of AMI when the morphology of sinus beats is not diagnostic.

To determine the significance of exercise-induced ST-segment elevation in patients with previous AMI, Fox and associates[5] from London, England, studied 156 patients a mean of 26 months after AMI. Each patient underwent 16 lead precordial ECG mapping before, during, and after exercise and in addition coronary arteriography was performed. There was no significant difference in the extent of CAD or abnormalities of LV function between patients with exercise-induced ST-segment elevation that was noted to occur in leads with Q waves and those with ST-segment elevation plus depression or those with ST-segment depression alone. Patients without exercise-induced ST-segment changes had fewer coronary arteries involved than those who developed ST-segment changes. Nineteen patients with exercise-induced ST-segment elevation alone underwent CABG; in 11 this resulted in complete abolition of the exercise-induced ST-segment elevation and was associated with symptomatic relief and patent grafts without alteration of LV function. Thus, exercise-induced ST-segment elevation in patients with previous AMI should be considered as important as ST-segment depression in terms of underlying myocardial ischemia, coronary anatomy, and LV function.

Persistent ST-segment elevation in the anterior precordial leads occurs occasionally after anterior AMI and is considered usually to be indicative of underlying LV aneurysm. Although myocardial ischemia does not appear to play a role in the genesis of chronic ST-segment elevation in these patients, the role of ischemia in exercise-induced additional or new ST-segment elevation is less clear. To study the hypothesis that myocardial ischemia is responsible for exercise-induced ST-segment elevation in patients with previous anterior wall AMI, Gewirtz and associates[6] from Providence, Rhode Island, performed exercise stress tests in conjunction with thallium imaging of the myocardium in 28 patients with previously documented anterior wall AMI. Thallium images were analyzed by computer for the presence of initial uptake defects and evidence of abnormal clearance of the isotope from the myocardium (that is, imaging evidence of ischemia). Total ST-segment elevation (ΣST) in precordial leads V_1–V_6 at rest was subtracted from ΣST at peak stress in order to quantitate the extent of ST elevation induced by stress (ΔST). Two groups of patients were identified; 1 with stress-induced ST elevation (group I, ΔST $\geq$ 4.0 mm) and 1 without this abnormality (group II, ΔST $\geq$ 4.0 mm). Evidence of abnormal thallium washout from myocardial scan segments occurred in 12 of 15 group I patients -vs- 9 of 13 group II patients (difference not significant). In addition, abnormal tracer washout from anterolateral or septal scan segments occurred in 5 patients in each group. Likewise, abnormal thallium clearance from inferior or posterior scan segments occurred in 8 of 15 group I patients -vs- 7 of 13 group II patients (difference not significant). The patient with the greatest amount of stress-induced ST elevation (11.5 mm) had no evidence of ischemia during the stress test. However, group I patients did have larger anterolateral plus septal initial thallium uptake defect scores than did those of group II (10 of 15 with defect score $\geq$350 in group I -vs- 1 of 13 in group II; p $<$ 0.002). Similarly, resting LV EF $\geq$30% was present in only 4 of 15 group I patients -vs- 13 of 13 in group II (p $<$ 0.001). Finally, multiple stepwise linear regression analysis demonstrated that ΔST correlated best with the extent of initial anterolateral plus septal thallium uptake defect score (F = 17.3; p $<$ 0.001) and to a lesser extent with resting EF (F = 5.2; p $<$ 0.05) and change in heart rate from rest to peak stress (F = 8.1; p $<$ 0.01. Corrected multiple correlation coefficient,

0.76; p < 0.001). Thus, in patients with previous anterior MI: 1) exercise-induced myocardial ischemia occurs as often with as without ST-segment elevation; 2) myocardial ischemia is not required for the production of stress-induced ST-segment elevation; and 3) stress-induced ST elevation primarily reflects the extent of previous anterior wall damage and to a lesser extent an increase in heart rate between rest and peak stress.

Camara and associates[7] from Baltimore, Maryland, evaluated 25 consecutive patients admitted with their first AMI with serial ECGs and 2-D echo to determine the time course and significance of reciprocal ST-segment changes. Reciprocal change was noted in all patients with inferior AMI and in 70% of patients with anterior AMI. Reciprocal change resolved within 24 hours in 59% of patients. Echocardiographic evidence of alterations in regional wall motion remote from the area of AMI was detected in 45% of patients, but the location of the wall motion abnormalities did not correlate with the location of reciprocal ST-segment change. Thus, these data do not support the hypothesis that reciprocal ST-segment depression during early transmural AMI reflects remote ischemia elsewhere. Rather, the ST-segment changes appear to be influenced by factors that determine the degree of ST-segment elevation, including infarct size, shape, and location.

Serum enzyme aids

Although increased serum creatine kinase (CK) activity in the presence of an increased level of myocardial-specific isoenzymes (CK-MB) has been strongly associated with AMI, the significance of an increased serum CK-MB level in the presence of a normal total CK level is uncertain. In 335 consecutive patients suspected of having an AMI and 71 control subjects, Heller and associates[8] from Boston, Massachusetts, correlated peak serum CK-MB and CK levels with the presence of other clinical criteria for AMI: 1) typical chest pain; 2) increased myocardial lactate dehydrogenase (LDH_1/LDH_2); 3) acute ECG changes (new or ST-T wave changes with evolution), and 4) an elevated CK-MB level on ≥ 2 determinations or a typical CK curve. No control subject had an increase in CK or CK-MB or any of the 4 criteria for AMI. Of the 176 subjects with normal CK and normal CK-MB (group 1), only 11% had more than a single criterion, and none had more than 2 criteria consistent with myocardial injury. In contrast, of the 83 with elevated CK and CK-MB levels (group 2), 93% had ≥ 2 and 81% had ≥ 3 of the 4 criteria. Of the 63 patients with elevated CK-MB but a persistently normal CK (group 3), 65% had ≥ 2 criteria for AMI and 77% had subendocardial ECG changes; these patients resembled those with both elevated CK and MB. The phenomenon of elevated CK-MB with normal CK occurred in 20% of the patients aged ≥ 70 years but in only 10% of the younger group (p < 0.01). These findings suggest that elevated CK-MB with normal CK likely represents definite myocardial injury, is more common in the elderly, and should be considered part of the spectrum of nontransmural AMI.

To document optimal sampling frequency, Fisher and associates[9] from Baltimore, Maryland, reviewed CK-MB results in 314 patients with suspected AMI. In 127 patients with elevated CK/CK-MB, peak CK observed using all samples (every 4-hour [Q4 h] method) was compared with results that would have been obtained had samples been taken on admission and either twice daily (every 12-hour [Q12 h] method) or once daily (every 24-hour

[Q24 h] method). Although average peak CK was statistically different (Q4 h > Q12 h > Q24 h), major underestimation of peak CK ($\geq$500 U/liter) was uncommon (3%) using the Q12 h method, suggesting that Q12 h sampling is a practical, cost-effective approach for patients with suspected AMI.

Distribution volume (DV) and disappearance rate (K_d) of native CK, parameters needed for enzymatic estimation of infarct size, have not been characterized in the human. In the past, values for these parameters have been obtained in experimental models and extrapolated for use in the human. Therefore Tommasini and associates[10] from Los Angeles, California, determined DV and K_d of CK in the clinical setting. During hemodynamic monitoring, 100–150 ml of enzyme-rich plasma was collected from 10 patients with AMI, stored at $-30°C$ for a maximum of 6 days, and then rapidly reinfused back into the same patient after return of CK serum activity to baseline levels. After reinfusion, blood samples were obtained at 5–15-minute intervals for 2 hours and at 30–60-minute intervals for an additional 10 hours. In each specimen, total CK activity and CK-MM and CK-MB concentrations were determined by spectrophotometry and radioimmunoassay. Data were analyzed by either nonlinear least squares approximation or the noncompartmental approach after baseline subtraction. Concentration of immunologically active molecules appeared to decline in parallel to enzymatic activity. In 3 patients, a double exponential decay was demonstrated. All others exhibited single exponential decay, with a K_d of 0.0023 ± 0.00057 (SD) minute^{-1}. The DV averaged 3284 ± 693 (SD) ml, 5% of body weight. There was no correlation between K_d estimated from terminal portions of CK time activity curves following infarction and K_d calculated after reinfused plasma. It was concluded that 1) a 1-compartment model using values for K_d and a DV compatible with plasma volume is suitable for clinical application and 2) true K_d cannot be determined from the terminal portion of CK time activity curves after AMI.

In a study carried out by Grenadier and associates[11] from Haifa, Israel, frequent blood samples were drawn for determination of serum myoglobin, CK, and CK-MB in 15 patients with AMI. Significantly elevated levels of myoglobin were present 1.5 hours following onset of chest pain and predated elevations of CK and CK-MB by 3 hours. No evidence was found of the previously described staccato phenomenon of intermittent myocardial necrosis. Due to very frequent blood sampling, a detailed picture of the evolution over time of these indices was obtained. Significant differences were found in the biochemical profile of anterior and diaphragmatic AMI (greater CK-MB elevation occurs earlier and disappears sooner in anterior AMI). A curve showing sensitivity of the assay at each time following onset of symptoms was obtained for myoglobin, CK, and CK-MB. It was concluded that 1) myoglobin is the most sensitive biochemical indicator of AMI in its early phase, and, since it decreases rapidly back to normal values, it can serve as an invaluable aid in the diagnosis of reinfarction and infarct extension; and 2) CK-MB is a less sensitive indicator of AMI but has the advantage of greater specificity.

To determine the cost effectiveness of routine use of serial aspartate aminotransferase (SGOT), lactic dehydrogenase (LDH) (upper limits equal 193 U/liter) and LDH isoenzyme determination in patients with suspected AMI, Fisher and associates[12] from Baltimore, Maryland, analyzed 166 consecutive patients admitted to a coronary care unit. Based on chest pain

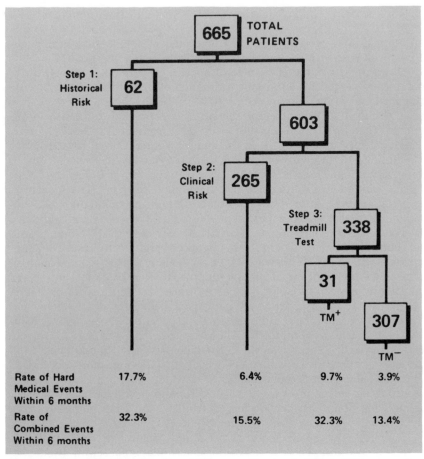

Fig. 2-1. Risk stratification procedure. TM$^+$ = positive treadmill test; TM$^-$ = negative treadmill test.

characteristics, ECG, and CK-MB results, patients were placed in categories of definite AMI (31%), possible AMI (34%), or AMI excluded (36%). The SGOT and/or LDH patterns were considered positive (i.e., suggestive of AMI) in 82% of the patients with definite AMI but only confirmed CK-MB results. Positive SGOT/LDH results yielded new clinically relevant information in only 14 patients (8%). Total charges for SGOT/LDH determinations in these 166 patients totaled $10,938, or approximately $780 for each additional clinically important positive result. When serial ECG and CK-MB results are available, routine serial SGOT/LDH determinations are not justified. These authors suggested the following approach: attain an admission sample followed by 8:00 a.m. and 8:00 p.m. samples over the next 24–36 hours. Promptly assay each sample for total CK, with an aliquot being stored frozen and the remainder stored at room temperature. After ≥2 total CK determinations, analyze the frozen aliquot from the sample with the highest total CK activity for CK-MB. When serial ECGs and CK/CK-MB results are not diagnostic, use the aliquots stored at room temperature for serial LDH/LDH isoenzyme

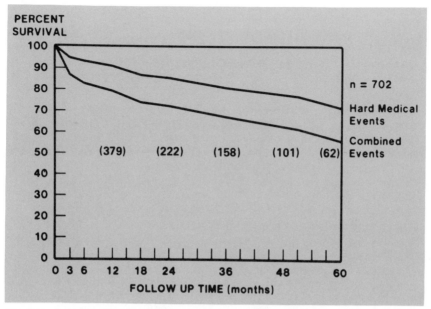

Fig. 2-2. Survival without events in the entire population during 60 month follow–up. Numbers in parentheses indicate patients being followed at each time point.

determinations if 1) the patient's symptoms occurred >12 hours before admission, or 2) the clinical history and/or ECG are still considered strongly suggestive of myocardial ischemia.

Exercise testing

DeBusk and associates[13] from Stanford, Redwood City, and Santa Clara, California, applied a stepwise risk stratification procedure sequentially combining history and clinical characteristics and treadmill exercise test results in 702 consecutive men aged ≤70 years who were alive 21 days after AMI (Fig. 2-1). History alone (prior AMI and prior angina or recurrence of pain in the coronary care unit) identified 10% of patients with the highest rate of reinfarction and death within 6 months (18%) (Fig. 2-2). Clinical contraindications to exercise testing identified another 40% of patients with an intermediate rate of cardiac events (6%) (Fig. 2-3). In the 50% of patients who underwent treadmill testing 3 weeks after AMI, the rate of cardiac events within 6 months was 4% in patients with a negative test and 10% in patients with a positive test (ischemic ST-segment depression ≥0.2 mV and a peak heart rate ≤135 beats/min). Patients with negative treadmill tests, who comprised 46% of patients ≤70 years and 53% of patients ≤60 years, had a cardiac death rate of <2% in the 6 months after AMI. The stepwise classification procedure correctly classified 72% of patients with cardiac events within 6 months. Thus, most patients who experience subsequent cardiac events are correctly classified on the basis of history and clinical risk characteristics. In patients without these risk characteristics, early treadmill testing is useful for further discriminating high risk from very low risk patients.

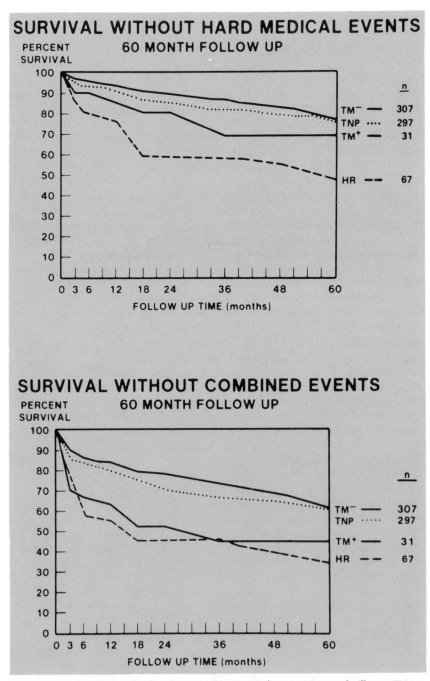

Fig. 2-3. Survival during the first 5 years after MI. TM$^+$ = positive treadmill test; TM$^-$ = negative treadmill test; TNP = treadmill not performed; HR = historical risk group.

DETERMINING INFARCT SIZE

Estimates of AMI size based on plasma creatine kinase (CK) are used widely for prognosis and in the assessment of therapy designed to salvage ischemic myocardium. If the initial plasma CK activity, however, is elevated, AMI size will be underestimated. To determine the impact of loss of early CK values on estimates of AMI size and to develop a procedure to compensate for it, estimates of AMI size based on complete and incomplete MB and total CK time activity curves from 120 patients were compared by Smith and associates[14] from St. Louis, Missouri, and from certain members of the Multicentered Investigation for Limitation of Infarct Size (MILIS). Estimates of AMI size based on data inclusion intervals beginning at 24, 12, 8, and 4 hours before peak CK were 11, 14, 23, and 47% smaller than values based on complete CK curves, but the correlation was good between complete and incomplete estimates of AMI size at any given interval, with r values ranging from 0.91–0.98. The derived correction factors were then prospectively applied to a new population (n, 25) with complete CK curves to compensate for purposely omitted early CK values. The corrected estimates of AMI size were within 7% of those based on the complete CK curves. Similar results were obtained for transmural and nontransmural and anterior or inferior AMI. Thus, if peak plasma CK is known, underestimation of AMI size can be compensated for despite the unavailability of early CK values. Since 90% of patients present before plasma CK has reached its peak (24 hours), AMI size can be obtained in nearly all patients. Thus, being able to correct for unavailable early CK values makes AMI size a more widely applicable end point for use in clinical trials and patient management.

Hirsowitz and associates[15] from Detroit, Michigan, evaluated 26 patients to determine the relations between CK enzyme release, radionuclide gated blood pool measurements, and thallium-201 scintigraphic measurements of AMI size. The CK estimates of AMI size correlated closely with the percent of abnormally contracting regions, LV EF, and thallium-201 estimates of percent abnormal perfusion area (r = 0.78, 0.69, and 0.74, respectively). Careful comparisons demonstrated a close correlation between the percent of abnormal perfusion area and the percent of abnormally contracting regions (r = 0.81) and LV EF (r = 0.69). Enzymatic AMI size was larger in anterior than inferior AMI and was associated with a more severely impaired LV function. These data suggest that each of the nuclear cardiology methods provides a reasonably accurate estimate of AMI size when CK estimates of AMI size are used as the gold standard.

Sederholm and coworkers[16] from Sandvika, Norway, compared the accuracy of the use of maximal QRS vector difference to estimate AMI size irrespective of AMI location with that of measurement of cumulative CK release. Sixty patients with AMI and a history of symptoms of <4 hour duration were followed for 24–72 hours with orthogonal vectorcardiography and CK release analysis. Spatial QRS vector differences were calculated between the first QRS complex recorded and subsequent QRS complexes at timed intervals. The QRS vector difference increased rapidly and reached a plateau at an average 12 hours after onset of symptoms, compared with 34 hours for the cumulated CK release. In 42% of the patients a stepwise

TABLE 2-1. *QRS scoring system.*

CATEGORY	LEAD	DURATION (MS)	AMPLITUDE RATIO (MS)	MAXIMUM POINTS
Criterion for IMI required for inclusion in study	aVF	Q $\geq$ 30 (1)		1
Additional criteria for IMI	II	Q $\geq$ 40 (2)		
		Q $\geq$ 30 (1)		2
	aVF	Q $\geq$ 50 (3)	R/Q $\leq$ 1 (2)	
		Q $\geq$ 40 (2)	R/Q $\leq$ 2 (1)	4
Criteria for posterior involvement	V_1	R $\geq$ 50 (2)		
		R $\geq$ 40 (1)	R/S $\geq$ 1 (1)	3
	V_2	R $\geq$ 60 (2)		
		R $\geq$ 50 (1)	R/S $\geq$ 1.5 (1)	3
Criteria for apical involvement	V_5	Q $\geq$ 30 (1)	R/Q or R/S $\leq$ 1 (2)	
			R/Q or R/S $\leq$ 2 (1)	3
	V_6	Q $\geq$ 30 (1)	R/Q or R/S $\leq$ 1 (2)	
			R/Q or R/S $\leq$ 3 (1)	3
Criteria for anterior and lateral involvement used for exclusion from this study	I	Q $\geq$ 30 (1)	R/Q $\leq$ 1 (1)	2
	aVL	Q $\geq$ 30 (1)	R/Q $\leq$ 1 (1)	2
	V_1	Any Q (1)		1
	V_2	Any Q or R $\leq$ 10 (1)		1
	V_3	Any Q or R $\leq$ 20 (1)		1
	V_4	Q $\geq$ 20 (1)	R/Q or R/S $\leq$ 0.5 (2)	
			R/Q or R/S $\leq$ 1 (1)	3

IMI = inferior myocardial infarction.

progression of AMI evolution was observed. Irrespective of AMI location the maximal spatial ST vector magnitude was related to the ultimate QRS vector difference and to the cumulative amount of CK release. Maximal QRS vector difference correlated well with the maximal cumulative CK release. Ten patients had possible AMI expansion, as indicated by recurrent QRS changes without concomitant CK release. Fifteen patients had AMI extension that was indicated by secondary CK release and that in 7 patients was associated with further QRS changes. Infarct extension caused an approximate 25% increase in AMI size. Spatial ST vector magnitude, QRS vector difference, and cumulative CK release are complementary measures in the quantification of evolving myocardial injury after acute coronary occlusion and in the determination of sequels to therapeutic interventions.

Albert and associates[17] from Durham, North Carolina, compared the development and regression of QRS changes associated with AMI occurring naturally and after CABG by a QRS scoring system for estimating AMI size. Only patients in both groups who had a baseline ECG with no evidence of previous myocardial infarction, ventricular hypertrophy, or BBB were included. Both groups attained similar peak QRS scores during the acute phase but different rates of resolution of scores were observed. During the subsequent 2 months, regression of QRS changes occurred more rapidly in the perioperative group than in the control group (43 -vs- 19%). Rates of regression were similar in both groups during the remainder of the follow-up period, attaining total decreases of 62% in the operative group and 37% in the nonoperative group by 18 months. These results could mean either that factors other than AMI are responsible for the perioperative QRS changes or that the infarct healing process in the 2 clinical settings are quite different.

Anderson and associates[18] from Durham, North Carolina, studied in 82 consecutive patients the evolution of changes in the QRS complex during the initial 3 days after onset of an initial inferior (posterior) AMI. Each patient's standard 12-lead ECG was assigned points (a QRS score) according to the absolute duration of the Q and R waves and the amplitude ratios of R/Q and R/S waves (Table 2-1). This QRS score has been demonstrated to correlate (r = 0.74) with the anatomic extent of single inferior AMI. By this system, 43 patients (53% of the study group) had an initial ECG that registered a score of 0 and developed QRS points only after admission. The QRS scores of 18 additional patients (22% of the study group) changed after admission. Forty-nine score changes were noted on Day 2 and 18, on Day 3. All of these changes resulted in an increased QRS score. Alteration of the QRS complex during initial inferior AMI evolves over 2–3 days in many patients. There is a distinct pattern to this evolution, which results in sequential increases in a QRS score based upon ECG indicators of the extent of myocardial necrosis. This QRS scoring system might be applied to evaluate clinical interventions aimed at limiting the extent of necrosis in patients with initial acute inferior AMI.

COMPLICATIONS

Arrhythmias

Although many patients with CAD and VT have transmural LV scars or LV aneurysms, few patients with LV aneurysms actually develop VT. To determine which factors are associated with the development of VT in patients with LV aneurysms, Cohen and associates[19] from New York City reviewed records of 154 patients with CAD and akinetic or dyskinetic segments, or both, on left ventriculography. Of the 154 patients, 85 had 24-hour Holter ECG monitoring or 48 consecutive hours of continuous ECG monitoring in an intensive care unit within 6 hours of catheterization. Ventricular tachycardia occurring ≥10 days after AMI or in the chronic phase was recorded in 19 patients (group I); the remaining 66 patients did not have VT (group II). Clinical, hemodynamic, and angiographic characteristics of these 2 groups showed no significant difference with respect to age, time from first transmural AMI to catheterization, CHF, EF, or presence of dyskinesia. Patients with VT had significantly larger LV aneurysms and a higher prevalence of septal akinesia or dyskinesia. However, stepwise discriminant analysis revealed septal akinesia or dyskinesia to be the only independently significant variable distinguishing the 2 groups. Thus, septal involvement appears to be a major determinant of VT in patients with CAD and LV aneurysm.

Richards and associates[20] from West Meade, Australia, assessed the frequency of ventricular electrical stability using a standardized protocol of programmed stimulation in 165 hemodynamically stable patients 6–28 days after AMI. Ventricular electrical instability was defined as induction at programmed stimulation of VF or VT lasting ≥10 seconds. Of 165 AMI survivors, 38 (23%) had ventricular electrical instability. No significant differences were noted between stable and unstable patients in terms of coronary prognostic index, elevation of serum creatine kinase, coronary anatomy, site of AMI, or frequency of VT within 48 hours of AMI. The mean follow-up period was 8 months (range, 0–12). There were 7 deaths in stable patients (5 from cardiogenic shock, 1 from septicemia, and 1 unwitnessed) and 10 deaths in unstable patients (8 instantaneous, 1 from cardiogenic shock, and 1 unwitnessed) during the subsequent year. In addition, 2 of 127 stable patients and 4 of 38 unstable patients had spontaneous VT from which they were satisfactorily resuscitated. Thus, the sensitivity of ventricular electrical instability as a predictor of instantaneous death or spontaneous VT was 86% and the specificity was 83%. The predictive accuracy of the absence of ventricular electrical instability as an indicator for the absence of instantaneous death or spontaneous VT was 98%. The predictive accuracy of the presence of ventricular electrical instability as a predictor of instantaneous death or spontaneous VT was 32%.

Sclarovsky and associates[21] from Petah Tikva and Tel Aviv, Israel, described findings in 13 patients with AMI with multiform accelerated idioventricular rhythm (AIVR) occurring during the first 12 hours of monitoring in the coronary care unit. This arrhythmia, similar to the more common uniform AIVR, was intermittent, did not cause hemodynamic compromise, and was not related to more serious ventricular arrhythmias. There was no correlation between the BBB pattern of the multiform AIVR and the ECG location of the AMI, but there was a perfect correlation between the frontal plane electrical axis of the multiform AIVR and the ECG location of the AMI. The presence of fusion beats between the different forms of AIVR suggests multifocality rather than multiformity. Intravenous verapamil (3–5 mg bolus) was administered to 6 patients with multiform AIVR in whom the arrhythmias were persistent enough to allow the evaluation of the effect of verapamil on the arrhythmia. Verapamil caused no change in the rate of AIVR in 1 patient, but in a second patient it decreased the rate by 20 beats/minute. In 4 patients, verapamil abolished the arrhythmia: in 2 patients carotid sinus pressure (induced sinus slowing) allowed the emergence of the AIVR at a lower rate, and in the remaining 2 patients the arrhythmia was not observed.

A relation between free fatty acids (FFA) and arrhythmias during AMI has been observed in some studies. Tansey and Opie[22] from Cape Town, South Africa, measured FFA plasma levels every hour in the first 12 hours after AMI in 35 patients admitted an average of 4.5 hours (range, 1–9) after onset of chest pain of AMI. There was a significant relation between arrhythmias and high mean FFA levels in the first 12 hours after AMI. A similar but weaker relation was observed for arrhythmias and high peak FFA levels but not high admission FFA levels. These results suggest that the arrhythmogenicity of FFA within the first 12 hours of AMI may depend partly on FFA levels that remain consistently high. Because of the rapid and wide fluctuation of FFA levels during this time, no single random value can be considered representative of the mean level, which may explain the conflicting results of previous studies.

Nordrehaug and Von Der Lippe[23] from Sweden determined serum potassium concentrations on admission and correlated them to the frequency of VF in 289 women and in 785 men with AMI, 92 of whom developed VF. Hypokalemia (serum potassium concentration ≤3.5 mmol/liter) was found in 122 patients (11%). The frequency of VF was significantly greater in patients with hypokalemia compared with normokalemia (serum potassium concentration ≥3.6 mmol/liter) (17% -vs- 7%). The increased risk of VF in the hypokalemic group was similar in women and men. While they were in the hospital, patients with hypokalemia developed VF significantly earlier than did normokalemic patients (median, 0.3 -vs- 7 hours). Hypokalemia was more common in women (17%) than in men (9%), and 55% of the hypokalemic patients had been treated with diuretics before admission compared with 22% of the normokalemic group. Hypokalemia on admission to the hospital predicts an increased likelihood and early occurrence of VF in patients with AMI.

Shock

Rosenkranz and colleagues[24] from Los Angeles, California, reviewed their initial clinical application of a cardioplegia system having as its basis the induction of cardioplegia with a warm (37°C) glutamate-enriched blood solution. Over 15 months 23 consecutive coronary patients requiring preoperative intraaortic balloon and inotropic drug support for cardiogenic shock underwent CABG. Twelve patients were given warm glutamate-enriched cardioplegic solution during the first 5 minutes of aortic clamping before multidose cold (4°C) glutamate blood cardioplegia was begun. Eleven patients received standard multidose cold blood cardioplegia without glutamate. All patients had comparably depressed LV performance preoperatively with extending AMI. There was no difference in the number of grafts, associated valve and aneurysm procedure, or cross-clamp time. All patients received warm blood cardioplegia reperfusion before aortic unclamping. The perioperative mortality was 2 of 23. Both patients who died received cold blood cardioplegia without glutamate. In addition to lower mortality, patients receiving warm glutamate blood cardioplegia exhibited better hemodynamics allowing earlier discontinuation of inotropic drug infusion (1.3 ± 0.5 -vs- 2.7 ± 0.8 days; p < 0.05) and intraaortic balloon support (1.2 ± 0.2 -vs- 3.6 ± 0.5 days; p < 0.05). Late mortality was 30%, resulting in a 65% overall survival rate. The operative principles evolving from this experience include the use of warm blood cardioplegic induction, glutamate enrichment, meticulous attention to cardioplegic distribution and grafting sequence, warm cardioplegic reperfusion before unclamping, and graft perfusion during construction of proximal anastomoses.

Right ventricular infarction

Although ischemic involvement of the ventricular septum (VS) occurs in patients with RV infarction, the potential functional significance of such involvement has not been previously explored. Mikell and colleagues[25] from Minneapolis, Minnesota, assessed ischemic involvement of the VS by measuring VS systolic thickening on M-mode echo in 10 patients with hemodynamically evident RV infarction. Six patients (group I) had decreased VS systolic thickening, an echo indicator of ischemia or infarction, but 4 (group II) did not. Group I had significantly higher RV filling pressures (19 ± 3 -vs- 12 ± 5 mmHg; p = 0.04) and RV end-diastolic echo dimensions (32 ± 8 -vs- 20 ± 3 mm; p = 0.02) than group II. Paradoxical septal motion was noted only in group I patients (p = 0.01). The LV filling pressures, LV end-diastolic dimensions, and systolic thickening of the LV posterior wall were not significantly different between the groups. Three group I patients died; all had decreased systolic thickening of both the VS and LV posterior wall. In each, necropsy confirmed infarction of the RV free wall, VS, and LV posterior wall. Thus, in patients with RV infarction, ischemic involvement of the VS has important consequences for both RV and LV function. Echo demonstration of ischemic abnormalities in both VS and LV posterior wall identifies a subset of patients with RV infarction with impaired prognosis.

The sensitivity and specificity of ST-segment elevation in the right precordial lead V_4R as an early indicator of RV infarction were examined by Klein and associates[26] from Tel-Aviv, Israel, in 110 patients admitted for inferior AMI. The sensitivity was 83%, the specificity, 77%, and the positive predictive value, 70% in 58 patients with RV infarction documented by necropsy or a combination of RNA and ≥1 of the following tests: echo, technetium-99m pyrophosphate scintigraphy, and hemodynamic monitoring. The negative predictive value was 88% because of its simplicity and its high sensitivity, and specificity recording of V_4R should be an intrinsic part of the early evaluation and ECG examination of inferior wall AMI.

Haupt and associates[27] from Baltimore, Maryland, studied 19 patients with proximal right coronary artery occlusions associated with AMI <30 days old. The RV infarct size, determined as a percentage of RV surface area, ranged from 0–19%. Correlation of 24 variables measuring infarct size, chamber size, and CAD did not demonstrate a significant correlation with the extent of RV infarction. However, estimates of the degree of obstruction to potential collateral flow into the right coronary arterial system from the LAD, especially through the moderator band artery, showed a significant positive correlation with infarct size. Among the 5 patients with >25% RV infarction, 4 had significant obstruction of the LAD system, resulting in potentially impaired collateral blood flow; the other patient had normal coronary arteries and embolic occlusion of the proximal right coronary artery with contraction band necrosis. The study suggests that collateral flow to the RV myocardium, especially through the moderator band artery, protects against massive RV infarction in the presence of proximal right coronary artery occlusion.

Thirty-seven patients with transmural inferior AMI were evaluated by Baigrie and associates[28] from Toronto, Canada, for evidence of RV damage. Hemodynamic criteria suggested that 29 patients (78%) had evidence of RV infarction, but only 5 (20%) of 25 patients had RV uptake of technetium pyrophosphate. Either 2-D echo or isotope nuclear ventriculography or both were performed in 32 patients; 20 studies (62%) showed evidence of global or RV wall motion alterations. These data suggest that RV involvement with transmural inferior AMI is common and includes not only infarction, but also dysfunction without detectable infarction. The RV dysfunction may be caused by previous AMI or myocardial ischemia.

To study the value of the ECG in diagnosing RV AMI in the presence of posterior or inferior LV AMI, ECG findings were analyzed by Braat and associates[29] from Maastricht, The Netherlands, in 67 patients who had had scintigraphy to pinpoint the location of the AMI. All 67 patients had inferior wall AMI. A 12-lead ECG with 4 additional right precordial leads (V_3R, V_4R, V_5R, and V_6R) was routinely recorded on admission and every 8 hours therafter for 3 consecutive days. Thirty-six to 72 hours after the onset of chest pain a technetium pyrophosphate scintigraphy and a dynamic flow study were performed to detect RV involvement, which was found in 29 of the 67 patients (43%). ST-segment elevation >1 mm in leads V_3R, V_4R, V_5R, and V_6R is a reliable sign of RV involvement. ST-segment elevation >1 mm in lead V_4R was found to have the greatest sensitivity (93%) and predictive accuracy (93%). The diagnostic value of a QS pattern in lead V_3R and V_4R or ST elevation >1 mm in lead V_1 was much lower. ST-segment elevation in the right precordial leads was short lived, having disappeared within 10 hours after the onset of chest pain in half of the patients with RV involvement. When ECGs are recorded in patients with an inferior AMI within 10 hours after the onset of chest pain, additional RV infarction can easily be diagnosed by recording lead V_4R.

Dell'italia and associates[30] from San Antonio, Texas, evaluated prospectively 53 consecutive patients with inferior (posterior) AMI by physical examination and right-sided cardiac catheterization within 36 hours of onset of symptoms to determine whether physical findings could separate such patients into those with and without associated RV AMI. Hemodynamic findings consistent with RV AMI were defined as RV pressure ≥ 10 mmHg and a RA/PA wedge pressure ratio ≥ 0.80. Eight patients (group 1) had hemodynamic evidence of RV AMI, whereas 45 patients (group 2) did not. Group 1, compared with group 2, had a lower cardiac index (1.8 ± 0.3 -vs- 2.6 ± 0.6 liters/min/M^2, and a lower RV stroke work index (4.1 ± 3.6 -vs- 7.3 ± 3.2 g/m/M^2). An elevated jugular venous pressure ≥ 8 cm H_2O was seen in 7 of 8 group 1 and 14 of 45 group 2 patients. In addition, a Kussmaul's sign, substantiated by hemodynamic findings, was seen in all 8 group 1 and in no group 2 patients. The absence of both an elevated jugular venous pressure and a Kussmaul's sign in patients with inferior AMI makes the presence of a hemodynamically signifcant RV AMI highly unlikely.

Angina pectoris

Williams and associates[31] from Seattle, Washington, determined the efficacy of surgical revascularization for postinfarction angina within 30 days of AMI. Eighty-four patients (82% were men and 18% women) with a mean age of 58 years underwent CABG following AMI because of postinfarction angina. Eleven patients (group A) had CABG within 24 hours of AMI, 21 patients (group B) within 7 days of AMI, and 71 patients (group C) within 30 days of AMI. Eighty-four patients (82%) had subendocardial AMI and 19 patients (18%) had transmural AMI. Most patients in group A had transmural AMI, whereas patients in groups B and C had a higher frequency of subendocardial AMI. There were 2 surgical deaths and both were in group C patients. It was necessary to use intraaortic balloon or inotropic support to treat major ventricular arrhythmias or to cope with perioperative AMI in 30 patients (29%), and 64% of these patients were in group A. Late follow-up (mean, 15 months) demonstrated no late AMI, and 93 patients (96%) were essentially free of angina. Thus, these data suggest that CABG within the first

30 days after AMI can be accomplished with an acceptable operative mortality in properly selected patients with postinfarction angina refractory to medical management.

Left ventricular thrombus

Keating and associates[32] from San Diego, California, studied 54 consecutive patients with anterior wall AMI to determine the frequency and natural history of mural thrombus formation. A 2-D echo was performed in the immediate post-AMI period. Multiple views were utilized. Standard criteria for defining mural thrombus formation and minimizing false positive readings were adhered to. Correlation with clinical data was obtained in all patients to define a subgroup at high risk for the development of a mural thrombus. Follow-up was obtained for all patients to assess the natural history of mural thrombus formation, treated and untreated, with regard to peripheral embolization. Seventeen patients (32%) had mural thrombus formation. Statistically significant ($p < 0.001$) correlation for mural thrombus formation was found with markedly elevated creatine kinase and lactate dehydrogenase levels and with apical dyskinesis. Ten patients with mural thrombi received anticoagulants. None has had clinically evident emboli at a mean of 11 months follow-up. Resolution of the mural thrombus was demonstrated with serial 2-D echo in 8 patients. Six of 7 patients who did not receive anticoagulation therapy had embolic events within 3 months (<0.001). None of the 36 patients without a mural thrombus has had a spontaneous clinical embolus.

To assess the relative diagnostic value of invasive and noninvasive cardiac techniques for the identification of LV mural thrombi in patients with LV aneurysms, Starling and associates[33] from San Antonio, Texas, evaluated 21 consecutive patients who had LV biplane cineangiography, 2-D echo, and equilibrium RNA completed within 1 week of surgery for aneurysmectomy or at necropsy. Thirteen (65%) of the 21 patients had a LV thrombus, and 6 of the 13 patients had a large thrombus (≥ 2 cm^2). Cineangiography detected a thrombus in 8 of the 13 patients (sensitivity, 62%); RNA detected a thrombus in 4 of the 13 patients (sensitivity, 31%). Compared with RNA, 2-D echo demonstrated a significantly higher sensitivity for thrombus (10 of 13 patients; $p < 0.01$). The other methods identified significantly more small thrombi compared with RNA ($p < 0.05$). No false positive diagnosis of thrombus was made by the 3 techniques.

AMI extension

To examine the prevalence, clinical significance, and problems in the diagnosis of AMI extension, 103 patients with AMI were studied by Buda and colleagues[34] from Toronto, Canada. Each patient underwent enzymatic infarct sizing in the initial 72 hours and then had quantitative creatine kinase (CK) MB analysis at 8-hour intervals over the remaining hospitalization. In addition, daily standard 12-lead ECGs and documentation of prolonged (>15 minutes) resting ischemic chest pain were recorded. An AMI extension, by CK-MB methods, occurred in 32 (31%) of 103 patients at 6 ± 0.3 days after initial AMI. Changes suggesting AMI extension on an ECG occurred in 14 (14%), but only 6 of these patients had extension by CK-MB. Similarly, recurrent chest pain following initial MI occurred in 28 (27%), but enzymatic extension was evident in only 11. Extension of AMI resulted in significantly greater early in-hospital mortality (16%) compared with those patients without AMI extension (2.8%, p < 0.05). Thus, AMI extension occurs commonly and may explain some early in-hospital deaths post-AMI. The usual clinical and ECG diagnostic parameters utilized are insensitive indicators of enzymatic AMI extension.

Rupture of left ventricular free wall, ventricular septum, or papillary muscle

Feneley and associates[35] from Darlinghurst, Australia, reviewed 49 patients with AMI in whom myocardial rupture occurred: 33 with rupture of the ventricular septum, 12 of the LV free wall, and 4 of a LV papillary muscle. Of the 19 patients with VSD, 9 underwent surgical repair of a postinfarction VSD and survived. The major determinant of survival was the preoperative hemodynamic status. Ten of 13 patients who developed cardiogenic shock preoperatively died, whereas none of the 6 patients who were not in cardiogenic shock died. Survival was not related to the site or size of infarction, extent of CAD, or magnitude of the left-to-right shunt. The 14 patients with isolated LV free wall rupture who developed mechanical cardiac arrest died at the onset of rupture, but 5 patients developed subacute heart rupture and 2 of these patients survived after emergency surgical repair. Two of the 4 patients with papillary muscle rupture underwent MVR, but both died in the early postoperative period; both patients who were not operated on died. Early detection and early surgical intervention are essential in the management of myocardial rupture complicating AMI. (I [WCR] do not understand why there were nearly 3 times as many ruptures of the ventricular septum as of the LV free wall.)

The results of 2-D echo, confirmed by oximetry, in 13 patients who had VSD after AMI were reported by Drobac and colleagues[36] from Toronto, Canada. Eight patients were men and 5, women; 5 had anterior and 8, inferior AMI. The 2-D echo revealed akinesis or dyskinesis of the ventricular septum (VS) in all 13 patients. In only 6 patients could a defect in the VS be directly visualized. The 2-D echo LV wall motion abnormalities correlated with ECG and angiographic site of AMI in all patients. Twelve patients had adequate saline contrast studies. Positive LV contrast (microbubbles entering the left ventricle through the VSD) was seen in 11 patients and negative RV contrast (washout of the RV bubbles by LV blood crossing the VSD) in 5 patients. At least 1 abnormality was present in every patient. The location of the VSD was determined by visualizing a VSD or by the site of the positive LV or negative RV contrast. Oximetry showed VSD shunts of 1.4/1–7/1, with no correlation between the degree of negative RV contrast and shunt size. Morphologic confirmation of VSD was obtained in 12 patients with agreement of VSD location by 2-D echo in all. Four of the 11 patients who underwent surgical repair died, and 2 patients died before surgery could be attempted. Thus, 2-D echo is a sensitive, rapid, and safe technique for diagnosing VSD after AMI. Positive LV contrast with or without negative RV contrast is more sensitive in diagnosis and localization of post-AMI VSD than direct echo visualization of the VSD.

The acute mechanical complications resulting from AMI are associated with a very high mortality. Recently an effort has been made to operate early in the course of patients having post-AMI VSD. Eight patients are reported by

Miyamoto and colleagues[37] from Los Angeles, California. These patients had VSD within 1–21 days of AMI and they were operated upon 8 hours to 18 days after septal rupture. All but 1 had low cardiac output syndrome necessitating intraaortic balloon pumping. The VSD was closed via a transinfarct ventriculotomy with an oversized folded double patch, the folded edge being incorporated into the ventriculotomy closure. Five patients also had CABG. There were no recurrent shunts. Six patients survived, 2 died postoperatively, 1 from an arrhythmia and the other while on biventricular bypass support. This report and others suggest that delay of operative intervention in the seriously ill patient produces no saluatory effect and may lead to irreversible subsystem dysfunction. Therefore early diagnosis and early operation appear indicated.

Nishimura and associates[38] from Rochester, Minnesota, reviewed the records of 17 patients (10 men and 7 women) in whom rupture of 1 LV papillary muscle occurred during AMI. Eight of the 17 patients underwent MVR and CABG during the AMI. The other 9 had the diagnosis of papillary muscle rupture confirmed at necropsy, and none of them had a cardiac operation. The ages of the 17 patients ranged from 44–80 years (mean, 64). The site of the AMI was inferior in 15 and anterior in 2. The onset of MR ranged from <24 hours to 28 days after AMI (mean, 6 days). Eleven patients presented with pulmonary congestion alone, and 6 of them remained stable and had subsequent MVP and CABG. Of these 11 patients, however, the condition in 5 initially remained stable with medical therapy alone and then suddenly deteriorated after 1–60 days, and all 5 died. Of the 6 patients who presented with shock plus pulmonary congestion, the 4 treated medically died, and 1 of the 2 treated operatively survived. The extent of the AMI at necropsy was small and limited to subendocardium in half the patients. Significant CAD was limited to 1 vessel in 7 of 14 patients. The unpredictable and rapid clinical deterioration and the limited extent of coronary atherosclerosis and AMI size suggest that early surgical repair should be strongly considered in patients with papillary muscle rupture during AMI.

PROGNOSTIC INDEXES

Age, sex, previous AMI, stroke, diabetes mellitus, past systemic hypertension, tachycardia at presentation, hypotension at presentation, and early arrhythmias

Patients registered by the 1971 Perth Coronary Register as having had an AMI were followed by Martin and colleagues[39] from Nedlands, Australia, for 9 years. Of the 1,078 patients studied, 77% survived the first 24 hours and 62%, the first 28 days; 0.3% were lost to follow-up. For the 666 patients alive at 28 days, the crude 1-, 5-, and 9-year survival rates were 88, 67, and 52%, respectively. The relation between 54 variables and the survival of patients alive 28 days after AMI was examined by life-table methods and the log-rank test, and then by fitting a proportional hazards model to the data. The important prognostic factors were age, sex, past history of AMI, stroke, diabetes mellitus, and systemic hypertension, tachycardia at presentation, hypotension at presentation, and the occurrence of arrhythmias as short-term complications. The most appropriate mathematical description of the joint effects of the prognostic factors was a multiplicative model with no interaction.

Q-wave -vs- non-Q-wave AMI

In this editorial Spodick[40] emphasizes, as have a number of others previously, that abnormal Q waves are not synonymous with transmural AMI and that non Q-wave or ST-T abnormalities are not necessarily synonymous with nontransmural or subendocardial AMI. In tables 2-2 and 2-3, Spodick summarizes some differences between Q-wave and non-Q-wave AMI.

Coll and associates[41] from Barcelona, Spain, prospectively assessed prevalence, prognosis, and coronary artery anatomy associated with non-transmural AMI in 458 consecutive men admitted to their coronary care unit with a first AMI. Cardiac catheterization was performed in 402 of the 436 survivors within 1 month of the acute event. Mean follow-up was 33 months (range 5–72). Nontransmural AMI was diagnosed in 28 patients (6%). These patients were younger (46 ± 10 versus 51 ± 7 years; $p < 0.001$) and had lower peak creatine kinase values (601 ± 319 -vs- 1,141 ± 923 U; $p < 0.01$) and better EF (63 ± 8 -vs- 46 ± 14; $p < 0.001$) than did their counterparts. Survivors of nontransmural AMI also had fewer affected arteries ($p < 0.001$) and a lower prevalence of total or subtotal occlusion (>90%) in the involved artery ($p < 0.01$). Mortality in the acute phase and long-term survival at 4 years (Kaplan-Meier) in patients with nontransmural AMI (94%) were similar to those in patients with transmural AMI (90%). The occurrence of new nonfatal coronary events was also similar in both groups of AMI

TABLE 2-2. *Q–wave infarction versus ST infarction: differences.*

	Q-WAVE INFARCT	S-T INFARCT*
Fresh thrombosis	More	Less
Collateral vessels	Fewer	More
Damage		
↑ Enzyme levels	Higher	Lower
↓ Tracer concentration (PET)	Homogeneous	Unequal
LV wall abnormality,†	More	Less
improved by bypass	Less or none	More
Tendency to expand	More	Less
Prodromal symptoms	Less	More
Vomiting	More	Less
Atrioventricular and intraventricular blocks	More	Fewer
Congestive failure	More	Less
Early mortality	More	Less
Recurrent infarction	Less	More

* Without QRS abnormality.
† Some studies differ.
PET = positron emission tomography.

TABLE 2-3. *Q–wave infarction versus ST infarction: similarities.*

Both either transmural or nontransmural
Number of diseased vessels
Degree of occlusion throughout coronary arteries
Ejection fraction*
Hypotension
Ventricular arrhythmia*
Late (>2 year) mortality

* Some studies differ.

survivors. Thus, in the absence of symptoms, more aggressive management to improve survival does not seem warranted after nontransmural AMI.

Krone and associates[42] from St. Louis, Missouri, presented follow-up results in 593 patients ≤7 years (mean, 4.7) after hospital discharge for their first AMI. Patients were grouped according to the presence or absence of Q waves on ECGs after the AMI and by peak serum glutamic oxalacetic transaminase (SGOT) level during hospitalization. Cardiac mortality varied. Patients with Q-wave infarcts and an SGOT level ≤240 IU/liter had a cardiac mortality of 3.1% a year, whereas patients with Q-wave AMI and an SGOT level >240 IU/liter had an 11% 6-month mortality and a 3.8% yearly cardiac mortality thereafter. However, patients with non-Q-wave (nontransmural) AMI had an excellent survival rate for 2 years (96.8%), which continued in patients aged ≤60 years thereafter. However, patients with non-Q-wave infarcts aged >60 years had a 12% yearly cardiac mortality in the third post-AMI year and an additional 12% died each year thereafter. Early mortality was related to enzyme level, whereas late mortality was a function of type (Q-wave or non-Q-wave) and age.

TABLE 2-4. *Coronary angiographic data.*

NUMBER OF SIGNIFICANTLY STENOSED VESSELS*	
Left main	3
3 vessels	2
2 vessels	19
1 vessel	49
0 vessel	13
Diameter reduction of IRV	
Occluded	33
>90 ≤99%	27
≥70 ≤90%	8
<70%	18
Collateral vessels present to IRV	38
Jeopardized collateral vessels† to IRV	17
Proximal LAD stenosis‡	20

* Luminal diameter reduction of ≥50% of LM or ≥70% of LAD, circumflex or right coronary arteries.
† Arising from a vessel which is itself ≥50% stenosed.
‡ LAD arterial diameter reduction by ≥90% before the first septal or diagonal branch, or both.
IRV = infarct–related vessel; LAD = left anterior descending artery.

Nicholson and associates[43] from Sydney, Australia, followed-up prospectively 86 consecutive hospital survivors aged ≤60 years of a first non-Q-wave AMI. Coronary arteriography was performed a median of 2 weeks after AMI. The size of the AMI was small (as judged by a mean peak creatine kinase level of 906 IU/liter); 90% were in Killip class I, and the mean LV EF was 60 ± 11% (±SD). Forty-nine patients had 1-vessel CAD (≥70% luminal diameter reduction), 19 had 2-vessel, 2 had 3-vessel, 3 had LM (≥50% luminal diameter reduction), and 13, minimal or no CAD (Table 2-4). Complete occlusion of the AMI-related artery was present in 33 patients. All 33 and an additional 5 patients had collateral vessels to the AMI area. During a mean follow-up of 25 months, 1 cardiac death and 4 recurrent infarcts (3 with non-Q-wave AMI) occurred. Angina occurred in 53 patients (62%) and responded medically in all but 7 who underwent coronary artery surgery. Angina after AMI occurred frequently in patients with severe proximal LAD CAD (≥90%), and in those with CAD (≥50%) in a vessel supplying collaterals to the infarct area. Because angina can be managed medically in most patients and the outcome is good, routine coronary angiography is not indicated in asymptomatic survivors ≤60 years of a first non-Q-wave AMI.

Serum enzymes

Davies and associates[44] from Preston, England, studied the response of total creatine kinase (CK) and CK-MB in 22 men, 3–6 months after AMI by a functional graded exercise test. Eleven patients (group A) completed the test without developing significant ECG abnormalities. Eleven subjects (group B) showed changes that necessitated premature termination of the test. No significant differences were observed before the functional graded exercise test between the groups in serum concentration of CK, CK-MB, and the percentage of CK-MB/CK (MB/CK%). The 2 groups were significantly different ($p < 0.01$) 24 hours after the graded exercise test in CK-MB and MB/CK%, but not in CK. In group B, CK and CK-MB rose significantly after the graded exercise test ($p < 0.05$), as did MB/CK% ($p < 0.01$). In group A only CK showed a significant rise ($p < 0.05$). It is probable that increases in CK-MB after exercise arise from myocardial tissue efflux, reflecting reversible ischemia. It is concluded from this study that CK-MB appears to be a specific indicator of myocardial ischemia and could, therefore, be of significant assistance in the clinical and functional assessment of the post-AMI patient.

Early noninvasive testing

When the course of an AMI has been complicated by angina pectoris, CHF, complex ventricular arrhythmias, or other serious cardiac problems, it is expected that the patient will undergo intensive evaluation and treatment before discharge. Cohn[45] from Stony Brook, New York, reviewed the role for cardiac testing by means of relatively new noninvasive procedures after AMI. This is true both for patients with initial AMI and for those who have had multiple AMI. These noninvasive tests, which are performed either before or very soon after hospital discharge, are safe, and their results are important not only in advising patients and their families about prognosis, but also in planning the best treatment program. Probably the single most important of these procedures is the low level exercise test performed 10–21 days after

AMI. This readily available procedure will greatly help the primary physician to determine which postinfarction patients without complications have an increased risk of dying in the subsequent year. This risk may be as high as 5–10 times that of patients with normal test responses. The risk is especially great when ST-segment depression is combined with hypotension or when the ST-segment depression is marked (>2 mm). Patients with these responses often require a particularly aggressive approach, including coronary arteriography and CABG. By contrast, patients with completely negative tests seldom require an aggressive approach. The role of RNA as a routine test is less well defined in the patient without complications. The exercise-thallium scintigram is important when the resting ECG is grossly abnormal, primarily because of the association between low EF and complex ventricular arrhythmias. The cost effectiveness of this test as a routine procedure in patients without complications is questionable, however, since many physicians order 24-hour ambulatory ECG for all post-AMI patients. The ambulatory ECG is much less expensive than RNA, and the results have both prognostic value and a direct influence on antiarrhythmic therapy.

Exercise testing

Ewart and associates[46] from Stanford, California, evaluated the effects of exercise testing 3 weeks after clinically uncomplicated AMI on subsequent physical activity in 40 consecutive men with a mean age of 52 ± 9 years. Patients' confidence in their ability to perform various physical activities was evaluated with self-efficacy scales that patients completed before and after a symptom-limited treadmill exercise test. Increases in confidence (self-efficacy) for activities similar to treadmill exercise (walking, stair climbing, and running) were greatest after treadmill exercise, whereas increases for dissimilar activities (sexual intercourse and lifting) were greatest after test results were explained by a physician and nurse. The intensity and duration of subsequent physical activity at home were more highly correlated with self-efficacy after treadmill exercise than with peak treadmill heart rate. Of the 8 patients whose treadmill tests were limited by angina pectoris, 7 had self-efficacy scores that remained low after treadmill testing or that decreased from initially high values after treadmill testing. These patients had lower peak heart rates and work loads than patients whose self-efficacy increased or remained high after treadmill testing. After AMI, patients' perception of their capacity for physical activity and their actual patterns of subsequent physical activity are influenced by early treadmill testing in a manner that is congruent with these patients' treadmill performance.

Cardiac catheterization studies have shown that patients with poor ventricular reserve show a marked increase in LV end-diastolic pressure and a decrease in LV stroke work with sustained static muscle contraction, whereas persons with relatively normal ventricular reserve show an increase in LV stroke work with little or no change in LV end-diastolic pressure. Based in part on these studies, it has been suggested that cardiac patients, especially those with more severe LV dysfunction, may be at risk for developing acute episodes of pulmonary congestion, dangerous arrhythmias, and myocardial ischemia with static exercise. In vocational and avocational activities, static exercise is often combined with dynamic exercise, thus adding a rapid-onset pressure load (afterload) to the myocardial demands of dynamic exercise. The effects of combining different levels of static work to dynamic exercise in patients after AMI have received minimal study. Consequently, activity guidelines given to post-AMI patients for this type of work are frequently tenuous, especially for patients with compromised LV function. Sheldahl and associates[47] from Milwaukee, Wisconsin, determined cardiovascular responses to carrying graded weight loads of 20–50 pounds in 52 patients after AMI ($\geq$2 months): 60% were stopped before completing the heaviest weight load because of an increase in diastolic BP to 120 mmHg (end point) or arm fatigue. Compared with symptom-limited graded dynamic exercise, peak systolic and diastolic BP were significantly greater (p < 0.05 and p < 0.01, respectively) with weight carrying, whereas peak heart rate, pressure-rate product, ventilation and oxygen consumption were significantly lower (p < 0.01). Ischemic responses were less frequent with weight carrying. Patients with severely reduced resting LV EF (<35%) tolerated the weight carrying test as well as patients with normal resting LV EFs (>50%). We conclude that 1) ischemic responses occur less frequently while carrying up to 50 pounds for 2 minutes than with symptom-limited dynamic exercise, 2) a significant number of patients have an increase in diastolic BP $\geq$120 mmHg while carrying objects that weigh 30–50 pounds for 2 minutes, and 3) a poor correlation exists between resting LV EF and tolerance for weight carrying.

Early radionuclide angiography

To assess the prognostic value of radionuclide ventriculography, Dewhurst and Muir[48] from Edinburgh, Scotland, followed 100 consecutive patients for 2 years after their first AMI. Ventricular performance was assessed by LV EF measured at rest 1 day before hospital discharge and again 1, 4, and 12 months later at rest and during submaximal exercise. The LV EF at discharge was below normal (<47%) in 74 patients and correlated well with abnormality of regional LV wall motion. Low LV EF (<30%) observed in 25 patients was poorly predicted either clinically, radiographically, or electrocardiographically. Peak serum creatine kinase correlated well with LV EF but there was a significant difference between anterior (46 patients) and inferior (54 patients) AMI with relative sparing of LV function after inferior AMI. The LV EF after inferior AMI was significantly higher both for transmural and subendocardial AMI, reflecting a variable degree of RV nephrosis. Within 2 years of first AMI, angina had developed in 32 patients, LV failure in 17, VT or VF in 4 patients, another AMI in 7, and 17 died suddenly. Low resting LV EF before discharge was associated with LV failure, ventricular arrhythmia, and sudden death (10 patients). Of the remaining patients, exercised 1 month after AMI, 27 showed a significant fall (>5%) in LV EF and 23 developed post-AMI angina, 4 had another nonfatal AMI, and 5 patients died. Radionuclide ventriculography with exercise testing thus identified 88% of patients who died suddenly in the first 2 years after AMI. This was superior to any other coronary prognostic indices currently in use and more predictive than the conventional end points of exercise testing (chest pain or ST-segment depression) used either separately or in combination.

Ong and associates[49] from New York City studied the relation of initial precordial ST-segment depression to anterior ischemia and eventual progno-

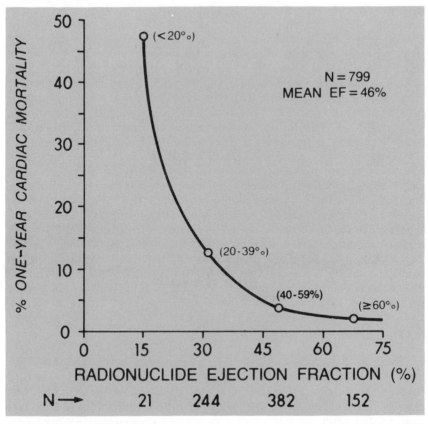

Fig. 2-4. Cardiac mortality rate in 4 categories of radionuclide ejection fraction (EF) determined before discharge. N = number of patients in total population and in each category. Of 811 patients in whom the EF was recorded, 12 were lost to follow–up during first year after hospitalization. Reproduced with permission from Multicenter Postinfarctionel Research Group.[52]

sis in 70 patients with inferior AMI. Early quantitative thallium-201 (^{201}Tl) scintigraphy and technetium-99m ventriculography were used to evaluate anterior ischemia. In comparison with patients without ST-segment depression, those with depression had lower global EF, 45 ± 10 -vs- 52 ± 7 (p < 0.01), lower inferoposterior regional EF, 40 ± 14 -vs- 52 ± 13 (p < 0.005), and larger ^{201}Tl defect index, 21 ± 7 -vs- 16 ± 6 (p < 0.005). In contrast, anteroseptal regional EFs were similar in the 2 groups, 54 ± 13 -vs- 56 ± 12 (p, NS), and the frequency of anteroseptal ^{201}Tl defects or redistribution abnormalities was not significantly different, 17 of 47 -vs- 5 of 23 and 8 of 31 -vs- 4 of 11 (p, NS). The predictive value of precordial ST-segment depression for mortality was low (21%) compared with the Killip class (75%), chest radiographs (67%), and EF (60%). Multiple logistic regression confirmed that the presence of ST-segment depression did not significantly improve the prediction of mortality when considered with these other risk factors. Thus, precordial ST-segment depression is a marker of larger MI size and not of

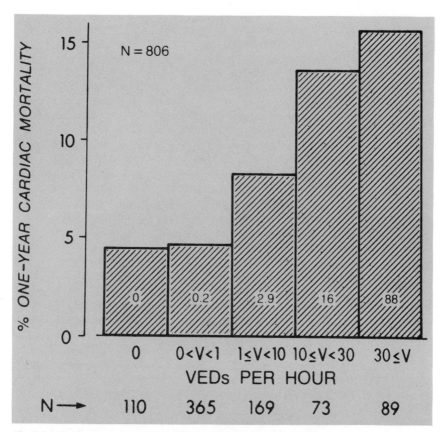

Fig. 2-5. Cardiac mortality rate in 5 categories for frequency of ventricular ectopic depolarizations (VEDs) determined by 24–hour Holter recording before discharge. N = patients in the total population and in each category. Of 819 patients with Holter recordings, 13 were lost to follow–up during the first year after hospitalization. Numbers within each of the boxes denote the median frequency of ventricular ectopy. Reproduced with permission from Multicenter Postinfarctionel Research Group.[52]

anterior ischemia. When examined with other variables reflecting MI size and LV function, precordial ST-segment depression was not a significant independent risk factor.

Botvinick and associates[50] from San Francisco, California, performed perfusion scintigraphy with ^{201}Tl, AMI scintigraphy with technetium-99m pyrophosphate (TcPYP), and equilibrium blood pool scintigraphy during the initial hospitalization for AMI in 25 patients without evidence of CHF. Each presented with advanced ECG rhythm and conduction disturbances requiring treatment. Scintigraphic findings during short-term hospitalization were related to the late clinical follow-up performed an average of 14 months later, when patients were grouped as asymptomatic, 8 patients; symptomatic, 9 patients; and deceased, 8 patients. Quantitation of perfusion abnormalities, TcPYP image abnormalities and LV EF revealed that the deceased group had significantly larger TcPYP abnormalities (36 ± 20 cm^2), absolute perfusion abnormalities (32 ± 16 cm^2), and perfusion abnormalities ex-

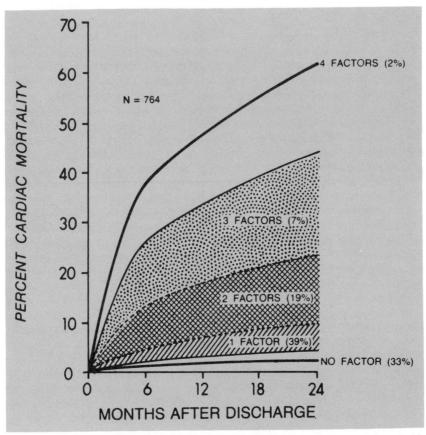

Fig. 2-6. Mortality curves after discharge and zones of risk, according to number of risk factors. Risk factors were NYHA functional class II–IV before admission, pulmonary rales, occurrence of 10 or more ventricular ectopic depolarizations per hour, and a radionuclide ejection fraction <0.40. Variation of risk within each zone reflects spectrum of relative risk for individual factors (Table 2) as well as range of multiplicative risks for combinations of 2 and 3 factors. Numbers in parentheses denote the percentage of the population with specified number of factors. See text for details. Reproduced with permission from Multicenter Postinfarction Research Group.[52]

pressed as a percentage of the projected LV area (42 ± 8%) than the asymptomatic group (13 ± 8 cm², 14 ± 6 cm², and 20 ± 9%). The percent perfusion abnormality was significantly larger in the deceased group (42 ± 8%) than in either the symptomatic group (35 ± 13%) or the asymptomatic group (20 ± 9%), and this parameter in the symptomatic group also differed from that in the asymptomatic group. The study indicates that patients with rhythm and conduction disturbances and without CHF during AMI may follow an uncomplicated late clinical course. Early scintigraphic measurements of AMI and perfusion correlate well with this outcome; however, EF could not differentiate among prognostic subgroups.

In patients who survive AMI, those with multivessel CAD generally have a worse prognosis than those with 1-vessel CAD. Some patients with significant

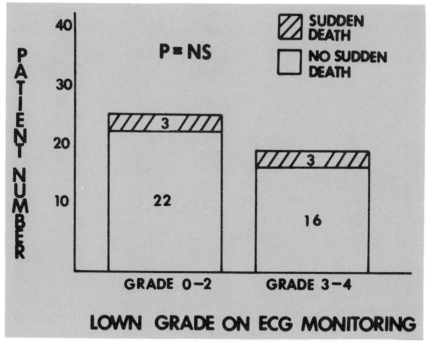

Fig. 2-7.   Relation of Lown grade of spontaneous ventricular arrhythmia noted during 24–hour ECG monitoring after MI is related to subsequent development of sudden cardiac death. Incidence of sudden cardiac death in patients with grade 0–2 ventricular arrhythmia does not differ from that in patients with grades 3 or 4. NS = not significant.

multivessel CAD, however, have a good prognosis, whereas some with significant 1-vessel CAD have a poor prognosis. Thus, although definition of coronary anatomy may be helpful, it is not a fail-safe prognosticator. In a retrospective analysis, Nicod and associates[51] from Dallas, Texas, assessed in patients with single and multivessel CAD the association of abnormalities at rest and during submaximal exercise testing with radionuclide ventriculography after AMI with major cardiac complications (death, recurrent AMI, severe angina, or CHF) in the ensuing 6 months. Coronary angiography and submaximal exercise testing with radionuclide ventriculography were performed within 3 months of each other in 42 patients. Eleven of the 16 patients with 1-vessel CAD had major cardiac complications. The subsequent course of these 16 patients was correctly predicted by LV EF ≤0.40 in 8 patients, by LV EF <0.55 in 7 patients, by failure of LV EF to increase by 0.05 units in 13 patients, and by an increase in LV end-systolic volume index (LV ESVI) during exercise >5% above baseline in 11 patients. Of the 26 patients with multivessel CAD, 24 had major cardiac complications. The subsequent course of these 26 patients was correctly predicted in 13 by LV EF ≤0.40, in 20 by LV EF <0.55, in 25 by a failure of LV EF to increase in LV ESVI by >5% during exercise. Thus, submaximal exercise testing with radionuclide ventriculography may provide valuable prognostic information concerning the occurrence of major cardiac events after AMI not only in patients with multivessel CAD, but also in those with 1-vessel CAD. Exercise-induced abnormalities of LV function may have greater prognostic importance than the delineation of coronary arterial anatomy or the assessment of residual LV function at rest.

Members of the Multicenter Postinfarction Research Group[52] assessed the role of physiologic measurements of heart function in predicting mortality after AMI. Most of the 866 patients enrolled in the multicenter study underwent 24-hour Holter monitoring and determination of the resting radionuclide ventricular EF before discharge. Univariate analyses showed a progressive increase in cardiac mortality during 1 year as the EF fell <0.40 (Fig. 2-4) and as the number of VPC exceeded 1/hour (Fig. 2-5). Only 4 risk factors among 8 prespecified variables were independent predictors of mortality (Fig. 2-6): an EF <0.40, VPC ≥10/hour, advanced New York Heart Association functional class before AMI, and rales heard in the upper two-thirds of the lung fields while the patient was in the coronary care unit. Various combinations of these 4 factors identified 5 risk subgroups with 2-year mortality rates ranging from 3% (no factors) to 60% (all 4 factors).

In 33 patients admitted with an extensive anterior AMI, Braat and associates[53] from Maastricht, The Netherlands, determined LV EF within 1 week after AMI using RNA. In 15 patients, sustained VT developed in the second and third week after AMI. Thirteen of the 15 patients had an LV EF <40%. Only 3 of 18 patients who did not develop late VT had an LV EF <40%. Of the 15 patients who developed VT, 8 had right BBB within 48 hours after the onset of chest pain. Right BBB was seen in only 3 of the 18 patients who did not develop VT. Thus, in patients with extensive anterior AMI, a radionuclide LV EF of <40% identifies a group at high risk of developing VT within a few weeks after AMI.

Abrams and associates[54] from San Antonio, Texas, evaluated 26 consecutive patients with acute clinical class II AMI to determine the ability of 2-D echo and gated equilibrium RNA to predict early morbidity and mortality. Within 48 hours of the onset of symptoms suggestive of AMI, right-sided heart catheterization, 2-D echo, and radionuclide ventriculography were performed. Important in-hospital complications developed in 7 patients, whereas the remaining 19 patients recovered uneventfully. The data obtained demonstrate that mean LV stroke work index was the only hemodynamic variable that differed significantly between patients who subsequently developed complications and those who did not. However, those patients with future complications had a significantly lower LV EF by 2-D echo (26 ± 5 -vs- 51 ± 10%; p < 0.001) and by radionuclide ventriculography (29 ± 9 -vs- 46 ± 12%; p < 0.001). Those patients with future complications also had greater extent of regional wall motion abnormalities than those patients without future events. Stepwise multiple regression analysis demonstrated that LV EF or wall motion index by 2-D echo or radionuclide ventriculography had additional predictive value in characterizing patients at risk for future complications.

Early electrophysiologic studies

Marchlinski and associates[55] from Philadelphia, Pennsylvania, compared the ability of programmed ventricular stimulation to identify risk of sudden death after AMI with 24-hour ECG assessment of ventricular ectopic activity and determination of LV dysfunction. Forty-six patients underwent pro-

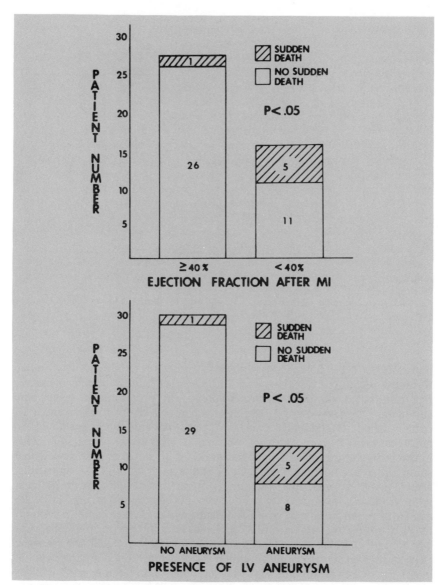

Fig. 2-8. Top, incidence of sudden cardiac death in patients with an EF of <40% after MI is significantly greater than in patients with an EF of ≥40%. Bottom, incidence of subsequent sudden cardiac death is significantly greater in patients who have a LV aneurysm after MI.

grammed stimulation 8–60 days (mean, 22) after AMI. Programmed stimulation consisted of single and double extrastimuli from the RV apex at 2 times diastolic threshold during ventricular pacing and normal sinus rhythm. Of the 46 patients, 44 underwent ECG monitoring ≥6 days after AMI. In 43 of the 46 patients, LV EF and the presence of LV aneurysm were determined. In response to programmed ventricular stimulation, 5 patients

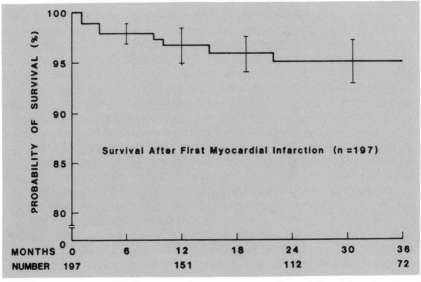

Fig. 2-9.   Cumulative life–table survival (±1 standard error of mean) for total study group of 197 survivors of a first MI aged ≤60 years.

had sustained VT, 5 had nonsustained VT (≥4 beats), 13 had intraventricular reentrant repetitive responses, and 23 had either bundle branch reentrant repetitive responses or no extra responses to programmed ventricular stimulation (negative study). During a mean follow-up of 18 months, 10 patients died, 6 suddenly. One of the 10 patients with sustained or nonsustained VT died suddenly, compared with 3 of 13 patients with intraventricular reentrant responses and 2 of 23 patients with a negative study (difference not significant). Of 25 patients with grades 0–2 ventricular ectopic activity, 3 died suddenly after AMI, compared with 3 of 19 patients with grades 3 or 4 activity (difference not significant) (Fig. 2-7). By comparison, the frequency of sudden death was greater in patients with an LV EF of <40% (5 of 16 -vs- 1 of 27 patients) or an LV aneurysm (5 of 13 -vs- 1 of 30 patients) (Fig. 2-8). Thus, using the described protocol, the response to programmed ventricular stimulation is not helpful in identifying patients at risk for sudden death after AMI. The presence of an LV aneurysm or EF of <40% appears to provide the greatest prognostic information with respect to risk for sudden cardiac death.

Early hemodynamic variables

To assess the hemodynamic monitoring in the coronary care unit for long-term prognosis after recovery from an AMI, Wolffenbuttel and associates[56] from Rotterdam, The Netherlands, reviewed the records of 2 groups of consecutive patients. From 254 patients, 32 (13%) died in the hospital and 9 patients had to be excluded from subsequent follow-up for various reasons. Four-year mortality among the 213 patients who were discharged from the

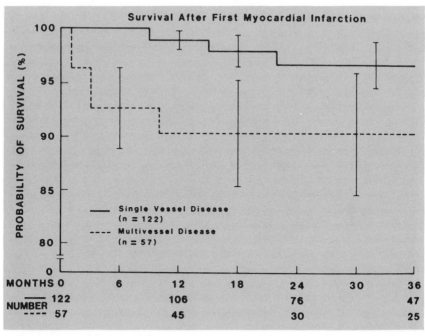

Fig. 2-10. Life–table survival (±1 standard error of mean) of patients with single– and multivessel disease.

hospital and could be followed up was 26%. Of the hemodynamic variables measured on admission a PA wedge pressure >18 mmHg and a mixed venous oxygen saturation <60% were not only associated with a high hospital admission rate but also with a high 4-year mortality, whereas a systolic BP <100 mmHg, an important prognosticator during admission to hospital, was only of minor significance thereafter. A negative value on admission of a specific index (0.24 times systolic BP [mmHg] minus 0.217 times PA wedge pressure [mmHg] plus 0.234 times mixed venous oxygen saturation [%] minus 13.1) developed for the prediction of short-term survival was also associated with a much higher 4-year mortality than a positive value. Low cardiac index on admission could be correlated with high mortality during the first 2 years after discharge, whereas only 9% of patients with a higher cardiac index died. Hemodynamic monitoring in the coronary care unit thus is not only relevant for the immediate prognosis, but a high mortality risk during hospital stay persists for several years after discharge.

Early coronary angiography

Roubin and colleagues[57] from Sydney, Australia, followed for a median of 24 months 229 hospital survivors of AMI aged ≤60 years who underwent coronary arteriography a median of 2 weeks after AMI. In 62% of the patients, AMI was the first presentation of CAD and 75% were in clinical

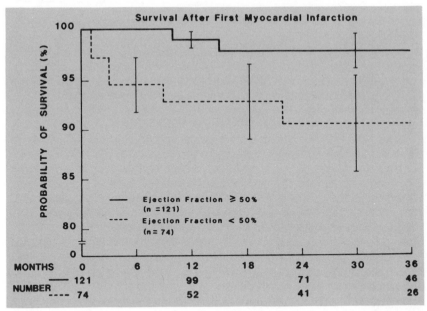

Fig. 2-11.   Life–table survival (±1 standard error of mean) for patients with EF ≥50% and <50%.

Killip class I. Overall outcome was good: 96% survival at 1 year, 95% survival at 2 years. This was due to the high prevalence of patients with 1-vessel CAD (58%) with a survival of 99% at 1 year and 96% at 2 years. Only 9% of patients had 3-vessel CAD and they had an 85% survival at 1 year. Eleven patients died and 23 had CABG. In this cohort of younger patients (mean age, 51 years), prophylactic therapy, such as beta blocking agents, may not be justified because of the lower mortality, and they might be reserved for identifiable high risk groups.

To relate coronary anatomy and LV function to prognosis, Abraham and associates[58] from Sydney, Australia, followed for a median of 24 months (range, 12–61) 197 of 269 consecutive survivors of a first AMI ≤60 years old, all of whom had undergone prospective cardiac catheterization a median of 2 weeks after initial hospitalization. Seventy-two patients were excluded from angiography because of early death (9 patients), severe non-CAD (44 patients), AMI complications (6 patients), or patient refusal (13 patients). The presence of multivessel CAD was only 30% and unrelated to the site of AMI or presence of Q waves but was increased in patients with previous angina pectoris or those in Killip class II or III. There were only 8 deaths from heart disease. The survival rate at 12 months was 97 ± 1% and at 24 and 36 months, 95 ± 2% (Fig. 2-9). Nineteen patients underwent coronary revascularization surgery. Because the number of deaths was small, the differences in survival between patients with single or multivessel CAD and normal or depressed EF did not reach significance (Fig. 2-10, 2-11). Survivors of a first AMI ≤60 years old have a low prevalence of multivessel CAD and a good prognosis.

TREATMENT

Intracoronary streptokinase

Goldberg and associates[59] from Philadelphia, Pennsylvania, studied the effects of coronary recanalization on arrhythmogenesis in patients undergoing intracoronary (IC) thrombolysis during the early hours of AMI. Catheterization, ventriculography, coronary angiography, and IC streptokinase (STK) infusion were performed in 22 patients. Twenty-one of 22 had thrombotic total occlusion of the infarct-related artery. Sixteen of the 21 had rapid persistent restoration of coronary flow. One patient had transient thrombolysis with reocclusion by the end of the procedure. In 12 of the 17 patients, restoration of antegrade coronary flow was accompanied by transient arrhythmia. In these 12 patients, coronary angiography within seconds of onset of arrhythmia showed artery patency in a previously totally occluded artery. Two additional patients developed arrhythmias during STK infusion but after reperfusion had already been established. Accelerated idioventricular rhythm was most often noted. Sinus bradycardia and AV block with hypotension occurred during restoration of flow in arteries supplying the LV inferoposterior wall. Thus, these arrhythmias are useful noninvasive markers of successful reperfusion during thrombolytic therapy in AMI.

Reflex hypotension and sinus bradycardia are commonly associated with AMI, especially of the inferior LV wall where most cardiac receptors with vagal afferents that are stimulated during coronary occlusion are located. To determine whether reperfusion of an acutely ischemic area can activate cardiac reflexes, changes in heart rate, arterial pressure and rhythm were correlated by Wei and coworkers[60] from Boston, Massachusetts, with the time course and location of IC thrombolytic therapy in 41 patients with AMI. Of the 27 patients with successful reperfusion, 17 developed significant transient bradycardia and hypotension and 1 became tachycardic and hypertensive at the time of recanalization. Spontaneous reversion of the bradycardia and hypotension occurred definitely in 6 patients and possibly in more (9 reverted after atropine and 2 after fluids). A positive correlation existed between the changes in heart rate and BP in contrast to the usual inverse relation when baroreceptors are stimulated. Two of the 3 patients in whom reperfusion was transient also developed hypotension and bradycardia. In contrast, all 11 patients with persistent occlusion demonstrated no reflex cardiovascular changes during IC thrombolytic therapy. Thus, successful reperfusion in AMI stimulates cardioinhibitory and vasodepressor (Bezold-Jarisch) reflexes. These observations raise the possibility that the transient hypotension and bradycardia observed during AMI, particularly inferior AMI, may sometimes reflect the occurrence of spontaneous reperfusion of the acutely ischemic myocardium.

Cowley and colleagues[61] from Richmond, Virginia, obtained serial coagulation studies in 25 patients treated with IC STK infusion for AMI (23 patients) or coronary insufficiency (2 patients) to determine the frequency of systemic fibrinolytic activity. Clotting studies were obtained before and after infusion and at 4-hour intervals until normalization. The IC thrombolysis was successful in 20 of 23 patients with AMI, and STK dosage in this study was 201,000. Systemic fibrinolytic activity defined as >70% reduction of fibrinogen using a functional assay occurred in 22 of 25 patients and was present at a mean STK dosage of 119,000 IU. Fibrinogen in the total population decreased from 342–87 mg/dl. In patients with systemic effect, the mean fibrinogen level after infusion was 17% of baseline, increased to 43% at 24 hours, and returned to normal at 30 hours. Plasminogen decreased to 7% of baseline activity after infusion, was 44% of baseline at 24 hours, and returned to normal at 48 hours. Intraprocedural sampling during infusion showed reduction of fibrinogen by 25% after 30,000 IU and by 71% at 120,000 IU; plasminogen decreased by 50% after 30,000 IU and by 84% at 120,000 IU. Prothrombin time increased from 12–22 seconds after infusion and returned to normal at a mean of 18 hours after infusion. Partial thromboplastin time was markedly prolonged, (>100 s) after infusion, returned to <2 times control at 5 hours and returned to normal at 9 hours after infusion. Fibrinogen degradation products were <10 μg/ml before infusion, increased to >40 μg/ml after infusion and remained >40 μg/ml in 40% of patients at 24 hours after infusion. These data demonstrate that systemic fibrinolytic activity occurs in a high percentage of patients with low dose IC STK infusion and that coagulation variables may be altered for 24–48 hours after infusion.

The effect of recanalization of the infarct artery on LV function was assessed by DeFeyter and colleagues[62] from Amsterdam, The Netherlands, 6 to 8 weeks after AMI in 2 groups: patients who had STK-induced recanalization during the acute phase and control patients who had spontaneous recanalization. The EF and severity of LV wall motion abnormalities in 100 patients with recanalization were compared with those in 78 patients with persistent occlusion of the infarct artery. Among patients with inferior AMI, LV function was significantly better in those with spontaneous and STK-induced recanalization than those with persistent occlusion of the infarct artery in the control group. Among anterior AMI patients, LV function was significantly better in those with STK-induced recanalization than in those with spontaneous recanalization or persistent occlusion in the control group. Thus, these investigators concluded that recanalization has a beneficial effect on LV function in patients with AMI.

From a prospective randomized trial, Khaja and associates[63] from Detroit and Ann Arbor, Michigan, compared IC administration of STK with dextrose placebo within 6 hours after the onset of symptoms of AMI in 40 patients. The baseline clinical, hemodynamic, and angiographic findings were similar in the control and STK-treated groups. Reestablishment of flow occurred in 12 of 20 patients treated with STK and in 2 of 20 given placebo (p < 0.05). The LV function, angiographic EF, and regional wall motion, measured before and immediately after intervention, and serial radionuclide EFs, measured at treatment, at 12 days, and at 5 months, were compared according to type of treatment (STK -vs- placebo) and outcome of therapy (reperfusion -vs- no reperfusion). No statistically significant differences between groups were found (Fig. 2-12). Thus, although STK was more effective than placebo in achieving reperfusion, no improvement of LV function as a result of reestablished coronary flow was detected. Several letters concerning the studies on coronary thrombolysis from IC STK were published in the November 3, 1983, issue of *The New England Journal of Medicine*.

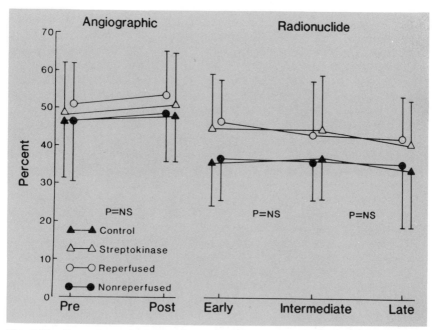

Fig. 2-12. Comparison of angiographic and radionuclide mean EF in the control and streptokinase groups, and in the reperfused and nonreperfused groups. NS = not significant; verticle bars represent standard deviations at each point. Reproduced with permission from Khaja et al.[63]

Anderson and associates[64] from Salt Lake City, Utah, randomly assigned 50 patients with AMI to receive either IC STK or standard (control) therapy within about 3 hours after the onset of chest pain. Coronary perfusion was reestablished in 19 of 24 patients receiving STK. The STK alleviated pain (as indicated by differences in subsequent morphine use), and the Killip class was significantly improved after therapy, as were changes in radionuclide EF between days 1 and 10 in surviving patients (+3.9 -vs- −3.0%; p < 0.01) (Fig. 2-13). The echo wall motion index also showed greater improvement after STK treatment (p < 0.01). The STK therapy was associated with rapid evolution of ECG changes, which were essentially complete within 3 hours after therapy, but loss of R waves, ST elevation, and development of Q waves in the convalescent period were greater in the control group (p < 0.01). The time required to reach peak plasma enzyme concentrations was significantly shorter after STK. The frequency of early and late ventricular arrhythmias was not affected by treatment. This article was followed by an editorial on this subject by Swan[65] from Los Angeles, California.

Schwarz and associates[66] from Heidelberg, West Germany, estimated a quantity of myocardium that can be salvaged by reperfusion in transmural AMI by serial analysis of creatine kinase (CK) activity in 41 consecutive patients with AMI who underwent IC thrombolysis. Enzymatic estimate of AMI size was calculated using an average (method A) and an individually determined elimination constant (method B). The LV EF 4 weeks after successful thrombolysis (cineangiogram) correlated inversely with AMI size

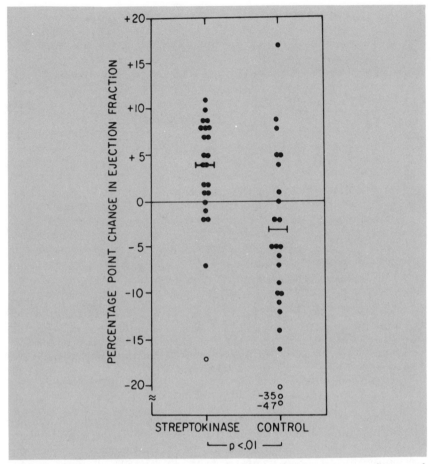

Fig. 2-13. Absolute percentage point change in EF (day 10 vs. day 1) in streptokinase and control groups, and mean EF in surviving patients (solid circles). Deaths are indicated by open circles, assuming a value of 0 on day 10. Reproduced with permission from Anderson et al.[64]

(method A: r = −0.85; method B: r = −0.76; both p < 0.001). Patients with recanalization within 4 hours after the onset of symptoms were assembled in group A_1 (n, 13, early reperfusion), and patients with successful recanalization after 4 hours in group A_2 (n, 16, late reperfusion). Group B consisted of 12 patients without reperfusion. The AMI size in group A_1 was 21 CK gram equivalents (g Eq) (method A) and 23 CK g Eq (method B), in group A_2 50 CK g Eq (method A) and 54 CK g Eq (method B), and in group B 73 CK g Eq (method A) and 63 CK g Eq (method B). Mean values in group A_1 were lower than in group A_2 and group B (p < 0.05) (Fig. 2-14). Thus, AMI size was significantly reduced to about one-third after early reperfusion compared with no reperfusion. In contrast, AMI size was not significantly reduced after late reperfusion.

Although IC thrombus may be important in transmural AMI, its occurrence in unstable angina and in nontransmural AMI has not been

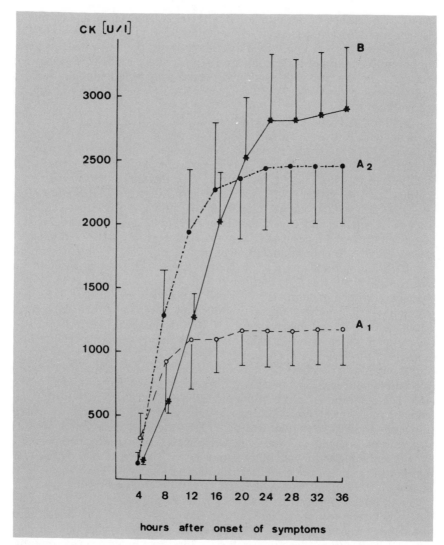

Fig. 2-14. Total appearance curves of creatine kinase (CK) activities which were averaged at 4 hourly intervals for 3 groups: group A_1 = reperfusion within 4 hours; group A_2 = reperfusion after 4 hours; group B = no reperfusion. The plateau of the curve of group A_1 was lower than that of both other groups (p < 0.05).

established. To determine whether IC thrombus does occur in these latter 2 syndromes, Mandelkorn and associates[67] from Philadelphia, Pennsylvania, performed coronary arteriography before, during, and after IC nitroglycerin and STK infusion in 17 patients. None of the 8 patients with nontransmural AMI and 1 of the 9 patients with unstable angina responded to IC nitroglycerin. Seven of 8 patients with nontransmural AMI and 4 of 9 patients with unstable angina responded to STK infusion with opening of the occluded artery, an increase in stenotic diameter, dissolution of an intracoronary filling defect, or a combination of these. Serial opening and closing of ischemia-related arteries occurred spontaneously and in response to STK in some patients in whom presumed thrombolysis was demonstrated. Evidence of presumed thrombolysis was not seen in any patient studied >1 week from the onset of the rest pain syndrome. Thus, these arteriographic findings suggest that a portion of the occlusion of the coronary artery is due to thrombus.

Smalling and colleagues[68] from Houston, Texas, prospectively studied 188 patients with AMI from August 1980 to September 1982: 136 were entered into an IC STK study; the remaining 52 patients, who either met exclusion criteria or refused to participate, served as a control group and were treated as those in the study group except that they did not undergo emergency cardiac catheterization. With successful reperfusion up to 18 hours after onset of chest pain, mean LV function in the study group improved (EF was 39% on admission and 46% at discharge). Mean EF in control patients and those not achieving reperfusion did not change from admission to discharge. Mean EF at 6-month follow-up was not significantly different than at discharge in the study group or the control group. Total cardiac mortality in the control group was 19% compared with 10% in the study group. When patients admitted in pulmonary edema or shock were excluded, total cardiac mortality in the study group was significantly lower (4%) than the control group (13%). The administration of IC STK during evolving AMI up to 18 hours after onset of chest pain may result in decreased mortality and sustained improvement in LV function.

The Bezold-Jarisch reflex, an inhibitory reflex characterized by bradycardia and hypotension, is induced by stimulation of receptors situated in the LV. These receptors signal in nonmyelinated vagal afferent fibers and respond to chemical, mechanical, or metabolic stimuli. In the cat, increased discharge from LV receptors was noted after coronary occlusion as well as reperfusion. Ischemia-activated vagal afferent receptors are located primarily in the inferoposterior wall of the canine heart. The exact location of similar receptors in man has not been determined experimentally. However, the high incidence of bradycardia-hypotension syndrome observed during the early phase of inferior myocardial infarction strongly suggests that in the human heart such receptors are situated in the inferoposterior LV wall. Esente and associates[69] from Syracuse, New York, reported the occurrence of bradycardia and hypotension (Bezold-Jarisch reflex) induced by myocardial reperfusion. Among 92 patients undergoing interventional catheterization for IC thrombolysis in an early phase of AMI, LAD, right coronary, and LC arteries were identified as the "infarct vessel" in 44, 41, and 7 cases, respectively. The Bezold-Jarisch reflex occurred in 15 of 23 patients (65%) after right coronary recanalization and in 1 of 34 patients after LAD recanalization. The reflex also was observed in 4 (22%) of 18 patients with nonoccluded or nonrecanalized right coronary arteries. The average time from onset of symptoms to right recanalization was significantly shorter (p < 0.01) among patients in whom the reflex did not develop. Atropine, postural changes, or temporary pacing, or all 3, were generally sufficient to control symptoms. The findings of this study are substantially parallel to those reported by others and confirm that reperfusion of the inferoposterior myocardium is capable of stimulating a cardioinhibitory reflex. Follow-up data available in 15 patients with occluded and recanalized right coronary arteries indicate that the occurrence of the Bezold-Jarisch reflex after reperfusion is not a reliable predictor of myocardial salvage.

Blanke and coworkers[70] from New York City assessed ECG changes in 15 patients in whom IC STK recanalized a totally occluded LAD coronary artery during AMI. These results were compared retrospectively with those in 22 comparable conventionally treated patients who underwent catheterization during AMI. Before angiography, no significant differences were found in the sum of ST elevation, the sum of R waves, or the number of Q waves in leads V_1–V_6. The sum of ST elevation was significantly lower in the STK group than in control groups at all times after angiography. The sum of R waves declined and the number of Q waves increased in both groups during the first 12 hours, but there was no further change in the control group, whereas in the STK group a significant increase in the sum of R waves and a decrease in the number of Q waves followed. There was a significant correlation between long-term ECG sum of R waves and number of Q waves and angiographic findings (EF and akinetic segment length). Thus, the Q-wave regression and increase in sum of R waves after STK suggests that jeopardized myocardium was salvaged by reperfusion.

Sheehan and associates[71] from Seattle, Washington, and Hamburg, West Germany, studied the ability of IC STK infused early in patients with AMI to salvage LV function in 62 patients who underwent contrast angiography immediately after STK and 6 ± 7 weeks later. Ten nonrevascularized patients had no lysis or reocclusion. Of 42 patients with thrombolysis, 22 with optimal reperfusion underwent CABG to prevent rethrombosis (STK + CABG group) and 20 did not (STK group). Motion was measured at 100 chords around the left ventricle and expressed in SD from the normal mean. Hypokinesia was computed as the mean motion of chords in the infarct artery territory and hyperkinesia on the opposite wall was similarly computed. Hypokinesia improved ≥1 SD/chord in 9 STK + CABG patients (41%), 8 STK patients (30%) (p, NS -vs- STK + CABG) and 0 nonrevascularized patients. However, the EF did not change because it was normal in AMI despite severe hypokinesia due to hyperkinesia on the opposite wall, and a subsequent decrease in hyperkinesia masked significant improvement in hypokinesia. Thus, regional wall motion must be measured to assess the effect of therapeutic interventions on LV function adequately. Early thrombolysis in AMI results in improved LV function. The main benefit of CABG is to prevent rethrombosis.

Schofer and associates[72] from Hamburg, West Germany, evaluated 31 patients with AMI undergoing IC thrombolysis. The IC thallium-201 scintigrams were obtained before and 30–60 minutes after thrombolysis and technetium-99m pyrophosphate scintigraphy simultaneously after thrombolysis in 16 of the 31 patients. Two patients with inferior AMI had a normal LV cineangiogram with no initial significant LV thallium defect. Eight patients had an improvement in regional EF and all 8 had substantial new thallium uptake after thrombolysis. In 5 patients, regional EF improved (20–40%; p < 0.01) and in 3 of these there was new thallium uptake, but large residual defects after thrombolysis. The remaining 2 patients had new thallium uptake, but technetium-99m pyrophosphate accumulation in the area of new thallium uptake. In 9 patients with no significant change in regional EF despite thrombolysis, the initial thallium defect remained unchanged in 7; 2 patients showed new thallium uptake with technetium-99m pyrophosphate accumulation in the same area. In 7 patients in whom thrombolysis failed, there was no change in thallium defect size or regional EF, and IC injection of technetium-99m pyrophosphate revealed a localized accumulation in the area of the thallium defect. These data suggest that combined IC thallium and technetium-99m pyrophosphate scintigraphy is helpful in predicting regions of myocardial salvage and in identifying areas of reversible cellular damage immediately after IC thrombolysis.

Serruys and associates[73] from Rotterdam, The Netherlands, described their experiences with IC STK infusion with or without associated PTCA during AMI over a 12-month period. Of 105 patients undergoing cardiac catheterization during AMI, 64 were recanalized with 250,000 units of STK, but in 25 patients recanalization was not achieved. In the remaining 16, the infarct-related artery was patent at the time of the procedure. Eighteen of the 78 who had a patent infarct-related artery at the end of the recanalization procedure underwent PTCA immediately afterward. Postlysis angiograms were analyzed quantitatively with a computerized measurement system. The contours of the relevant arterial segments were detected automatically. Reference diameter, minimal obstruction diameter, length of the narrowings, and percentage diameter reduction were averaged from multiple views. In 31% of our patients a diameter stenosis of <50% was found, whereas ⩾70% was seen in only 19%. Eleven stenotic lesions, recanalized at the acute stage, reoccluded in the short term, and in the long term 8 other patients sustained a reinfarction in the same myocardial territory. Seventeen of the 19 recanalized lesions had a diameter stenosis ⩾58%. Thus, combining recanalization and angioplasty may be useful. In these patients, the mean diameter stenosis decreased from 59–30% and mean pressure gradient from 41–8 mmHg. Late follow-up showed reocclusion in 1 patient. Although PTCA does not seem to be mandatory at the acute stage in most patients, it is feasible to undertake in one sitting and seems to prevent reocclusion in patients selected on the basis of quantitative angiographic criteria.

The rate and form of CK-MB enzyme release following reflow to ischemic myocardium has not been examined previously. In an investigation by Shell and colleagues[74] from Los Angeles, California, they examined the combined CK-MB time activity curves during transmural AMI in a group of patients receiving conventional therapy (CAMI) (n, 109), and in a group of 9 patients with successful reperfusion by fibrinolytic therapy (RAMI). The average time of reflow in the latter group was 4.2 ± 1.7 hours (mean ± SD) following the onset of symptoms. The average time to peak CK-MB for the CAMI group was 18.3 ± 5.5 hours and for RAMI it was 9.9 ± 1.1 (p < 0.001). At hour 4 (about the time of reflow), the 2 groups had similar CK-MB elevations (CAMI, 11 ± 7; RAMI, 13 ± 11 IU/liter). By hour 6 (reflow + 2 hours), the RAMI CK-MB values were significantly higher (55 ± 33 -vs- 20 ± 15 IU/liter; p < 0.02) than the CAMI group, demonstrating an increase in the release rate of CK-MB associated with reperfusion. It was concluded that in the human reflow to the ischemic myocardium significantly augments the release rate of CK-MB.

Cribier and associates[75] from Rouen, France, utilized IC STK in 80 patients during AMI. The average delay between onset of symptoms and STK infusion was 3.6 hours. Thrombolysis was successful in 64% of the 80 patients. No serious complications related to the procedure occurred. Of 12 patients in cardiogenic shock, recanalization was achieved in 4, of whom 2 survived. To evaluate the LV salvage resulting from early recanalization, the last 58 patients had a second LV angiogram and further coronary angiograms 21 ± 10 days later and 16 patients had a third study 3 months later. From the LV angiogram in the right anterior oblique projection, the EF and 2 graphic variables of regional wall motion were computed quantifying the hypokinetic zone. Patients were divided into 2 groups, according to the patency of the infarct-related artery at the second control: group 1 consisted of 28 patients with successful recanalization confirmed, and group 2 of 30 patients in whom no recanalization was achieved or secondary reocclusion had occurred. At the second study the EF was unchanged in group 1 but had significantly decreased in group 2. Regional wall motion improved in group 1 and worsened in group 2, more so in patients without recanalization than in those in whom secondary reocclusion had occurred. The third study showed a further decrease in EF in group 2. A progressive decrease in percentage residual stenosis was observed in group 1. This sequential angiographic study confirms the partial myocardial salvage resulting from early coronary recanalization during AMI.

To evaluate the relative thrombolytic efficacy and complications of IC -vs-high dose short-term intravenous (IV) STK infusion in patients with AMI, Rogers and colleagues[76] from Birmingham, Alabama, performed baseline coronary arteriography and then randomly allocated 51 patients with AMI to receive either IC (n, 25) or IV (n, 26) STK. Patients getting the drug by the IC route received 240,000 IU of STK into the infarct-related artery over 1 hour, and those getting the drug by the IV route received STK 500,000 IU over 15 minutes (n, 10) or 1,000,000 IU over 45 minutes (n, 16). Angiographically observed thrombolysis occurred in 76% of the patients receiving IC STK, in 10% of the patients receiving 500,000 IU of IV STK and in 44% of the patients receiving 1 million IU of IV STK. Among patients in whom thrombolysis was observed, mean elapsed time from onset of STK infusion until lysis was 31 minutes in patients receiving IC STK and 38 minutes in those receiving IV STK. Among patients in whom IV STK "failed," IC STK in combination with IC guidewire manipulation recanalized only 7%. Fibrinogen levels within 6 hours after STK were significantly lower in the patients receiving IV STK than the levels in those receiving IC STK, but were similar 24 hours after STK in both groups. Bleeding requiring transfusion occurred in 1 patient in each group. Hemorrhagic complications were few. Although the thrombolytic efficacy of IC STK was superior to that of high dose, short-term IV STK, the higher dose IV regimen achieved thrombolysis in 44% of patients.

Kennedy and associates[77] from Seattle, Washington, studied the efficacy of IC STK thrombolysis in AMI in 250 patients enrolled in a multicenter community-based study: 134 were randomly assigned to STK therapy and 116 were controls. All patients underwent LV angiography and coronary arteriography before the random assignment. The mean time from the onset of symptoms to hospitalization was 134 ± 144 minutes (SD), and the mean time to random assignment was 276 ± 185 minutes. Coronary reperfusion was achieved in 68% of the STK-treated group. The overall 30-day mortality was 18 (7%); there were 5 deaths in the STK-treated group (4%) and 13 in the control group (11%; p < 0.02). Fifteen of the 18 deaths occurred in patients with anterior AMI. Therapy with IC STK resulted in a nearly 3-fold reduction in the 30-day mortality after hospitalization for AMI.

Intravenous streptokinase

Schroder and coinvestigators[78] from Berlin, West Germany, performed short-term intravenous (IV) infusion of STK in 93 patients within 6 hours after the onset of AMI: 26 patients underwent angiography in the acute phase (group A) and 52 underwent angiography in the fourth week only (group B); 15 patients had no angiography. Seven patients died in the hospital and 6 had a nonfatal reinfarction. There were no bleeding complications during the study. In 11 of 21 group A patients, occluded coronary arteries were opened within 1 hour after the STK infusion was started. In 84% of groups A and B, the infarct-related coronary artery was patent in the fourth week. In 75% of the patent arteries, the residual luminal diameter stenosis was <70%. According to serial serum creatine kinase MB curves, recanalization was achieved mostly within 1–2 hours. Myocardial salvage was indicated by improvement in local contraction disorders in the recanalized group A patients and by the significant relation between infarct size and time from symptom onset to treatment in group B. These data suggest that a high dose short-term IV infusion of STK is a safe and efficient method of restoring coronary blood flow. Expeditious initiation of IV STK infusion is a critical determinant for early recanalization and salvage of myocardium. Patients with thrombotically subtotal occlusion probably receive the most benefit.

Percutaneous transluminal coronary angioplasty

In a study carried out by Hartzler and colleagues[79] from Kansas City, Missouri, successful PTCA was performed during evolving AMI in 41 patients. Catheterization was performed within 1 hour of presentation, from 1–12 hours (mean, 3.3) following symptom onset. In 17 of 29 patients with a total occluded coronary artery, successful thrombolytic therapy was followed by PTCA of a residual high grade atheromatous stenosis. Successful PTCA without prior thrombolytic therapy was employed in 11 of 12 subtotal coronary stenoses producing AMI syndromes and in 2 patients having critical coronary stenoses not immediately responsible for AMI. Three patients had early in-hospital reocclusion with reinfarction. One death occurred in a patient presenting with cardiogenic shock. All remaining patients had prompt pain relief, subsequent stable clinical courses, and no clinical or late angiographic evidence of coronary reocclusion. Dramatic improvement of regional and global LV function was evident in 22 of 27 patients undergoing late LV angiography. At follow-up, 94% of patients remained free of angina, although 3 required repeat dilation of recurrent stenoses. Thus, PTCA may be performed with or without thrombolytic therapy in selected patients with AMI and may reduce the likelihood of late reocclusion following successful thrombolytic therapy.

Coronary artery bypass grafting

Restoration of blood flow distal to the point of coronary occlusion may protect marginally perfused ischemic areas as well as myocardium that might otherwise progress to infarction. Successful early reperfusion may be accompanied by improvement in global and regional wall motion. For large patient groups little is known regarding the in-hospital and long-term fate of

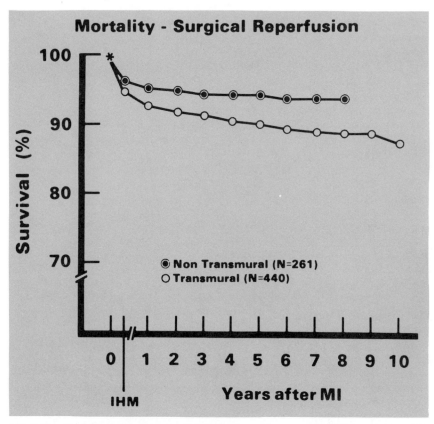

Fig. 2-15. Mortality in the 2 groups. Mortality for nontransmural group was 3.1%, while mortality for the transmural group was 5.2%. Reproduced with permission from DeWood et al.[80]

patients after surgical reperfusion for AMI. DeWood and colleagues[80] from Spokane, Washington, report on 701 patients who underwent CABG as treatment for AMI within 24 hours of symptom onset. This included 444 patients with transmural and 261 patients with nontransmural AMI. The hospital mortality was 5% in the transmural group and 3% in the nontransmural group (Fig. 2-15). Over the 10-year study period, total late mortality of the transmural group was 13% and the nontransmural group, 7%. For the transmural group, the major predictor of in-hospital mortality was presurgical cardiogenic shock, whereas LM CAD was the major factor associated with mortality in the nontransmural group. For the transmural group in those receiving early reperfusion, that is, within 6 hours from symptom onset, the short-term mortality was significantly lower than in the group receiving later reperfusion (>6 hours); (11 of 291, 4%; 12 of 149, 8%; p = 0.05) (Fig. 2-16). Furthermore the long-term outlook was less favorable in the patient group receiving late reperfusion. The total mortality between the groups was significantly different (24 of 291, 8%; 31 of 149, 21%; p < 0.01). The major cause of in-hospital mortality was presurgical cardiogenic shock that occurred in 12 of the 23 patients who died. These data are observational and

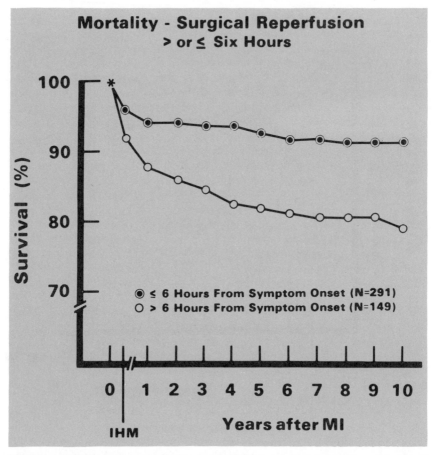

Fig. 2-16. Mortality for transmural MI group divided into subgroups receiving early (within 6 hr) or late (longer than 6 hr) reperfusion. The in–hospital mortality for early reperfusion group was significantly lower than that for late reperfusion group. This trend continued in the 10 year follow–up period. See text for details. Reproduced with permission from DeWood et al.[80]

not derived from a controlled or randomized trial. However, the findings suggest that early reperfusion for both transmural and nontransmural myocardial infarction is associated with low early and late mortality. Early reperfusion is associated with significantly lower short- and long-term mortality than is late reperfusion.

Nitrates

Nelson and associates[81] from Leeds, England, compared the immediate hemodynamic effects of intravenous furosemide (1 mg/kg) and intravenous isosorbide dinitrate (50–200 µg/kg/hr) in a prospective, randomized, between-group study in 28 men with radiographic and hemodynamic evidence of CHF after AMI. The diuresis induced by furosemide reduced the LV filling pressure and cardiac output and transiently raised systemic BP. In contrast, isosorbide dinitrate was accompanied by a reduction in systemic BP and peripheral resistance with the result that the cardiac output was not decreased despite a large fall in the pulmonary vascular and LV filling pressures. These results indicate that reduction of excessive preload by venodilation may be hemodynamically superior to that induced by diuresis in terms of both reducing myocardial oxygen consumption and maintaining peripheral perfusion.

Glyceryl trinitrate has been said to be contraindicated in patients with AMI. Its intravenous administration during AMI, however, has been associated with a beneficial effect as determined by ST-segment mapping. Jaffe and associates[82] from St. Louis, Missouri, administered intravenous glyceryl trinitrate and observed its effect on infarct size as determined by enzyme levels. Of the 85 patients studied with AMI, the 43 treated patients received glyceryl trinitrate within 10 hours of onset of symptoms (mean, 6 hours) and the dose was titrated to preset limits for changes in heart rate and BP. In patients with inferior wall AMI, infarct size estimated by enzymes in the treated group was 12 ± 2 -vs- 19 ± 4 creatine kinase (CK) gram equivalents per meter squared in the placebo group. A similar but statistically insignificant trend was observed for subendocardial AMI but no difference was observed for anterior wall AMI. Ventricular arrhythmias determined from 24-hour tapes were insignificantly more frequent in treated patients. Lidocaine requirements in treated and control patients were similar, as were requirements for morphine. These results indicate that intravenous glyceryl trinitrate can be administered safely during evolving AMI without invasive monitoring and it reduces the size of inferior wall AMI.

A prospective randomized study of intravenous (IV) nitroglycerin (NTG) administered 48 hours after AMI was undertaken by Flaherty and colleagues[83] from Baltimore, Maryland, to determine whether clinical improvement and/or evidence of preservation of ischemic myocardium could be demonstrated: 104 patients were randomly assigned to NTG and placebo groups. The NTG was infused at a rate sufficient to lower mean arterial pressure 10%, monitored noninvasively. When all NTG- and placebo-treated patients were compared, no significant differences in clinical or laboratory outcomes could be demonstrated. Placebo- and NTG-treated patients were retrospectively subdivided into early and late treatment groups (treatment begun < or > 10 hours after onset of symptoms). Early NTG treatment was associated with a lower incidence of infarct complications within the first 10 days, defined by new CHF, infarct extension, or cardiac death (15% in early NTG compared with a 39% in the other 3 groups). Mortality at 3 months was lower in the group treated early with NTG (15%) compared with a mean of 25% in the other 3 subgroups. No significant differences were found in peak CK blood levels, CK infarct size, or preservation of precordial R waves by serial ECG mapping. Among 49 patients with pretreatment and day 7–14 post-treatment LV EF measurements, improvement of >10% occurred in 35% of the NTG patients treated early compared with 6% of those treated late with NTG, 11% of those treated early with placebo, and 0% of those treated late with placebo. Similarly, in 68 patients in whom paired thallium scintigrams were taken, a decrease of >75% in the computer-determined thallium defect score was seen in 48% of NTG patients treated early, compared with 14% of NTG patients treated late, 33% of placebo patients treated early, and 0% of placebo patients treated late. Patients demonstrating significant scintigraphic improvement were treated earlier, tended to have less severe initial scintigraphic abnormalities, inferior rather than anterior location of AMI, a longer history of angina, and no prior history of CHF. Thus, IV NTG could not be shown to result in significant improvement in clinical or scintigraphic outcomes when the patient population was analyzed as a whole. After retrospective subgroup analysis, IV NTG protected ischemic myocardium in the subset of patients with small- to moderate-sized AMI when treatment was begun ≤10 hours of the onset of symptoms. The results of this trial also suggest that future clinical trials designed to show a reduction in the infarct size might limit patient entry to those admitted early after symptom onset and those with significant abnormalities in their admission scintigraphic studies.

To determine whether early NTG infusions in patients with AMI decreased the extent of LV asynergy, Jugdutt and coworkers[84] from Edmonton, Canada, used 2-D echo to measure asynergy segments either akinetic or dyskinetic at 4 serial short axis levels from base to apex in 22 patients with a first AMI. Patients were randomized between infusions of NTG or 5% dextrose in water within 6 hours after the onset of pain. NTG infusion rates were titrated to lower mean arterial pressure to an average level of 7% below control but not <80 mmHg and were maintained at this level for the duration of the infusions for 39 hours. After NTG, LV function improved as LV filling pressure decreased and the summation ST on precordial ST-segment mapping decreased. Computed CK infarct size was smaller in the NTG group than in the control group. Before the infusions, the mean extent of LV asynergy were similar in both groups: mitral 18 -vs- 21%; chordal 22 -vs- 23%; midpapillary 26 -vs- 24%; lower papillary 32 -vs- 29%. In addition, the computed total LV asynergy also was similar for these 2 groups before therapy. There was no change in LV asynergy from pretreatment values at 1 hour and 10 days among control subjects. In contrast, there was a significant decrease in LV asynergy from pretreatment values at 1 hour and 10 days with NTG: mitral 21 -vs- 10 -vs- 8%; chordal 23 -vs- 12 -vs- 10%, midpapillary 24 -vs- 13 -vs- 9%, lower papillary 29 -vs- 14 -vs- 10%; total, 25 -vs- 12 -vs- 9%. Thus, the prompt decrease in LV asynergy in the NTG group persisted for at least 10 days or 7–9 days after NTG infusions were stopped. These effects on hemodynamics, summation of ST segment, CK infarct size, and asynergy suggest that careful early and prolonged low dose NTG infusion might reduce the extent of infarction.

Beta blockers

Braunwald and associates[85] from Boston, Massachusetts, summarized beneficial effects of beta adrenergic blockade on ischemic myocardium, both in experimental animals and in patients. They concluded that there is substantial evidence that beta blockade, when induced promptly after coronary occlusion, is capable of limiting the size of experimentally produced AMI. Its mechanism is unclear, but it appears that beta blockade reduces the severity of myocardial ischemia by reducing myocardial oxygen demands. Both intravenous and oral therapy with beta blockers is safe and invasive hemodynamic monitoring is usually not necessary for safe use of these drugs. The authors caution, however, that before early beta blockade is recommended as standard therapy for uncomplicated AMI that the experimental findings should be confirmed in rigorously controlled clinical trials utilizing several techniques for assessment of AMI size. These drugs, however, clearly improve survival when administered to patients on a long-term basis after AMI. Although the mechanism of this protective effect is not understood, the results are clear enough to warrant the routine administration of a beta blocker to patients who have had an AMI and who have no contraindication to such therapy.

During a double-blind trial in which patients with suspected AMI received metoprolol or placebo, Ryden and associates[86] from Gothenburg, Sweden, analyzed the occurrence of ventricular tachyarrhythmias. Metoprolol (15 mg intravenously) was given as soon as possible after admission, and thereafter 200 mg was given daily for 3 months. Antiarrhythmic drugs were given only for VF and sustained VT ($>$60 beats/s). Definite AMI developed in 809 of the 1,395 participants, and probable AMI, in 162. Metoprolol did not influence the occurrence of VPC or short bursts of VT. However, there were 17 cases of VF in the placebo group (697 patients) and only 6 in the metoprolol group (698 patients; $p < 0.05$). During the hospital stay significantly fewer patients receiving metoprolol (16) than placebo (38) ($p < 0.01$) required lidocaine. In a separate analysis of 145 patients, metoprolol did not influence the occurrence of VPC or short bursts of VT during the first 24 hours of treatment. Despite a lack of effect on less serious ventricular tachyarrhythmias, metoprolol had a prophylactic effect against VF in AMI.

Gundersen[87] from Stavanger, Norway, examined the influence of heart size on the effect of long-term timolol treatment on mortality and reinfarction after AMI in 1,881 patients randomized to either active or placebo treatment. The patients were followed for 12–33 months. At baseline, heart size was determined by x ray in 2 projections: 1,199 patients had normal-sized hearts, 262 had borderline hearts, and 420 had enlarged hearts. The frequency of total cardiac deaths was 3 times greater in the patients with enlarged hearts than in those with normal-sized hearts. The frequency of nonfatal reinfarction, however, was independent of heart size at baseline. The timolol-related reduction of total cardiac death compared with placebo was 41% in patients with normal heart size, 48% in patients with borderline heart size, and 38% in patients with enlarged hearts at baseline (intention to treat approach). The reduction of first nonfatal reinfarctions in the timolol group compared with placebo was, respectively, 32, 41, and 26%. Thus, timolol treatment appears to reduce cardiac death and nonfatal reinfarctions after AMI independent of heart size at baseline. Timolol treatment may be of special importance in patients with cardiomegaly, because of the high incidence of cardiac mortality in this group of patients, and consequently a larger number of cardiac deaths may be prevented.

In a double-blind randomized trial, Herlitz and associates[88] from Guttenberg, Sweden, investigated 1,395 patients with suspected AMI to evaluate the possibility of limiting indirect signs of the size and severity of AMI with the beta$_1$ selective adrenoceptor antagonist metoprolol. Metoprolol (15 mg) was given intravenously and followed by oral administration for 3 months (200 mg daily). Placebo was given in the same way. The size of the AMI was estimated by heat stable lactate dehydrogenase analyses and precordial ECG mapping. Lower maximal enzyme activities compared with placebo were seen in the metoprolol group (11.1 ± 0.5 μkat-liter^{-1}) when the patient was treated within 12 hours of the onset of pain (13.3 ± 0.6 μkat-liter^{-1}; n, 936; $p = 0.009$). When treatment was started later than 12 hours, no difference was found between the 2 groups. Enzyme analyses were performed in all but 20 patients. Precordial mapping with 24 chest electrodes was performed in patients with anterior wall AMI. The final total R-wave amplitude was higher and the final total Q-wave amplitude lower in the metoprolol group than in the placebo group. Patients treated with metoprolol ≤12 hours also showed a decreased need for furosemide, a shortened hospital stay, and a significantly reduced 1-year mortality compared with the placebo group, whereas no difference was observed among patients treated later on. After 3 months, however, there was a similar reduction in mortality among patients in whom therapy was started ≤12 hours and >12 hours after the onset of pain. The results support the hypothesis that intravenous metoprolol followed by oral treatment early in the course of suspected AMI can limit infarct size and improve long-term prognosis.

Turi and Braunwald[89] from Boston, Massachusetts, reviewed several studies showing the effectiveness of several beta blockers in reducing total mortality during the extended recovery period after AMI. The rate of occurrence of reinfarction and sudden death also is reduced. Although the exact mechanisms of this beneficial effect are unknown, it appears to result from a "class" effect, i.e., secondary to beta blockade, since neither cardioselectivity, intrinsic sympathomimetic activity, nor membrane-stabilizing activity appears to be a requisite. The reduction in mortality is seen in all age groups, for all types of AMI, and in all risk groups. On the basis of presently available evidence, in patients without contraindication to beta blockade, prophylactic treatment with beta blockers should be initiated between 1 and 4 weeks after AMI. The dosage should be sufficient to blunt the heart rate response to exercise, and therapy should be continued for at least 2 years. This article was followed by an unsigned editorial[90].

Systemic hypertension is frequent during the early stage of AMI, and it is associated with a higher frequency of complications. Labetalol, which combines alpha and beta adrenoceptor blockade, is an effective drug in managing this type of hypertension. In 11 patients with systolic BP >150 mmHg during AMI, Renard and associates[91] from Brussels, Belgium, infused labetalol to lower systolic BP to <130 mmHg. The optimal rate was then maintained for 1 hour (mean rate, 2.3 mg/min). Hemodynamic variables were measured before, during, and after labetalol infusion. Labetalol lowered BP in all patients; this effect was related to a decrease both in total systemic resistance (18–14 IU) and in cardiac index (3.1–2.7 liters/min/M^2); the stroke index remained unchanged and the heart rate was reduced (94–81 beats/min). There was no significant change in the mean PA wedge pressure; it was decreased, however, in the 6 patients with an initial pressure >15 mmHg. The double product was greatly decreased (16,497–8,598 mmHg times beats/min), which is favorable in AMI. The authors concluded that labetalol was superb for treatment of hypertension in AMI and that its hemodynamic effects are likely to reduce myocardial oxygen requirements. It does not worsen moderate left-sided CHF, although it may reduce the cardiac output.

The Beta-Blocker Heart Attack Trial (BHAT) was a placebo-controlled, randomized, double-blind clinical trial of the long-term administration of propanolol hydrochloride to persons who had had ≥1 confirmed AMI[92]. A total of 3,837 patients in 31 centers were randomly placed into 2 groups

(1,916 to propranolol and 1,921 to placebo) and followed for an average of 25 months. A previously published report of the BHAT described a 26% reduction of total mortality in survivors of AMI assigned to propranolol therapy compared with similar patients assigned to placebo therapy. Cause-specific mortality analysis indicated that both sudden and nonsudden CAD mortality was decreased in the propranolol group. This study dealt with the effect of propranolol therapy on CAD incidence, defined as recurrent nonfatal AMI and CAD mortality. Coronary incidence, i.e., recurrent nonfatal definite reinfarction plus fatal CAD, in the propranolol group was 10% compared with 13% in the placebo group, a reduction of 23%. The incidence of definite nonfatal reinfarction was lower by 16%, and that of definite or probable nonfatal reinfarction by 15%. Among patients with a history of CHF, 15% of the propranolol-treated patients had definite CHF during the study, as did 13% of the placebo-treated patients. Among patients without history of CHF, the percentages experiencing CHF were 5%. In patients with no history of angina, the incidence of angina was 36% in the propranolol group and 34% in the placebo group. Among those who had a history of angina, the incidence was 66% in both groups. The BHAT analyses of nonfatal events reinforce the previous recommendation for the use of propranolol in the treatment of patients who have had a recent AMI and who have no contraindications to beta blockers.

Dopamine and dobutamine

In 8 mechanically ventilated patients in cardiogenic shock, Richard and colleagues[93] from Le Kremlin Bicetre, France, assessed the hemodynamic effects of an infusion of dopamine and dobutamine and evaluated the role of this combination in preventing the deleterious effects that occur when each amine is administered alone. Each patient received 3 infusions in a randomly assigned order: dopamine, 15 mg/kg/minute; dobutamine, 15 mg/kg/minute; and a combination of dopamine 7.5 mg/kg/minute and dobutamine 7.5 mg/kg/minute. Stroke volume index increased similarly with the 3 infusions, but dopamine alone increased oxygen consumption. The dopamine-dobutamine combination increased mean arterial pressure, maintained PA wedge pressure within normal limits, and prevented the worsening of hypoxemia induced by dopamine. The dopamine-dobutamine combination appears to be useful in the management of mechanically ventilated patients in cardiogenic shock.

Combined nitroglycerin and dobutamine

The immediate therapy of severe LV failure after AMI frequently requires simultaneous preload reduction, pump output augmentation, and maintenance of systemic BP. The effects of intravenous nitroglycerin (NTG) and dobutamine (DB) were evaluated in 12 patients with severe LV failure following AMI by Awan and colleagues[94] from Davis, California. Nitroglycerin achieved salutary lowering of abnormally elevated LV filling pressure (23–14 mmHg; p < 0.001), whereas dobutamine markedly augmented LV pump function (cardiac index rose from 1.7–2.5 liters/min/M^2; p < 0.005). Notably, the combined infusion of NTG plus dobutamine simultaneously decreased preload (LV filling pressure, 23–14 mmHg; p < 0.001) and markedly enhanced LV pump performance (cardiac index increased from 1.7–2.4 liters/min/M^2; p < 0.001). Minor decline in mean systemic BP with NTG (72–66 mmHg; p < 0.05) was rapidly reversed by dobutamine addition (69 mmHg; p > 0.05). Both agents were well tolerated without clinical or ECG evidence of myocardial ischemia or dysrhythmias. Thus, in LV failure due to AMI, the infusion of NTG (venodilator) plus dobutamine (positive inotrope) together provide the complementary beneficial actions of substantially decreasing abnormally raised LV filling pressure in concert with maintenance of systemic perfusion pressure and marked elevation of low cardiac index.

Nitroprusside

In an investigation carried out by Shah and associates[95] from Los Angeles, California, to evaluate the effects of nitroprusside infusion on LV EF, RV EF, and LV regional wall motion, RNA with simultaneous hemodynamic assessment was performed before and during nitroprusside infusion in 20 patients with AMI complicated by LV failure and/or systemic arterial hypertension. Nitroprusside produced significant reductions in PA wedge pressure (21 ± 6–13 ± 5 mmHg; −38%; p < 0.001), mean arterial pressure (107 ± 19–90 ± 13 mmHg; −15.9%; p < 0.001), LV end-diastolic volume index (84 ± 28–75 ± 23 ml/M^2; −10.7%; p < 0.001), and RV end-diastolic volume index (77 ± 30–67 ± 27 ml/M^2; −13.0%; p < 0.007); and significant increases in LV EF (0.32 ± 0.12–0.37 ± 0.13; +15.6%; p < 0.0001), RV EF (0.37 ± 0.11–0.45 ± 0.14; +21.6%; p < 0.001), and stroke volume index (25 ± 7–27 ± 7 ml/beat M^2; +8.0%; p < 0.03). These beneficial changes in global ventricular performance were accompanied by no change in the regional contractile function of 90% of the abnormally contracting infarct-related LV segments, and improved regional wall motion in 34% of noninfarcted but abnormally contracting LV segments. It was concluded that nitropursside-induced reduction of elevated preload and afterload in AMI results in salutary effects on global ventricular function and improved regional function of noninfarcted LV segments but with less prominent effects on regional function of infarcted segments.

Cessation of smoking

The beneficial effects of stopping cigarette smoking after AMI are well known. In studies with short follow-ups, cessation of cigarette smoking reduces the cardiovascular mortality rate in half and the rate of nonfatal recurrence of AMI in half. The death rate after AMI is higher in those who continue to smoke cigarettes compared with those who do not. To reaffirm these findings after longer periods of observation, Aberg and associates[96] from Gothenburg, Sweden, followed to 10 years 10 annual cohorts of men after their first AMI: 1,023 men of the group were cigarette smokers. Three months after AMI, 55% had stopped smoking cigarettes and 45% had not. These 2 groups were then compared and followed with regard to a nonfatal second AMI and death. Pre-AMI characteristics were similar in the 2 groups. In different age groups, life-table technique analysis disclosed that those who stopped smoking had a considerably higher survival rate and lower cumulative frequency of recurrence AMI.

RELATED TOPICS

Angiography of infarct-related artery in healed or healing AMI

There is a high prevalence of total coronary occlusion during AMI. Pichard and associates[97] from New York City reported the angiographic appearance of the infarct-related artery (IRA) in 130 patients with healed AMI who underwent cardiac catheterization 2 weeks to >12 months afterward. The IRA was the LAD in 47%, the right in 50%, and the LC in 3%. Total coronary occlusion was found in 80% of patients studied 2–4 weeks after AMI and decreased gradually, reaching 40% of those studied after 12 months of MI. In those patients with a patent IRA, severe stenosis remained: 99% obstruction at 2–4 weeks, decreasing to 86% obstruction after 12 months ($p < 0.005$). The prevalence of total coronary occlusion and the severity of stenosis in those without total occlusion was similar in those with transmural or nontransmural AMI and in those with 1-, 2-, or 3-vessel CAD.

AMI in young adults

In an investigation carried out by Uhl and Farrell[98] from Lackland Air Force Base, Texas, the risk factors and clinical course of 165 patients <40 years of age (mean age, 35) having an initial AMI (group I) were compared with 100 patients >40 (mean age, 50) (group II). Six risk factors were analyzed: smoking 20 pack-years, hyperlipidemia, systemic hypertension, family history of CAD, diabetes mellitus, and obesity. Only 2 patients in group I and 6 patients in group II had no risk factors, but the mean number of risk factors in group I (3) differed from group II (2) ($p < 0.05$). Group I had only 18% of patients without either obesity, hyperlipidemia, hypertension, or diabetes mellitus as risk factors, whereas group II had 41 patients with similar findings ($p < 0.001$). Group I had hyperlipidemia, obesity, and family history more commonly than did group II, whereas hypertension was more frequent in the older patients. A prior history of angina was present in nearly half of groups I and II, but physical exertion just prior to AMI was more common in group I (32%) than in group II (20%) ($p < 0.05$). Death at the time of AMI was more frequent in group II ($p < 0.001$), but CHF occurred in 17% of both groups. On follow-up, 45% of both groups had no complications, and the rates of subsequent AMI and angina pectoris were similar in both groups. Late death was less frequent in group I than in group II. Thus, patients <40 with AMI have more risk factors than those >40. Physical exertion at the time of AMI is more common in younger patients. The complication rate is similar in both young and older MI patients, but the mortality rate, both early and late, is lower in young adult AMI patients.

AMI in women <50 years of age

Rosenberg and associates[99] from Cambridge, Massachusetts, Rockville, Maryland, and Philadelphia, Pennsylvania, evaluated risk factors for first nonfatal AMI in women < age 50 years in a case control study of 255 women with AMI and 802 controls. The relative risk of AMI increased with the number of cigarettes smoked daily. The estimated risk of AMI for current

TABLE 2-5. *Total plasma cholesterol levels among cases of MI and controls by high-density lipoprotein (HDL) levels. Reproduced with permission from Rosenberg et al.[99]*

PLASMA HDL, MG/DL	TOTAL PLASMA CHOLESTEROL, MG/DL	NO. (%)		RELATIVE RISK ESTIMATE*	95% CONFIDENCE INTERVAL
		CASES	CONTROLS		
<40	<200	45 (30)	141 (53)	1.5	0.9–2.4
	200–249	59 (40)	90 (34)	3.1	1.9–5.0
	250–299	31 (21)	25 (9)	5.2	2.6–10
	≥300	14 (9)	8 (3)	5.2	2.3–12
≥40	<200	27 (26)	264 (50)	0.5	0.3–1.0
	200–249	45 (43)	203 (38)	(1.0)†	. . .
	250–299	20 (19)	49 (9)	2.0	1.0–4.1
	≥300	12 (12)	13 (2)	5.5	2.3–14

* Allowance made for age and cigarette smoking.
† Reference category.

smokers of ≥35 cigarettes/day was 10 times that of women who had never smoked cigarettes; an estimated 65% of AMIs were attributable to cigarette smoking. The relative risk of AMI increased markedly with increasing levels of plasma total cholesterol and decreasing levels of HDL cholesterol and the effects of the 2 factors appeared to be independent (Table 2-5). Other factors significantly associated with AMI were systemic hypertension, angina pectoris, diabetes mellitus, blood group A, and a history of AMI or stroke before age 60 years in a mother or sibling. Factors not significantly associated with AMI were obesity, history of preeclamptic toxemia, and type A personality. Women who were postmenopausal appeared to have a lower risk of AMI than premenopausal women of similar ages. Thus, in this study of women <50 years of age, 84% of those with AMI were current cigarette smokers. The authors estimated that about 65% of nonfatal first AMI among women younger than age 50 might not occur if they did not smoke.

Relation of AMI in women to sexual activity

Although successful rehabilitation of cardiac patients should include consideration of their sexuality, a paucity of data regarding the sexual activity of women who have had AMI is available. Papadopoulos and associates[100] from Baltimore, Maryland, interviewed 130 such patients. Sexual concern soon developed in 30% of those sexually active before AMI. Fear of resumption of sexual activity was expressed by 51% of the women and 44% of their husbands. Sexual activity was not resumed by 27%, was unchanged in 27%, and decreased in 44%. Only 45% of the total group received sexual instructions before discharge, and in only 18% of cases did the physician raise the topic. Symptoms during intercourse were reported by 57% of the patients. Thus, AMI had a negative impact on the sexuality of women and although many patients who have had AMI desire sexual counseling, their desires are still not being met. Accurate and complete sexual instructions of both partners with specific attention to the woman's concerns and needs should be part of cardiac rehabilitation.

AMI with coronary artery spasm

In a report by Cipriano and colleagues[101] from Stanford, California, 12 patients with AMI were documented in 11 of 39 patients who had coronary artery spasm that was observed by angiography either before AMI (3 patients), after AMI (5 patients), or both before and after AMI (3 patients). The AMI corresponded in location to sites of ECG changes of myocardial ischemia during spontaneous angina pectoris in 7 of 7 patients and to the region of myocardium supplied by the artery in which spasm was observed by angiography in each patient. The AMI occurred in the distribution of the right coronary artery in 8 patients and of the left coronary artery in 4 patients. Of 12 arteries that supplied infarcted regions of myocardium, 7 vessels had ≥50% fixed diameter narrowing, but the remaining 5 had minimal (10%) or no fixed narrowing. In those patients who were studied after AMI coronary angiography demonstrated that only 3 of 9 vessels in the distribution of infarcted regions of myocardium were completely occluded. Clinical follow-up for an average of 1.3 years after AMI showed that 7 patients continued to have chest pain, 2 patients were asymptomatic, and 2 patients died suddenly 9 weeks and 1 year after AMI. Therefore among these patients with coronary spasm demonstrated by angiography, AMI 1) was frequent (28%); 2) occurred in the distribution of observed coronary spasm; 3) was frequently (5 of 12 arteries) in the distribution of arteries having minimal or no fixed narrowing; and 4) was often (6 of 9 arteries) in the distribution of arteries that were demonstrated to be patent after AMI.

Length of hospitalization and risk calculation

The feasibility of the use of a Cox model for risk assessment of individualized hospital discharge after AMI was evaluated by Madsen and coworkers[102] from San Diego, California. First, a previously developed prognostic index computed at the fifth day after admission was tested on a new population of 1,140 patients. After 5 days 52% of patients could be discharged with low risk. A new competing risk variant of the Cox model that updates prognosis according to the occurrence of complications was developed that describes the risk of death, cardiac arrest, and cardiogenic shock within 44 days after hospital admission. With a risk of one of these events being <2% during a 14-day period after proposed discharge, 453 (47%) of 966 survivors could be discharged after only 5 days. A longer stay of ≤30 days was proposed for 338 patients (35%) to achieve the same level of risk. The savings in hospitalization days would be 15%. These results were confirmed in a new sample of 197 patients from the same institution who were discharged according to the proposed system. Of the 169 day 5 survivors, 67% were discharged on days 6 through 15, and this resulted in only 2 unexpected deaths and a 20% savings in hospitalization days. The investigators concluded that individually determined discharge time is feasible without increased risk of death or severe complications after early discharge.

Hyperglycemia during AMI

Hyperglycemia is common in patients admitted to hospitals with suspected AMI. The meaning of this hyperglycemia and carbohydrate intolerance seen in patients with AMI is controversial. Impaired oral and intravenous glucose tolerance has frequently been reported to return to normal after recovery from AMI. It has been assumed that this applies equally to hyperglycemia occurring without an exogenous glucose load, and that this hyperglycemia is induced by stress. When diabetes mellitus (DM) persists after recovery from AMI, it has been proposed that the AMI precipitated the DM. Husband and associates[103] from Newcastle upon Tyne, England, studied 26 patients not previously known to have DM with blood glucose values ≥10 mmol/liter on admission to a coronary care unit: 16 survived for 2 months at which time a 75 g oral glucose tolerance test (GTT) showed DM in 10 (63%) and impaired glucose tolerance in 1. All those with abnormal glucose tolerance at 2 months had had raised glycosylated hemoglobin (HbA_1) (>7.5%) on admission, indicating preexisting DM. All those with a HbA_1 level >8% had abnormal glucose tolerance. Seven of the 10 who died or did not have an oral GTT also had raised HbA_1 at admission. An admission blood glucose ≥10 mmol/liter in patients with severe chest pain is more likely to indicate previously undiagnosed diabetes than "stress" hyperglycemia. There is no evidence that AMI precipitates diabetes. The glycosylated hemoglobin concentration can be used to distinguish between stress hyperglycemia and hyperglycemia caused by DM.

Mortality in first year

The mortality rate after AMI has generally been modeled by single exponential function. Gilpin and associates[104] from San Diego and La Jolla, California, and Vancouver, Canada, undertook to determine in 3 different populations whether or not periods exist during the first year after AMI that have mortality distributions that differ from this pattern. The 3 patient populations included San Diego (346 patients, 71 deaths), Vancouver (704 patients, 146 deaths), and Copenhagen (1,140 patients, 262 deaths). Hospital admission was within 24 hours of the onset of symptoms, and patients dying within the first 24 hours after hospital admission or of noncardiac or unknown causes were not analyzed. The mortality between 2 and 21 days in the combined data base was 11% and from 3 weeks to 1 year, 11%. A high degree of similarity was noted among the shapes of the 3 survival curves. The hypothesis of an exponential mortality rate during the entire first year was rejected. Using a special statistic, change points at days 17, 23, and 24 in the 3 populations (21 days for the combined data base) were identified and used thereafter to divide the year into 2 separate periods of mortality within which exponentiality for the mortality rate was not rejected. The point by which exactly 50% of deaths had occurred was day 19, with 75% of deaths occurring by day 100. These data further define the natural history after AMI and indicate optimal follow-up periods for short- and long-term management strategies based on risk assessment or trials of risk reduction after AMI.

Most important factors affecting survival after AMI

Rapaport and Remedios[105] from San Francisco, California, evaluated the risk of recurrent AMI or death after recovery from an AMI in 139 patients discharged from the San Francisco General Hospital between July 1978 and September 1981. Multivariate stepwise discriminant analysis of 20 variables contributing to sudden and total death identified complex ventricular ectopic rhythm as the most important variable followed by age. The presence of an initial anterior AMI and impaired LV function were independent variables contributing to sudden death. Twenty-four hour ambulatory ECG monitoring, RNA, and submaximal exercise stress tests performed during the second week after recovery from an AMI also provided insight into a high risk group of patients.

Symposium on post-AMI patient

This symposium was published in the October 1, 1983, issue of *The American Journal of Cardiology* and consisted of 6 articles edited by Sniderman.[106–111] The first 3 articles dealt with the identification of the high-risk patient while hospitalized during the period of AMI. Another article reviewed the use of beta blockers after AMI, and finally an overview of an integrated approach to patient management was outlined. Although this symposium does not provide new information, it makes recently acquired information easily obtainable.

References

1. Rude RE, Poole WK, Muller JE, Turi Z, Rutherford J, Parker C, Roberts R, Raabe DS, Gold HK, Stone PH, Willerson JT, Braunwald E, MILIS Study Group: Electrocardiographic and clinical criteria for recognition of acute myocardial infarction based on analysis of 3,697 patients. Am J Cardiol 52:936–942, Nov 1983.

2. Warner RA, Reger M, Hill NE, Mookherjee S, Smulyan H: Electrocardiographic criteria for the diagnosis of anterior myocardial infarction: importance of the duration of precordial R waves. Am J Cardiol 52:690–692, Oct 1983.

3. Warner RA, Hill NE, Mookherjee S, Smulyan H: Electrocardiographic criteria for the diagnosis of combined inferior myocardial infarction and left anterior hemiblock. Am J Cardiol 51:718–722, March 1983.

4. Dash H, Ciotola TJ: Morphology of ventricular premature beats as an aid in the electrocardiographic diagnosis of myocardial infarction. Am J Cardiol 52:458–461, Sept 1983.

5. Fox KM, Jonathan A, Selwyn A: Significance of exercise–induced ST segment elevation in patients with previous myocardial infarction. Br Heart J 49:15–19, Jan 1983.

6. Gewirtz H, Sullivan M, O'Reilly G, Winter S, Most AS: Role of myocardial ischemia in the genesis of stress–induced ST segment elevation in previous anterior myocardial infarction. Am J Cardiol 51:1289–1283, May 1983.

7. Camara EJN, Chandra N, Ouyang P, Gottlieb SH, Shapiro EP: Reciprocal ST change in acute myocardial infarction: assessment by electrocardiography and echocardiography. J Am Coll Cardiol 2:251–257, Aug 1983.

8. Heller GV, Blaustein AS, Wei JY: Implications of increased myocardial isoenzyme level in the presence of normal serum creatine kinase activity. Am J Cardiol 51:24–27, Jan 1983.

9. Fisher ML, Carliner NH, Becker LC, Peters RW, Plotnick GD: Serum creatine kinase in the diagnosis of acute myocardial infarction: optimal sampling frequency. JAMA 249:393–394, Jan 21, 1983.

10. Tommasini G, Karlsberg RP, Tamagni F, Berra R, Oddone A, Orlandi M, Raimondi W, Malusardi R: Direct determination of distribution volume and disappearance rate of native creatine kinase in humans. Am Heart J 105:402–407, March 1983.

11. Grenadier E, Keidar S, Kahana L, Alpan G, Marmur A, Palant A: The roles of serum myoglobin, total CPK, and CK–MB isoenzyme in the early phase of myocardial infarction. Am Heart J 105:408–416, March 1983.

12. Fisher ML, Kelemen MH, Collins D, Morris F, Moran GW, Carliner NH, Plotnick GD: Routine serum enzyme tests in the diagnosis of acute myocardial infarction: cost effectiveness. Arch Intern Med 143:1541–1543, Aug 1983.

13. Debusk RF, Kraemer HC, Nash E, Berger WE, Lew H: Stepwise risk stratification soon after acute myocardial infarction. Am J Cardiol 52:1161–1166, Dec 1983.

14. Smith JL, Ambos HD, Gold HK, Muller JE, Poole WK, Raabe DS, Rude RE, Passamani E, Braunwald E, Sobel BE, Roberts R, MILIS Study Group: Enzymatic estimation of myocardial infarct size when early creatine kinase values are not available. Am J Cardiol 51:1294–1300, May 1983.

15. Hirsowitz GS, Lakier JB, Marks DS, Lee TG, Goldberg AD, Goldstein S: Comparison of radionuclide and enzymatic estimate of infarct size in patients with acute myocardial infarction. J Am Coll Cardiol 1:1405–1412, June 1983.

16. Sederholm M, Grottum P, Erhardt L, Kjekshus J: Quantitative assessment of myocardial ischemia and necrosis by continuous vectorcardiography and measurement of creatinine kinase release in patients. Circulation 68:1006–1012, Nov 1983.

17. Albert DE, Califf RM, Lecocq DA, McKinnis RA, Ideker RE, Wagner GS: Comparative rates of resolution of QRS changes after operative and nonoperative acute myocardial infarcts. Am J Cardiol 51:378–381, Feb 1983.

18. Anderson CI, Harrison DG, Stack NC, Hindman NB, Ideker RE, Palmeri ST, Selvester RH, Wagner GS: Evaluation of serial QRS changes during acute inferior myocardial infarction using a QRS scoring system. Am J Cardiol 52:252–256, Aug 1983.

19. Cohen M, Wiener I, Pichard A, Holt J, Smith H, Gorlin R: Determinants of ventricular tachycardia in patients with coronary artery disease and ventricular aneurysm: clinical, hemodynamic, and angiographic factors. Am J Cardiol 51:61–64, Jan 1983.

20. Richards DA, Cody DV, Denniss AR, Russell PA, Young AA, Uther JB: Ventricular electrical instability: a predictor of death after myocardial infarction. Am J Cardiol 51:75–80, Jan 1983.

21. Sclarovsky S, Strasberg B, Fuchs J, Lewin RF, Arditi A, Klainman E, Kracoff OH, Agmon J: Multiform accelerated idioventricular rhythm in acute myocardial infarction: electrocardiographic characteristics and response to verapamil. Am J Cardiol 52:43–47, July 1983.

22. Tansey MJB, Opie LH: Relation between plasma–free fatty acids and arrhythmias within the first 12 hours of acute myocardial infarction. Lancet 2:419–421, Aug 20, 1983.

23. Nordrehaug JE, Von Der Lippe G: Hypokalaemia and ventricular fibrillation in acute myocardial infarction. Br Heart J 50:525–529, Dec 1983.

24. Rosenkranz ER, Buckbery GD, Laks H, Mulder DG: Warm induction of cardioplegia with glutamate–enriched blood in coronary patients with cardiogenic shock who are dependent on inotropic drugs and intraaortic balloon support: initial experience and operative strategy. J Thorac Cardiovasc Surg 86:507–518, Oct 1983.

25. Mikell FL, Asinger RW, Hodges M: Functional consequences of interventricular septal involvement in right ventricular infarction: echocardiographic, clinical, and hemodynamic observations. Am Heart J 105:393–401, March 1983.

26. Klein HO, Tordjman T, Ninio R, Sareli P, Oren V, Lang R, Gefen J, Pauzner C, Di Segni E, David D, Kaplinsky E: The early recognition of right ventricular infarction: diagnostic accuracy of the electrocardiographic V_4R lead. Circulation 67:558–565, March 1983.

27. Haupt HM, Hutchins GM, Moore GW: Right ventricular infarction: role of the moderator band artery in determining infarct size. Circulation 67:1268–1272, June 1983.

28. Baigrie RS, Haq A, Morgan CD, Rakowski H, Drobac M, McLaughlin P: The spectrum of

right ventricular involvement in inferior wall myocardial infarction: a clinical, hemodynamic and noninvasive study. J Am Coll Cardiol 1:1396–1404, June 1983.

29. BRAAT SH, BRUGADA P, DE ZWAAN C, COENEGRACHT JM, WELLENS HJJ: Value of electrocardiogram in diagnosing right ventricular involvement in patients with an acute inferior wall myocardial infarction. Br Heart J 49:368–372, Apr 1983.

30. DELL'ITALIA LJ, STARLING MR, O'ROURKE RA: Physical examination for exclusion of hemodynamically important right ventricular infarction. Ann Intern Med 99:608–611, Nov 1983.

31. WILLIAMS DB, IVEY TD, BAILEY WW, IREY SJ, RIDEOUT JT, STEWART D: Postinfarction angina: results of early revascularization. J Am Coll Cardiol 2:859–864, Nov 1983.

32. KEATING EC, GROSS SA, SCHLAMOWITZ RA, GLASSMAN J, MAZUR JH, PITT WA, MILLER D: Mural thrombi in myocardial infarctions: prospective evaluation by 2–dimensional echocardiography. Am J Med 74:989–985, June 1983.

33. STARLING MR, CRAWFORD MH, SORENSEN SG, GROVER FL: Comparative value of invasive and noninvasive techniques for identifying left ventricular mural thrombi. Am Heart J 106:1143–1149, Nov 1983.

34. BUDA AJ, MACDONALD IL, DUBBIN JD, ORR SA, STRAUSS HD: Myocardial infarction extension: prevalence, clinical significance, and problems in diagnosis. Am Heart J 105:744–749, May 1983.

35. FENELEY MP, CHANG VP, O'ROURKE MF: Myocardial rupture after acute myocardial infarction: 10 year review. Br Heart J 49:550–556, June 1983.

36. DROBAC M, GILBERT B, HOWARD R, BAIGRIE R, RAKOWSKI H: Ventricular septal defect after myocardial infarction: diagnosis by 2–dimensional contrast echocardiography. Circulation 67:335–341, Feb 1983.

37. MIYAMOTO AT, LEE ME, KASS RM, CHAUX A, SETHNA D, GRAY R, MATLOFF JM: Post–myocardial infarction ventricular septal defect: improved outlook. J Thorac Cardiovasc Surg 86:41–46, July 1983.

38. NISHIMURA RA, SCHAFF HV, SHUB C, GERSH BJ, EDWARDS WD, TAJIK AJ: Papillary muscle rupture complicating acute myocardial infarction: analysis of 17 patients. Am J Cardiol 51:373–377, Feb 1983.

39. MARTIN CA, THOMPSON PL, ARMSTRONG BK, HOBBS MST, DE KLERK N: Long–term prognosis after recovery from myocardial infarction: a nine year follow–up of the Perth Coronary Register. Circulation 68:961–969, Nov 1983.

40. SPODICK DH: Q–wave infarction versus ST infarction: nonspecificity of electrocardiographic criteria for differentiating transmural and nontransmural lesions. Am J Cardiol 51:913–915, March 1983.

41. COLL S, CASTANER A, SANZ G, ROIG E, MAGRINA J, NAVARRO–LOPEZ F, BETRIU A: Prevalence and prognosis after a first nontransmural myocardial infarction. Am J Cardiol 51:1584–1588, June 1983.

42. KRONE RJ, FRIEDMAN E, THANAVARO S, MILLER JP, KLEIGER RE, OLIVER GC: Long–term prognosis after first Q–wave (transmural) or non–Q–wave (nontransmural) myocardial infarction: analysis of 593 patients. Am J Cardiol 52:234–239, Aug 1983.

43. NICHOLSON MR, ROUBIN GS, BERNSTEIN L, HARRIS PJ, KELLY DT: Prognosis after an initial non–Q–wave myocardial infarction related to coronary arterial anatomy. Am J Cardiol 52:462–465, Sept 1983.

44. DAVIES B, WATT DAL, DAGGETT A: Serum creatine kinase and creatine kinase MB isoenzyme responses of postinfarction patients after a graded exercise test. Br Heart J 50:65–69, July 1983.

45. COHN PF: The role of noninvasive cardiac testing after an uncomplicated myocardial infarction. N Engl J Med 309:90–93, July 14, 1983.

46. EWART CK, TAYLOR B, REESE LB, DEBUSK RF: Effects of early postmyocardial infarction exercise testing on self perception and subsequent physical activity. Am J Cardiol 51:1076–1080, Apr 1983.

47. SHELDAHL LM, WILKE NA, TRISTANI FE, KALBFLEISCH JH: Response of patients after myocardial infarction to carrying a graded series of weight loads. Am J Cardiol 52:698–703, Oct 1983.

48. DEWHURST NG, MUIR AL: Comparative prognostic value of radionuclide ventriculography at

rest and during exercise in 100 patients after first myocardial infarction. Br Heart J 49:111–21, Feb 1983.

49. ONG L, VALDELLON B, COROMILAS J, BRODY R, REISER P, MORRISON J: Precordial ST segment depression in inferior myocardial infarction: evaluation by quantitative thallium–201 scintigraphy and technetium–99m ventriculography. Am J Cardiol 51:734–739, March 1983.

50. BOTVINICK EH, PEREZ–GONZALES JF, DUNN R, PORTS T, CHATTERJEE K, PARMLEY W: Late prognostic value of scintigraphic parameters of acute myocardial infarction size in complicated myocardial infarction without heart failure. Am J Cardiol 51:1045–1051, Apr 1983.

51. NICOD P, CORBETT JR, FIRTH BG, LEWIS SE, RUDE RE, HUXLEY R, WILLERSON JT: Prognostic value of resting and submaximal exercise radionuclide ventriculography after acute myocardial infarction in high–risk patients with single and multivessel disease. Am J Cardiol 52:30–36, July 1983.

52. THE MULTICENTER POSTINFARCTION RESEARCH GROUP: Risk stratification and survival after myocardial infarction. N Engl J Med 309:331–336, Aug 11, 1983.

53. BRAAT SH, ZWAAN C, BRUGADA P, WELLENS HJJ: Value of left ventricular ejection fraction in extensive anterior infarction to predict development of ventricular tachycardia. Am J Cardiol 52:686–689, Oct 1983.

54. ABRAMS DS, STARLING MR, CRAWFORD MH, O'ROURKE RA: Value of noninvasive techniques for predicting early complications in patients with clinical class II acute myocardial infarction. J Am Coll Cardiol 2:818–825, Nov 1983.

55. MARCHLINSKI FE, BUXTON AE, WAXMAN HL, JOSEPHSON ME: Identifying patients at risk of sudden death after myocardial infarction: value of the response to programmed stimulation, degree of ventricular ectopic activity and severity of left ventricular dysfunction. Am J Cardiol 52:1190–1196, Dec 1983.

56. WOLFFENBUTTEL BHR, VERDOUW PD, SCHEFFER MG, BOM HPA, BIJLEVELD RE, HUGENHOLTZ PG: Significance of haemodynamic variables in coronary care unit for prediction of survival after acute myocardial infarction. Br Heart J 50:266–272, Sept 1983.

57. ROUBIN GS, HARRIS PJ, BERNSTEIN L, KELLY DT: Coronary anatomy and prognosis after myocardial infarction in patients 60 years of age and younger. Circulation 67:743–749, Apr 1983.

58. ABRAHAM RD, ROUBIN GS, HARRIS PJ, BERNSTEIN L, KELLY DT: Coronary and left ventricular angiographic anatomy and prognosis of survivors of first acute myocardial infarction. Am J Cardiol 52:257–260, Aug 1983.

59. GOLDBERG S, GREENSPON AJ, URBAN PL, MUZA B, BERGER B, WALINSKY P, MAROKO PR: Reperfusion arrhythmia: a marker of restoration of antegrade flow during intracoronary thrombolysis for acute myocardial infarction. Am Heart J 105:26–32, Jan 1983.

60. WEI JY, MARKIS JE, MALAGOLD M, BRAUNWALD E: Cardiovascular reflexes stimulated by reperfusion of ischemic myocardium in acute myocardial infarction. Circulation 67:796–801, Apr 1983.

61. COWLEY MJ, HASTILLO A, VETROVEC GW, FISHER LM, GARRETT R, HESS ML: Fibrinolytic effects of intracoronary streptokinase administration in patients with acute myocardial infarction and coronary insufficiency. Circulation 67:1031–1038, May 1983.

62. DEFEYTER PJ, VAN EENIGE MJ, VAN DER WALL EE, BEZEMER PD, VAN ENGELEN CLJ, FUNKE–KUPPER AJ, KERKKAMP HJJ, VISSER FC, ROOS JP: Effects of spontaneous and streptokinase–induced recanalization on left ventricular function after myocardial infarction. Circulation 67:1039–1044, May 1983.

63. KHAJA F, WALTON JA, BRYMER JF, LO E, OSTERBERGER L, O'NEILL WW, COLFER HT, WEISS R, LEE T, KURIAN T, GOLDBERG AD, PITT B, GOLDSTEIN S: Intracoronary fibrinolytic therapy in acute myocardial infarction: report of a prospective randomized trial. N Engl J Med 308:1305–1311, June 2, 1983.

64. ANDERSON JL, MARSHALL HW, BRAY BE, LUTZ JR, FREDERICK PR, YANOWITZ FG, DATZ FL, KLAUSNER SC, HAGAN AD: A randomized trial of intracoronary streptokinase in the treatment of acute myocardial infarction. N Engl J Med 308:1312–1318, June 2, 1983.

65. SWAN HJC: Thrombolysis in acute evolving myocardial infarction: a new potential for myocardial salvage. N Engl J Med 308:1354–1355, June 2, 1983.

66. SCHWARZ F, FAURE A, KATUS H, VON OLSHAUSEN K, HOFMANN M, SCHULER G, MANTHEY J, KUBLER W: Intracoronary thrombolysis in acute myocardial infarction: an attempt to quantitate its effect by comparison of enzymatic estimate of myocardial necrosis with left ventricular ejection fraction. Am J Cardiol 51:1573–1578, June 1983.

67. MANDELKORN JB, WOLF NM, SINGH S, SHECHTER JA, KERSH RI, RODGERS DM, WORKMAN MB, BENTIVOGLIO LG, LAPORTE SM, MEISTER SG: Intracoronary thrombus in nontransmural myocardial infarction and in unstable angina pectoris. Am J Cardiol 52:1–6, July 1983.

68. SMALLING RW, FUENTES F, MATTHEWS MW, FREUND GC, HICKS CH, REDUTO LA, WALKER WE, STERLING RP, GOULD KL: Sustained improvement in left ventricular function and mortality by intracoronary streptokinase administration during evolving myocardial infarction. Circulation 68:131–138, July 1983.

69. ESENTE P, GIAMBARTOLOMEI A, GENSINI G, DATOR C: Coronary reperfusion and Bezold–Jarisch reflex (bradycardia and hypotension). Am J Cardiol 52:221–224, Aug 1983.

70. BLANKE H, SCHERFF F, KARSCH DR, LEVINE RA, SMITH H, RENTROP P: Electrocardiographic changes after streptokinase–induced recanalization in patients with acute left anterior descending artery obstruction. Circulation 68:406–412, Aug 1983.

71. SHEEHAN FH, MATHEY DG, SCHOFER J, KREBBER HJ, DODGE HT: Effect of interventions in salvaging left ventricular function in acute myocardial infarction: a study of intracoronary streptokinase. Am J Cardiol 52:431–438, Sept 1983.

72. SCHOFER J, MATHEY DG, MONTZ R, BLEIFELD W, STRITZKE P: Use of dual intracoronary scintigraphy with thallium–201 and technetium–99m pyrophosphate to predict improvement in left ventricular wall motion immediately after intracoronary thrombolysis in acute myocardial infarction. J Am Coll Cardiol 2:737–744, Oct 1983.

73. SERRUYS PW, WIJNS W, VAN DEN BRAND M, RIBEIRO V, FIORETTI P, SIMOONS ML, KOOIJMAN CJ, REIBER JHC, HUGENHOLTZ PG: Is transluminal coronary angioplasty mandatory after successful thrombolysis? Quantitative coronary angiographic study. Br Heart J 50:257–267, Sept 1983.

74. SHELL W, MICKLE DK, SWAN HJC: Effects of nonsurgical myocardial reperfusion on plasma creatine kinase kinetics in man. Am Heart J 106:665–669, Oct 1983.

75. CRIBIER A, BERLAND J, CHAMPOUD O, MOORE N, BEHAR P, LETAC B: Intracoronary thrombolysis in evolving myocardial infarction: sequential angiographic analysis of left ventricular performance. Br Heart J 50:401–410, Nov 1983.

76. ROGERS WJ, MANTLE JA, HOOD WP JR, BAXLEY WA, WHITLOW PL, REEVES RC, SOTO B: Prospective randomized trial of intravenous and intracoronary streptokinase in acute myocardial infarction. Circulation 68:1051–1061, Nov 1983.

77. KENNEDY JW, RITCHIE JL, DAVIS KB, FRITZ JK: Western Washington randomized trial of intracoronary streptokinase in acute myocardial infarction. N Engl J Med 309:1477–1482, Dec 15, 1983.

78. SCHRODER R, BIAMINO G, LEITNER, ER, LINDERER T, BRUGGEMANN T, HEITZ J, VOHRINGER HF, WEGSCHEIDER K: Intravenous short-term infusion of streptokinase in acute myocardial infarction. Circulation 67:536–548, March 1983.

79. HARTZLER GO, RUTHERFORD BD, MCCONAHAY DR, JOHNSON WL JR, MCCALLISTER BD, GURA GM JR, CONN RC, CROCKETT JE: Percutaneous transluminal coronary angioplasty with and without thrombolytic therapy for treatment of acute myocardial infarction. Am Heart J 106:965–973, Nov 1983.

80. DEWOOD MA, SPORES J, BERG R, KENDALL RW, GRUNWALD RP, SELINGER SL, HENSLEY GR, SUTHERLAND KI, SHIELDS JP: Acute myocardial infarction: a decade of experience with surgical reperfusion in 701 patients. Circulation 68 (suppl II), II-8–II-16, Sept 1983.

81. NELSON GIC, AHUJA RC, SILKE B, HUSSAIN M, TAYLOR SH: Hemodynamic advantages of isosorbide dinitrate over frusemide in acute heart failure following myocardial infarction. Lancet 1:730–732, Apr 2, 1983.

82. JAFFE AS, GELTMAN EM, TIEFENBRUNN AJ, AMBOS HD, STRAUSS HD, SOBEL BE, ROBERTS R: Reduction of infarct size in patients with inferior infarction with intravenous glyceryl trinitrate: a randomised study. Br Heart J 49:452–460. May 1983.

83. FLAHERTY JT, BECKER LC, BULKLEY BH, WEISS JL, GERSTENBLITH G, KALLMAN CH, SILVERMAN KJ, WEI JY, PITT B, WEISFELDT ML: A randomized prospective trial of intravenous nitroglycerin in patients with acute myocardial infarction. Circulation 68:576–588, Sept 1983.

84. JUGDUTT BI, SUSSEX BA, WARNICA JW, ROSSALL RE: Persistent reduction in left ventricular asynergy in patients with acute myocardial infarction by intravenous infusion of nitroglycerin. Circulation 68:1264–1273, Dec 1983.

85. BRAUNWALD E, MULLER JE, KLONER RA, MAROKO PR: Role of beta–adrenergic blockade in the therapy of patients with myocardial infarction. Am J Med 74:113–123, Jan 1983.

86. RYDEN L, ARINIEGO R, ARNMAN K, HERLITZ J, HJALMARSON A, HOLMBERG S, REYES C, SMEDGARD P, SVEDBERG K, VEDIN A, WAAGSTEIN F, WALDENSTROM A, WILHELMSSON C, WEDEL H, YAMAMOTO M: A double–blind trial of metoprolol in acute myocardial infarction: effects on ventricular tachyarrhythmias. N Engl J Med 308:614–618, March 17, 1983.

87. GUNDERSEN: Influence of heart size on mortality and reinfarction in patients treated with timolol after myocardial infarction. Br Heart J 50:135–139, Aug 1983.

88. HERLITZ J, ELMFELDT D, HJALMARSON A, HOLMBERG S, MALEK I, NYBERG G, RYDEN L, SWEDBERG K, VEDIN A, WAAGSTEIN F, WALDENSTROM A, WALDENSTROM J, WEDEL H, WILHELMSEN L, WILHELMSSON C: Effect of metoprolol on indirect signs of the size and severity of acute myocardial infarction. Am J Cardiol 51:1282–1288, May 1983.

89. TURI ZG, BRAUNWALD E: The use of beta–blockers after myocardial infarction. JAMA 249:2512–2516, May 13, 1983.

90. UNSIGNED EDITORIAL: Implications of recent beta–blocker clinical trials for patients after myocardial infarction. JAMA 249:2482–2483, May 13, 1983.

91. RENARD M, RIVIERE A, JACOBS P, BERNARD R: Treatment of hypertension in acute stage of myocardial infarction: hemodynamic effects of labetalol. Br Heart J 49:522–527, June 1983.

92. BETA-BLOCKER HEART ATTACK TRIAL RESEARCH GROUP: A randomized trial of propranolol in patients with acute myocardial infarction: morbidity results. JAMA 250:2814–2819, Nov 25, 1983.

93. RICHARD C, RICOME JL, RIMAILHO A, BOTTINEAU G, AUZEPY P: Combined hemodynamic effects of dopamine and dobutamine in cardiogenic shock. Circulation 67:620–626, March 1983.

94. AWAN NA, EVENSON MK, NEEDHAN EK, BEATTIE JM, MASON DT: Effect of combined nitroglycerin and dobutamine infusion in left ventricular dysfunction. Am Heart J 106:35–40, July 1983.

95. SHAH PK, ABDULLA A, PICHLER M, SHELLOCK F, BERMAN D, SINGH BN, SWAN HJC: Effects of nitroprusside–induced reduction of elevated preload and afterload on global and regional ventricular function in acute myocardial infarction. Am Heart J 105:531–542, Apr 1983.

96. ABERG A, BERGSTRAND R, JOHANSSON S, ULVENSTAM G, VEDIN A, WEDEL H, WILHELMSSON C, WILHELMSEN L: Cessation of smoking after myocardial infarction: effects on mortality after 10 years. Br Heart J 49:416–422, May 1983.

97. PICHARD AD, ZIFF C, RENTROP P, HOLT J, BLANKE H, SMITH H: Angiographic study of the infarct–related coronary artery in the chronic stage of acute myocardial infarction. Am Heart J 106:687–692, Oct 1983.

98. UHL GS, FARRELL PW: Myocardial infarction in young adults: risk factors and natural history. Am Heart J 105:548–553, Apr 1983.

99. ROSENBERG L, MILLER DR, KAUFMAN DW, HELMRICH SP, VAN DE CARR S, STOLLEY PD, SHAPIRO S: Myocardial infarction in women under 50 years of age. JAMA 250:2801–2806, Nov 25, 1983.

100. PAPADOPOULOS C, BEAUMONT C, SHELLEY SI, LARRIMORE P: Myocardial infarction and sexual activity of the female patient. Arch Intern Med 143:1528–1530, Aug 1983.

101. CIPRIANO PR, KOCH FH, ROSENTHAL SJ, BAIM DS, GINSBURG R, SCHROEDER JS: Myocardial infarction in patients with coronary artery spasm demonstrated by angiography. Am Heart J 105:542–547, Apr 1983.

102. MADSEN EB, HOUGAARD P, GILPIN E, PEDERSEN A: The length of hospitalization after acute myocardial infarction determined by risk calculation. Circulation 68:9–16, July 1983.

103. HUSBAND DJ, ALBERTI KGMM, JULIAN DG: "Stress" hyperglycaemia during acute myocardial infarction: an indicator of preexisting diabetes? Lancet 2:179–205, July 23, 1983.

104. GILPIN EA, KOZIOL JA, MADSEN EB, HENNING H, ROSS J: Periods of differing mortality distribution during the first year after acute myocardial infarction. Am J Cardiol 52:240–244, Aug 1983.

105. RAPAPORT E, REMEDIOS P: The high risk patient after recovery from myocardial infarction: recognition and management. J Am Coll Cardiol 1:391–400, Feb 1983.

106. SNIDERMAN AD, BEAUDRY JP, RAHAL DP: Early recognition of the patient at late high risk: incomplete infarction and vulnerable myocardium. Am J Cardiol 52:669–673, Oct 1983.

107. MOSS AJ: Prognosis after myocardial infarction. Am J Cardiol 52:667–669, Oct 1983.

108. THEROUX P, MARPOLE DGF, BOURASSA MG: Exercise stress testing in the post–myocardial infarction patient. Am J Cardiol 52:664–667, Oct 1983.

109. PRATT CM, ROBERTS R: Chronic beta blockade therapy in patients after myocardial infarction. Am J Cardiol 52:661–664, Oct 1983.

110. WENGER NK: Uncomplicated acute myocardial infarction: long–term management. Am J Cardiol 52:658–660, Oct 1983.

111. SNIDERMAN A: Symposium on the patient postinfarction: new knowledge and new therapeutic strategies: introduction. Am J Cardiol 52:657, Oct 1983.

3

Arrhythmias, Conduction Disturbances, and Cardiac Arrest

To determine the frequency of arrhythmias and conduction disturbances in trained athletes and the level of physical training at which they occur, Pilcher and associates[1] from Atlanta, Georgia, obtained 24-hour ambulatory ECG recordings in 80 healthy runners during both exercise and free activity. Subjects were grouped according to the number of miles per week (mpw) they had regularly run during the previous 3 months: Group I: 0 to ≤5 mpw (≤8 km); group II: >5 to ≤15 mpw (>8 to ≤24 km); group III: >15 to ≤30 mpw (>24 to ≤48 km); and group IV: >30 mpw (>48 km). In 41 of 80 subjects VPC occurred and ectopic supraventricular complexes occurred in 33 (41%). There were 2 episodes of paired VPC and a 5-beat run of VT with exercise. The study revealed no significant differences in the occurrence of arrhythmias or conduction disturbances in the different groups, although the 2 episodes of paired ventricular ectopic activity and 5-beat run of VT are of concern.

Northcote and associates[2] from Glasgow, Scotland, carried out ambulatory ECG in 21 healthy, fit, male squash players aged 23–43 years before, during, and after match play. The ECGs were analyzed for heart rate and changes in rhythm. The heart rate increased to 80% of the individual's predicted maximum heart rate for the duration of a game. Ventricular arrhythmias were detected in 7 subjects during play and in 7 in the immediate postexercise period, a frequency that was not reproduced on subsequent maximal treadmill exercise testing. The maximal recorded heart rate for the group during play was 170 ± 16 beats/minute with a range of 144–197. The mean heart rate through the 40-minute period of play was 149 $\pm$ 18 beats/minute. Of the 14 patients who had an arrhythmia during or shortly after play, 3 had an episode of VP, 1 had coupled VPC and a prolonged run of VT lasting 9 cycles. The other players had $\geqslant 1$ VPC or atrial premature contraction.

Caffeine has long been implicated in the causation of arrhythmias, but studies in human beings have been limited. Dobmeyer and associates[3] from Columbus, Ohio, performed electrophysiologic study before and after the administration of oral coffee or intravenous caffeine citrate in 7 normal volunteers aged 20–30 years (mean, 24) and in 12 patients with noncoronary types of cardiac disease. The maximum serum concentration of caffeine was reached in 30 minutes in the patients receiving coffee orally and in 10 minutes in those who received caffeine citrate intravenously. Caffeine did not significantly change sinoatrial, interatrial, intraatrial, AV node, or His-Purkinje conduction intervals or sinus node recovery times. Caffeine did significantly shorten the effective refractory period of the right atrium, the AV node, and the right ventricle. Caffeine also increased the effective refractory time of the left atrium. Two patients had unsustained VT in response to programmed ventricular stimulation after caffeine. Three of the controls had sustained AF in response to atrial extrastimuli only after administration of caffeine. Before receiving caffeine, only 1 of the 12 patients had sustained atrial tachycardia, whereas 6 had sustained AF after receiving caffeine. The production of tachyarrhythmias in controls and patients after administration of caffeine suggests that these rhythms may occur in a spontaneous fashion. The observation of tachycardia in all 5 patients who had arrhythmic symptoms after administration of caffeine lends credence to this supposition and such patients should avoid caffeine. This article was followed by an editorial by Graboys and Lowe[4] from Boston, Massachusetts.

Montague and associates[5] from Halifax, Canada, studied 45 subjects, aged 2 weeks to 62 years, who presented with frequent (>100/day) VPC and without evidence of underlying cardiac disease. The spectrum of ventricular arrhythmia was assessed by 24-hour ambulatory ECG and exercise tolerance test. Sinus rhythm was the prevailing rhythm in all subjects. The VPC frequency averaged 444 ± 454/hour (range, 0–1,863) over the 24-hour monitoring period and was not significantly different during waking or sleeping periods. There was no simple correlation of VPC frequency with prevailing sinus rate ($r = -0.0006$; p, NS). The prevalence of complex VPC (multiform, R-on-T, and repetitive) was relatively high (18 of 45 patients) and was equally distributed about the median VPC frequency of 314 VPC/hour (7 of 18 -vs- 11 of 18; p, NS). Of the 43 subjects who had exercise tests, 37 had VPC during the preexercise rest phase, compared with only 11 at peak exercise (p < 0.0001). To assess the short-term natural history of the VPC, 27 subjects had repeat clinical examinations and 24-hour ECGs at a mean interval of 8 months. All remained well. Although there was considerable individual temporal variability of VPC frequency in this subgroup, there was no significant change in group mean values (415 ± 409 VPC/hour initially -vs- 401 ± 383 VPC/hour at follow-up study; p, NS). The relative temporal constancy of VPC frequency in the group as a whole also was reflected in a high linear correlation of VPC frequency at initial and follow-up studies (r = 0.816; p < 0.001). Follow-up in 2 other patients revealed that 1 died suddenly (age 4 months) of indeterminate cause in the setting of sudden infant death syndrome, and the other (age 36 years) had symptomatic, sustained VT. The other 16 subjects remain well a mean of 22 months after the initial study. Thus, patients who present with frequent VPC and no evidence of underlying anatomic cardiac disease have a high prevalence of complex VPC. Despite marked individual temporal variability of VPC frequency in these patients, the VPC tend to persist over the short-term period. Most, however, remain asymptomatic and clinically well, and the risk of clinical progression of their disease, although present, appears small.

ATRIAL FIBRILLATION/FLUTTER

There is wide beat-to-beat variability in cycle length and LV performance in patients with AF. Schneider and associates[6] from New Haven and New Britain, Connecticut, evaluated LV EF and relative LV volumes on a beat-to-beat basis with the computerized nuclear probe, an instrument with sufficiently high sensitivity to allow continuous evaluation of the radionuclide time activity curve. Of 18 patients with AF, 5 had MS, 6 had MR, and 7 had CAD. Fifty consecutive beats were analyzed in each patient. The mean LV EF ranged from 17–51%. There was substantial beat-to-beat variation in cycle length and LV EF in all patients, including those with marked LV dysfunction. In 14 patients who also underwent multigated cardiac blood pool imaging, there was an excellent correlation between mean EF derived from the nuclear probe and gated EF obtained by gamma camera imaging (r = 0.90). Based on beat-to-beat analysis, LV function was dependent on relative end-diastolic volume and multiple preceding cycle lengths, but not preceding end-systolic volumes. This study demonstrates that a single value for LV EF does not adequately characterize LV function in patients with AF. Furthermore, both the mean beat-to-beat and the gated EF may underestimate LV performance at rest in such patients.

Engel and Luck[7] from Philadelphia, Pennsylvania, evaluated 11 alcohol abusers without cardiomyopathy or overt CHF to determine their vulnerability to AF and flutter. Atrial extrastimulation was performed with rapid pacing to facilitate induction of atrial vulnerability seen in 4 alcohol abusers. The remaining 7 patients were retested 30 minutes after drinking 60–120 ml of 86 proof whiskey and AF or flutter was induced in 3 drinkers. Three nondrinkers, symptomatic with sinus bradycardia but not CHF, were found not to be vulnerable to AF or flutter, but flutter was induced in 2 of the 3 after drinking whiskey. Whiskey did not increase atrial functional refractory periods or widen dispersion among 3 disparate right atrial sites. Thus, these data suggest that whiskey enhances vulnerability to AF and flutter in patients without CHF or cardiomyopathy.

Lowenstein and associates[8] from Denver, Colorado, reviewed retrospectively 40 patients with new onset AF to establish the frequency of its various causes. Alcohol intoxication caused or contributed to the development of AF in 14 cases (35%), CAD in 23%, and pulmonary disease in 23%. Among patients <65 years old, alcohol caused or contributed to 63% of the cases of AF. Thyrotoxicosis was the cause in only 1 of the 40 patients and none of the 40 patients had MS, pulmonary embolism, or pericarditis. None of the alcoholic patients with AF had complications; 89% converted spontaneously to normal sinus rhythm within 24 hours. Thus, alcohol intoxication should be considered early in the differential diagnosis of new onset AF.

Panidis and associates[9] from Philadelphia, Pennsylvania, evaluated the safety and efficacy of oral verapamil to control exercise tachycardia in 27 patients with AF and 3 with atrial flutter receiving digitalis. The study was performed in a double-blind, randomized, crossover manner. The heart rate in patients who received verapamil compared with placebo group was lower at rest (mean 69 ± 13 -vs- 87 ± 20 beats/min; $p < 0.01$), as was the degree of tachycardia at the end of 3 minutes of a standardized exercise test (104 ± 14 -vs- 136 ± 23 beats/min; $p < 0.01$). Doses of verapamil required to achieve suppression of tachycardia were 240 mg/day in 18 patients, 320 mg/day in 6 patients, and 480 mg/day in 3 patients. Only 3 patients complained of adverse effects from verapamil during the double-blind phase of the study. Two patients were discontinued from the study because of adverse reactions. No clinically significant changes during verapamil therapy were observed on the electrocardiogram, chest roentgenogram, echo, or in the laboratory evaluation. Digoxin blood levels were higher in patients who received concomitant verapamil compared with placebo (1.23 ± 0.59 -vs- 0.85 ± 0.46 ng/ml; $p < 0.01$), but no patient had signs or symptoms of digitalis toxicity. Thus, oral verapamil given in addition to digitalis is a safe and effective agent in the treatment of patients with chronic AF or flutter to decrease exercise-induced tachycardia.

Tommaso and associates[10] from Chicago, Illinois, in 17 patients (9 with atrial flutter and 8 with AF) examined the safety and efficacy of intravenous verapamil in controlling the ventricular response or converting to sinus rhythm. The patients had been difficult to control by other medications. All patients at the time of study were receiving digoxin. Either verapamil or placebo was chosen randomly and a bolus of 0.075 mg/kg (up to 5 mg) was administered. Twelve patients had a marked reduction in their ventricular response after intravenous administration of verapamil (7 with atrial flutter and 5 with AF). None of these 12 patients converted (nonconverters). The average reduction in heart rate was from 120 ± 6 beats/minute to a minimum of 83 ± 13 beats/minute within 20 minutes after drug administration. Verapamil was found to convert 5 patients with atrial arrhythmias to sinus rhythm (2 with atrial flutter and 3 with AF) (converters). In addition, 3 patients with atrial arrhythmias of less than 1 month who did not convert with parenteral drug therapy converted within 24 hours while receiving the oral drug. Converters had their supraventricular arrhythmias of significantly shorter duration (median, 3 hours -vs- 30 days) and tended to have smaller left atrial size (3.8 ± 0.7 cm -vs- 4.3 ± 1.3 cm) compared with the nonconverters. We conclude that verapamil is safe and effective when administered intravenously to patients with atrial flutter and AF for control of ventricular response. In short duration atrial arrhythmias, conversion to sinus rhythm is likely once the ventricular response is controlled.

Pozen and associates[11] from Miami, Florida, studied 18 men age 49–71 years (mean, 59) who were electrically cardioverted for pure atrial flutter to determine factors influencing the maintenance of regular sinus rhythm or reversion to atrial flutter. Of the 18 patients, 12 had underlying heart disease (valvular in 6, CAD in 4, and dilated cardiomyopathy in 3) and the other 6 had no evidence of underlying heart disease. Six months after successful cardioversion, 10 patients (55%) had recurrent atrial flutter and 8 patients (45%) were still in sinus rhythm. The 2 groups were not significantly different with respect to age, symptomatology, abnormalities on the 12-lead electrocardiogram (during sinus rhythm), or the administration of digoxin and a class Ia antiarrhythmic agent (after cardioversion). There was a trend for those patients with recurrent atrial flutter to have a higher incidence of underlying heart disease and previous episodes of atrial flutter than the nonrecurrent group. There were statistically significant differences between the recurrent and nonrecurrent groups with respect to echocardiographically determined LA size and LV EF. Patients with a LA size >45 mm or with an EF <45% were all at high risk for recurrent atrial flutter after successful cardioversion.

SUPRAVENTRICULAR TACHYCARDIA WITH OR WITHOUT SHORT P-R INTERVAL SYNDROMES

Benson and associates[12] from Minneapolis, Minnesota, and Durham, North Carolina, used programmed atrial stimulation with an esophageal electrode in 12 children aged 1–13 years with either ECG documented SVT (7) or recurrent palpitations (5). Atrial stimulation initiated and terminated SVT in all 7 patients with a previously documented tachycardia prior to quinidine therapy but could not be initiated after therapy with quinidine. In addition, atrial stimulation initiated SVT in 4 of 5 patients with a history of palpitations. These studies document the usefulness of this approach for diagnosis and treatment of SVT. This approach can be extremely useful for evaluating therapy and attempting to document the abnormality in patients with persistent occurrence of palpitations with inability to document whether or not SVT is present.

In patients with WPW syndrome, observations during BBB in reciprocating tachycardia are of value in accessory pathway localization. Most importantly, an increase in the ventriculoatrial (VA) interval of ≥35 ms has indicated an ipsilateral free wall location and excluded a septal location. Broughton and associates[13] from Durham, North Carolina, examined whether data collected in the presence of type I antiarrhythmic drugs retained localizing value. Review of retrospective data showed that observations in the drug-free state were precluded by the need to suppress atrial arrhythmia during electrophysiologic study in 20% of patients with WPW syndrome who underwent preoperative workup. Prospectively, in 15 patients with left free wall or posteroseptal pathways, we observed transient left BBB during tachycardia before and after administration of procainamide, disopyramide, or quinidine. Serum drug levels ranged from 4.6–6.9 mg/liter, except in 1 patient with a serum procainamide level of 18 mg/liter. Drugs increased the VA interval during narrow QRS tachycardia by 17% (p < 0.01). However, the change in the VA interval with left BBB was not significantly affected. The baseline and drug values averaged 73 ms (range, 39–94) and 70 ms (range, 39–90), respectively, for left free wall pathways (n, 8), and 19 ms (range, 0–28) and 21 ms (range, 2–35), respectively, for posteroseptal pathways (n, 7). Among the latter, the interval increased <30 ms during left BBB except in the patient with the high serum procainamide level, in whom the increase was 35 ms. Thus, the VA interval change that accompanied left BBB remained of localizing value with moderate blood levels of type I drugs, and an increase ⩾35 ms indicated a left free wall rather than posteroseptal pathway.

Intermittent loss of the delta wave in the WPW syndrome may result from precarious conduction over the accessory pathway and, as such, would predict a benign prognosis in the event of the occurrence of AF. Klein and Gulamhusein[14] from Ottawa, Canada, evaluated 52 consecutive patients for the assessment of the WPW syndrome and determined the prevalence of intermittent preexcitation using review of serial ECGs, ambulatory monitoring, and treadmill testing. All patients subsequently had electrophysiologic testing using standard techniques to determine the properties of the accessory pathway. Of the 52 patients, 26 (50%) had intermittent preexcitation as defined by loss of the delta wave with concomitant prolongation of the P-R interval on ⩾1 occasion. These patients had longer effective refractory periods of the accessory pathway (356 ± 114 -vs- 295 ± 29 ms, mean ± SD, p < 0.05) and longer shortest cycle lengths maintaining 1/1 antegrade conduction (426 ± 171 -vs- 291 ± 63 ms; p < 0.02) than their counterparts with constant preexcitation. During AF, 15% of patients with intermittent preexcitation had shortest R-R intervals between preexcited beats <250 ms -vs- 50% of patients with constant preexcitation (p < 0.01). These data support the hypothesis that intermittent preexcitation suggests a benign prognosis in the event of AF.

Morady and associates[15] from San Francisco, California, did electrophysiologic testing in 20 patients with WPW syndrome and ⩾1 episode of symptomatic AF due to rapid antegrade bypass tract conduction. The mean ventricular rate during spontaneous AF was 242 ± 56 beats/minute (± SD) and the shortest preexcited R-R interval was 194 ± 40 ms. Six patients underwent surgical bypass tract ablation and 14 were treated medically, based on the results of electropharmacologic testing. Over a mean follow-up period of 35 ± 19 months, only 1 patient treated medically had a recurrence of minimally symptomatic AF. The successful chemoprophylaxis of symptomatic AF was associated with the inability to induce AF and AV reciprocating tachycardia during drug testing (7 patients) or with the induction of AF with a ventricular rate <200 beats/minute and a shortest preexcited R-R interval of >250 ms (7 patients). Electrophysiologic testing can identify a subgroup of patients with WPW and AF in whom medical therapy is a suitable alternative to bypass tract ablation.

Spontaneous variability in the occurrence of paroxysmal arrhythmias has made it difficult to apply objective and quantitative methods to describe their clinical course. Pritchett and associates[16] from Durham, North Carolina, used the "tachycardia-free interval" of paroxysmal atrial tachycardia (PAT) as a quantitative measure of drug efficacy during treatment with oral verapamil. The tachycardia-free interval is the time a patient remains free from an episode of tachycardia after drug treatment is begun. Recurrent PAT was documented by telephone transmission of the ECG. Improvement caused by increasing the drug dose (360 -vs- 480 mg/day) or by comparing verapamil with placebo treatment was demonstrated by upward shifts in the cumulative tachycardia-free interval curves. The tachycardia-free interval is an easily measured clinical variable that has substantial promise in the study of paroxysmal arrhythmias.

Jedeikin and associates[17] from Houston, Texas, studied the antegrade effective refractory period of the accessory connection in 21 patients with WPW. The mean age was 10 ± 2 years (range, 1 month to 31 years). A change in the antegrade refractory period of the accessory connection of ≥10 ms after ouabain administration was found in 11 of 21 patients. Refractory period decreased in 9 of 21 and increased in 2 of 21. In patients aged ≤3 years, refractory period decreased in 4 of 6. These data indicate that digitalis can enhance conduction through the accessory pathway in children just as it does, as has previously been reported, in adults. Because pediatric patients rarely develop AF or flutter, rapid ventricular rates due to conduction antegrade over the accessory pathway is probably less likely to occur in infants and children than in adults. Thus, digoxin should be used with caution in children with WPW. Patients with WPW and a history suggestive of atrial flutter or AF or rapid clinical deterioration with the onset of tachycardia deserve electrophysiologic study and assessment of the effect of digitalis before such therapy is used.

Smith and associates[18] from Durham, North Carolina, studied the pharmacokinetic and pharmacodynamic effects of diltiazem in 8 patients with a history of paroxysmal atrial tachycardia (PAT) after a short intravenous infusion (20 mg over 10 minutes), a single oral dose (60 or 90 mg), and repeated oral administration (60 or 90 mg every 6 hours for 16 doses). Diltiazem levels decreased in a triexponential manner after intravenous infusion. Terminal half-lives after intravenous, single oral, and repeated oral administration were not significantly different (4.5 ± 1.3, 3.7 ± 0.6, and 4.9 ± 0.4 hours, respectively). The kinetic effects of oral diltiazem were nonlinear. With repeated oral administration, there was accumulation of both diltiazem and its metabolite, deacetyldiltiazem. The diltiazem area under the time -vs- concentration curve increased by a factor of 2.39 ± 0.42 (p = 0.00002). Most patients showed a double peaked time -vs- concentration curve after oral administration, indicating possible enterohepatic recirculation. After intravenous administration, there was a substantial increase in the P-R interval (14.3 ± 5.4%). Although only small changes in P-R interval were seen with a single oral dose, with chronic administration there was persistent P-R interval prolongation, peaking at 17.3 ± 5.6% over control. Counterclockwise hysteresis was present in the P-R interval -vs- plasma diltiazem concentration curve after intravenous administration. Only small changes were seen in heart rate and BP.

Walker and associates[19] from Dallas, Texas, described 6 patients who had frequent episodes of AV junctional rhythm during long-term oral verapamil therapy. In no patient was this rhythm associated with symptoms or adverse effects nor did it force a discontinuation of therapy or a reduction in verapamil dosage. Thus, in the patient receiving oral verapamil therapy AV junctional rhythm should not be considered a manifestation of drug toxicity.

Chang and associates[20] from Taipei, Taiwan, evaluated 15 patients with recurrent SVT to determine the efficacy of antiarrhythmic therapy with oral nadolol. Eight patients had AV nodal reentrant tachycardia and 7 had AV reciprocating tachycardia involving an accessory AV pathway. Electrophysiologic studies were performed before and after IV infusion of propranolol and repeated 5–8 days after oral nadolol therapy at a daily dose of 80–160 mg. Beta adrenergic blockers (IV propranolol and oral nadolol) caused significant prolongation of the sinus cycle length and depressed AV nodal but not accessory AV pathway conduction. Ten patients (7 with AV nodal reentry and 3 with AV reciprocation) who responded to IV propranolol also responded to oral nadolol with loss of inducibility of sustained tachycardia. In the remaining 5 patients (1 with AV nodal reentry and 4 with AV reciprocation) who did not respond to IV propranolol, there was no response to oral nadolol and SVT persisted. Thus, IV propranolol testing may be used to predict the therapeutic efficacy of oral nadolol therapy in the long-term treatment of SVT.

German and associates[21] from Durham, North Carolina, studied the effects of exercise and isoproterenol on AF in 17 patients with WPW to assess the risk of developing a rapid ventricular response. Mean cycle length (R-R interval) and shortest R-R interval between both preexcited and nonpreexcited QRS complexes were recorded, as well as the percentage of preexcited complexes during control periods, during bicycle exercise, and during isoproterenol infusion. Exercise resulted in significantly shorter mean cycle length and the shortest R-R interval between nonpreexcited complexes. Exercise also resulted in a significantly lower percentage of preexcited complexes during AF, but had no effect on the R-R intervals between preexcited complexes. Isoproterenol had a variable effect on the percentage of preexcited QRS complexes, but resulted in significant shortening of mean cycle length and the shortest R-R interval between both normal and preexcited complexes. With isoproterenol, 12 of 17 patients had shortest preexcited R-R intervals ≤215 ms, compared with 6 of 17 in the control state. Isoproterenol infusion increased the rate of conduction over the accessory pathway during AF and allowed better assessment of the risk of excessively rapid rates occurring during AF. Exercise is not an adequate test for this purpose.

Intravenous flecainide acetate was administered by Hellestrand and associates[22] from London, England, to 33 patients undergoing routine electrophysiologic study: 18 patients had a direct accessory atrioventricular (AV) pathway and 15 patients had functional longitudinal A-H dissociation (dual A-H pathways). Flecainide was given to 14 patients during sustained AVRT and in 9 patients during sustained intra-AV nodal reentrant tachycardia. The AVRT was successfully terminated in 12 of 14 patients. Tachycardia termination was due to retrograde accessory pathway block in 11 patients and AV nodal block in 1. During flecainide administration, tachycardia cycle lengths increased (327 ± 55–426 ± 84 ms) principally because of retrograde conduction delay in the accessory pathway (127 ± 34–197 ± 67 ms). After flecainide administration, tachycardia reinitiation was not possible in 6 patients. In all 18 patients with accessory AV pathway conduction, flecainide significantly increased both antegrade and retrograde accessory pathway effective refractory periods, with antegrade accessory pathway block in 3 patients and retrograde accessory pathway block in 8. Intra-AV nodal reentrant tachycardia was successfully terminated in 8 of 9 patients. Tachycardia termination was due to retrograde "fast" A-H pathway block in 7 patients and antegrade "slow" A-H pathway block in 1 patient. During flecainide administration, tachycardia cycle lengths increased (326 ± 50–433 ± 64 ms) due to both antegrade, A-H and H-V (AV 242 ± 97–343 ± 75 ms), and retrograde, earliest ventricular to earliest atrial (51 ± 14–70 ± 23 ms) conduction delay. After flecainide administration, reinitiation of intra-AV nodal reentrant tachycardia was not possible in 4 patients. In all 15 patients with dual A-H pathways, flecainide selectively prolonged the retrograde effective refractory period of the fast A-H pathway, having little effect on antegrade fast A-H pathway refractoriness or on antegrade and retrograde slow A-H pathway refractoriness. Antegrade fast A-H pathway block occurred in 1 patient and retrograde fast A-H pathway block occurred in 6 patients. No serious adverse effects were encountered during the study. Flecainide acetate is an effective agent for the acute termination of both orthodromic AV and intra-AV nodal reentrant tachycardias. This antiarrhythmic action appears to be mediated through a predominant effect on either accessory AV pathway or retrograde fast A-H pathway refractoriness.

Kasper and associates[23] from Mainz, West Germany, studied the electrophysiologic effects of lorcainide, a class I antiarrhythmic agent with local anesthetic properties, in 20 patients with WPW syndrome. After intravenous administration of lorcainide (2 mg/kg), the sinus cycle length decreased in all patients from 705 ± 117–636 ± 94 ms (p < 0.001). The atrioventricular conduction time lengthened from 84 ± 22–94 ± 22 ms (p < 0.01) and the QRS duration increased from 92 ± 19–120 ± 29 ms (p < 0.001). The effective refractory period of the atrium increased from 230 ± 27–243 ± 35 ms (p < 0.05), whereas the ventricular refractoriness was unaffected. Retrograde conduction over the accessory pathway was blocked in 5 of 18 patients after lorcainide; in the remaining 13 patients a prolongation from 107 ± 32–162 ± 57 ms (p < 0.001) was found. Antegrade conduction over the accessory pathway was blocked in 6 patients, and in all other patients it increased considerably. Circus movement tachycardia could be induced in 14 patients before and in 10 patients after the drug. The shortest R-R interval during tachycardia lengthened from 326 ± 40–364 ± 67 ms (p < 0.05). The tachycardia zone was unaffected by lorcainide. In 15 patients AF was induced. After lorcainide, antegrade conduction during AF was blocked (n, 5). The shortest R-R interval over the accessory pathway during induced AF increased from 228 ± 35–304 ± 103 ms (p < 0.05). Intravenous administration of lorcainide produced a pronounced negative dromotropic effect on the conduction properties of the accessory pathway. Lorcainide appears to be a promising new antiarrhythmic agent in patients with the WPW syndrome.

In patients with the WPW syndrome, intravenous ajmaline (50 mg administered over 3 minutes) or procainamide (10 mg/kg body weight administered over 10 minutes) is helpful in defining the duration of the antegrade effective refractory period of the accessory pathway. Brugada and associates[24] from Maastricht, The Netherlands, assessed the value of the ajmaline-procainamide test to predict the effects on the antegrade effective refractory period of the accessory pathway of long-term oral amiodarone.

Thirty-six patients with the WPW syndrome were studied: 24 (group A) had a negative result of the ajmaline-procainamide test and a mean duration of the antegrade effective refractory period of the accessory pathway of 237 ± 24 ms; 12 (group B) had a positive result (disappearance of preexcitation during sinus rhythm after administration of ajmaline and procainamide) and a duration of the antegrade effective refractory period of the accessory pathway of 284 ± 25 ms (p < 0.05 -vs- values in group A). Amiodarone prolonged the antegrade effective refractory period of the accessory pathway by 53 ± 35 ms in patients in group A to 290 ± 37 ms (p < 0.001) and by 100 ± 85 ms in patients in group B to 384 ± 94 ms (p < 0.001). The difference in mean increase between both groups was not significant. In most patients (83%) in group A amiodarone prolonged the antegrade effective refractory period of the accessory pathway to 260–330 ms. However, in most patients (83%) in group B, amiodarone prolonged the antegrade effective refractory period of the accessory pathway to ≥330 ms (p < 0.01). Thus, an ajmaline-procainamide test is of value in predicting the results of oral amiodarone on the antegrade effective refractory period of the accessory pathway.

RELATED TOPICS

Sleep apnea syndrome

Guilleminault and associates[25] from Stanford, California, presented the first study of cardiac arrhythmia and conduction disturbances in a large group (400 patients) with sleep apnea syndrome studied between 1974 and 1979 with 24-hour Holter ECG and a simultaneously recorded polygraph during late afternoon or nocturnal sleep. Of the 400, 193 patients (48%) had cardiac arrhythmias during the recorded night (Table 3-1). The mean number of apneic events, age, weight, and lowest oxygen saturation during

TABLE 3-1. *Cardiac arrhythmias and conduction abnormalities seen during sleep in association with sleep apnea syndrome.*

ARRHYTHMIA OR CONDUCTION ABNORMALITY	PERCENT OF TOTAL POPULATION	PATIENTS (N)
Sinus arrest (2.5 to 13 s)	11	43
Second-degree atrioventricular cardiac block		
Mobitz type I	5	19
Mobitz type II	3	12
Ventricular tachycardia	3	12
Atrial tachycardia	7	28
Sinus bradycardia		
(<30 beats/min for at least 10 s)	7	29
Paroxysmal atrial fibrillation	3	10
Paroxysmal atrial flutter	1	3
Frequent premature ventricular contractions (>2/min)	20	75*

* Only 40 patients had premature ventricular contractions not associated with other arrhythmia during sleep.

sleep were not significantly different in those with arrhythmias. The most significant abnormalities were unsustained VT in 8 patients, sinus arrest that lasted for 2.5–13 seconds in 43 patients, and second degree AV conduction block in 31. Seventy-five had frequent (>2 beats/min) VPC during sleep. Fifty patients with significant arrhythmias had a tracheostomy and were monitored again after surgery. No arrhythmia was present in these patients except for VPC contractions.

Sleep is usually associated with a reduction in the frequency of ventricular arrhythmias. Rosenberg and colleagues[26] from Chicago, Illinois, analyzed 1,260 24-hour Holter recordings exhibiting ventricular ectopic activity and identified 50 patients who had significant increases in such sleep-related ectopic activity. This study group was compared with an age, sex, and 24-hour ventricular ectopic frequency matched control group. There were 21 females and 29 males with a mean age of 64 years in each group. During sleep, the study patients had more frequent ventricular ectopic activity per hour than did controls (mean ± SEM; 143 ± 31 -vs- 63 ± 16; $p < 0.005$). The study group had fewer daytime VPC per hour than did the control patients (45 ± 14 -vs- 68 ± 14; $p < 0.05$). The study patients also exhibited a significant sleep-related increase in complexity of ventricular arrhythmias and the control group, a decrease. Nocturnal heart rates were slower than daytime rates in both the study (69 ± 15 -vs- 79 ± 12 beats/min; $p < 0.005$) and control groups (76 ± 16 -vs- 83 ± 16 beats/min; $p < 0.005$), without significant differences between the 2 groups. No significant differences in clinical and ECG characteristics of the study and control groups were found regarding presence or type of organic heart disease, pulmonary disease, hypertension, medication use, intraventricular conduction delay, abnormal Q waves, ventricular hypertrophy, or QT prolongation. Neurologic abnormalities (60 -vs- 28%; $p < 0.005$), in particular cerebrovascular disease (30 -vs- 14%; $p < 0.01$), were significantly more common in the study group. This investigation identified a subgroup of individuals with ventricular ectopic activity who increased the frequency and complexity of VPC during sleep. The higher prevalence of neurologic disease in these individuals suggests a neurologic or neurohumoral mediation of these arrhythmias.

Effects of alcohol

Although the "holiday heart syndrome," highlighted by rhythm disturbances after acute alcohol ingestion, is well known, the potential arrhythmogenic effects of alcohol in patients with habitual alcoholism have not been studied. Greenspon and Schaal[27] from Columbus, Ohio, studied 14 patients (2 with dilated cardiomyopathy) with a history of rhythm disturbances and alcohol consumption. By electrophysiologic studies, 1 patient had nonsustained VT, 1 had nonsustained AF, 1 had paired ventricular responses, and the remainder had no response to the extrastimulus technique. After 90 ml of 80 proof whiskey, 10 of the 14 patients developed sustained or nonsustained atrial or ventricular tachyarrhythmias. Significant prolongation of His ventricular conduction was seen after alcohol intake; 1 patient previously had Mobitz II AV block after acute alcohol consumption. Alcohol in modest doses has the potential to produce rhythm disturbances in patients with a history of chronic alcohol consumption and heart disease.

Fetal arrhythmias by echo

Allan and coworkers[28] from London, England, studied 23 fetuses whose mothers were referred because of abnormal fetal rate or rhythm. Ten had atrial or ventricular extrasystoles with no associated perinatal morbidity or mortality. Seven patients had complete heart block with ventricular rates of 60–80 beats/minute with no associated intrauterine or perinatal problems. Six patients had SVT or flutter, 5 of whom had successful treatment and 1 delivered prematurely. Maternal digoxin was used successfully in 4 or 5 patients. One patient with hydrops had a ventricular rate of 240 beats/minute and required maternal digoxin, verapamil, and furosemide therapy. This infant was delivered in sinus rhythm at 39 weeks gestation with only minimal ascites. It appears that maternal therapy with digoxin is the drug of first choice with verapamil a possible second drug. This is the first report of furosemide therapy for the mother to help in the treatment of fetal hydrops.

VENTRICULAR ARRHYTHMIAS

Ventricular tachycardia in coronary heart disease

Lam and associates[29] from Chicago, Illinois, reported angiographic studies of 53 consecutive patients with CAD and recurrent sustained VT occurring ≥6 weeks after AMI. Triple-vessel CAD was present in 25 patients (47%), 2-vessel CAD in 19 patients (36%), and 1-vessel CAD in 9 patients (17%). All patients with 1-vessel CAD had LAD CAD. Patients <50 years old had significantly fewer diseased arteries than those >50 years old (1.4 -vs- 2.4 arteries; $p < 0.025$). The LV EF ranged from 0.15–0.61 (mean, 0.34 ± 0.11) and was ≤0.25 in 14 patients (26%). All patients had regional wall motion abnormalities. There was akinesia and/or dyskinesia in 49 patients (92%). Akinesia or dyskinesia was inferior in 17 patients (32%), anteroapical in 14 patients (26%), inferoapical in 10 patients (19%), and anteroapicoinferior in 6 patients (11%). Involvement of the septum was noted in 19 patients (36%) and of basal segments in 26 patients (49%). An average of 2.7 (of 7) segments per patient were dyskinetic or akinetic. Thus, multivessel CAD markedly reduced LV EF, and severe and extensive regional wall motion abnormalities are generally present with chronic VT complicating CAD. Although both medical and/or surgical therapy may be successful in abating the immediate problem of VT, the long-term prognosis is influenced by the underlying CAD and LV dysfunction.

Marchlinski and associates[30] from Philadelphia, Pennsylvania, evaluated 40 patients with sustained VT occurring 3–65 days after AMI to determine its prognostic importance for survival. These patients were characterized clinically by a complicated initial 48 hours of hospitalization following AMI (85% of the patients studied) and the development of a BBB in association with AMI in 32% of them. Programmed electrophysiologic stimulation was performed and VT similar in configuration to spontaneous arrhythmia was induced in 33 (85%) patients. In 45% of the patients, additional morphologically different VT not seen clinically was caused by the programmed stimulation. Only 50% of these patients were alive after a mean follow-up period of 20 ± 15 months. Twelve of the 20 patients died suddenly. Sixteen of the 33 patients with inducible VT died; 8 of the 16 deaths were sudden. Four of the 7 patients with no inducible VT also died suddenly. Thus, the data suggest that patients with sustained VT occurring >48 hours after AMI are at high risk for sudden death. Furthermore, the prognosis for survival is poor irrespective of whether such ventricular arrhythmias are induced by programmed stimulation.

Of left bundle branch morphology

Reiter and associates[31] from Durham, North Carolina, evaluated 29 patients with apparent VT of left BBB morphology. The VT was associated with an organic basis in 24 of the 29 patients: 7 had Mahaim fibers of the nodoventricular type, 7 had arrhythmogenic RV dysplasia, 5 had CAD, 3 had cardiomyopathy, and 2 had associated congenital heart disease. In many patients the underlying cardiac disease was not readily apparent. In the patients with a Mahaim fiber, the ECG taken during sinus rhythm was frequently normal. A reentry tachycardia with antegrade conduction over the nodoventricular fiber could mimic VT as diagnosed by the usual criteria; nodoventricular fibers were therefore often unsuspected before electrophysiologic evaluation. In patients with arrhythmogenic RV dysplasia, cineangiography demonstrated RV abnormalities, but only minor or no LV abnormalities. Clinical and electrocardiographic features were not distinctive. Of the 29 patients, 22 had serious symptoms accompanying the tachyarrhythmia or had required cardioversion. Patients were followed for an average of 20 months: 4 patients died. Thus, VT exhibiting a left BBB morphology often occurs and is frequently associated with organic heart disease, serious symptoms, and significant mortality. A RV angiography and electrophysiologic study may clarify the diagnosis in these patients.

Exercise-induced VT

To elucidate electrophysiologic mechanism of exercise-induced VT, Sung and associates[32] from San Francisco, California, performed electrophysiologic studies in 12 patients in whom sustained VT had developed during treadmill exercise testing. Six patients had arteriosclerotic CAD, 3 had cardiomyopathy, and 3 had no clinical evidence of organic heart disease. All patients had had documented episodes of sustained VT related to exertion and had experienced dizziness, syncope, or both. In addition, 3 patients had had nonfatal cardiac arrest. Electrophysiologic studies provoked paroxysms of sustained VT identical to those observed during treadmill exercise testing in 10 patients and provoked VF in 1. Seven patients had VT suggestive of a reentrant mechanism, since VT could be readily initiated with programmed ventricular extrastimulation or terminated by ventricular overdrive pacing, or both. Three patients had VT suggestive of catecholamine-sensitive automaticity. The VT could not be initiated with programmed electrical stimulation, but it could be provoked by intravenous isoproterenol infusion; furthermore, VT could not be terminated with ventricular overdrive pacing, but it could be abolished by discontinuing isoproterenol infusion. Reproduction of VT in these 10 patients allowed serial pharmacologic testing in selecting an effective antiarrhythmic regimen. Thus, exercise-induced VT can be caused by either reentry or catecholamine-sensitive automaticity, and electrophysiologic studies are of use in defining the underlying mechanism of exercise-induced sustained VT.

Determinants of survival

Swerdlow and associates[33] from Stanford, California, analyzed data from 239 patients with sustained VT or VF to determine prognosis, predictors of survival, and prognostic value of inducing arrhythmia and assessing therapy at the time of electrophysiologic study. Therapy predicted to be effective on the basis of electrophysiologic study was administered over a sustained period. There were 71 cardiac deaths, including 44 sudden deaths, during a mean (±SD) follow-up period of 15 ± 14 months (range, 1 day to 67 months). At 1, 2, and 3 years, the actuarial incidence of sudden death was 17 ± 3, 25 ± 4, and 34 ± 6%, and that of cardiac death was 28 ± 3, 37 ± 4, and 50 ± 6% (Fig. 3-1). Multivariate regression analyses demonstrated that the 2 strongest predictors of both sudden death and cardiac death were a higher New York Heart Association functional class (p < 0.0001 for sudden death and p < 0.0001 for cardiac death) and the failure of any therapy to be

Fig. 3-1. Actuarial curves for sudden death and cardiac death in patients with ventricular tachyarrhythmias. Standard errors of cumulative percentages are shown. Dashed lines indicate extensions of curves beyond the last event to longest duration of follow–up. Arrows indicate that longest duration of follow–up is 2,020 days. Numbers adjacent to circles represent number of patients remaining at various follow–up intervals. Reproduced with permission from Swerdlow et al.[33]

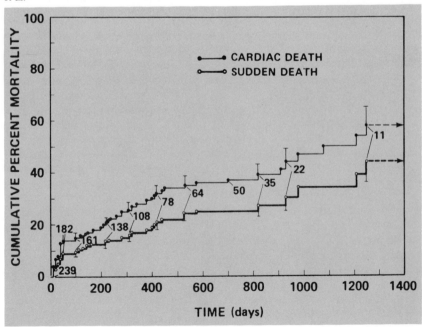

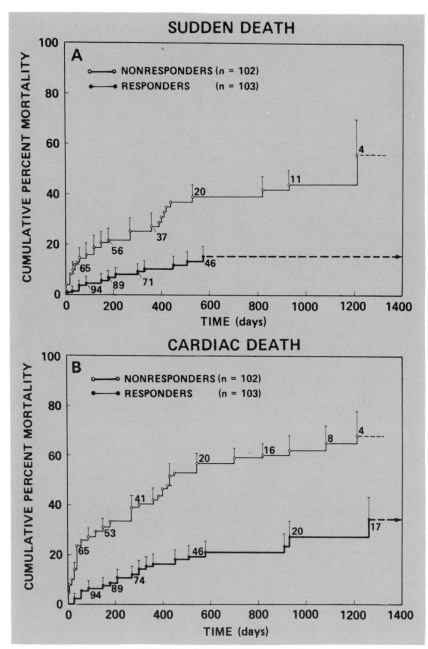

Fig. 3-2. Actuarial curves for sudden death (A) and cardiac death (B) in responders and nonresponders to therapy as assessed by electrophysiologic study. The differences between curves for sudden death are significant at the level p = 0.0011; the differences between curves for cardiac death are significant at p < 0.0001. Arrow indicates extension of follow-up to 2,020 days. See Figure 3-1 legend for explanation of format. Reproduced with permission from Swerdlow et al.[33]

identified as potentially effective on the basis of electrophysiologic study (p = 0.0019 and p = 0.0003) (Fig. 3-2). Most deaths in patients with VT were sudden, but the severity of CHF was the strongest independent predictor of mortality. Response to therapy during electrophysiologic study was also an independent predictor of survival.

Right BBB pattern and left axis deviation

Lin and associates[34] from Taipei, Taiwan, and Los Angeles, California, performed electrophysiologic evaluation before and after the serial administration of verapamil, lidocaine, propranolol, and procainamide in 4 young asymptomatic patients with recurrent, sustained VT. No patient had obvious organic heart disease. The ECG during sinus rhythm showed ST depression and T-wave inversion over the inferior and lateral precordial leads in 3 patients. QRS morphologic characteristics during episodes of VT showed a pattern of right BBB and left axis deviation. In all 4 patients, VT could be both induced and terminated with electrical stimulation. Verapamil terminated VT and prevented the induction of sustained VT in 3 patients, and markedly slowed the rate of VT in 1 patient. Procainamide effectively prevented the induction of sustained VT in 2 patients and, although ineffective in preventing induction in 2 patients, it slowed the rate of tachycardia in both. Lidocaine and propranolol did not prevent the induction of VT in any patient. These findings suggest that slow-response tissues may be involved in the genesis of VT in these patients, and that VT in these patients may represent a unique clinical entity with distinct electrocardiographic, electrophysiologic, and electropharmacologic properties.

Syncope and ventricular preexcitation

Lloyd and associates[35] from Indianapolis, Indiana, described 4 patients with ventricular preexcitation in whom syncope initially was attributed to an arrhythmia utilizing the accessory pathway. At electrophysiologic study, however, the electrophysiologic characteristics of the accessory pathways were considered unlikely to support a tachycardia of a rate sufficient to result in syncope. Programmed RV stimulation, however, reproducibly induced VT to which the syncope was subsequently attributed in 3 patients.

Torsade de pointes

Kay and associates[36] from Birmingham, Alabama, evaluated 32 patients with torsade de pointes. Thirty-one patients had underlying cardiac disease and 30 had a previous important cardiac arrhythmia. Antiarrhythmic medications, often in association with hypokalemia or hypomagnesemia, were the most common precipitating factors. In 22 of 26 patients receiving antiarrhythmic agents, the serum drug levels were within the therapeutic range before the administration of antiarrhythmic agents known to prolong the Q-T interval; 20 of the 32 patients had either a prolonged Q-T interval, hypokalemia, or hypomagnesemia. A characteristic long-short ventricular cycle length as the initiating sequence for torsade de pointes was found in 41 of 44 episodes. Cardiac pacing was the only consistently effective therapeutic intervention.

In young adults

Morady and colleagues[37] from San Francisco, California, studied 31 patients 16–40 years of age (mean ± SD, 31 ± 7 years) with ≥1 episode of sustained VT or VF. Underlying cardiac abnormalities consisted most commonly of cardiomyopathy (9 patients), long Q-T syndrome (LQTS) (5 patients), and MVP (5 patients); no identifiable heart disease was found in 4 patients. Programmed ventricular stimulation induced VT in only 1 of 4 patients with the LQTS but induced VT in 64% of 22 patients with other abnormalities. Chronic drug treatment was based either on serial electropharmacologic testing or was empiric when electrophysiologic testing failed to provoke an arrhythmia. Using this approach, there was a 13% incidence of recurrent VT and a 10% mortality over a follow-up period of 18 ± 14 months. In young adults with VT or VF, an underlying cardiac abnormality can usually be found. Extensive evaluation should be performed to uncover the underlying cardiac abnormality, since this may influence chronic management.

Programmed electrical stimulation in CAD

The frequency and significance of inducible arrhythmia in patients with stable CAD who do not have a history of serious arrhythmia are unknown. Kowey and associates[38] from Boston, Massachusetts, studied 32 such patients (31 men; mean age, 55 years) with programmed electrical stimulation (PES) at the same time of cardiac catheterization. Fourteen patients (group I) manifested ≥3 extraventricular responses when challenged with 1–3 propagated RV extrastimuli during ventricular pacing. Twelve (86%) of the 14 had evidence of LV dysfunction, defined by a global EF of <50% or regional wall motion abnormalities. The remaining 18 patients (group II) manifested ≤2 responses to extrastimulation. Only 4 (22%) of these 18 had LV dysfunction. Proximal 3-vessel CAD was more frequent in group I patients (10 of 14, 71%) than in group II (7 of 18, 39%). Only 5 patients (4 from group I and 1 from group II) demonstrated complex arrhythmia during exercise testing or ambulatory monitoring. The induction of extraventricular responses during PES may serve as an independent marker of electrical instability in the coronary population and is a much more common finding in those with LV dysfunction.

Nonsustained VT as a guide to antiarrhythmic therapy

From a population of 260 patients with malignant ventricular arrhythmia (VF or VT with syncope), Podrid and associates[39] from Boston, Massachusetts, identified 52 (20%) who had infrequent VPC during exercise testing and 48 hours of ambulatory monitoring. These patients underwent invasive electrophysiologic study utilizing programmed premature stimulation with ≤3 extrastimuli at currents of 2 and 3 times mid-diastolic threshold. The end point for testing was nonsustained VT defined as 3–20 propagated responses resulting from the last premature stimulus. A multiple response was obtained in 45 patients consisting of reproducible nonsustained VT in 36 and sustained VT in 9. The 36 patients with nonsustained VT underwent 540 electrophysiologic tests with 18 antiarrhythmic agents. Suppression of the repetitive response was achieved in 31 (86%) of the 36 patients. After an average follow-up of 21 months, 1 of 31 patients in whom the repetitive response had been abolished had recurrent arrhythmia. This contrasted with recurrence in 2 of the 5 patients in whom nonsustained VT was still provoked. During the extensive testing, VF was not induced. Sustained VT occurred in 27 (5%) of the 540 tests, but cardioversion was required in only 12 (2%). It was concluded that nonsustained VT constitutes a safe electrophysiologic end point for selecting an effective antiarrhythmic program in patients who have experienced malignant ventricular arrhythmia but in whom monitoring and exercise testing are inadequate to guide therapy.

Predictors of successful therapy

Spielman and associates[40] from Philadelphia, Pennsylvania, evaluated predictors of the success or failure of medical therapy in the treatment of chronic, recurrent, sustained VT in 84 patients with this arrhythmia. Using univariate analysis, 4 factors were associated with successful medical therapy: age <45 years, EF >50%, hypokinesia as the only contraction abnormality, and the absence of organic heart disease. Four findings correlated with the failure of medical therapy, including: the induction of VT with a single ventricular extrastimulus, an H-V interval >60 ms, the presence of a LV aneurysm, and Q waves on a baseline ECG. None of these findings accurately predicted treatment results in >75% of patients. However, 75% of patients could be classified into groups with a high or low probability of success where accuracy increased to 90%. Thus, these data allow the physician to select a group of patients likely to respond to medical therapy with appropriate electrophysiologic drug testing and a group with low probability of responding to medical therapy, thus allowing electrophysiologic studies to be avoided and alternate forms of therapy to be explored.

Swerdlow and associates[41] from Stanford, California, evaluated 142 patients with sustained VT or VF to determine if clinical variables might be used to predict response to antiarrhythmic drugs during electrophysiologic study. Effective antiarrhythmic drugs were identified for 43 patients (30%). Stepwise logistic regression analysis identified 3 variables independently predictive of drug response: fewer coronary arteries with 70% or greater diameter narrowing, female sex, and fewer episodes of arrhythmia. A function incorporating these 3 variables was constructed to predict the probability of drug response and subsequent accuracy of prediction corresponding to high, intermediate, and low probabilities of drug response were identified. When the predictor function was applied prospectively to 25 additional patients, response rates in the 3 probability ranges were consistent with what had been predicted. Thus, an analysis of clinical variables may be used to estimate the probability of benefit from electrophysiologic-pharmacologic study in patients with sustained VT or VF.

Diagnostic and prognostic significance of exercise-induced premature complexes

Nair and associates[42] from Omaha, Nebraska, evaluated 280 patients with chest pain and normal rest ECG and no history of previous AMI to determine whether exercise-induced VPC were important prognostic indicators of significant CAD. The frequency of exercise-induced VPC was not significantly different in patients without CAD compared with those with 1-artery and multiartery CAD. At a mean follow-up of 47 months, exercise-induced VPC did not predict subsequent cardiac death or nonfatal AMI in either men or women.

Value of 3 and 4 extrastimuli

Mann and associates[43] from Houston, Texas, analyzed initiation of VT by RV extrastimulation in 142 consecutive patients, 53 with ECG documented episodes of spontaneous VT or VF and 68 without spontaneous VT or VF; 21 patients with a history of nonfatal cardiac arrest but no documented arrhythmia were excluded. All patients received 1–4 extrastimuli (S_2, S_3, S_4, and S_5) during pacing at fixed cycle lengths of 600 or 500 ms at 1 or 2 RV sites. Clinical VT was reproduced by extrastimulation in 28 of 43 patients (65%) with sustained VT and in 0 of 10 patients with nonsustained VT. Clinical VT was induced by S_2 or S_3 in 16 patients and by S_4 or S_5 in 12 patients. Ventricular burst pacing reproduced clinical VT in 3 other patients. Nonclinical VT, which was most often polymorphic and nonsustained, was induced in 24 of 121 patients (20%), in 11 by S_2 or S_3 and in 13 by S_4 or S_5. Ventricular burst pacing induced nonclinical VT in 4 other patients. In patients with spontaneous sustained VT, the use of S_4 and S_5 in the RV increases the yield of inducible clinical VT compared with use of S_2 and S_3 alone, but at a cost of increased induction of nonclinical VT. Frequent induction of nonclinical VT limits the interpretation of the results of such stimulation in patients without previously documented VT.

Platia and colleagues[44] from Baltimore, Maryland, studied 117 consecutive patients with a history of sudden cardiac death (group I, 62 patients) or recurrent symptomatic VT (group II, 55 patients) and 11 control subjects (group III) with programmed electrical stimulation during 1 year. Programmed RV stimulation included premature stimulation during atrial pacing (A_1, V_2 mode) and during ventricular pacing (V_1V_2 mode), double ventricular extrastimuli during ventricular pacing ($V_1V_2V_3$), and brief bursts of rapid ventricular pacing (V_{burst}). Repetitive ventricular responses were defined as ≥ 2 ventricular premature beats produced by the final ventricular pacing stimulus occurring by intraventricular reentry. All but 13 patients were on antiarrhythmic therapy at the time of study. The incidence of repetitive ventricular responses induced by A_1V_2 pacing mode was 22% (22 of 104 patients) and that of sustained VT was 1%. The sensitivity of inducing repetitive ventricular responses with V_1V_2 stimulation was 44% and that of sustained VT was 7%; the sensitivity with $V_1V_2V_3$ pacing mode was significantly higher at 77% and 25%, respectively. When $V_1V_2V_3$ and V_{burst} stimulation were directly compared, the incidence of induction of repetitive ventricular responses and sustained VT were comparable. The incidence of induction of repetitive ventricular responses and sustained VT in groups I and II was similar; no repetitive ventricular responses were induced in group III patients. There was no significant difference in the sensitivity of either repetitive ventricular response or sustained VT induction in patients with CAD compared with those with the diagnosis of noncoronary disease. It was concluded that the incidence of induction of repetitive ventricular responses to single ventricular extrastimuli during atrial pacing is low in patients with a history of sudden death or recurrent VT. The incidence of induction of repetitive ventricular responses and sustained VT is highest using the $V_1V_2V_3$ and V_{burst} modes of stimulation.

Nonsustained VT without organic heart disease

Buxton and associates[45] from Philadelphia, Pennsylvania, performed electrophysiologic studies in 83 patients with spontaneous episodes of nonsustained VT. The clinical arrhythmia was reproduced in 63% (in 42 patients by programmed stimulation and in 10 by isoproterenol infusion). In 15 patients sustained VT could be reproducibly induced by programmed stimulation. Inducibility was related to the associated heart diseases: programmed stimulation induced VT in 25 (75%) of 33 patients with CAD, 6 (33%) of 18 patients with cardiomyopathy (dilated in 16, hypertrophic nonobstructive in 2), in 4 of 8 patients with MVP, and in 7 (29%) of 24 patients without structural heart disease. Isoproterenol infusion induced VT in no other patient with CAD, 1 other patient with MVP, 3 patients with cardiomyopathy, and in 6 of 24 patients without structural heart disease. Sustained VT was induced only in patients with structural heart disease, and correlated with the presence of LV aneurysms: sustained VT was induced in 9 of 13 patients with LV aneurysms. The study demonstrates that electrophysiologic techniques can reproduce episodes of nonsustained VT in most patients with spontaneous arrhythmias. Some patients who demonstrate only nonsustained VT spontaneously have inducible, sustained VT, most often in the setting of CAD and LV aneurysms.

Stimulation at a second right ventricular site

Doherty and associates[46] from Philadelphia, Pennsylvania, subjected to stimulation at the RV outflow track 100 patients without VT initiated from their RV apex. Sixty-two patients had no clinical arrhythmias, and 38 had sustained VT, VF, or cardiac arrest. Of the 38 patients with clinical arrhythmias, 22 (58%) had VT or VF induced from the RV outflow tract. Among the 62 patients without arrhythmias, 5 (13%) had polymorphic nonsustained VT or VF induced, which occurred with 3 extrastimuli in all 5 patients. The 22 patients with VT initiated at the RV outflow tract were a heterogeneous group; 10 (45%) patients had cardiac diagnoses other than CAD. In contrast were patients whose VT was initiated at the RV apex (n, 84); in this group, 20 patients (22%) had diagnoses other than CAD (p < 0.05). These 22 patients also were younger (mean age, 46 years) than patients whose VT was initiated at the RV apex (mean age, 58; p < 0.01). Of the 16 patients with clinical VT and no induced arrhythmia from either RV site, 7 had CAD (4 with cardiac arrest), 5 had the long Q-T syndrome, 3 had dilated cardiomyopathy, and 1 had valvular heart disease. In conclusion, stimulation at a second RV site increases the sensitivity of RV stimulation in patients with known VT and seldom initiates VT in patients without clinical VT.

Four ventricular stimuli

Brugada and associates[47] from Maastricht, The Netherlands, assessed in a prospective study the results of an aggressive ventricular stimulation protocol in 52 nonmedicated patients without documented or suspected ventricular arrhythmia (VA): 36 patients had no structural heart disease; 8, CAD; 6, HC; 2, mitral valve disease; and 1, dilated cardiomyopathy. The patients were 12–72 years old. One to 4 VPC (twice diastolic threshold, 2 ms in duration) were given during sinus rhythm and during ventricular pacing at 100 beats/minute at the RV apex. End points were initiation ≥6 beats of VA or every extrastimulus brought to its refractory period. In 31 (60%) of 52 patients, a VA was initiated (nonsustained polymorphic VT in 24 patients, nonsustained monomorphic VT in 2, and VF requiring countershock in 5). Repetitive ventricular responses (RVR) (1–5 beats) were initiated in 46 patients. In 15 patients only RVRs were initiated. In 6 patients RVRs or VA were not initiated. At the end of the follow-up period (mean, 14 months), no patient had spontaneous VA and all were alive. This study shows that ventricular stimulation can result in initiation of VA in patients without clinical VA. Interpretation of results of programmed ventricular stimulation in patients without clinically documented VA should be made with caution.

Right ventricular tachycardia

Surgical cure of RV tachycardia has been recently described in patients with arrhythmogenic RV dysplasia, a disease characterized by abnormal electrical activation of the right ventricle and localized or generalized angiographic RV wall motion abnormalities. Pietras and colleagues[48] from Chicago, Illinois, searching for a selective RV cardiomyopathy complicated by chronic recurrent RV tachycardia, studied 38 consecutive patients (mean age, 31 ± 12 years) with RV tachycardia and no CAD clinically, noninvasively, and by cardiac catheterization, including LV and RV angiography. The RV volumes were as follows: end-systolic volume ranged from 23–103 (mean ± SD, 46 ± 20) cc/M^2 and was abnormal in 14 patients (37%); end-diastolic volume ranged from 57–138 (90 ± 26) cc/M^2 and was abnormal in 15 patients (39%); EF ranged from 0.18–0.64 and was decreased in 5 patients (13%). Seventeen patients (45%) had abnormal RV volumes, EF, and/or RV end-diastolic pressure (EDP), 5 (13%) of whom had abnormal LV volumes, EF, and/or LV EDP, and 12 (32%) patients with abnormal RV EDP had no abnormal LV EDP. Twenty-one patients (55%) had no abnormal RV EDP, 2 of whom had abnormal LV EDP. Only 2 of the 17 patients had RV regional wall motion abnormalities, 1 with and 1 without abnormal LV EDP. Most patients with elevated LV EDP, 5 of 7, also had elevated RV EDP while 12 (39%) of 31 patients with no LV EDP elevation had increased RV EDP. It was concluded that <50% of patients with RV tachycardia have selective RV cardiomyopathy, and >50% of patients have normal RV hemodynamics and angiography.

Buxton and coinvestigators[49] from Philadelphia, Pennsylvania, described clinical and electrophysiologic characteristics of 30 patients without myocardial disease who had VT with the morphologic characteristics of left BBB and inferior axis. The tachycardias were nonsustained in 24 patients, sustained (>30 s) in 6 patients, and provocable by exercise in 14 of 23 patients undergoing a standard Bruce protocol. A VT was induced during electrophysiologic study in 22 of 30 patients. Programmed stimulation induced tachycardia in 10 of 30 patients, most frequently by rapid atrial or ventricular pacing. Isoproterenol infusion facilitated tachycardia induction in 13 of 23 patients. Endocardial activation mapping, performed in 10 patients, confirmed that earliest ventricular activation during tachycardia occurred at the RV outflow tract on the ventricular septum. These tachycardias were unique in their responsiveness to a wide variety of antiarrhythmic drugs, including type I drugs and propranolol. During a mean follow-up of 30 months, no patient died or experienced cardiac arrest. Two patients appeared to be in spontaneous remission, and no patient has developed additional signs of cardiac disease.

Treatment with quinidine

DiMarco and associates[50] from Boston, Massachusetts, evaluated quinidine during serial electrophysiologic testing with programmed ventricular stimulation in 89 patients with life-threatening ventricular arrhythmias. In 30 of the 89 patients quinidine therapy prevented the initiation of VT during programmed ventricular stimulation. In 8 additional patients no single drug tested was effective, and quinidine in combination with either mexiletine (7 patients) or propranolol (1 patient) prevented the initiation of VT during electrophysiologic testing. The mean serum concentrations of quinidine in the patients who responded and those who failed to respond were 2.9 ± 0.8 and 2.8 ± 1.1 µg/ml, respectively; nonresponders were characterized by more severe congestive heart failure and an increased incidence of digitalis use. During chronic therapy (24 ± 3 months) with quinidine either alone or in combination with a second antiarrhythmic drug in the 38 patients whose arrhythmia had been suppressed during electrophysiologic testing, 32 (84%) remain symptom-free, 3 have had recurrent arrhythmia, and 3 discontinued quinidine because of adverse effects. These data demonstrate that quinidine, when selected on the basis of electrophysiologic testing, provides effective long-term prophylaxis against recurrent ventricular arrhythmia and that approximately 40% of patients tested are likely to respond either to quinidine alone or quinidine in combination with another antiarrhythmic agent.

Flecainide -vs- quinidine

In a randomized placebo-controlled double-blind trial, Salerno and associates[51] from Minneapolis, Minnesota, compared flecainide to quinidine for treatment of VPC in 19 patients. The mean percent suppression of total VPC was 95% for flecainide and 56% for quinidine. A >80% reduction of total VPC was obtained in 8 of 9 patients given flecainide and in 5 of 10 given quinidine. After the randomized protocol, the patients who had received quinidine were given flecainide: 9 of the 10 patients had >80% reduction of total VPC. Flecainide produced 100% suppression of nonsustained VT and 100% suppression of paired VPC. Flecainide prolonged the P-R in QRS intervals; Quinidine prolonged the P-R and J-T$_c$ intervals. Side effects were more common with quinidine than flecainide. Three patients were unable to complete the protocol because of serious adverse experiences.

Digoxin

The ventricular antiarrhythmic properties of oral digoxin were examined by Gradman and associates[52] from West Haven and New Haven, Connecticut, in 13 patients with chronic ventricular ectopic activity using serial 24-hour ECG monitoring. Mean VPC frequency per 1,000 normal beats decreased from 56 ± 47 during the placebo period to 40 ± 27 (p, NS) and 25 ± 17 (p $<$ 0.05) during daily administration of digoxin, 0.25 and 0.375 mg. Digoxin had no significant effect on the qualitative occurrence of complex ventricular arrhythmia patterns (multiformity, bigeminy, couplets, ventricular tachycardia). Radionuclide LV EF was measured during the placebo period. Seven patients had normal (EF $>$ 50%) and 6 abnormal global LV performance. In the normal group, the mean VPC frequency decreased from 69 ± 58–20 ± 18 (p $<$ 0.05) and the mean couplet frequency decreased from 0.59 ± 0.85–0.07 ± 0.06 (p $<$ 0.04) during the placebo and 0.375 mg digoxin dosing periods, respectively. In contrast, no significant changes in either variable occurred after digoxin in subjects with depressed LV function. This study indicates that oral digoxin is moderately effective in suppressing VPC, and that its effects are greatest in patients with normal overall LV performance.

Lidocaine

To determine whether prophylactic lidocaine could decrease the incidence of advanced ventricular arrhythmias, Sprung and associates[53] from Miami, Florida, studied 62 patients undergoing 67 PA catheterizations, and each was given lidocaine or placebo before and during catheterization. Advanced ventricular arrhythmias occurred in 42 (63%) of 67 catheterizations. In 18 (58%) of 31 patients receiving lidocaine arrhythmias developed, whereas 24 (67%) of 36 patients who received placebo had evidence of arrhythmias (p, NS). Patients with catheterization times of $<$20 minutes who were treated with lidocaine had less ectopic activity (25%) than patients treated with placebo (68%) (p $<$ 0.05). Two patients had sustained VT and both were receiving placebo. No complications of lidocaine prophylaxis were noted. Prophylactic lidocaine appears to decrease the incidence of mechanically induced arrhythmias in critically ill patients undergoing catheterization that is not prolonged.

Flecainide

Anderson and associates[54] from Salt Lake City, Utah, evaluated the efficacy of flecainide in 15 patients with ventricular tachyarrhythmias previously unsuccessfully treated with multiple antiarrhythmic agents. Flecainide resulted in an increase in cardiac conduction time, A-H intervals, H-V intervals, P-R intervals, and QRS duration. Ventricular refractory period increased by 10% and corrected sinus node recovery time lengthened 153 ms. Flecainide prevented tachycardia induction by programmed stimulation in 9 of 15 patients and improved the response in 2. Cycle length of induced ventricular ectopic rhythms increased by 141 ms after drug administration. The antiarrhythmic response rate was higher in patients without important CAD. Follow-up experience in 10 patients for a mean of 6.5 months demonstrated that flecainide has been well tolerated and generally efficacious. Thus, these data suggest that flecainide may be a useful antiarrhythmic agent for the management of inducible ventricular tachyarrhythmias.

Oetgen and associates[55] from Washington, D.C., and Bethesda, Maryland, gave flecainide acetate to 4 patients with recurrent, symptomatic VT refractory to conventional antiarrhythmic agents. Ventricular stimulation studies were performed in all patients before and 1–2 weeks after initiation of oral flecainide therapy. Before flecainide, all patients had easily inducible VT that was morphologically identical to their spontaneously occurring arrhythmia. Flecainide increased the mean P-R interval (from 0.17–0.23 second), mean QRS duration (from 0.08–0.12 s), and mean ventricular effective refractory period (from 235–270 ms). Mean corrected Q-T interval did not change (0.51 s). In 2 patients, VT could not be induced during follow-up stimulation studies. One patient has been treated successfully for 10 months with no clinically apparent episodes of VT. One patient had recurrent nonsustained VT and was withdrawn from the study as a treatment failure after 6 months of therapy. Two patients had inducible, polymorphous VT that degenerated into VF that required 2 countershocks before the successful restoration of sinus rhythm. One of these patients had VT stimulation by atrial pacing at a cycle length of 320 ms in the postflecainide electrophysiologic study. The VT was not inducible by atrial pacing during this patient's preflecainide study. Thus, sustained oral flecainide administration may precipitate serious electrical instability in susceptible patients, and ventricular stimulation studies and other clinical variables may be useful in selecting patients with recurrent VT who may benefit or may be endangered by oral flecainide therapy.

Encainide

Winkle and associates[56] from Stanford, California, gave encainide for 1 year to 12 patients with encainide-responsive frequent complex ventricular ectopic activity to establish long-term efficacy and the relation between drug plasma concentration and antiarrhythmic response. Twenty-four-hour ambulatory ECG was obtained at baseline and every 2 months. Drug withdrawal with concomitant plasma sampling and electrocardiographic monitoring was performed at 6 and 12 months. Average group premature VPC suppression during the year was 97–99%, with nearly total suppression of pairs and salvos. The most common adverse effects were transient visual disturbances and dizziness or lightheadedness. During a dose interval (6–12 hours), the concentration of encainide metabolites exceeded that of encainide by severalfold. The median time of arrhythmia return after drug withdrawal was 12–14 hours. At the time of arrhythmia return encainide was generally no longer detectable, but the average concentration of O-demethylencainide and 3 methoxy-O-demethylencainide was 72 ± 49 and 172 ± 74 ng/ml, respectively. It is concluded that encainide therapy is extremely effective for continuous long-term suppression of complex ventricular arrhythmias and its metabolites contribute significantly to its antiarrhythmic action during chronic oral therapy.

Chesnie and associates[57] from Boston, Massachusetts, studied 80 patients with sustained VT or VF in whom encainide, a new antiarrhythmic agent, was administered. Drug efficacy was evaluated by ambulatory monitoring and exercise testing in 63 patients who had frequent or repetitive VPC and by means of electrophysiologic testing in 17 patients who did not have significant arrhythmia during a 48-hour control period. Encainide was effective in 36 of 63 patients (57%) as judged by ambulatory monitoring and in 35 of 51 patients (69%) who had exercise tests while taking the drug. Overall, 34 patients (54%) responded to encainide when evaluated by both monitoring and exercise testing. The drug was effective in 7 of 16 patients (44%) who underwent electrophysiologic studies. Daily doses and blood levels of encainide were comparable in responders and nonresponders. Toxicity occurred in 24 patients (30%) and included nausea, vomiting, headaches, lethargy, tremors, and conduction disturbances. In 18 patients (23%) arrhythmia was aggravated. An increase in arrhythmia correlated with larger daily doses of encainide and higher serum blood levels of encainide and its metabolite O-demethylencainide, but did not correlate with QRS- or Q-T-interval widening. Of the 27 patients who were discharged on encainide, 23 were maintained on the drug for an average of 21 months (range, 12–44). Three patients died suddenly. Thus, encainide is a useful agent for suppression of malignant ventricular arrhythmias. However, it has a high potential for worsening arrhythmias and careful evaluation by both monitoring and exercise testing is necessary to judge its effect.

Gated cardiac scanning was used by Sami and associates[58] from Montreal, Canada, to evaluate the hemodynamic effects of encainide in 19 patients with complex ventricular arrhythmia and depressed LV EF (<45%). Patients were 36–80 years old (average, 61). All were candidates for long-term encainide therapy after having failed with currently available antiarrhythmic agents. Sixty-three percent had CHF before they received encainide. All were evaluated in the hospital before encainide therapy by a gated cardiac scan performed at least 3 days after discontinuing all antiarrhythmic drugs. Patients received oral encainide in doses of 75–200 mg. Gated cardiac scans were repeated 1–2 weeks later when an 80% reduction in frequency of VPC was observed on a 24-hour Holter recording. No patient had worsening of CHF during encainide therapy. Encainide did not significantly affect EF, which averaged 22 ± 10% before and 25 ± 14% (SD) after encainide (difference not significant). Other hemodynamic variables, including heart rate, BP, stroke volume, and end-diastolic volume, remained unchanged during encainide therapy. Digoxin blood levels in 10 patients averaged 1.04 ± 0.43 before and 1.22 ± 0.47 mg/ml (NS) during encainide therapy. Thus, encainide given orally in clinically effective doses does not appear to have significant hemodynamic effects in patients with ventricular arrhythmia and depressed LV function.

Lorcainide

Echt and colleagues[59] from Stanford, California, compared the electrophysiologic effects of intravenous lorcainide (2.2 mg/kg) in 10 patients with the electrophysiologic effects of oral lorcainide (mean dose, 400 mg/day for 8 days) in 11 patients, all with recurrent VT that could be induced with programmed stimulation. Intravenous and oral lorcainide resulted in similar prolongation of the QRS, Q-T, and H-V intervals, but only oral lorcainide resulted in prolongation of the A-H interval and atrial and ventricular effective refractory periods. After both oral and intravenous lorcainide, VT could still be induced, but the arrhythmia was slower and better tolerated hemodynamically. The mean plasma lorcainide level during a maintenance intravenous infusion was 1,254 ng/ml compared with lorcainide level of 562 ng/ml and a norlorcainide level of 1,212 ng/ml after oral dosing. No norlorcainide was detected in plasma after intravenous lorcainide. These data suggest that the short-term electrophysiologic effects of intravenous lorcainide may be different from those of short-term therapy with the oral drug and these differences should be considered during short-term studies of lorcainide.

Procainamide

Waxman and colleagues[60] from Philadelphia, Pennsylvania, assessed 126 patients with inducible sustained ventricular tachyarrhythmias to determine whether the response to procainamide during electrophysiologic study could predict responses to other conventional antiarrhythmic agents and combinations of agents. Thirty of 42 patients in whom VT was not inducible after the administration of procainamide and 69 of 84 patients in whom VT could be induced after procainamide underwent serial studies. Forty-three of 67 antiarrhythmic regimens (64%) tested in the patients in whom VT could not be induced after procainamide prevented induction of VT compared with 10 of 145 regimens (7%) tested in the patients in whom VT could be induced after procainamide. Sixty of 69 patients in whom VT remained inducible after procainamide had VT induced on all other conditional antiarrhythmic regimens tested. By comparison, of the 30 patients in whom VT became noninducible after procainamide, 25 had no VT inducible on at least one other antiarrhythmic regimen tested. Thus, the response to procainamide accurately predicts the response to other conventional antiarrhythmic agents during the electrophysiologic study.

Mexiletine

Waspe and associates[61] from Philadelphia, Pennsylvania, evaluated the antiarrhythmic efficacy of mexiletine in 44 patients with drug-resistant ventricular tachyarrhythmias. In 33 of these patients, the efficacy of mexiletine was assessed on the basis of the results of programmed ventricular stimulation. Mexiletine did not alter the ventricular effective refractory period, the Q-Tc interval, or the methods of tachyarrhythmia induction and termination during programmed stimulation. The mean cycle length of VT increased from 270 ± 49–313 ± 80 ms in 21 patients in whom VT remained inducible on mexiletine alone ($p < 0.002$). Overall, VT remained inducible with methods similar to control (no drugs) inductions in 25 patients receiving mexiletine alone or in combination with a type I agent. Induction of VT was prevented in only 8 patients, 3 on mexiletine alone and 5 receiving mexiletine combined with another drug. Mexiletine alone (in 2 patients) or with another agent (in 3) suppressed clinical recurrence of VT in another 5 of 11 patients who did not undergo electrophysiologic study. These 13 patients were discharged on mexiletine alone (5 patients) or in combination with other drugs (8 patients) and remained arrhythmia-free over a mean follow-up period of 7.7 ± 4.1 months. Adverse effects occurred in 27 of 44 patients (61%) and were gastrointestinal in 17 and/or neurologic in 22. The drug was discontinued because of adverse effects in 6 patients (14%). Thus, mexiletine has limited efficacy when used alone, but when combined with other drugs it may be useful in up to 30% of patients with drug-resistant ventricular arrhythmias. Adverse effects are relatively common.

Duff and associates[62] from Nashville, Tennessee, used mexiletine, an orally active lidocaine congener, to treat 21 patients in whom ventricular arrhythmias were not responsive to conventional antiarrhythmic therapy or in whom therapy produced limiting side effects. Of the 21 patients, 17 had CAD, 5 had episodes of VF, 6 had recurrent, sustained VT requiring cardioversion, and the remainder had episodic nonsustained VT. As the dosage of mexiletine was gradually increased, only 3 patients' arrhythmias were controlled without limiting side effects. One patient continued to have episodic VF during mexiletine therapy and was excluded. The other 17 patients had a partial antiarrhythmic response and 10 continued to have VT, but dose-related side effects limited therapy. These 17 patients had not responded to or did not tolerate quinidine. With the maximum well-tolerated dosage of quinidine, the mean suppression of VPC was 59%. Of the 17 patients, 11 continued to have VT with quinidine and therapy was limited by side effects in 11. In the group of 17 patients, the addition of a previously well-tolerated dosage of quinidine to a well-tolerated but only partially effective dose of mexiletine produced a significantly greater antiarrhythmic response. The mean suppression of VPC during combination therapy increased to 86%. Only 1 patient continued to have VT and limiting side effects occurred in 12% of the patients. Continuation of quinidine and withdrawal of mexiletine was associated with recurrence of complex ventricular arrhythmias and documented the need for combination treatment in 9 patients. The coupling interval of the predominant ectopic beat prolonged during mexiletine therapy and further prolonged with the addition of quinidine. After withdrawal of mexiletine from the combination treatment in 9 patients, the Q-Tc intervals significantly prolonged. Thus, mexiletine limited the quinidine-induced increase in Q-Tc interval. During 18 months of follow-up, 3 patients died. The addition of quinidine, which prolongs repolarization of the action potential in vitro, enhanced the antiarrhythmic efficacy of mexiletine, which shortens the action potential duration in vitro. Combinations of drugs with different electrophysiologic properties may enhance antiarrhythmic efficacy.

Acebutolol

The antiarrhythmic efficacy of oral acebutolol, a new cardioselective beta-blocking agent, was assessed in a randomized double-blind, placebo-controlled study by Lui and associates[63] from Davis, California. Twenty-five patients with ≥30 VPC per hour on 3 control ambulatory monitorings were studied. Mean VPC reduction from the control period was 35% with placebo and 45% and 50% with the use of acebutolol 200 mg and 400 mg, respectively. Eleven patients had ≥70% reduction in VPC with acebutolol and 9 of them had ≥90 VPC reduction. Among these 11 patients, the mean VPC suppression was 51% after placebo but significantly higher following the 2 doses of acebutolol at 71% (p < 0.05) and 86% (p < 0.01). The mean reduction of paired VPC compared with placebo was 71% (p < 0.05) and 75% (p < 0.01) following 200 mg and 400 mg of acebutolol and only 49% after placebo. Complete suppression of paroxysmal VT was also noted in 5 patients. Mean P-R interval only increased slightly when patients took 400 mg of acebutolol, but there was no significant change in either the QRS or Q-Tc intervals. A significant decrease in heart rate from that during control periods was noted after acebutolol. No significant adverse reactions were noted during the study. Acebutolol appears to be an effective and well-tolerated antiarrhythmic agent in the treatment of VPC and higher grades of ventricular ectopic activity.

Disopyramide

Lerman and associates[64] from Philadelphia, Pennsylvania, evaluated the efficacy of disopyramide in the management of sustained VT or VF in 50 patients by programmed ventricular stimulation: 38 had CAD (16 with LV aneurysm), 8 had other cardiac diseases, and 4 had no apparent heart disease. Disopyramide was administered orally for 72 hours (dosage, 400–1,600 mg/day), resulting in a plasma level of 3.6 ± 1.2 μg/ml (mean ± SD). Disopyramide prevented induction of sustained ventricular tachyarrhythmias in 17 patients (34%) and failed to prevent induction in 33 patients (66%). Plasma levels were not significantly different regardless of response to disopyramide. The VT cycle length in patients responding to disopyramide was shorter than in nonresponding patients (225 ± 51 ms -vs- 281 ± 70 ms; p = 0.005). Disopyramide increased VT cycle length in those patients in whom it was ineffective (failed to prevent induction) from 281 ± 70–347 ± 64 ms (p < 0.001). Ventricular refractory periods, QRS, and Q-Tc durations significantly increased after disopyramide administration. Of the 17 patients in whom tachyarrhythmias were noninducible on disopyramide, 11 were discharged on disopyramide and followed for 19 ± 9 months; 9 of them remained free of VT. Heart failure developed in 2 of these patients. One other patient in whom disopyramide was ineffective had irreversible CHF and died. It was concluded that disopyramide: 1) prevents induction of ventricular tachyarrhythmias in one-third of patients studied and remains clinically effective in approximately 80%; 2) is more frequently effective in rapid tachycardias; 3) prolongs the VT cycle length when ineffective, and 4) may produce marked hemodynamic embarrassment in patients with significant LF dysfunction.

Ethmozine

Pratt and associates[65] from Houston, Texas, reported on a total of 1,677 patient days of ethmozine use to suppress VPC. A total of 39 patients were studied on 3 placebo-controlled protocols. Ethmozine, given at a mean total daily dose of 830 mg ± 318 mg on a dosing schedule of every 8 hours, resulted in a mean plasma ethmozine level of 0.42 ± 0.28 μg/ml. In addition to reducing VPC from 11,049/24 hours during placebo to 2,231/24 hours during ethmozine therapy (80% reduction), the drug also resulted in 95% reduction in paired forms and 99% reduction in total runs of VT. Ethmozine was well tolerated with only mild side effects of dizziness, perioral tingling, and euphoria, with no serious toxicity requiring discontinuation of therapy. Therefore ethmozine (a phenothiazine derivative) demonstrates great potential as an effective drug in suppressing VPC with minimal side effects or toxicity.

Pirmenol

Reiter and associates[66] from Durham, North Carolina, tested a 3-stage concentration-maintaining intravenous infusion regimen of pirmenol, a new antiarrhythmic agent, for efficacy and safety in 8 patients with chronic stable VPC. The regimen, which consisted of a priming bolus of 50 mg over 2 minutes followed by a rapid loading infusion of 2.5 mg/minute for 1 hour and a maintenance infusion of 0.25 mg/minute, rapidly achieved and maintained stable plasma pirmenol levels from 0.94–2.75 μg/ml, during infusions lasting up to 48 hours. Therapeutic efficacy was evaluated during 4-hour infusions in 5 patients utilizing a randomized, double-blind, placebo-controlled study design. Pirmenol suppressed average VPC frequency 93 ± 6% compared with control values ($p = 0.03$). Pirmenol infusions were unassociated with toxicity. There were slight but significant increases in diastolic BP, QRS duration, and corrected Q-T interval. No significant changes occurred in systolic BP, heart rate, P-R interval, or laboratory variables. Pirmenol is a promising therapeutic agent that warrants further evaluation. The 3-stage infusion satisfactorily achieves and maintains therapeutic plasma pirmenol levels.

Propafenone

Connolly and associates[67] from Stanford, California, treated 16 patients with VT or nonfatal cardiac arrest with propafenone, 900 mg/day. Electrophysiologic studies were performed before and during therapy with propafenone. All patients had inducible sustained VT at the baseline study. During propafenone therapy, VT was not inducible in 1 patient, was unsustained in 1, and was more difficult to induce in 2 patients. Propafenone increased the cycle length of VT from 307 ± 67–382 ± 107 ms. Five patients began outpatient therapy with propafenone, including 2 in whom VT was slowed to <125 beats/minute. Two are arrhythmia-free during follow-up of 2 and 8 months. Propafenone significantly increased intraatrial conduction time (from 44 ± 12–72 ± 22 ms), A-H interval (from 115 ± 36–152 ± 45 ms), H-V interval (from 55 ± 18–92 ± 42 ms), QRS duration (from 140 ± 36–180 ± 48 ms) and Q-T interval (from 402 ± 30–459 ± 60 ms). Propafenone increased atrial (from 247 ± 36–288 ± 38 ms) and ventricular (from 249 ± 20–277 ± 32 ms) effective refractory periods. Sinus cycle length did not change, but the corrected sinus node recovery time increased (from 162 ± 85–821 ± 1,607 ms). Propafenone aggravated arrhythmias in 4 patients. The plasma propafenone concentration, measured either at the time of electrophysiologic studies or when therapy was discontinued, was 753 ± 428 ng/ml. Propafenone suppressed ventricular ectopic beats in 33% and increased them in 1 patient. Propafenone has antiarrhythmic activity against VT similar to that of other antiarrhythmic drugs and has potential for serious adverse effects in some patients.

N-Acetylprocainamide

To define electrophysiologic properties and antiarrhythmic mechanisms of N-acetylprocainamide (NAPA), Sung and colleagues[68] from Miami, Florida, studied 16 patients with symptomatic ventricular arrhythmias.

Electrophysiologic studies were performed before and after intravenous infusion of NAPA at 20 mg/kg over 20 minutes, achieving plasma concentrations of 24 ± 3.2–35.5 ± 4.5 µg/ml; NAPA did not significantly change sinus cycle length or AV conduction times (P-A, A-H, H-V, and QRS), but it lengthened the Q-Tc interval ($p < 0.001$) during sinus rhythm. Programmed atrial stimulation revealed that NAPA had no discernible effects on AV nodal conduction; however, it exerted depressive effects on the His-Purkinje system in 9 of 16 patients. In 7 of 16 patients who manifested frequent VPC, NAPA abolished VPC in only 3 of them; NAPA induced progressive prolongation of the premature coupling interval before complete abolition of VPC. In 8 of 16 patients who had inducible repetitive ventricular response (RVR) because of reentry within the His-Purkinje system, NAPA narrowed or abolished the RVR zone in 3 patients and slowed the RVR rate with widening of the RVR zone in the remaining 5 patients. In 2 of 16 patients with slow VT, NAPA had no antiarrhythmic effects. By contrast, in the other 2 of 16 patients in whom sustained VT could be reproducibly elicited with programmed ventricular stimulation, NAPA slowed the rate of VT and suppressed VT inducibility. Thus, the electrophysiologic properties of NAPA are slightly different from those of procainamide and NAPA is not uniformly effective for suppressing ventricular arrhythmias, but its antiarrhythmic mechanisms are similar to those of procainamide.

Beta blockers

Pratt and associates[69] from Houston, Texas, examined the extent of suppression of VPC that can be achieved with metoprolol, a semiselective beta-adrenergic blocking agent, at doses of 100–200 mg daily, utilizing a single-blind placebo-controlled 10-day protocol with continuous ambulatory ECG recording of 20 patients with cardiac disease and complex ventricular arrhythmias. Metoprolol (200 mg/day) resulted in suppression of 60% of total VPC, with couplets (pairs) and VT decreased 84 and 94%, respectively (all $p < 0.01$). Exercise-induced VPC, especially VT, were effectively suppressed. The peak plasma metoprolol level to achieve these results was 72 ± 34 ng/ml (mean ± 1 SD). At this plasma concentration, the mean 24-hour heart rate during normal activity was reduced from 78 ± 8 beats/minute (placebo) to 62 ± 4 (metoprolol 200 mg/day) ($p < 0.001$). Beta blockade also was demonstrated by a 20% reduction in heart rate during maximal Bruce exercise testing with metoprolol 200 mg/day. Although resting LV function was not affected by metoprolol, pulmonary function tests show a statistically significant decrease in forced vital capacity, forced expiratory volume in 1 second, and forced expiratory flow rates (25–75) reversible with a beta-2 agonist.

Glasser and associates[70] from Tampa, Florida, designed a study to assess the relative antiarrhythmic activity of fixed doses of 2 beta-adrenergic blocking agents, propranolol and acebutolol, in a prospective double-blind crossover trial. Twenty-one patients who had ≥30 VPC per hour while receiving placebo were entered into the study. Ten patients were randomized to receive propranolol 40 mg every 8 hours initially, and 11 were assigned to receive acebutolol 300 mg every 8 hours. After 6 weeks of treatment, patients were weaned off medication for 1 week and then placed on placebo for 1 week. Eighteen patients were available and eligible for crossover to the alternative regimen for an additional 6 weeks. All 21 patients completed courses with propranolol and 17 completed courses with acebutolol. The mean number of VPC per hour during placebo, propranolol, and acebutolol treatment were 267, 87, and 119, respectively. Both propranolol and acebutolol significantly reduced the number of VPC per hour compared with placebo, whereas similar analysis revealed no significant difference in the antiarrhythmic effect. With the current sample size, the power of the test is too low for the latter conclusion to be stated with confidence. Side effects were mild and infrequent, requiring discontinuation of acebutolol in 2 patients and discontinuation of propranolol in 1. Thus, acebutolol is a safe and effective antiarrhythmic agent and compares favorably with propranolol.

Calcium channel blockers

Mason and associates[71] from Stanford, California, gave verapamil, 0.25 mg/kg, to 24 patients with chronic, recurrent VT whose clinical tachyarrhythmias were reproduced at electrophysiologic study. Seven patients (29%) had a short-term response to verapamil: VT was not inducible in 5 and spontaneously terminated within 5 seconds of induction in 2 patients in whom it was previously sustained. Four of the 7 responders had no identifiable structural heart disease and 3 had CAD. Responders were younger and had better LV function than did nonresponders. Long-term therapy with verapamil, attempted in 5 of the 7 responders, was effective in 3, ineffective in 1, and of uncertain efficacy in 1. Verapamil therapy was discontinued because of worsened CHF in 2 patients. The short-term efficacy of verapamil in these patients compares favorably with the efficacy of other antiarrhythmic agents against VT induction in patients with long-term, recurrent, drug-refractory VT. The short-term efficacy of verapamil correlated with its long-term efficacy. These observations provide preliminary evidence that verapamil may be useful in the treatment of some patients with recurrent VT. When standard drugs are not effective, verapamil should be given a trial, especially in young patients with good LV function.

Yeh and associates[72] from Taipai, Taiwan, performed electrophysiologic studies before and 2 hours after the oral administration of 270 mg of diltiazem in 3 divided doses at 8-hour intervals in 36 patients with paroxysmal SVT. Before diltiazem, all 36 patients had induction of sustained SVT: 24 with AV reentrance incorporating an accessory pathway (group 1) and 12 with AV nodal reentrance (group 2). After diltiazem, 20 patients in group 1 lost the ability to induce or sustain SVT because of increased antegrade normal pathway refractoriness in 19 patients and increased retrograde accessory pathway refractoriness in 1. Eight patients in group 2 could no longer induce or sustain SVT because of increased antegrade slow pathway refractoriness in 2 patients and increased retrograde fast pathway refractoriness in 6. Diltiazem concentration in the blood, measured in 29 patients, was 156 ± 75 ng/ml (mean $\pm$ SD). Fifteen patients, 2 with and 13 without induction of sustained SVT after diltiazem, were discharged on the same dosage of diltiazem and followed 5 ± 3 months. The former 2 patients had attacks of sustained SVT, whereas the latter 13 have been free of sustained SVT. In conclusion, oral diltiazem prevents induction and sustenance of paroxysmal SVT in most patients and may be used as an alternative agent for the prophylaxis of SVT.

Amiodarone

Morady and associates[73] from San Francisco, California, reported on 15 patients with recurrent symptomatic VT refractory to at least 2 conventional antiarrhythmic drugs, all of whom had organic heart disease with a mean EF of 30%, 12 had overt CHF and 5 had BBB. Before treatment with intravenous amiodarone, the patients had had 6–40 episodes of symptomatic VT over 1–8 days of hospitalization. All patients received an initial bolus of 5 mg/kg amiodarone over 15 minutes. Seven patients also received a continuous infusion of 600–1,000 mg of amiodarone over 12–24 hours. Additional doses depended on the patient's clinical response. In 11 of 15 patients, antiarrhythmic drugs that had failed to suppress VT were continued during administration of amiodarone. In 12 of 15 patients acute control of VT was obtained with intravenous administration of amiodarone either alone or in combination with previously ineffective drugs. Three patients continued to have frequent episodes of VT while being treated with intravenous amiodarone. Mobitz type 1 AV block developed in 1 patient. No patient had high degree AV block, symptomatic hypotension, or a clinically apparent worsening of CHF. The use of intravenous amiodarone represents a significant advance in the acute treatment of frequent life-threatening VT refractory to other drugs. With appropriate monitoring, it can be used safely in patients with CHF, BBB, or AMI.

Heger and associates[74] from Indianapolis, Indiana, studied the clinical antiarrhythmic efficacy of amiodarone treatment in 196 patients with recurrent VT or VF resistant to other antiarrhythmic drugs. Patients had received a mean of 4.4 ± 1.9 unsuccessful drug trials over a mean of 15 months before amiodarone treatment of recurrent VF in 57 patients; recurrent sustained VT in 95 patients; and recurrent nonsustained VT in 44 patients. Amiodarone dosage during the first 2–4 weeks of treatment was 800–1,600 mg/day. During long-term follow-up, amiodarone dosage was reduced to 200–600 mg/day, based on the control of arrhythmia and patient tolerance. Electrophysiologic studies were performed prior to and after 2 or more weeks of amiodarone treatment. After a mean follow-up of 16 ± 13 months, 126 (64%) of 196 patients continued successful treatment with amiodarone. At electrophysiologic study, amiodarone prevented VT induction in 13 patients, and although VT was induced in 101 patients, 80 patients continued treatment for 14 months without recurrence of spontaneous VT. Amiodarone treatment was discontinued because of recurrent VT in 22 patients, sudden cardiac death in 15 patients, adverse effects in 12 patients, and noncardiac death in 21 patients. In 9 patients, recurrent VT/VF appeared related to amiodarone-induced exacerbation of arrhythmia. Pulmonary toxicity occurred in 7 patients, and 19 patients developed blue skin discoloration. Other adverse effects were usually dosage related. In conclusion, amiodarone is a highly effective antiarrhythmic drug, but at the dosages necessary, the risk of significant adverse effects warrants careful surveillance during treatment.

Morady and associates[75] from San Francisco, California, administered amiodarone to 154 patients with sustained, symptomatic VT (n, 118) or cardiac arrest (n, 36) and who were refractory to conventional antiarrhythmic drugs. The loading dose was 800 mg/day for 6 weeks and the maintenance dose was 600 mg/day. Sixty-nine percent of patients continued treatment with amiodarone and had no recurrence of symptomatic VT or VF over a follow-up of 6–52 months (mean ± SD, 14 ± 8). Six percent of the patients had a nonfatal recurrence of VT and were successfully managed by continuing amiodarone at a higher dose or by the addition of a conventional antiarrhythmic drug. One or more adverse drug reactions occurred in 51% of patients. Adverse effects forced a reduction in the dose of amiodarone in 41% and discontinuation of amiodarone in 10% of patients. The most common symptomatic adverse reactions were tremor or ataxia (35%), nausea and anorexia (8%), visual halos or blurring (6%), thyroid function abnormalities, (6%) and pulmonary interstitial infiltrates (5%). Although large-dose amiodarone is highly effective in the long-term treatment of VT or VF refractory to conventional antiarrhythmic drugs, it causes significant toxicity in approximately 50% of patients. However, when the dose is adjusted based on clinical response or the development of adverse effects, 75% of patients with VT or VF can be successfully managed with amiodarone.

Treatment with ultrarapid stimulation or countershock

Termination of VT with single programmed extrastimuli or slow underdrive competitive pacing is often possible. The usefulness of these techniques is limited because the zone in the cardiac cycle during which programmed stimuli are effective may be narrow, with significant time elapsing until termination of the VT, and the zone may vary markedly between episodes, rendering preset extrastimuli ineffective. Ultrarapid trains of stimuli beginning during the refractory period and of a duration sufficient to cause only a single capture should terminate all tachycardias whose termination zone begins just after the refractory period. To test this hypothesis, Fisher and associates[76] from New York City performed single programmed extrastimuli in trains of 10 bipolar stimuli at 25, 50, and 100 Hz in 21 patients with 371 well-tolerated episodes of VT. The VT was terminated 1 or more times in 18 of the 21 patients with programmed extrastimuli or trains, or both. Forty-eight percent of 290 episodes were terminated with programmed stimulation, compared with 56% of 120 episodes with trains (difference not significant). In 98 episodes, the effects of trains and programmed stimulation could be matched (same patient, date, tachycardia morphology, rate, and drug therapy); the results were concordant (both techniques either terminated the VT or failed) in 92 and discordant in 6. With only 2 possible exceptions, the termination zone always began just after the refractory period; thus, for tachycardias terminating with single captures, the first train to achieve capture was effective, minimizing the duration of the VT.

Waspe and associates[77] from New York City evaluated the practicality and safety of using a single catheter system for transvenous countershock, programmed stimulation, and ventricular pacing during electrophysiologic tests in 13 patients with inducible sustained VT or VF. The efficacy and patient toleration of transvenous countershock were compared with other methods of arrhythmia termination. The same lead was used for programmed stimulation at the RV apex and for VT termination by pacing methods during serial testing (20 ± 15 days [mean ± SD]). Synchronized countershock using energies that patients found tolerable (0.01–5 J) terminated 31 of 50 episodes (62%) of induced VT. Episodes of VT cardioverted with these low energies were distinguished from other episodes by a longer cycle length (352 ± 62 ms -vs- 297 ± 50 ms; p < 0.004). Among paired episodes of VT matched for patient, date of induction, morphologic characteristics, cycle length, and drugs administered, pacing methods (single extrastimuli and bursts of rapid pacing) were just as effective as low-energy countershock for VT termination (25 of 25 -vs- 21 of 25, difference not significant). Transvenous countershock was uniformly effective for termination of ventricular flutter and VF when sufficient energy was used (range, 5–30 J; mean, 20.4 ± 7.7). This required interfacing leads to a defibrillation unit. Acceleration of VT occurred during 7 of 50 synchronized low-energy cardioversion attempts (14%). There was no evidence of myocardial injury as a result of shocks as high as 30 J, but patients required increasing sedation when energy exceeded 0.5 J. Thus, a single catheter system can be used for programmed stimulation, ventricular pacing, and countershock during electrophysiologic tests. Low-energy countershock (0.01–5 J) is no more effective than pacing methods for VT termination and is tolerated less well. The most practical use of this catheter system, including any implantable unit, may be for slightly higher energy (5–30 J) countershock termination of repeated episodes of very rapid VT or VF, for which pacing techniques are ineffective. This method may be safer and less traumatic than conventional transthoracic countershock.

Internal automatic cardioverter-defibrillator

Reid and associates[78] from Baltimore, Maryland, evaluated an R-wave synchronous implantable automatic cardioverter-defibrillator (IACD) in 12 patients with repeated episodes of cardiac arrest who remain refractory to medical and surgical therapy. Seven men and 5 women, average age of 61 years, surgically received a complete IACD system. Coronary artery disease was found in 11 and the prolonged Q-T syndrome in 1. The average EF was 34%, and 6 patients had severe CHF (New York Heart Association class III or IV). The IACD is a completely implantable unit consisting of 2 bipolar lead systems. One system uses a lead in the superior vena cava and on the LV apex through which the cardioverting pulse is delivered. The second system employs a close bipolar lead implanted in the ventricle for sensing rate. After the onset of VT or fibrillation, the IACD automatically delivers approximately 25 J. Postoperative electrophysiologic study in 10 and spontaneous VT in 1 patient demonstrated appropriate IACD function and successful conversion in all with an average of 18 ± 4 seconds. The induced arrhythmias were VT (160–300 beats/min) in 9 and VF in 1. These data demonstrate that VT, not VF, was the preventricular stimulation in these survivors of cardiac arrest and that the IACD effectively responded to a wide range of VT rates as well as VF. Use of the IACD offers an effective means of therapy for some patients who otherwise may not have survived.

Dulk and associates[79] from Maastricht, The Netherlands, described results of insertion of an externally activated pacemaker system in 13 patients to control their drug-resistant tachycardias. Four patients had VT, 2 had AV nodal reentrant tachycardia, 3 had tachycardias due to left-sided concealed accessory pathway, and 4 had WPW syndrome. Nine patients were paced from the right ventricle, 2 from the right atrium, and 2 from the coronary sinus. The pacing system consisted of an implantable pacemaker, an external pacemaker activator, and a prescription formulator. The pacemaker can signal sensing by way of radiofrequency signals to the pacemaker activator or prescription formulator. Either of the latter 2 devices then determines whether the sensed rhythm fulfills the tachycardia detection criteria and, if so, controls the delivery of the selected stimulation treatment by the pacemaker. With this bidirectional radiofrequency coupling, tachycardias were noninvasively initiated by the prescription formulator after implantation and at follow-up visits to test and eventually reprogram the pacemaker activator. During a follow-up of 116 patient-months, 624 episodes of tachycardia were effectively terminated by the patients. Incidental failure to terminate occurred in 3 patients because of a defective activator, changes in the electrophysiologic substrate, and inappropriate use of the device. These problems were solved by reprogramming, replacement of the activator, and education of the patient. Hospital admissions for termination of tachycardia decreased from an average of 2.6/patient-month (in the 3 months before implantation) to 0.03/patient-month after implantation (follow-up, 4–16 months). It is concluded that this programmable externally activated pacemaker system 1) effectively manages drug-resistant tachycardia; 2) has the advantage of easy testing, multiple pacing modes, and ready reprogrammability; and 3) is cost effective because of marked reduction in hospital admissions.

The first-generation automatic implantable defibrillator sensed arrhythmias by monitoring a transcardiac ECG signal. This sensing system reliably detected VF and sinusoidal VT but failed to sense all nonsinusoidal VT. To solve this problem, Winkle and associates[80] from Stanford, California, developed a new VT detection scheme using a local ventricular bipolar electrogram and electronic circuits using rate averaging and automatic gain control to permit sensing of electrograms as low as 0.1 mV. This detection scheme was tested during electrophysiologic studies in 11 patients with VT and fibrillation. All 22 episodes of induced VT with a rate higher than the selected cutoff were detected after an average of 5.1 ± 1.8 seconds. No episodes below the rate cutoff were detected. The bipolar circuits also reliably detected VF. Arrhythmia detection and signal quality in 9 patients receiving automatic defibrillators using the new bipolar rate detection circuit were compared with the findings in 5 patients previously receiving units that sensed arrhythmias using the transcardiac ECG signal. Compared with the transcardiac monitoring units, the newer bipolar units had shorter and more uniform sense times (5.5 ± 1.4 -vs- 12.2 ± 7.1 seconds). It is concluded that malignant VT can be sensed accurately using bipolar rate detection and that this system has numerous advantages over the previously used transcardiac ECG signal.

Surgery

Kienzle and associates[81] from Philadelphia, Pennsylvania, evaluated 36 patients after endocardial resection for medically refractory VT to determine the prognostic importance of inducibility of VT by programmed stimulation and then the predictive ability of drug suppression of VT occurring following electrical stimulation. Postoperatively, VT was noninducible in 25 patients and inducible in 11. After administration of antiarrhythmic agents, VT could no longer be induced in 4 patients and remained inducible in the other 7 patients. Most postoperative patients had repetitive forms of ventricular arrhythmia and there was no difference between patients with inducible and noninducible VT postoperatively in regard to Holter monitoring characteristics. There was also no significant difference in postoperative EF between patients with inducible and noninducible VT. The VT recurred in 2 of 29 patients without inducible tachycardia at the time of hospital discharge and in 1 of 7 patients in whom it was inducible at the time of hospital discharge during a mean follow-up of 7 months to 1 year. These data suggest: 1) subendocardial resection does not affect the level of ventricular ectopic activity; 2) ventricular ectopic activity measured by postoperative 24-hour ECG monitoring is not related to postoperative inducibility of VT; and 3) inducible VT despite antiarrhythmic therapy or high grade ectopic activity does not preclude a good outcome after subendocardial resection for refractory VT.

Garan and associates[82] from Boston, Massachusetts, performed electrophysiologic studies with programmed cardiac stimulation on 17 patients with severe proximal CAD involving ≥2 major coronary arteries and with an LV EF >30% who were undergoing CABG after prehospital cardiac arrest or VT unassociated with AMI. Before surgery and without antiarrhythmic drug therapy, programmed cardiac stimulation induced VF in 4 patients, and VT (≥5 beats) in 11 patients. Inducible VT or VF was suppressed by antiarrhythmic drugs in 7 of 13 patients in whom they were tried. Patients underwent CABG unassociated with perioperative AMI. When studied again an average of 19 days after surgery, 10 patients had no inducible VT or VF without antiarrhythmic drug therapy; 6 had induced VT. One patient had spontaneous VT. An effective antiarrhythmic regimen that suppressed inducible or spontaneous VT, or both, was defined by serial electrophysiologic studies in 4 patients, whereas 3 patients continued to manifest electrically inducible VT with all antiarrhythmic regimens tested. All but 1 patient, in whom postoperative VT could not be suppressed, are free of arrhythmias after a mean follow-up period of 23 months (range, 6–53). It was concluded that CABG alone may improve the abnormal electrophysiologic findings in certain patients; however, this effect of CABG is unpredictable, and pre- and postoperative electrophysiologic studies are recommended as part of the evaluation of these patients.

Page and associates[83] from Birmingham, Alabama, evaluated early postoperative epicardial programmed ventricular stimulation after electrophysiologically guided surgery for ventricular arrhythmias in 34 patients undergoing epicardial stimulation within 7–30 days after surgery and with a follow-up for ≥6 months. Endocardial ventriculotomy or endocardial resection or a combination of these 2 procedures was used in these patients. Temporary epicardial electrodes were placed at the time of surgery and were used to perform the pacing. In 19 patients, no ventricular arrhythmia was produced, whereas 15 patients had VT induced by epicardial pacing. In 4 patients, no major arrhythmias occurred during a mean follow-up of 20 months, whereas 7 important arrhythmias occurred in patients in whom ventricular arrhythmias could be induced by pacing postoperatively. In these latter patients, the arrhythmic events included sudden death in 5 patients and sustained tachycardia in 2 patients. Therefore these data suggest that temporary epicardial pacing may be used to determine the risk for future life-threatening arrhythmias in patients following cardiac surgery for correction of ventricular tachyarrhythmias.

CARDIAC ARREST

Benson and associates[84] from Minneapolis, Minnesota, examined clinical, hemodynamic, and electrophysiologic findings in 11 patients aged 15 months to 29 years who are survivors of a cardiac arrest. All patients previously were in good health, and cardiac arrest was the initial manifestation of cardiac disease in all. Overt clinical and hemodynamic abnormalities were not as common as previously reported, and in some instances apparent cardiac abnormalities failed to provide a link to cardiac arrest. No patient had congenital heart disease or HC. However, during multicatheter electrophysiologic study, sustained tachyarrhythmia was reproducibly initiated in 8 of 11 patients (73%). Young, ostensibly healthy patients who survive cardiac arrest form a diverse group. Diligent programmed intracardiac electrical stimulation may demonstrate life-threatening tachycardias in these patients. Treatment to prevent recurrence of cardiac arrest is difficult in this group of patients. However, the ability to initiate tachycardia in the electrophysiologic laboratory may be useful in the management of these patients.

Ventricular fibrillation is a frequent terminal cardiac electrical activity in adults, but frequency data in pediatric patients were unavailable until Walsh and Krongrad[85] from New York City determined terminal cardiac electrical activity in 100 pediatric patients (Fig. 3-3). Bradycardic arrest throughout the death process occurred in 88% of the newborn, 67% of infants, and 64% of children. Although bradycardic arrest was more common, the frequency of ventricular tachyarrhythmias was higher in patients who had congenital heart disease, who had received cardiopulmonary resuscitation, who were beyond the neonatal period, and/or who weighed >2.23 kg. No definite associations could be established between arterial blood gases, electrolyte values, and type of terminal cardiac electrical activity. The development of VF may be related to cardiac mass and the developing autonomic nervous system and therefore is less likely to occur in patients with a small heart.

Morady and associates[86] from San Francisco, California, performed programmed ventricular stimulation in 45 patients who survived cardiac arrest due to either VT or VF. While the patients were taking no antiarrhythmic medications, sustained VT was induced in 26 patients (58%) and nonsustained VT in 8 (18%). With treatment aimed at the underlying heart disease (plus empiric antiarrhythmic therapy in 2 patients), the 11 patients who had no inducible VT have had no recurrence of symptomatic VT or cardiac arrest over a follow-up period of 19 ± 9 months (mean ± SD). Conventional antiarrhythmic drugs suppressed the induction of VT and were used for chronic treatment in 9 of 34 patients (26%) with inducible VT. Three of these 9 patients had recurrent VT or sudden death, whereas 6 have had no recurrence over a follow-up of 20 ± 7 months. In 25 of 34 patients in

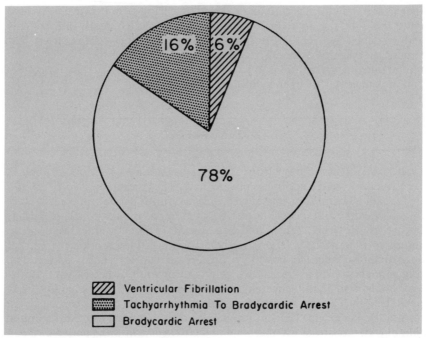

Fig. 3-3. Summary of terminal cardiac electrical activity in 100 patients. Bradycardic arrest occurred throughout the death process in 78% of patients. Sixteen percent had episodes of VT or VF, with bradycardic arrest as the final electrical event. Unremitting VF was seen in 6%.

whom the induction of VT was not suppressed by conventional antiarrhythmic drugs, 23 were treated with amiodarone (daily dose, 550 ± 120 mg) and 2 underwent CABG with either aneurysmectomy or map-directed endocardial resection. One of the latter 2 patients died suddenly 12 months after surgery. Among the 23 patients treated with amiodarone, 2 had fatal VT or sudden death and 21 (91%) did not at 18 ± 14 months of follow-up. In survivors of a cardiac arrest, the chief value of electrophysiologic testing is in identifying patients without inducible VT who appear to have a low risk of recurrent sudden death with treatment directed at the underlying heart disease. Serial electropharmacologic testing with conventional antiarrhythmic drugs is disappointing, with low incidence of arrhythmia suppression.

To develop a model that would forecast neurologic recovery after out-of-hospital cardiac arrest, Longstreth and associates[87] from Seattle, Washington, reviewed charts of 389 consecutive patients who were not awake on admission to the hospital after resuscitation from asystole or VF. The outcome variable was "awakening," which was defined as having comprehensible speech or the ability to follow commands. Predictor variables considered included both preadmission and admission data. Using discriminant analysis, models were derived from a 60% random sample of cases and tested on the remaining 40%. The best model contained 4 variables from the admission examination: motor response, pupillary light response, spontaneous eye movements, and blood glucose (<300 mg/dl predicted awakening). Overall correct classification was 80% in the derivation sample and 77% in the test sample. In a simplified form, the model's predictions of awakening had a sensitivity of 0.92, a specificity of 0.65, a positive predictive value of 0.80, and a negative predictive value of 0.84. This rule should be clinically useful in estimating the neurologic prognosis of patients resuscitated after out-of-hospital cardiac arrest.

Little is known about prognostic factors that determine outcomes after in-hospital cardiopulmonary resuscitation. Bedell and associates[88] from Boston, Massachusetts, studied prospectively 294 consecutive patients who were resuscitated in a university teaching hospital. Forty-one patients (14%) were discharged from the hospital; 75% were still alive 6 months later. A multivariate analysis revealed that pneumonia, hypotension, renal failure, cancer, and a homebound lifestyle before hospitalization were significantly associated with in-hospital mortality ($p < 0.05$). None of the 58 patients with pneumonia and none of the 179 in whom resuscitation took >30 minutes survived to be discharged. Of the patients who survived for 24 hours after resuscitation, 42% left the hospital. At discharge from the hospital and again 6 months later, 93% of the survivors were mentally intact. Although depression was generally present at the time of discharge, it tended to resolve subsequently. All patients reported some decrease in functional capacity, which persisted at 6 months after discharge. Age alone did not appear to influence the prognosis for survival after cardiopulmonary resuscitation or the adjustment to chronic illness after discharge from the hospital.

Panidis and Morganroth[89] from Philadelphia, Pennsylvania, evaluated 15 patients with cardiac arrest occurring during ambulatory ECG monitoring in the hospital. Eleven of these patients had heart disease and 7 of the patients were admitted to the hospital with chest pain before sudden death occurred. The terminal event at the time of cardiac arrest in 3 of the 15 patients was a bradyarrhythmia expressed as complete heart block and none of these patients survived. In the remaining 12 patients, a ventricular tachyarrhythmia was the precursor of sudden cardiac death; 2 of these patients had slow VT and both died. Five had polymorphous VT associated with a prolonged Q-T interval (torsade de pointes) and 3 were receiving a class I antiarrhythmic agent. This rhythm degenerated into VF in 1 patient and 4 of the 5 patients survived after electrical cardioversion. One patient had VT followed by asystole. Four patients had rapid VT (rate >250/min) that degenerated into VF in 1 patient. Thus, these data suggest that a ventricular tachyarrhythmia is usually found on Holter monitoring during sudden cardiac death in hospitalized patients and that VF is almost always preceded by VT.

Previous studies have suggested that a number of factors may influence the ability to defibrillate: the transthoracic resistance and resultant current flow, the paddle electrode size, the duration of preshock VF and cardiopulmonary resuscitation, metabolic abnormalities, body weight, the shock energy selected, and whether the patient was receiving lidocaine. To examine the effect of these variables, Kerber and associates[90] from Iowa City, Iowa, conducted a prospective study of 183 patients who received direct current shocks for VF. Overall defibrillation rates approached 90%, even in patients with secondary VF, but rates of successful resuscitation and survival were much lower. Patients who never defibrillated despite multiple shocks had a prolonged duration of cardiopulmonary resuscitation preceding the first shock (21 ± 14 minutes) and systemic hypoxia and acidosis. These conditions tended to occur in patients who initially had cardiac arrest from causes other than VF: asystole, severe bradycardia, and electromechanical dissociation. In such patients, VF developed only as a late event, which was then often unresponsive to attempted defibrillation. The other factors examined were not major determinants of defibrillation.

Ruskin and associates[91] from Boston, Massachusetts, used standard electrophysiologic techniques to evaluate 6 patients taking an antiarrhythmic drug (5 patients, to suppress ventricular premature beats and 1 to control recurrent atrial flutter) who were without evidence of drug toxicity at the time of cardiac arrest. When antiarrhythmic drugs were withheld, no arrhythmia could be induced by programmed cardiac stimulation. When the 6 patients were rechallenged with the same drug at therapeutic levels, VT was initiated by programmed cardiac stimulation in 4 of the 6, and high grade AV block developed in a fifth patient. Without antiarrhythmic drugs, 5 patients were alive and free of recurrent arrhythmia after a follow-up of 8–50 months. These observations suggest that antiarrhythmic drugs may contribute to the occurrence of cardiac arrest in some patients.

Roy and associates[92] from Philadelphia, Pennsylvania, performed electrophysiologic studies in 119 survivors of cardiac arrest. Sustained ventricular arrhythmias were initiated by programmed ventricular stimulation in 72 patients (61%). In CAD patients with induced sustained ventricular arrhythmias a higher frequency of prior AMI (95 -vs- 72%) and ventricular aneurysm (59 -vs- 28%) occurred, and there was a lower EF (37 -vs- 50%) than in those with no inducible sustained ventricular arrhythmias. Of the 72 patients with inducible ventricular arrhythmias, 11 (15%) died suddenly during a mean follow-up of 18 months (range, 15 days to 58 months). In this group, 6 (15%) of 41 patients discharged on a successful antiarrhythmic regimen and 5 (19%) of 27 patients discharged on an unsuccessful regimen or without a predischarge study died suddenly. Of these 27 patients, 1 of 12 patients treated with amiodarone and 4 (27%) of 15 with conventional antiarrhythmic therapy died suddenly. The remaining 4 patients died of nonarrhythmic causes in the postoperative period. Of 47 patients without inducible sustained ventricular arrhythmias, 15 (32%) died suddenly at a mean follow-up of 20 months, 10 (34%) with and 15 (28%) without empiric therapy. It is concluded that sustained ventricular arrhythmias can be initiated in most patients resuscitated from cardiac arrest. Patients with inducible arrhythmias have greater LV dysfunction than those without inducible arrhythmias. Medical or surgical therapy that prevented the induction of sustained ventricular arrhythmias was predictive of a successful outcome in 85% of the patients. Patients with persistence of inducible sustained ventricular arrhythmias despite conventional drug therapy and patients without inducible arrhythmias in whom therapy cannot be guided by electrophysiologic testing have a higher incidence of recurrent sudden death.

Pratt and associates[93] from Houston, Texas, evaluated 15 patients who developed VF during ambulatory ECG monitoring. Quantitative analysis of ECG alterations in the hours prior to VF revealed an increase in frequency of VPC and VT, especially in the 2 hours immediately before VF. The VF was initiated by VT in all 15 patients. Preceding runs of VT were characterized by a relatively long length and rapid rate; occasional R-on-T VPC were documented but the mean prematurity index of the initiating VPC was not early. Q-T prolongation was present in only 3 of the 15 patients. The mean LV EF was 34.9 ± 9.9% and CAD was nearly always present. The cardiac medications most frequently associated with these arrhythmias were digitalis and quinidine.

Lewis and associates[94] from Boston, Massachusetts, evaluated the ambulatory ECG recordings in 12 patients who developed VF or torsade de pointes. Common ambulatory ECG features in these 12 patients experiencing VF or torsade de pointes included increasing frequency or complex ventricular arrhythmias or both, R-on-T beats, and repolarization abnormalities present for several hours before the electrical event. Thus, ventricular arrhythmias resulting in sudden death in an ambulatory population are preceded by a period of increased or more complex ventricular ectopic activity.

Benditt and associates[95] from Minneapolis, Minnesota, evaluated the usefulness of serial provocative electropharmacologic testing for predicting the efficacy of prophylactic antiarrhythmic treatment regimens in patients resuscitated from sudden cardiac death in the absence of AMI. Thirty-four consecutive patients who had required cardiopulmonary resuscitation (CPR) and direct current countershock for treatment of primary VF (28 patients), VT (5 patients), or excessively rapid heart rate during AF with preexcitation (1 patient) were evaluated. Drug testing was not feasible in 8 patients because of the absence of inducible arrhythmias or was incomplete because of patient withdrawal; 3 of these 8 patients had recurrent sudden cardiac arrest within 10–19 months. In 5 more patients, treatment regimens failed to prevent sustained ventricular tachyarrhythmias in the cardiac catheterization laboratory and 2 of these 5 patients had cardiac arrest recurrences subsequently. The remaining 21 patients had a drug regimen or surgical treatment or both that prevented inducible life-threatening tachyarrhythmias in the laboratory. Only 1 of these patients died suddenly during 7–38 months of follow-up. These data confirm that electropharmacologic testing is useful in predicting response to therapy in survivors of sudden cardiac arrest.

Clark and associates[96] from New York City analyzed ambulatory ECG recordings of 6 patients with CAD who died during monitoring. In 4 patients sinus rhythm was interrupted by sinoatrial, AV, nodal, or infra-His conduction abnormalities leading to bradyarrhythmic sudden death. Two patients died of sustained VT or VF. These data emphasize that the arrhythmias involved in the sudden death syndrome may be more heterogenous than currently appreciated.

Cardiac arrest may be due to weakening or slowing of the normal heart beat, to asystole, or to VF. The first successful CPR outside an operating room was described in 1956 and the method of closed-chest massage in 1960. With modern CPR techniques and portable direct-current cardioversion equipment, of course, almost any patient may be a candidate for resuscitation. Most reports on this subject have dealt largely with cardiac arrest calls on general wards and in intensive care units, and these success rates have ranged from 2–14%. There is general agreement that CPR should not be attempted when a patient has terminal or incurable disease, but should age alone be an excluding factor? Because little is known of the outcome of CPR in older people, Gulati and associates[97] from Oldham, England, in a prospective study attempted CPR in 52 patients aged 64–91 years (mean, 76). Of the 14 who were resuscitated initially, 5 died in the first week; of the 9 still alive at 1 month, none appeared to have adverse effects in terms of mental status or physical dependence from the episode of cardiac arrest and resuscitation and 7 left the hospital. Thus, the nature of the cardiac arrhythmia is a strong predictor of outcome, but age, sex, and time of arrest are not.

This article on CPR in older persons was followed by an unsigned editorial entitled "Should Dying be a Diagnosis?"[98] The following are quotations from the unsigned editorial. "Although age alone is not a reason for excluding patients from active medical treatment, there is a stage when clinical facts and common sense dictate that living has become dying. This stage can be reached at any age—in the unborn child; in the comatose teenage motorcyclist; in the mature patient who has cancer; and most frequently in the old. . . . With the known incidence of mental impairment in the elderly and the susceptibility of this group of patients to the deleterious effects of cardiovascular collapse, these results (those of Gulati and associates) are remarkably, and perhaps freakishly, good. . . . Attempts were made to resuscitate 38 patients who did not survive. The report of Gulati and associates poses the ethical question, 'Is CPR in these circumstances good medical practice?' Two other important questions arise: Can sudden and inevitable dying in old age be recognized to avoid unwarranted resuscitative attacks on patients; and when should dying and old age be accepted and

Fig. 3-4. Thoracic structures punctured by clinical intracardiac injections. Reproduced with permission from Sabin et al.[99]

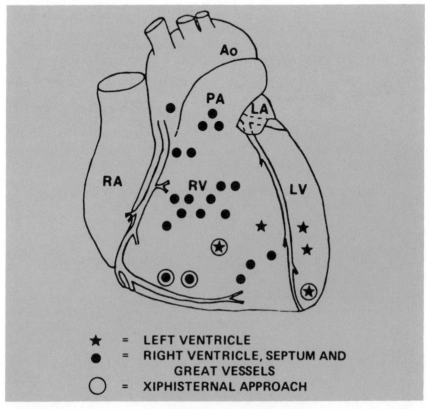

granted dignity? Those who may feel moved to repeat this work would do well to consider that, difficult though it is to assess intellectual impairment, especially in the elderly, the reckoning should include assessment of the life-quality of the survivors, to be weighed against stresses on fellow patients and the unpeaceful departure of those in whom the procedures are unsuccessful."

Sabin and associates[99] from Dundee, New Zealand, traced intracardiac injection sites at necropsy in 18 patients who died after unsuccessful CPR. In only 13 patients (72%) was the heart punctured (Fig. 3-4). Of the 46 injections, 5 (11%) pierced the left ventricle and 13 (28%) the right ventricle. Other structures punctured included the pulmonary trunk, the aorta, and the lung. The fourth intercostal space just lateral to the sternal edge was the most common injection site, and only 5 injections were subxiphoid. Postmortem injections on another 20 cadavers confirmed that the RV wall was the most frequent puncture site whichever approach is used.

SYNCOPE

Kapoor and associates[100] from Pittsburgh, Pennsylvania, prospectively evaluated and followed 204 patients with syncope to determine how often a cause of syncope could be established and to define the prognosis of such patients. A cardiovascular cause was established in 53 patients and a noncardiovascular cause in 54 (Tables 3-2 and 3-3). The cause remained

TABLE 3-2. *Findings on prolonged electrocardiographic monitoring. Reproduced with permission from Kapoor et al.[100]*

FINDING*	NO. OF PATIENTS	CAUSE OF SYNCOPE ASSIGNED
NSR, rare VPC, rare PAC	54	0
Sinus pauses (>2 s)	8	8
Sinus bradycardia	25	1
Frequent PACs	15	0
Ventricular arrhythmias		
Frequent, 100/hr	20	0
Multifocal	31	0
Couplets	24	0
Ventricular tachycardia	18	14†
Atrial fibrillation with ventricular responses less than 30 beats/min	2	2
Supraventricular tachycardia		
Unsustained short runs	15	0
Symptomatic and sustained	2	2
Mobitz II AV block	2	2
Complete heart block	3‡	0

* NSR denotes normal sinus rhythm. PAC premature atrial contraction, and AV atrioventricular.
† One patient was diagnosed as having drug-induced syncope, and in three other patients, VT had already been diagnosed from the initial ECG.
‡ Complete heart block had already been diagnosed from the initial ECG.

TABLE 3-3. *Causes of syncope. Reproduced with permission from Kapoor et al.*[100]

CAUSE	NO. OF PATIENTS
Cardiovascular	53
VT	20
Sick sinus syndrome	10
Bradycardia	2
SVT	3
Complete heart block	3
Mobitz II AV block	2
Pacemaker malfunction	1
Carotid sinus syncope	1
Aortic stenosis	5
Myocardial infarction	2
Dissecting aortic aneurysm	1
Pulmonary embolus	1
Pulmonary hypertension	2
Noncardiovascular	54
Vasodepressor syncope	9
Situational syncope	15
Drug-induced syncope	6
Orthostatic hypotension	14
Transient ischemic attacks	3
Subclavian-steal syndrome	2
Seizure disorder	3
Vagal reaction with trigeminal neuralgia	1
Conversion reaction	1
Unknown	97

unknown in 97 patients. At 12 months, the overall mortality was 14 ± 3%. The mortality rate (30 ± 7%) in patients with a cardiovascular cause of syncope was significantly higher than the rate (12 ± 4%) in patients with a noncardiovascular cause (p = 0.02) and the rate (6 ± 3%) in patients with syncope of unknown origin (p < 0.0001) (Figs. 3-5 and 3-6). The incidence of sudden death was 24 ± 7% in patients with a cardiovascular cause, compared with 4 ± 3% in patients with a noncardiovascular cause (p = 0.005) and 3 ± 2% in patients with syncope of unknown origin (p = 0.0002). Patients with syncope can be separated into diagnostic categories that have prognostic importance. Patients with a cardiovascular cause have a strikingly higher frequency of sudden death than patients with a noncardiovascular or unknown cause.

Fifty-three patients with recurrent syncope were evaluated by Morady and associates[101] from San Francisco, California, to determine the etiology for this clinical problem when it remained unexplained despite a thorough neurologic and noninvasive cardiac evaluation. Fifteen patients had no structural heart disease, 9 had MVP, and 29 had structural heart disease other than MVP. Nonsustained VT was induced in 15 patients (28%), sustained VT in 9 (17%), VF in 4 (8%), and sinus node function was abnormal in 2 (4%). Patients with inducible VT or VF were treated with antiarrhythmic agents selected on the basis of the results of electrophysiolog-

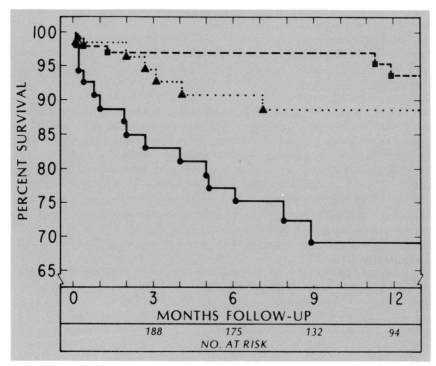

Fig. 3-5. Cumulative survival of patients with syncope due to cardiovascular cause (circles), syncope due to noncardiovascular cause (triangles), and syncope of unknown origin (squares) (Kaplan–Meier estimates). There was no significant difference between mortality in patients with a noncardiovascular cause and patients with syncope of unknown origin (p = 0.16). Reproduced with permission from Kapoor et al.[100]

ic testing. Recurrence rates for syncope were: 1) 43% during a 31 ± 10 month period (mean ± SD) of follow-up in patients with a negative electrophysiologic study; 2) 40% during a 22 ± 6 month period in patients with inducible nonsustained VT; 3) 0% during a 30 ± 12 month period in patients with inducible sustained VT; and 4) 25% during a 21 ± 10 month period in patients with inducible VF. These data suggest that inducible VT followed by selection of an antiarrhythmic agent that prevents such an event is associated with a very low incidence of recurrent syncope during the next several years. Polymorphic nonsustained VT or VF induced by electrical stimulation is a nonspecific response and syncope may recur despite treatment based on results of electropharmacologic testing.

Benditt and associates[102] from San Francisco, California, assessed both acute electrophysiologic actions of intravenously administered theophylline and clinical effects of chronic oral theophylline therapy in 10 patients aged 9–41 years without clinically significant cardiac disease in whom recurrent symptoms of syncope and dizziness were attributed to transient bradyarrhythmias (sinus pauses, marked sinus bradycardia, or paroxysmal AV block). Intravenous theophylline infusion (serum concentration range, 9.5–12.0 mg/liter) shortened means sinus cycle length (control 973 ± 285 ms -vs- theophylline 880 ± 226 ms; p < 0.005) and decreased both the estimated sinoatrial conduction time (control 169 ± 56 ms -vs- theophylline 143 ± 55

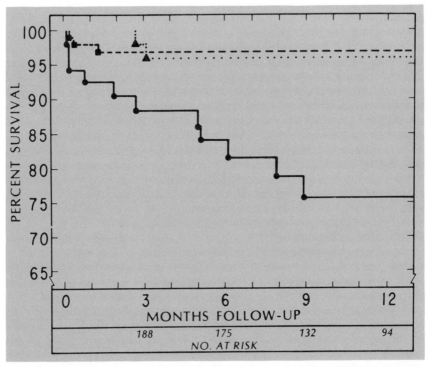

Fig. 3-6. Cumulative incidence of sudden death in patients with syncope due to cardiovascular cause (circles), syncope due to noncardiovascular cause (triangles), and syncope of unknown origin (squares) (Kaplan–Meier estimates). Reproduced with permission from Kapoor et al.[100]

ms; p < 0.05) and the maximum corrected sinus node recovery time (control 442 ± 251 ms -vs- theophylline 255 ± 146 ms; p < 0.05). In addition, theophylline infusion shortened the minimum atrial paced cycle length with sustained 1/1 AV conduction (control 414 ± 86 ms -vs- theophylline 379 ± 97 ms; p < 0.05) and consistently reduced AV node functional refractory periods. Subsequent chronic oral theophylline therapy (serum levels, 9–12 mg/liter) was tolerated in 8 patients (80%). During a follow-up of 5–24 months, suppression of symptoms was achieved in 6 of the 8 patients. Thus, theophylline exhibits positive chronotropic and dromotropic effects in man at serum concentrations in the usual therapeutic range (10–15 mg/liter). Furthermore, suppression of symptoms during follow-up suggests that theophylline treatment may be a useful therapeutic consideration in some patients with recurrent symptomatic bradyarrhythmias.

SICK SINUS SYNDROME

Gillett and coworkers[103] from Houston, Texas, reported on 51 patients aged 2–29 years (mean, 11 years) who had permanent pacing for sick sinus syndrome (SSS): 30 had previous surgery for congenital heart disease, with 50% having had TGA repair. Forty-eight had electrophysiologic studies before pacemaker implantation, of whom 35 had abnormal sinus node recovery time and 9 had a prolonged sinoatrial conduction time. The AV conduction in the 51 patients was normal in 30, mildly abnormal in 9, and severely abnormal in 12. Twenty had epicardial ventricular pacing, 12 had epicardial atrial implants, 7 had endocardial atrial pacing, 6 had epicardial AV sequential pacing, 4 had epicardial universal pacing, and 2 had endocardial universal pacing. None died with pacemaker implantation, and 45 of 49 had symptomatic relief. Eleven patients with associated tachyarrhythmia had amelioration of the tachycardia. There were 2 late deaths unrelated to the pacemakers. Seven patients during a mean follow-up period of 26 months required reoperation for pacing lead or sensing problems.

These authors have an extensive experience with pacing in children. They have moved from ventricular demand toward atrial pacing and then to a fully automatic AV sequential pacemaker during the time of these studies. The problem of pacemaker reciprocating tachycardia, which is a potential problem with this type of pacing in patients with intact retrograde conduction, did not occur in this series. The authors currently prefer transvenous implantation in children weighing >15 kg. Their current recommendation is for atrial demand pacing in patients with SSS and intact AV conduction and a fully automatic and AV conduction abnormalities. Further long-term follow-up data on the reliability and problems with atrial pacemakers in children is needed to evaluate optimal therapy for these patients.

Asseman and coworkers[104] from Lille, France, used a transvenous electrode catheter technique for direct recording of bipolar sinus node ECG during postpacing atrial pauses. Multiple repetitive local sinus node ECG during atrial quiescence validate sinus node ECGs. Such atrial pauses with sinus node ECGs are due to sinoatrial block; atrial pauses without sinus node ECGs are due to overdrive suppression or improper recording. Eight consecutive patients were prospectively selected on the basis of a corrected sinus node recovery time >1500 ms during diagnostic electrophysiologic evaluation. Six patients had atrial pauses with sinus node ECGs; 3 patterns of sinus node ECGs during atrial pauses were observed. The investigators concluded that 1) sinus node ECG recording is of value in understanding the mechanism of underlying postpacing atrial pauses; 2) atrial pauses are usually caused by sinoatrial block; 3) 3 patterns of sinus node ECGs are observed, thus making indirect interpretation unreliable.

In a review of 3,259 consecutive patients who had 24-hour Holter ECG studies, Mazuz and Friedman[105] from New York City found 84 patients (2.6%) to have prolonged (≥2.0 s) sinoatrial pauses. Pauses averaged 2.6 ± 1.5 seconds (±SD) (range, 2.0–15.2). In 17 (20%) no underlying heart disease was found and in 8 (10%) prolonged pauses appeared to be drug induced. No relation was found between length of pauses and presence of symptoms or risk of death. Twenty patients received a pacemaker. Pacemaker recipients were older and more likely to be male and to have symptoms, although 7 were asymptomatic. Patients who received a permanent pacemaker were not different from nonrecipients with respect to average longest pause, mechanisms of pause, underlying heart condition, or average time of follow-up. The survival rate was not improved by permanent pacemaker implantation. Of the 17 patients who died, only 3 died of cardiac causes; none had a recognizable bradycardic cause. Thirteen who initially had syncope did not receive a pacemaker; 2 died of noncardiac causes and none had a subsequent syncopal episode. Ten patients with a syncopal episode received a permanent pacemaker; 3 subsequently died and 3 survivors continued to complain of dizziness. Of the 37 patients who did not have any symptoms on initial examination, only 1 subsequently had a syncopal episode. Thus, length of sinoatrial pauses correlates poorly with symptoms and does not predict sudden death. Unless prolonged sinoatrial pauses are shown to cause symptoms, such pauses per se are not an indication for permanent pacemaker implantation.

BUNDLE-BRANCH BLOCK, HEMIBLOCK, OR BIFASCICULAR BLOCK

Sohi and colleagues[106] from Louisville, Kentucky, analyzed total body surface maps from 15 subjects with left BBB and normal axis (LBBB-NA) and 10 subjects with left BBB and left axis (LBBB-LA) and compared maps from normal subjects. In 19 of the 25 subjects with LBBB, the timing of early upper sternal positivity was similar to that of normal subjects, indicative of timely but oppositely directed septal activation. The RV breakthrough was normally located in all but was earlier after the onset of QRS than expected in some. The initial portion of the positivity produced by LV activation was located in the upper anterior chest in both LBBB-NA and LBBB-LA, but its onset was generally delayed compared with that in normal subjects, presumably because of the time taken by right to left septal activation. Also, the total duration of this positivity was longer than in normal subjects and extended considerably beyond 90 ms, indicating prolonged activation of the anterior free wall of the left ventricle. In LBBB-NA, this upper anterior positivity remained anterior throughout depolarization, but in LBBB-LA it moved toward the left shoulder and the left upper back, presumably due to the posterior orientation of the terminal portion of depolarization. This terminal orientation in patients with LBBB-LA was thought to be due to the additional delay in activation of the anterobasal LV portion caused by the selective involvement of the left anterior fascicle.

Hamby and associates[107] from Stony Brook, New York, examined clinical, coronary arteriographic, and hemodynamic studies in 55 patients with left BBB and CAD and compared them with 110 patients consecutively matched for age and sex with CAD but without left BBB. No significant differences were found in duration of symptoms or frequency of prior AMI, systemic hypertension, or diabetes mellitus; however, the left BBB patients had a significantly ($p < 0.001$) higher frequency of CHF (38 -vs- 12%) and cardiomegaly (64 -vs- 26%). An evaluation of severity of CAD on the basis of subtotal -vs- total obstructive lesions, number of arteries involved, total coronary score, and individual coronary arteries involved revealed no significant differences between the groups. The left BBB patients had significantly ($p < 0.001$) greater impairment of LV function as reflected by end-diastolic volume (107 ± 43 -vs- 79 ± 30 ml/M²), EF (0.35 ± 0.19 -vs- 0.59 ± 0.18), and frequency of abnormal contractile pattern (91 -vs- 61%). Evaluating the left

BBB patients on the basis of QRS width and axis revealed no significant intragroup differences in clinical profile, severity of CAD, or LV dysfunction. A prolonged (≥0.20 s) P-R interval was associated with more CAD and an enlarged heart. This study indicates that CAD associated with left BBB identifies patients with severe LV dysfunction.

To investigate changes in LV function during exercise in patients with left BBB, 22 patients without a history of physical findings of previous AMI or LV dysfunction were studied by gated RNA at rest and during bicycle exercise by Rowe and associates[108] from Houston, Texas. Coronary arteriography demonstrated >75% diameter narrowing of ≥1 coronary artery in 9 patients. Of the remaining 13 patients, RNA demonstrated LV wall motion abnormalities in 7 patients either at rest or with exercise. During exercise, mean EF did not increase in patients without CAD. Patients with CAD had a 12-point fall in mean EF with exercise. It was concluded that LV reserve, as demonstrated by ability to increase EF with exercise, is impaired in patients with left BBB even in the absence of CAD or other underlying cardiac disease and that standard gated RNA criteria to exclude the presence of CAD (>5-point increase in EF with exercise and normal wall motion) are not strictly applicable in screening patients with left BBB.

Bramlet and colleagues[109] from Durham, North Carolina, subjected 7 subjects with rate-dependent left BBB and 13 subjects with normal conduction (control group) to upright bicycle exercise RNA to determine the effects of the development of rate-dependent left BBB on global and regional LV function. Six of 7 patients had atypical chest pain syndrome; none had evidence of cardiac disease. The development of rate-dependent left BBB was associated with an abrupt decrease in LV EF in 6 of 7 patients and no overall increase in LV EF between rest and maximal exercise. In contrast, LV EF in the control group was 62% at rest and increased to 72% at intermediate and 78% at maximal exercise. The onset of left BBB was associated with the development of asynchronous LV contraction in each patient and hypokinesis in 4 of 7 patients. All patients in the control group had normal wall motion at rest and exercise. Thus, these data indicate that the development of rate-dependent left BBB is associated with changes in global and regional ventricular motion function that may be confused with development of LV ischemia during exercise.

Exercise-induced BBB is poorly understood. Wayne and associates[110] from Worcester, Massachusetts, investigated its occurrence in 16 patients, aged 59 ± 9 years, 11 of whom had left BBB and 5 of whom had right BBB. Fourteen had a preexisting baseline ECG abnormality; 11 had either incomplete BBB or nonspecific intraventricular conduction delay. Heart rates at onset of exercise BBB varied from 70–166 beats/minute and in 9 patients the rates at BBB onset and offset appeared to be related, occurring within 8 beats/minute of each other. Coronary artery disease was diagnosed in 10 patients, cardiomyopathy in 2, and probable coronary spasm in 2. One patient had ventricular arrhythmias of uncertain origin, and 1 appeared to have no cardiac disease. Three patients had reversible thallium perfusion defects consistent with ischemia concurrent with developing BBB. The 3 patients in whom exercise BBB persisted all had CAD. Over a mean of 28 months of follow-up, only 1 patient had a morbid cardiac event, a nonfatal AMI, and 2 died from noncardiac causes. Thus, exercise BBB primarily occurs in the context of cardiac disease, most commonly CAD, and concurrent ischemia may be demonstrable; the presence of "rate relation" does not militate against CAD.

Left BBB is associated with a prolongation of the interval from the QRS onset to the onset of LV ejection. The locus and prevalence of specific sites of delay were examined by Hultgren and associates[111] from Palo Alto, California, and Chapel Hill, North Carolina, in 56 patients with complete left BBB using echocardiography, phonocardiography, and external pulse recordings. The results were compared with those in 52 control subjects without left BBB. The onset of the QRS complex was used as the initial reference point of measurement of time intervals. The following abnormalities were found in patients with left BBB: 1) delayed mitral valve closure (Q-MC > 0.08 s) was the major site of delay in 23% of patients; 2) prolongation of the LV isovolumetric contraction time (>0.06 s) was the major site of delay in 41%; 3) both Q-MC and LV isovolumetric contraction time were prolonged in 18%; and 4) in 26% of patients the onset of ventricular contraction determined by the onset of the increase of the apex impulse was delayed (Q-VC > 0.07 s). The most common cause of delayed ejection was a prolonged LV isovolumetric contraction time, which occurred in 59% of patients. A control group of 20 patients with abnormal LV function but without left BBB had a low incidence of the 3 types of delay in LV ejection (0–15%). Thus, the major abnormalities in the cardiac cycle in left BBB are due to the conduction defect and not to LV dysfunction. The results of this study suggest the presence of variable abnormalities of conduction in complete left BBB.

Warner and associates[112] from Syracuse, New York, proposed new ECG criteria for the diagnosis of left anterior hemiblock. The proposed criteria are based upon the relation between portions of the vectorcardiographic (VCG) QRS loop in the frontal plane and the corresponding portions of the ECG QRS complexes recorded by the limb leads. The application of the proposed criteria requires that the tracings be obtained with 3-channel ECG machines so that the temporal relation between the QRS complexes in simultaneously recorded limb leads can be inspected. This type of analysis of the ECG permits prediction of features of the VCG QRS loop that are important for the diagnosis of left anterior hemiblock. The proposed ECG criteria for the diagnosis of left anterior hemiblock are 1) the QRS complexes in leads aVR and aVL each end in an R wave (terminal R wave); and 2) the peak of the terminal R wave in lead aVR occurs later than the peak of the terminal R wave in lead aVL. The sensitivity and specificity of the proposed criteria were empirically evaluated using series of ECGs obtained under clinical circumstances during which the occurrence of left anterior hemiblock was, respectively, likely and unlikely. The performance of the proposed criteria was statistically superior to that of 2 sets of frontal plan QRS axis criteria.

Thirteen patients with syncope and bifascicular block were evaluated by electrophysiologic study, including programmed stimulation in an investigation carried out by Ezri and associates[113] from Philadelphia, Pennsylvania. The mean age was 62 years. Six patients had CAD, 3 had cardiomyopathy, and 4 showed no evidence of organic heart disease. Holter monitoring and neurologic evaluation were nondiagnostic in all patients. Electrophysiologic study demonstrated inducible VT in 4 patients, an H-V interval ≥70 ms in 4, intra- and infra-His block with atrial pacing in 1, and was nondiagnostic in 4 patients. Four of 6 patients with an H-V interval ≥70 ms or pacing-induced infranodal block were treated with permanent pacemakers, 4 of 4 patients with VT received antiarrhythmic therapy, and 3 of 4 patients with nondiagnostic studies received no therapy (1 patient received a permanent pacemaker). During a mean follow-up period of 19 months (range, 3–60 months) all but 3 patients have been free of syncope. One patient with VT did not take prescribed antiarrhythmic therapy, another patient with VT died suddenly; the remaining patient had a normal study and basilar migraines were subsequently diagnosed. It was concluded that: 1) VT may be a significant cause of syncope in patients with bifascicular block and was induced by programmed stimulation in approximately one-third of patients studied; 2) electrophysiologic study, including programmed stimulation, is helpful in delineating both the etiology of syncope and appropriate treatment in patients with bifascicular block. A negative study may also be of prognostic value.

SECOND AND THIRD DEGREE HEART BLOCK

Transient asystole is often noted during the course of permanent pacemaker implantation in patients with complete heart block. Since subcutaneous lidocaine is frequently used as the local anesthetic agent for permanent pacemaker implantation, Kosowsky and associates[114] from Boston, Massachusetts, studied the effect of this drug on ventricular escape intervals in 9 patients with complete heart block before and 10, 30, and 45 minutes after subcutaneous lidocaine administration for permanent pacemaker implantation. The total lidocaine dose ranged from 170–400 mg (1.9–9.5 mg/kg of body weight). Therapeutic blood levels were achieved in 7 patients. The mean ventricular escape interval before lidocaine was 1.83 ± 0.32 seconds, which increased to 2.58 ± 1.24, 2.96 ± 1.06, and 2.68 ± 1.27 seconds at 10, 30, and 45 minutes after lidocaine (p < 0.02). The mean maximal escape interval before lidocaine was 2.06 ± 0.30 seconds, which increased to 3.80 ± 1.44 seconds (p < 0.01), a mean increase of 84%. The percent increase in maximal escape interval was related directly to the peak lidocaine level achieved. After lidocaine administration, 5 patients had asystole >4 seconds and 1 required resumption of pacing. Thus, subcutaneous lidocaine contributes to the occurrence of asystole seen during permanent pacemaker implantation. It is advisable to limit the amount of lidocaine administered during permanent pacemaker implantation to the minimum necessary to achieve adequate local anesthesia. Strong consideration should be given to the use of a temporary pacemaker in patients with complete heart block during permanent pacemaker implantation even in the absence of previous asystole.

Woelfel and associates[115] from Chapel Hill, North Carolina, identified 3 patients with 1/1 AV conduction at rest who developed fixed 2/1 or 3/1 AV block during treadmill exercise testing. Electrophysiologic study documented the block distal to the AV node in all 3 patients and suggested that the exercise-induced block occurred because of increased atrial rate and abnormal refractoriness of the His-Purkinje conduction system. Thus, these observations suggest that high grade AV block may develop during exercise and reflects conduction disease in the His-Purkinje system rather than in the AV node. Patients with this abnormality should be considered for permanent cardiac pacing.

PROLONGED Q-T INTERVAL SYNDROMES

Parasympathetic blockade shortens the duration of the Q-T interval and ventricular effective refractory period independent of heart rate change. Since relative parasympathetic effect increases during sleep, Browne and associates[116] from Indianapolis, Indiana, determined whether sleep was associated with a change in the Q-T interval. Fifteen patients receiving no drugs underwent 3–6 days of continuous ECG recordings. Tracings were sampled every 30 minutes and recorded at a paper speed of 25 mm/s. This provided 12,000 Q-T and R-R intervals that were measured. Comparison of R-R intervals that had similar durations during sleep and awake states revealed that the duration of the Q-T interval was longer during sleep in all 15 patients (p < 0.001). Eight patients had sufficient range of overlap of R-R intervals to compare linear regression lines of Q-T intervals recorded while awake with Q-T intervals recorded while asleep. The regression lines during sleep exhibited a mean intercept change of 38 ± 37 ms and mean slope change of −0.021 ± 0.040 ms when compared with the regression lines during the awake state. The difference in Q-T interval between awake and sleep states was 19 ± 7 ms when calculated at a heart rate of 60 beats/minute. These statistical comparisons of the relationship of the Q-T interval to R-R interval indicate that the Q-T interval is longer during sleep than during the awake state at the same heart rate. Prolongation of the Q-T interval during sleep may reflect increased vagal tone or sympathetic withdrawal. These changes in repolarization may be related to the diurnal variation of some ventricular arrhythmias.

PACEMAKERS

In a recent health research report (Greenberg A, Kowey PR, Bargmann E, Wolfe SM. Permanent pacemakers in Maryland. Report by Health Research Group, Washington, D.C., July 7, 1982) face sheet data were utilized to determine whether permanent pacemakers had been inserted for appropriate reasons in the State of Maryland during 1979 and 1980. After reviewing data from 2,222 permanent pacemaker insertions, it was concluded that 23% were unnecessary and an additional 13% were questionable. Scherlis and Dembo[117] from Baltimore, Maryland, utilized the same indications and reviewed both the complete medical records and the face sheets for those patients who had been classified as having permanent pacemakers inserted for inappropriate or questionable reasons. In 32 hospitals, 75% of the records were reviewed (610 of 817 patients). Although coded as having received permanent pacemakers, 16% had received temporary pacemakers, battery change, and the like. Diagnoses justifying permanent pacemaker insertion had.been omitted in 53% of the face sheets, and coding errors were found in

39%. Although none of the 610 medical records reviewed had a valid indication for permanent pacemaker insertion listed on the face sheet, complete medical record review demonstrated valid indications in 95%. Inherent difficulties arise in attempting to list rigid indications for permanent pacemaker insertion. The face sheet does not provide adequate data for assessing the appropriateness of permanent pacemaker insertion.

In the March 15, 1983, issue of *The American Journal of Cardiology*, Kowey and associates[118] wrote a long letter defending their position regarding the comments of Scherlis and Dembo. Although Kowey and associates acknowledged that while some of Scherlis and Dembo's points were valid and were mentioned in the initial report of Kowey and associates,[118] the latter authors were astonished to learn that in only 53% of the charts surveyed did the physicians fail to include on the summary face sheet a diagnosis that would justify the need for a device and procedure costing >$7,000. Scherlis and Dembo[119] replied to the letter by Kowey and associates and simply concluded that "The track record of the Health Research Group is not one which encourages cooperation or confidence in its ability to participate in health research where a knowledge of technical terminology, chart problems, or face sheet data is concerned."

The DDD pacemaker allows sensing and pacing in both chambers and can therefore maintain AV synchrony. This pacemaker, however, creates an additional antegrade conduction system between the atrium and ventricle and, in the presence of ventriculoatrial (VA) conduction, the possibility of pacemaker-mediated tachycardia exists. Littleford and associates[120] from Orlando and Gainesville, Florida, devised a simple bedside technique that does not require catheterization or expensive equipment to detect VA conduction (Fig. 3-7). Just after DDD pacer implantation, an attempt was made to detect VA conduction in 31 patients. Ambulatory monitoring (Holter) was done for 24 hours after implantation and at 2–4 and 6–8 weeks after implantation to detect pacemaker-mediated tachycardia. Attempts to induce pacemaker-mediated tachycardia were made using a special programmable external stimulator at follow-up after implantation. It was found that 1) all the 17 patients with detectable VA conduction had pacemaker-mediated tachycardia when the atrial refractory period was less than the VA conduction time; 2) pacemaker-mediated tachycardias were not inducible or detected spontaneously when atrial refractory period was equal to or greater than VA conduction time +50 ms; and 3) VA conduction was not detectable in 9 of the 17 patients at a later visit. Six of these 9 received antiarrhythmic therapy or had developed CHF. Ventriculoatrial conduction has important implications in patients with DDD pacemakers and can be readily evaluated at the bedside.

Rubin and associates[121] from Augusta, Georgia, summarized the results in 20 adults who had undergone implantation of an automatic (DDD) pacemaker (Medtronic model 7000, Versatrax I) for treatment of symptomatic bradyarrhythmias. Only 9 patients had optimal DDD mode pacing during 78 paced months. In 3 patients, the DDD mode was changed to AV sequential (DVI) early because of risk imposed by sustained tachycardia upon underlying myocardial ischemia. The remaining 8 had had tachycardia due to pacemaker reentry, and 7 had neurologic and cardiovascular symptoms. DDD pacing was abandoned in 5 when reentry could not be interrupted by digitalis administration or reprogramming. Three continue to be paced

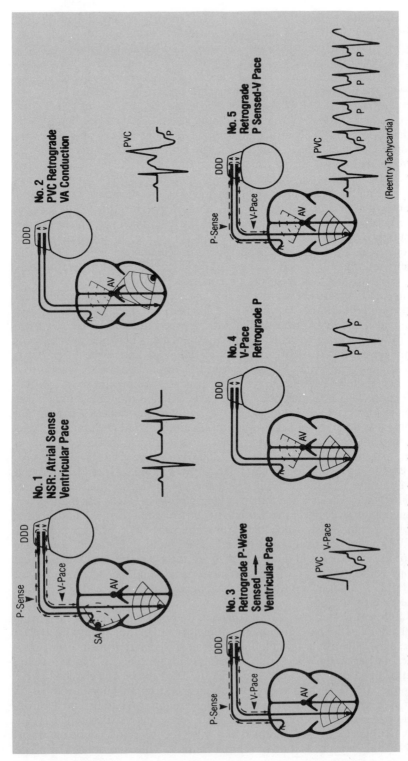

Fig. 3-7. Sequence that initiates pacemaker–mediated tachycardia by a VPC. AV = atrioventricular node; NSR = normal sinus rhythm; P-Sense = P wave sensed by atrial section of pacer; SA = sinoatrial node; VA = ventriculoatrial; V-Pace = ventricular activation sensed by ventricular section of pacer.

in DDD mode despite intermittent reentrant tachycardias, with digitalis diminishing episodes of reentry in only 1. Mean VA conduction time was 229 ± 34 ms. Reentrant pacemaker tachycardia developed in 7 of 12 with normal or nearly normal AV conduction, but in only 1 of 5 with complete heart block. Preimplantation electrophysiologic study did not reliably detect and initial postoperative Holter monitoring did not predict reentrant tachycardia. The risk of reentry caused by a short, fixed atrial refractory period combined with the high occurrence of slow retrograde AV conduction, particularly in patients with normal or nearly normal antegrade conduction, renders the Versatrax I and other similar pacemakers unsuitable for DDD mode pacing in many patients.

References

1. PILCHER GF, COOK AJ, JOHNSTON BL, FLETCHER GF: Twenty–four–hour continuous electrocardiography during exercise and free activity in 80 apparently healthy runners. Am J Cardiol 52:859–861, Oct 1983.

2. NORTHCOTE RJ, MACFARLANE P, BALLANTYNE D: Ambulatory electrocardiography in squash players. Br Heart J 50:372–377, Oct 1983.

3. DOBMEYER DJ, STINE RA, LEIER CV, GREENBERG R, SCHAAL S: The arrhythmogenic effects of caffeine in human beings. N Engl J Med 308:814–816, Apr 7, 1983.

4. GRABOYS TB, LOWN B: Coffee, arrhythmias, and common sense. N Engl J Med 308:835–836, Apr 7, 1983.

5. MONTAGUE TJ, MCPHERSON DD, MACKENZIE R, SPENCER CA, NANTON MA, HORACEK BM: Frequent ventricular ectopic activity without underlying cardiac disease: analysis of 45 subjects. Am J Cardiol 52:980–984, Nov 1983.

6. SCHNEIDER J, BERGER HJ, SANDS MJ, LACHMAN AB, ZARET BL: Beat–to–beat left ventricular performance in atrial fibrillation: radionuclide assessment with the computerized nuclear probe. Am J Cardiol 51:1189–1195, Apr 1983.

7. ENGEL TR, LUCK JC: Effect of whiskey on atrial vulnerability and "holiday heart." J Am Coll Cardiol 1:816–818, March 1983.

8. LOWENSTEIN SR, GABOW PA, CRAMER J, OLIVA PB, RATNER K: The role of alcohol in new–onset atrial fibrillation. Arch Intern Med 143:1882–1885, Oct 1983.

9. PANIDIS IP, MORGANROTH J, BAESSLER C: Effectiveness and safety of oral verapamil to control exercise–induced tachycardia in patients with atrial fibrillation receiving digitalis. Am J Cardiol 52:1197–1201, Dec 1983.

10. TOMMASO C, MCDONOUGH T, PARKER M, TALANO JV: Atrial fibrillation and flutter: immediate control and conversion with intravenously administered verapamil. Arch Intern Med 143:877–881, May 1983.

11. POZEN RG, PASTORIZA J, ROZANSKI JJ, KESSLER KM, MYERBURG RJ: Determinants of recurrent atrial flutter after cardioversion. Br Heart J 50:92–96, July 1983.

12. BENSON DW, DUNNIGAN A, STERBA R, BENDITT DG: Atrial pacing from the esophagus in the diagnosis and management of tachycardia and palpitations. J Pediatr 102:40–46, Jan 1983.

13. BROUGHTON A, GALLAGHER JJ, GERMAN LD, GUARNIERI T, TRANTHAM JL: Differentiation of septal from free wall accessory pathway location: observations during bundle branch block in reciprocating tachycardia in the presence of type I antiarrhythmic drugs. Am J Cardiol 52:751–754, Oct 1983.

14. KLEIN GJ, GULAMHUSEIN SS: Intermittent preexcitation in the Wolff–Parkinson–White syndrome. Am J Cardiol 52:292–296, Aug 1983.

15. MORADY F, SLEDGE C, SHEN E, SUNG RJ, GONZALES R, SCHEINMAN MM: Electrophysiologic testing

in the management of patients with the Wolff–Parkinson–White syndrome and atrial fibrillation. Am J Cardiol 51:1623–1628, June 1983.

16. PRITCHETT ELC, HAMMILL SC, REITER MJ, LEE KL, McCARTHY EA, ZIMMERMAN JM, SHAND DG: Life–table methods for evaluating antiarrhythmic drug efficacy in patients with paroxysmal atrial tachycardia. Am J Cardiol 52:1007–1012, Nov 1983.

17. JEDEIKIN R, GILLETTE PC, GARSON A, PORTER CJ, BEDER F, BARON T, ZINNER AJ: Effect of ouabain on anterograde effective refractory period of accessory atrial–ventricular connections in children. J Am Coll Cardiol 1:869–872, March 1983.

18. SMITH MS, VERGHESE CP, SHAND DG, PRITCHETT ELC: Pharmacokinetic and pharmacodynamic effects of diltiazem. Am J Cardiol 51:1369–1374, May 1983.

19. WALKER WS, WINNIFORD MD, MAURITSON DR, JOHNSON SM, HILLIS LD: Atrioventricular junctional rhythm in patients receiving oral verapamil therapy. JAMA 249:389–390, Jan 21, 1983.

20. CHANG MS, SUNG RJ, TAI TY, LIN SL, LIU PH, CHIANG BN: Nadolol and supraventricular tachycardia: an electrophysiologic study. J Am Coll Cardiol 2:894–904, Nov 1983.

21. GERMAN LD, GALLAGHER JJ, BROUGHTON A, GUARNIERI T, TRANTHAM JL: Effects of exercise and isoproterenol during atrial fibrillation in patients with Wolff–Parkinson–White syndrome. Am J Cardiol 51:1203–1206, Apr 1983.

22. HELLESTRAND KJ, NATHAN AW, BEXTON RS, SPURRELL RAJ, CAMM JA: Cardiac electrophysiologic effects of flecainide acetate for paroxysmal reentrant junctional tachycardias. Am J Cardiol 51:770–776, March 1983.

23. KASPER W, TREESE N, MEINERTZ T, JAHNCHEN E, POP T: Electrophysiologic effects of lorcainide on the accessory pathway in the Wolff–Parkinson–White syndrome. Am J Cardiol 51:1618–1622, June 1983.

24. BRUGADA P, DASSEN WR, BRAAT S, GORGELS AP, WELLENS HJJ: Value of the ajmaline–procainamide test to predict the effect of long–term oral amiodarone on the anterograde effective refractory period of the accessory pathway in the Wolff–Parkinson–White syndrome. Am J Cardiol 52:70–72, July 1983.

25. GUILLEMINAULT C, CONNOLLY SJ, WINKLE RA: Cardiac arrhythmia and conduction disturbances during sleep in 400 patients with sleep apnea syndrome. Am J Cardiol 52:490–494, Sept 1983.

26. ROSENBERG MJ, URETZ E, DENES P: Sleep and ventricular arrhythmias. Am Heart J 106:703, Oct 1983.

27. GREENSPON AJ, SCHAAL SF: The "holiday heart": electrophysiologic studies of alcohol effects in alcohol. Ann Intern Med 98:135–139, Feb 1983.

28. ALLAN LD, ANDERSON RH, SULLIVAN ID, CAPITAL S, HOLT DW, TYNAN M: Evaluation of fetal arrhythmias by echocardiography. Br Heart J 50:240–245, Sept 1983.

29. LAM W, PIETRAS R, BAUERNFEIND R, SWIRYN S, STRASBERG B, PALILEO E, ROSEN KM: Angiographic correlates of recurrent sustained ventricular tachycardia in chronic ischemic heart disease. Am Heart J 105:928–934, June 1983.

30. MARCHLINSKI FE, WAXMAN HL, BUXTON AE, JOSEPHSON ME: Sustained ventricular tachyarrhythmias during the early postinfarction period: electrophysiologic findings and prognosis for survival. J Am Coll Cardiol 2:240–250, Aug 1983.

31. REITER MJ, SMITH WM, GALLAGHER JJ: Clinical spectrum of ventricular tachycardia with left bundle branch morphology. Am J Cardiol 51:113–121, Jan 1983.

32. SUNG, RJ, SHEN EN, MORADY F, SCHEINMAN MM, HESS D, BOTVINICK EH: Electrophysiologic mechanism of exercise–induced sustained ventricular tachycardia. Am J Cardiol 51:525–530, Feb 1983.

33. SWERDLOW CD, WINKLE RA, MASON JW: Determinants of survival in patients with ventricular tachyarrhythmias. N Engl J Med 308:1436–1442, June 16, 1983.

34. LIN FC, FINLEY CD, RAHIMTOOLA SH, WU D: idiopathic paroxysmal ventricular tachycardia with a QRS pattern of right bundle branch block and left axis deviation: a unique clinical entity with specific properties. Am J Cardiol 52:95–100, July 1983.

35. LLOYD EA, HAUER RN, ZIPES DP, HEGER JJ, PRYSTOWSKY EN: Syncope and ventricular tachycardia in patients with ventricular preexcitation. Am J Cardiol 52:79–82, July 1983.

36. KAY GN, PLUMB VJ, ARCINIEGAS JG, HENTHORN RW, WALDO AL: Torsade de Pointes: the long–

short initiating sequence and other clinical features: observations in 32 patients. J Am Coll Cardiol 2:806–817, Nov 1983.

37. MORADY F, SCHEINMAN MM, HESS DS, CHEN R, STANGER P: Clinical characteristics and results of electrophysiologic testing in young adults with ventricular tachycardia or ventricular fibrillation. Am Heart J 106:1306–1314, Dec 1983.

38. KOWEY PR, FOLLAND ED, PARISI AF, LOWN B: Programmed electrical stimulation of the heart in coronary artery disease. Am J Cardiol 51:531–536, Feb 1983.

39. PODRID PJ, SCHOENEBERGER A, LOWN B, LAMPERT S, MATOS J, PORTERFIELD J, RAEDER E, CORRIGAN E: Use of nonsustained ventricular tachycardia as a guide to antiarrhythmic drug therapy in patients with malignant ventricular arrhythmia. Am Heart J 105:181–188, Feb 1983.

40. SPIELMAN SR, SCHWARTZ JS, McCARTHY DM, HOROWITZ LN, GREENSPAN AM, SADOWSKI LM, JOSEPHSON ME, WAXMAN HL: Predictors of the success or failure of medical therapy in patients with chronic recurrent sustained ventricular tachycardia: a discriminant analysis. J Am Coll Cardiol 1:401–408, Feb 1983.

41. SWERDLOW CD, GONG G, ECHT DS, WINKLE RA, GRIFFIN JC, ROSS DL, MASON JW: Clinical factors predicting successful electrophysiologic pharmacologic study in patients with ventricular tachycardia. J Am Coll Cardiol 1:409–416, Feb 1983.

42. NAIR CK, ARONOW WS, SKETCH MH, PAGANO T, LYNCH JD, MOOSS AN, ESTERBROOKS D, RUNCO V, RYSCHON K: Diagnostic and prognostic significance of exercise–induced premature ventricular complexes in men and women: a 4 year follow–up. J Am Coll Cardiol 1:1201–1206, May 1983.

43. MANN DE, LUCK JC, GRIFFIN JC, HERRE JM, LIMACHER MC, MAGRO SA, ROBERTSON NW, WYNDHAM CRC: Induction of clinical ventricular tachycardia using programmed stimulation: value of third and fourth extrastimuli. Am J Cardiol 52:501–506, Sept 1983.

44. PLATIA EV, GREENE HL, VLAY SC, WERNER JA, GROSS B, REID PR: Sensitivity of various extrastimulus techniques in patients with serious ventricular arrhythmias. Am Heart J 106:698, Oct 1983.

45. BUXTON AE, WAXMAN HL, MARCHLINSKI FE, JOSEPHSON ME: Electrophysiologic studies in nonsustained ventricular tachycardia: relation to underlying heart disease. Am J Cardiol 52:985–991, Nov 1983.

46. DOHERTY JU, KIENZLE MG, WAXMAN HL, BUXTON AE, MARCHLINSKI FE, JOSEPHSON ME: Programmed ventricular stimulation at a second right ventricular site: an analysis of 100 patients, with special reference to sensitivity, specificity and characteristics of patients with induced ventricular tachycardia. Am J Cardiol 52:1184–1189, Dec 1983.

47. BRUGADA P, ABDOLLAH H, HEDDLE B, WELLENS HJJ: Results of a ventricular stimulation protocol using a maximum of 4 premature stimuli in patients without documented or suspected ventricular arrhythmias. Am J Cardiol 52:1214–1218, Dec 1983.

48. PIETRAS RJ, LAM W, BAUERNFEIND R, SHEIKH A, PALILEO E, STRASBERG B, SWIRYN S, ROSEN KM: Chronic recurrent right ventricular tachycardia in patients without ischemic heart disease: clinical, hemodynamic, and angiographic findings. Am Heart J 105:357–366, March 1983.

49. BUXTON AE, WAXMAN HL, MARCHLINSKI FE, SIMSON MB, CASSIDY D, JOSEPHSON ME: Right ventricular tachycardia: clinical and electrophysiologic characteristics. Circulation 68:917–927, Nov 1983.

50. DiMARCO JP, GARAN H, RUSKIN JN: Quinidine for ventricular arrhythmias: value of electrophysiologic testing. Am J Cardiol 51:90–95, Jan 1983.

51. SALERNO DM, HODGES M, GRANRUD G, SHARKEY P: Comparison of flecainide with quinidine for suppression of chronic stable ventricular ectopic depolarizations. Ann Intern Med 98:455–460, Apr 1983.

52. GRADMAN AH, CUNNINGHAM M, HARBISON MA, BERGER HJ, ZARET BL: Effects of oral digoxin on ventricular ectopy and its relation to left ventricular function. Am J Cardiol 51:765–769, March 1983.

53. SPRUNG CL, MARCIAL EH, GARCIA AA, SEQUEIRA RF, POZEN RG: Prophylactic use of lidocaine to prevent advanced ventricular arrhythmias during pulmonary artery catheterization: prospective double–blind study. Am J Med 75:906–910, Dec 1983.

54. ANDERSON JL, LUTZ JR, ALLISON SB: Electrophysiologic and antiarrhythmic effects of oral flecainide in patients with inducible ventricular tachycardia. J Am Coll Cardiol 2:105–114, July 1983.

55. OETGEN WJ, TIBBITS PA, ABT MEO, GOLDSTEIN RE: Clinical and electrophysiologic assessment of oral flecainide acetate for recurrent ventricular tachycardia: evidence for exacerbation of electrical instability. Am J Cardiol 52:746–750, Oct 1983.

56. WINKLE RA, PETERS F, KATES RE, HARRISON DC: Possible contribution of encainide metabolites to the long–term antiarrhythmic efficacy of encainide. Am J Cardiol 51:1182–1188, Apr 1983.

57. CHESNIE B, PODRID P, LOWN B, RAEDER E: Encainide for refractory ventricular tachyarrhythmia. Am J Cardiol 52:495–500, Sept 1983.

58. SAMI MH, DERBEKYAN VA, LISBONA R: Hemodynamic effects of encainide in patients with ventricular arrhythmia and poor ventricular function. Am J Cardiol 52:507–511, Sept 1983.

59. ECHT DS, MITCHELL B, KATES RE, WINKLE RA: Comparison of the electrophysiologic effects of intravenous and oral lorcainide in patients with recurrent ventricular tachycardia. Circulation 68:392–399, Aug 1983.

60. WAXMAN HL, BUXTON AE, SADOWSKI LM, JOSEPHSON ME: The response to procainamide during electrophysiologic study for sustained ventricular tachyarrhythmias predicts the response to other medications. Circulation 67:30–37, Jan 1983.

61. WASPE LE, WAXMAN HL, BUXTON AE, JOSEPHSON ME: Mexiletine for control of drug–resistant ventricular tachycardia: clinical and electrophysiologic results in 44 patients. Am J Cardiol 51:1175–1181, Apr 1983.

62. DUFF HJ, RODEN D, PRIMM RK, OATES JA, WOOSLEY RL: Mexiletine in the treatment of resistant ventricular arrhythmias: enhancement of efficacy and reduction of dose–related side effects by combination with quinidine. Circulation 67:1124–1128, May 1983.

63. LUI HK, LEE G, DHURANDHAR R, HUNGATE EJ, LADDU A, DIETRICH P, MASON DT: Reduction of ventricular ectopic beats with oral acebutolol: a double–blind, randomized crossover study. Am Heart J 105:722–726, May 1983.

64. LERMAN BB, WAXMAN HL, BUXTON AE, JOSEPHSON ME: Disopyramide: evaluation of electrophysiologic effects and clinical efficacy in patients with sustained ventricular tachycardia or ventricular fibrillation. Am J Cardiol 51:759–764, March 1983.

65. PRATT CM, YEPSEN SC, TAYLOR AA, MASON DT, MILLER RR, QUINONES MA, LEWIS RA: Ethmozine suppression of single and repetitive ventricular premature depolarizations during therapy: documentation of efficacy and long–term safety. Am Heart J 106:85–91, July 1983.

66. REITER MJ, HAMMILL SC, SHAND DG, VERGHESE C, MCCARTHY E, PRITCHETT ELC: Efficacy, safety, and pharmacokinetics of a concentration–maintaining regimen of intravenous pirmenol. Am J Cardiol 52:83–87, July 1983.

67. CONNOLLY SJ, KATES RE, LEBSACK CS, ECHT DS, MASON JW, WINKLE RA: Clinical efficacy and electrophysiology of oral propafenone for ventricular tachycardia. Am J Cardiol 52:1208–1213, Dec 1983.

68. SUNG RJ, JUMA Z, SAKSENA S: Electrophysiologic properties and antiarrhythmic mechanisms of intravenous N-acetylprocainamide in patients with ventricular dysrhythmias. Am Heart J 105:811–819, May 1983.

69. PRATT CM, YEPSEN SC, BLOOM K, TAYLOR AA, YOUNG JB, QUINONES MA: Evaluation of metoprolol in suppressing complex ventricular arrhythmias. Am J Cardiol 52:73–78, July 1983.

70. GLASSER SP, CLARK PI, LADDU AR: Comparison of the antiarrhythmic effects of acebutolol and propranolol in the treatment of ventricular arrhythmias. Am J Cardiol 52:992–995, Nov 1983.

71. MASON JW, SWERDLOW CD, MITCHELL LB: Efficacy of verapamil in chronic, recurrent ventricular tachycardia. Am J Cardiol 51:1614–1617, June 1983.

72. YEH SJ, KOU HC, LIN FC, HUNG JS, WU D: Effects of oral diltiazem in paroxysmal supraventricular tachycardia. Am J Cardiol 52:271–278, Aug 1983.

73. MORADY F, SCHEINMAN MM, SHEN E, SHAPIRO W, SUNG RJ, DiCARLO L: Intravenous amiodarone in the acute treatment of recurrent symptomatic ventricular tachycardia. Am J Cardiol 51:156–159, Jan 1983.

74. HEGER JJ, PRYSTOWSKY EN, ZIPES DP: Clinical efficacy of amiodarone in treatment of recurrent ventricular tachycardia and ventricular fibrillation. Am Heart J 106:887–894, Oct 1983.

75. MORADY F, SAUVE MJ, MALONE P, SHEN EN, SCHWARTZ AB, BHANDARI A, KEUNG E, SUNG RJ, SCHEINMAN MM: Long–term efficacy and toxicity of high–dose amiodarone therapy for ventricular tachycardia or ventricular fibrillation. Am J Cardiol 52:975–979, Nov 1983.

76. FISHER JD, OSTROW E, KIM SG, MATOS JA: Ultrarapid single–capture train stimulation for termination of ventricular tachycardia. Am J Cardiol 51:1334–1338, May 1983.

77. WASPE LE, KIM SG, MATOS JA, FISHER JD: Role of a catheter lead system for transvenous countershock and pacing during electrophysiologic tests: an assessment of the usefulness of catheter shocks for terminating ventricular tachyarrhythmias. Am J Cardiol 52:477–484, Sept 1983.

78. REID PR, MIROWSKI M, MOWER MM, PLATIA EV, GRIFFITH LSC, WATKINS L, BACH SM, IMRAN M, THOMAS A: Clinical evaluation of the internal automatic cardioverter–defibrillator in survivors of sudden cardiac death. Am J Cardiol 51:1608–1613, June 1983.

79. DULK K, BERTHOLET M, BRUGADA P, BAR FW, RICHARDS D, DEMOULIN JC, WALEFFE A, BAKELS N, LINDEMANS FW, BOURGEOIS I, KULBERTUS HE, WELLENS HJJ: A versatile pacemaker system for termination of tachycardias. Am J Cardiol 52:731–738, Oct 1983.

80. WINKLE RA, BACH SM, ECHT DS, SWERDLOW CD, IMRAN M, MASON JW, OYER PE, STINSON EB: The automatic implantable defibrillator: local ventricular bipolar sensing to detect ventricular tachycardia and fibrillation. Am J Cardiol 52:265–270, Aug 1983.

81. KIENZLE MG, DOHERTY JU, ROY D, WAXMAN HL, HARKEN AH, JOSEPHSON ME: Subendocardial resection for refractory ventricular tachycardia: effects on ambulatory electrocardiogram, programmed stimulation and ejection fraction, and relation to outcome. J Am Coll Cardiol 2:853–858, Nov 1983.

82. GARAN H, RUSKIN JN, DiMARCO JP, DERKAC WM, AKINS CW, DAGGETT WM, AUSTEN WG, BUCKLEY MJ: Electrophysiologic studies before and after myocardial revascularization in patients with life–threatening ventricular arrhythmias. Am J Cardiol 51:519–524, Feb 1983.

83. PAGE PL, ARCINIEGAS JG, PLUMB VJ, HENTHORN RW, KARP RB, WALDO AL: Value of early postoperative epicardial programmed ventricular stimulation studies after surgery for ventricular tachyarrhythmias. J Am Coll Cardiol 2:1046–1052, Dec 1983.

84. BENSON DW, BENDITT DG, ANDERSON RW, DUNNIGAN A, PRITZKER MR, KULIK TJ, ZAVORAL JH: Cardiac arrest in young, ostensibly healthy patients: clinical, hemodynamic, and electrophysiologic findings. Am J Cardiol 52:65–69, July 1983.

85. WALSH CK, KRONGRAD E: Terminal cardiac electrical activity in pediatric patients. Am J Cardiol 51:557–561, Feb 1983.

86. MORADY F, SCHEINMAN MM, HESS DS, SUNG RJ, SHEN E, SHAPIRO W: Electrophysiologic testing in the management of survivors of out–of–hospital cardiac arrest. Am J Cardiol 51:85–89, Jan 1983.

87. LONGSTRETH WT, DIEHR P, INUI TS: Prediction of awakening after out–of–hospital cardiac arrest. N Engl J Med 308:1378–1382, June 9, 1983.

88. BEDELL SE, DELBANCO TL, COOK EF, EPSTEIN FH: Survival after cardiopulmonary resuscitation in the hospital. N Engl J Med 309:569–576, Sept 8, 1983.

89. PANIDIS IP, MORGANROTH J: Sudden death in hospitalized patients: cardiac rhythm disturbances detected by ambulatory electrocardiographic monitoring. J Am Coll Cardiol 2:798–805, Nov 1983.

90. KERBER RE, JENSEN SR, GASCHO JA, GRAYZEL J, HOYT R, KENNEDY J: Determinants of defibrillation: prospective analysis of 183 patients. Am J Cardiol 52:739–745, Oct 1983.

91. RUSKIN JN, McGOVERN B, GARAN H, DiMARCO JP, KELLY E: Antiarrhythmic drugs: a possible cause of out–of–hospital cardiac arrest. N Engl J Med 309:1302–1306, Nov 24, 1983.

92. ROY D, WAXMAN HL, KIENZLE MG, BUXTON AE, MARCHLINSKI FE, JOSEPHSON ME: Clinical characteristics and long–term follow–up in 119 survivors of cardiac arrest: relation to inducibility at electrophysiologic testing. Am J Cardiol 52:969–974, Nov 1983.

93. Pratt CM, Francis MJ, Luck JC, Wyndham CR, Miller RR, Quinones MA: Analysis of ambulatory electrocardiograms in 15 patients during spontaneous ventricular fibrillation with special reference to preceding arrhythmic events. J Am Coll Cardiol 2:789–797, Nov 1983.

94. Lewis BH, Antman EM, Graboys TB: Detailed analysis of 24–hour ambulatory electrocardiographic recordings during ventricular fibrillation or Torsade de Pointes. J Am Coll Cardiol 2:426–436, Sept 1983.

95. Benditt DG, Benson DW, Klein GJ, Pritzker MR, Kriett JM, Anderson RW: Prevention of recurrent sudden cardiac arrest: role of provocative electropharmacologic testing. J Am Coll Cardiol 2:418–425, Sept 1983.

96. Clark MB, Dwyer EM, Greenberg H: Sudden death during ambulatory monitoring: analysis of 6 cases. Am J Med 75:801–806, Nov 1983.

97. Gulati RS, Bhan GL, Horan MA: Cardiopulmonary resuscitation of old people. Lancet 2:267–269, July 30, 1983.

98. Unsigned Editorial: Should dying be a diagnosis. Lancet 2:261, July 30, 1983.

99. Sabin HI, Khunti K, Coghill SB, McNeill GO: Accuracy of intracardiac injections determined by a post–mortem study. Lancet 2:1054–1055, Nov 5, 1983.

100. Kapoor WN, Karpf M, Wieand S, Peterson JR, Levey GS: A prospective evaluation and follow–up of patients with syncope. New Engl J Med 309:197–204, July 28, 1983.

101. Morady F, Shen E, Schwartz A, Hess D, Bhandari A, Sung RJ, Scheinman MM: Long–term follow–up of patients with recurrent unexplained syncope evaluated by electrophysiologic testing. J Am Coll Cardiol 2:1053–1059, Dec 1983.

102. Benditt DG, Benson W, Kreitt J, Dunnigan A, Pritzker MR, Crouse L, Scheinman MM: Electrophysiologic effects of theophylline in young patients with recurrent symptomatic bradyarrhythmias. Am J Cardiol 52:1223–1229, Dec 1983.

103. Gillette TC, Shannon C, Garson A, Porter CJ, Ott D, Cooley DA, McNamara DG: Pacemaker treatment of sick sinus syndrome in children. J Am Coll Cardiol 1:1325–1329, May 1983.

104. Asseman P, Berzin B, Desry D, Vilarem C, Durand P, Delmotte C, Sarkis EH, Ledieffre J, Thery C: Persistent sinus nodal electrograms during abnormally prolonged postpacing atrial pauses in sick sinus syndrome in humans: sinoatrial block vs. overdrive suppression. Circulation 68:33–41, July 1983.

105. Mazuz M, Friedman HS: Significance of prolonged electrocardiographic pauses in sinoatrial disease: sick sinus syndrome. Am J Cardiol 52:485–489, Sept 1983.

106. Sohi GS, Flowers NC, Horan LG, Sridharan MR, Johnson JC: Comparison of total body surface map depolarization patterns of left bundle branch block and normal axis with left bundle branch block and left axis deviation. Circulation 67:660–664, March 1983.

107. Hamby RI, Weissman RH, Prakash MN, Hoffman I: left bundle branch block: a predictor of poor left ventricular function in coronary artery disease. Am Heart J 106:471–477, Sept 1983.

108. Rowe DW, De Puey EG, Sonnemaker RE, Hall RJ, Burdine JA: Left ventricular performance during exercise in patients with left bundle branch block: evaluation by gated radionuclide ventriculography. Am Heart J 105:66–71, Jan 1983.

109. Bramlet DA, Morris KG, Coleman RE, Albert D, Cobb FR: Effects of rate–dependent left bundle branch block on global and regional left ventricular function. Circulation 67:1059–1065, May 1983.

110. Wayne VS, Bishop RL, Cook L. Spodick DH: Exercise–induced bundle branch block. Am J Cardiol 52:283–286, Aug 1983.

111. Hultgren HN, Craige E, Fujii J, Nakamura T, Bilisoly J: Left bundle branch block and mechanical events of the cardiac cycle. Am J Cardiol 52:755–762, Oct 1983.

112. Warner RA, Hill NE, Mookherjee S, Smulyan H: Improved electrocardiographic criteria for the diagnosis of left anterior hemiblock. Am J Cardiol 51:732–726, March 1983.

113. Ezri M, Lerman BB, Marchlinski FE, Buxton AE, Josephson ME: Electrophysiologic evaluation of syncope in patients with bifascicular block. Am Heart J 106:693–697, Oct 1983.

114. Kosowsky BD, Mufti SI, Grewal GS, Moon RHS, Cashin WL, Pastore JO, Ramaswamy K: Effect of local lidocaine anesthesia on ventricular escape intervals during permanent pacemaker implantation in patients with complete heart block. Am J Cardiol 51:101–104, Jan 1983.

115. Woelfel AK, Simpson RJ, Gettes LS, Foster JR: Exercise–induced distal atrioventricular block. J Am Coll Cardiol 2:578–581, Sept 1983.

116. Browne KF, Prystowsky E, Heger JJ, Chilson DA, Zipes DP: Prolongation of the Q–T interval in man during sleep. Am J Cardiol 52:55–59, July 1983.

117. Scherlis L, Dembo DH: Problems in health data analysis: The Maryland permanent pacemaker experience in 1979 and 1980. Am J Cardiol 51:131–136, Jan 1983.

118. Kowey PR, Greenberg A, Bargmann E, Wolfe SM: Letter. Am J Cardiol 51-1042–1043, March 1983.

119. Scherlis L, Dembo DH: Reply. Am J Cardiol 51:1043, March 1983.

120. Littleford PO, Curry C, Schwartz KM, Pepine CJ: Pacemaker–mediated tachycardias: a rapid bedside technique for induction and observation. Am J Cardiol 52:287–291, Aug 1983.

121. Rubin JW, Frank MJ, Boineau JP, Ellison RG: Current physiologic pacemakers: a serious problem with a new device. Am J Cardiol 52:88–91, July 1983.

4

Systemic Hypertension

Simultaneous direct and indirect measurement of BP

Vardan and associates[1] from Syracuse, New York, simultaneously measured indirectly by the cuff-mercury sphygmomanometer (cuff) and directly by intraarterial recording from a brachial artery the BP in each of 26 patients with systolic systemic hypertension. The systolic BP recorded by the 2 methods were comparable, indicating that systolic hypertension can be reliably diagnosed by readings from the cuff alone. The average diastolic BP, however, was significantly overestimated by the cuff. This error in turn led to an underestimation by the cuff of the pulse pressure and overestimation of the mean arterial pressure. Thus, the low intraarterial (true) diastolic BP and wide pulse pressure make increased arterial stiffness a plausible contributing factor in the pathophysiology of systolic hypertension.

Miscuffing

For the accurate indirect measurement of BP, the American Heart Association (AHA) now recommends that cuff size should be based solely on limb circumference. Manning and coworkers[2] from Pittsburgh, Pennsylvania, studied prevailing cuffing habits and compared them with newly revised AHA guidelines. Monitoring their staff's cuff applications, the investigators found that "miscuffing" occurred in 65 (32%) of 200 BP determinations on

167 unselected adult outpatients, including 61 (72%) of 85 readings taken on "nonstandard" sized arms. Undercuffing large arms was the most frequent error, accounting for 84% of the miscuffings. Considering that miscuffing distorts BP readings by an average of 8.5 mmHg systolic and 4.6 mmHg diastolic, the investigators concluded the accuracy of BP determinations can be improved by marking cuffs and using the new AHA guidelines

Elevated BP in children

In the Minneapolis Children's BP Study carried out by Gillum and associates[3] from Minneapolis, Minnesota, 10,301 children aged 6 to 9 years were surveyed in 1978 and the prevalence of BP >130/90 mmHg at first screen was 1.22% (126 children). Only 0.25% (26 children) still had BP at this level (essential hypertension) on repeat measurement obtained on a separate day within 1 week. The BP remained elevated in this group over a 2.5-year follow-up period. Eleven of these 26 children (group 1) were intensively studied in comparison with 19 normal children with BP below the fifth percentile for age and sex (group 2) and 15 age-, sex-, and height-matched normal children (group 3). Maximal treadmill testing used a modified Balke protocol. M-mode echo and thoracic impedance cardiography also were performed. Group I showed a significantly shorter duration of exercise than group 2 ($p < 0.05$) independent of age, sex, or height (15 -vs- 19 minutes). Group 1 had significantly greater LV posterior wall thickness on echo than group 2 or 3, independent of age and height ($p < 0.02$). Echo and impedance measures of contractility did not differ significantly between groups, although there was a tendency for greater resting cardiac performance in group 1. Group 1 was much more obese than group 2 or 3, independent of age and height. Although the independent roles of obesity, cardiac function, and cardiopulmonary fitness as correlates of children's BP require clarification, this investigation reveals that school children with elevated BP differ from their normotensive peers by having greater obesity, lesser maximal exercise duration, and greater LV mass.

Improved detection and control

Folsom and associates[4] from Minneapolis, Minnesota, compared BP from a 1980–1981 survey of 1,656 adults in Minneapolis-St. Paul to BP from a similar community survey of 3,475 adults conducted in 1973–1974. Mean age-adjusted BP in 1980–1981 was 3 mmHg lower for men and 2 mmHg lower for women than in 1973–1974. Hypertension prevalence, defined as diastolic BP of ≥95 mmHg and/or use of antihypertensive medication, was essentially unchanged. In 1973–1974, however, only 40% of hypertensive persons had adequately controlled BPs, 14% were treated but had conditions that were uncontrolled, 20% had known hypertension but were untreated, and 26% had previously undetected hypertension. In 1980–1981, the respective percentages were 76, 9, 9, and 7. These impressive changes in hypertension detection and control may have contributed to the recent decline in cardiovascular disease mortality in this community. The article by Folsom and associates was followed by an editorial by Paul[5] from Boston, Massachusetts.

Response to isometric stress

Isometric exercise causes transient systemic hypertension, but with individual differences. Chaney and Arndt[6] from Notre Dame, Indiana, attempted to delineate predictors of those differences by analyzing the BP response in terms of variables readily measured in clinical practice. For each of 270 office patients, they determined BP, heart rate (HR), ECG findings, and symptoms in response to maximal isometric and maximal dynamic exercise. For systolic BP response as the predicted measure, 4 predictor variables in combination, including age, sex, resting systolic BP, and maximal treadmill systolic BP, yielded 70% predictability. For diastolic BP, 5 predictors in combination, including handgrip strength, resting diastolic BP, treadmill heart rate, systolic BP, and diastolic BP, allowed 66% prediction. Not predictive of either were resting heart rate, abnormality of treadmill test, presence of heart disease, and certain other medical diagnoses.

Response to treadmill exercise

Criqui and coinvestigators[7] from San Diego, California, in the Lipid Research Clinics Program for Prevalence Study used multiple linear regression to examine predictors of systolic BP response, that is, the increase in pressure above baseline after 3, 6, and 9 minutes of treadmill exercise in 4,262 men and women. Predictors were usual systolic BP, the difference in systolic BP between resting systolic BP and systolic BP immediately before exercise, age, education, obesity index, alcohol consumption, cigarette smoking, preexercise heart rate, and, in women, gonadal hormone use. In men, age, obesity index, and cigarette smoking were positively associated with systolic BP response and in women 20–49 years old, age, obesity index, and alcohol consumption were positively associated with systolic BP response. In women ≥50 years old, usual systolic BP was negatively associated with systolic BP response. In both men and women a larger difference in systolic BP was associated with a smaller systolic BP response. These results help explain the considerable variation in systolic BP response and the difference in systolic BP result, and the difference in systolic BP results suggest that potential systolic BP response may, to a certain extent, have a specific finite range. The similarity of predictor variables for systolic BP response to predictor variables for hypertension is concordant with the previous observation that a high systolic BP response may foreshadow subsequent hypertension.

The early detection of hypertension is of foremost concern. Dlin and associates[8] from Tel-Aviv, Israel, examined the possibility that individuals who are normotensive at rest but who show an exaggerated BP response to exercise are at greater risk of developing hypertension in the future. From exercise tests, a group (ER) of healthy young males who were normotensive at rest (BP ≤140/90 mmHg) but showed an exaggerated BP response to exercise (systolic BP ≥200 mgHg and/or diastolic BP increased by ≥10 mmHg to >90 mmHg) were selected. A control group (NR) with exercise BP values less than these were matched for age, weight/height, skinfold thickness, resting BP ≤140/90, resting heart rate, aerobic fitness level, physical activity, smoking history, and family history of hypertension. After a follow-up period of 5.8 years (range, 3–14 years), 8 individuals from the ER group were found to be hypertensive, whereas none of the NR group were hypertensive. Stepwise multivariate regression showed the exercise BP to be the best predictor of future BP of the parameters reviewed in this study. Thus exaggerated BP response to exercise may serve as an additional risk marker for hypertension.

Predictive value of systolic BP in young for elevation later

Systolic BP was determined by Froom and colleagues[9] from Tel Hashomer, Israel, annually for 12–15 years in 719 men 18–30 years old at entry into the study. Systolic BP values at entry were compared with those measured in the same individuals at the end of the follow-up period. The cutoff separating "normal" from "elevated" systolic BP was arbitrarily set at 140 mmHg. The highest systolic BP recorded at entry was 170 mmHg. Elevated systolic BP on follow-up was 2.3 times more common among subjects with elevated systolic BP at entry. Yet, 89% of the subjects with elevated systolic BP at entry had a normal systolic BP on follow-up. A normal systolic BP at entry did not reduce the risk of elevated systolic on follow-up.

Circadian variation

Mann and coworkers[10] from Middlesex, England, monitored ambulant intraarterial BP with the Oxford system in 6 subjects with autonomic failure who exhibited postural hypotension. Plotting pooled hourly mean values they demonstrated a consistent circadian trend in BP that was the inverse of the normal pattern, with the highest pressures at night and the lowest in the morning. In 4 subjects, confinement to bed did not substantially alter this pattern. Heart rate variability was much reduced in 4 of the subjects, but relatively normal in 2 in whom BP variation also was less abnormal. There was a correlation of the nadir of the BP measurements with the reported time of peak incidence of orthostatic symptoms.

EFFECTS OF VARIOUS NATURAL STATES

Measurement of BP by physician

Blood pressure measurements obtained by a doctor are often greater during the early than the later part of the visit. This phenomenon has been ascribed to the occurrence of a transient pressor response triggered by an alarm reaction of the patient to the visit. By introducing an error in estimating the patient's usual BP, this response may make less reliable the diagnosis of systemic hypertension. Because BP values measured during the doctor's visit have never been compared with those obtained before the visit, the pressor response to the widespread procedure for BP assessment has never been adequately characterized. Accordingly, Mancia and associates[11] from Milan, Italy, measured BP by the cuff method and also by continuous intraarterial recorder during 10 or 15 minute periods during which a doctor repeatedly measured BP by cuff. In almost all the 48 normotensive and hypertensive subjects tested, the doctor's arrival at the bedside induced immediate rises in systolic and diastolic BP, peaking within 1–4 minutes (mean, 27 ± 2 mmHg and 15 ± 2 mmHg above previsit values). There were large differences between individuals in the peak response (range, 4–75 mmHg systolic and 1–36 mmHg diastolic) unrelated to age, sex, baseline BP, or BP variability. There was concomitant tachycardia (average peak response, 16 ± 2 beats/min; range, 4–45 beats/min) which was only slightly correlated with the BP rise. After the peak response, BP declined and at the end of the visit was only slightly above the previsit level. A second visit by the same doctor did not change the average size of the early pressor response or the slope of its subsequent decline.

Obesity

Since obesity and essential hypertension frequently coexist, Messerli and associates[12] from New Orleans, Louisiana, analyzed some of their cardiovascular effects. Twenty-eight obese patients, half of whom where normotensive and half with established hypertension, were matched for mean arterial pressure with 28 corresponding lean subjects. Systemic and renal hemodynamics, intravascular volume, plasma renin activity, and circulating catecholamine levels were measured. Obese patients had increased cardiac output, stroke volume, central blood volume, plasma and total blood volume, and decreased total peripheral resistance. In contrast, cardiac output, central blood volume, and stroke volume of hypertensive patients were normal, but they had increased total peripheral and renal vascular resistance and a contracted intravascular volume. The LV stroke work was elevated to a similar level in obesity and hypertension, but the increase was caused by an expanded stroke volume in the former and by an increase in systolic pressure in the latter. It is concluded that the disparate effects of obesity and hypertension on total peripheral resistance and intravascular volume counteract and may even offset each other. Thus, obesity may mitigate the effects of chronically elevated total peripheral resistance (and therefore end-organ damage) in essential hypertension. Since both entities affect the heart through different mechanisms, their presence in the same patient results in a double burden to the left ventricle, thereby gently enhancing the long-term risk of CHF.

Cigarette smoking and oral contraceptives

To study the factors associated with malignant systemic hypertension in young women, Petitti and Klatsky[13] from Oakland, California, reviewed the medical records of all women aged 15–44 years who had been hospitalized in any of 15 affiliated hospitals from 1971–1980 with malignant systemic hypertension. There were 15 new patients in this period, an incidence of 0.5/100,000 women of these ages per year. Four women had underlying renal disease. All of the remaining 11 used oral contraceptives, smoked cigarettes, or both. Nine were white, and 6 women had normal BP in the 24 months before hospitalization. These findings support a relation of oral contraceptive use and cigarette smoking to an increased risk of malignant systemic hypertension in young women.

In a retrospective cohort study to investigate the association between cigarette smoking and renal stenosis, Nicholson and associates[14] from New York City compared 71 patients with documented renovascular hypertension and 308 age-matched control patients with essential hypertension: 94% (30 of 32) men and 74% (29 of 39) of women with renal artery stenosis had smoked cigarettes compared with only 43% (64 of 150) of men and 41% (65 of 158) of women in the control group. This striking relation was true for both patients with fibromuscular disease (71% smokers; 15 of 21) and patients with atherosclerotic lesions (88% smokers; 44 of 50). All renal artery stenosis groups had significantly higher systolic and diastolic BP than the relevant control group. When the groups were stratified according to BP, there were significantly more smokers in the renal artery stenosis group at every level of BP.

Coffee

Lang and associates[15] from Paris, France, studied the relation between coffee drinking and BP in a cross-sectional epidemiologic survey of 6,325 adults in the Paris, France, region. Systolic and diastolic BP levels were higher among the 5,430 coffee drinkers than among the 891 nondrinkers ($p < 0.001$ and $p < 0.01$). The BP levels adjusted for age by covariance analysis increased gradually from the noncoffee consumption category ($126/80 \pm 15/11$ mmHg [mean $\pm$ SD]) to the highest consumption category ($\geqslant 5$ cups/day) ($128/81 \pm 16/10$ mmHg) ($p < 0.001$ for systolic BP and $p < 0.002$ for diastolic BP). The positive association between coffee consumption and systolic, but not diastolic, BP remained significant in a multivariate analysis after controlling for age, sex, body mass index, alcohol consumption, tobacco consumption, and socioeconomic category ($p < 0.02$ for systolic BP and $p = 0.16$ for diastolic BP). It was concluded that coffee consumption is a significant but not strong contributor to the variation in BP levels.

Izzo and associates[16] from Rochester, New York, examined the effects of age and chronic caffeine use (300 mg/day) on the cardiovascular and humoral responses to 250 mg of oral caffeine (the equivalent of 2–3 cups of coffee). Older subjects had greater increases in BP than younger subjects and caffeine nonusers had greater BP increases than caffeine users, regardless of age. Caffeine increased the product of systolic BP and heart rate (an estimate of myocardial oxygen demand) in older caffeine nonusers, but this effect was absent in older caffeine users ($p < 0.01$). Cardiovascular effects of caffeine could not be related temporally to changes in plasma epinephrine, which were greater in caffeine nonusers and younger subjects, or to plasma norepinephrine, renin activity, or vasopressin, which did not change. Thus, age accentuates and moderate prior caffeine use attenuates the cardiovascular effects of oral caffeine; these effects are not mediated solely through the sympathoadrenal system.

Epinephrine

It is well known that increased catecholamines during AMI may contribute to the development of arrhythmias. Struthers and associates[17] from Glasgow and Lanarkshire, Scotland, infused epinephrine intravenously in 9 normal volunteers to levels similar to those seen during AMI. Epinephrine increased systolic BP, decreased diastolic BP, and increased heart rate. It also produced a decrease in T-wave amplitude and an increase in the Q-T interval. The serum potassium fell dramatically during the infusion from a control value of 4.06–3.22 mmol/liter. Thus, circulating epinephrine may increase the frequency of arrhythmias both directly via changes in ventricular repolarization and indirectly via epinephrine-induced hypokalemia. This fact must be kept in mind because hypokalemia during AMI is associated with an increased frequency of ventricular arrhythmias.

Older age

To disassociate the cardiovascular adaptations to high BP from those of aging, Messerli and associates[18] from New Orleans, Louisiana, matched 30 patients with essential systemic hypertension aged >65 years with 30 patients <42 years of age for mean arterial BP, race, sex, height, and weight. Cardiac output, heart rate, stroke volume, intravascular volume, renal blood flow, and plasma renin activity were significantly lower in the elderly, whereas total peripheral (and renal vascular) resistance, LV posterior wall and septal thicknesses, and LV mass were higher. Intravascular volume correlated inversely with total peripheral resistance in both groups and in all patients. Pathophysiologic findings of essential hypertension in the elderly are characterized by a hypertrophied heart of the concentric type with a low cardiac output resulting from a smaller stroke volume and a slower heart rate. Renal blood flow is disproportionally reduced and total peripheral and renal vascular resistance, elevated.

Offspring of hypertensive subjects

Watt and associates[19] from Middlesex, England, compared the BP, body weight, mean 24-hour urinary electrolyte excretion, and plasma renin activity in offspring whose parents both belonged to the top third of the distribution of BP in their 5-year age group to those in offspring whose parents belong to the bottom third. Altogether, 116 offspring, aged 10–43 years, took part in the study. Systolic BP was higher in the offspring with a family history of high BP, but there was no difference in 24-hour urinary electrolyte excretion or plasma renin activity. The study had a power of >80% to detect a 20 mmol difference in sodium excretion, and it provides evidence against the hypothesis that hypertensive patients have an avidity for sodium.

Postprandial state

Lipsitz and associates[20] from Boston, Massachusetts, evaluated the effects of a meal on systolic BP and heart rate in elderly institutionalized subjects (mean age, 87 ± 1) with and without histories of syncope and in young normal subjects (Fig. 4-1). Pulse and BP were measured before the test meal and at intervals for up to 60 minutes afterward. By 35 minutes, mean systolic BP had declined a maximum of 25 ± 5 mmHg in 10 elderly subjects with syncope and 24 ± 9 mmHg in 10 elderly subjects without syncope ($p < 0.03$); the level then stabilized without further change until 60 minutes. There were no changes in BP in 11 young subjects or in elderly subjects not given a meal.

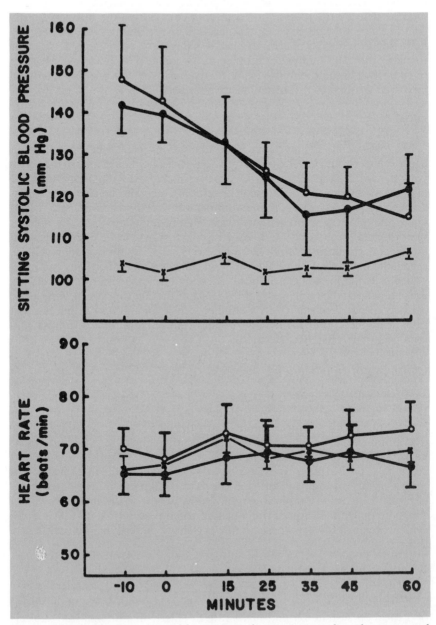

Fig. 4-1. Systolic blood pressure and heart rate in the 60 minute studies. The upper panel shows mean systolic pressure (±SEM) in the sitting position at intervals before and after the start of the meal (0 time) in 10 elderly subjects with syncope (●), and 10 elderly subjects without syncope (○) (p > 0.05), and 11 young normal subjects (X) (p < 0.001 compared with either elderly group). The lower panel shows mean heart rates (±SEM) at the same intervals. Reproduced with permission from Lipsitz et al.[20]

The postprandial change in systolic pressure was not related to medications or diagnoses. Compensatory cardioacceleration was minimal in the elderly, suggesting impaired baroreflexes. Our observations show that postprandial reductions in BP may predispose the elderly to symptomatic hypotension.

LEFT VENTRICULAR HYPERTROPHY: PATHOGENESIS

Echo studies

Culpepper and associates[21] from New Orleans, Louisiana, and Chicago, Illinois, did a prospective M-mode echo study to look for early cardiovascular changes in children prone to hypertension with BP between the 75th and 95th percentiles for age. Average systolic/diastolic BP in 27 children with borderline systemic hypertension was 137/89 mmHg compared with 110/68 mmHg for the 26 controls. Echo measurements were normalized for comparison using 2 methods. The borderline group mean values were significantly greater than controls for LV wall thickness, LV mass, and LV wall thickness to radius ratio. Echo estimates of LV function were lower in the hypertensive group. This study suggests that cardiac hypertrophy can be shown by noninvasive means in some children before arterial pressure becomes elevated. To assess the incidence and possible consequences of early target organ changes, more extensive clinical evaluation of borderline hypertension in children is recommended.

Left ventricular hypertrophy and dysfunction in patients with systemic hypertension are often poorly related to the level of the systemic BP. To evaluate the reasons for this, Devereux and associates[22] from New York City and Framingham, Massachusetts, studied 100 untreated patients with essential hypertension using cuff BP and quantitative echo to measure LV mass index and end-diastolic relative wall thickness of 2 indexes of LV hypertrophy. The LV hypertrophy, as measured by either LV mass index or end-diastolic relative wall thickness, correlated weakly with all indexes of BP, including systolic, diastolic, and mean BP ($r = 0.16$–0.32). In contrast, end-diastolic relative wall thickness, an index that assesses the severity of concentric LV hypertrophy, showed a closer direct relation with total peripheral resistance ($r = 0.52$, $p < 0.001$) and a significant inverse relation with cardiac index ($4 = -0.47$, $p < 0.001$). The LV performance as assessed by fractional systolic shortening of LV internal dimensions was not significantly related to LV mass index, BP, or peak systolic wall stress, but declined significantly with increasing mean systolic wall stress ($r = 0.42$, $p < 0.001$) and even more with increasing end-systolic wall stress ($r = -0.71$, $p < 0.001$). Thus, in patients with hypertension 1) LV hypertrophy correlates only modestly with measurements of resting BP; and 2) the classic pattern of concentric LV hypertrophy, as measured by relative wall thickness, is more closely related to the "typical" hypertensive abnormality of elevated peripheral resistance.

To determine whether BP measured under basal or stress conditions more closely determines LV hypertrophy, Devereux and associates[23] from

New York City compared echo LV mass index and relative wall thickness with clinical BP and with 24-hour recordings at home, work, and sleep in 19 normal subjects and 81 patients with mild hypertension. Only a weak correlation was observed in the entire group between LV mass index and clinical measurements of systolic and diastolic BP, which was only slightly improved by use of systolic and diastolic BP readings in the home. Sleep and total 24-hour BP also related poorly to LV mass index. In contrast, substantially higher correlations existed between LV mass index and systolic and diastolic BP measured by portable recorder in 60 subjects at work. Similarly, work diastolic BP bore the closest relationship to relative wall thickness. Home BP readings taken on a workday also showed a moderate relationship with indices of LV hypertrophy, whereas weaker correlations were found in employed subjects whose BP was recorded on a nonworkday, and no relation between BP and LV hypertrophy existed in subjects who were not employed. The investigators concluded that hypertensive LV hypertrophy is poorly related to clinical or home measurements of BP but that a substantially close relation exists between LV hypertrophy and BP during recurrent stress at work and between LV hypertrophy and home BP on a workday.

Drayer and associates[24] from Long Beach and Irvine, Californa, examined the relation between casual BP and LV hypertrophy derived from the ECG and also from M-mode echo. The ECG and echo measurements of LV muscle mass were related to various measures of BP obtained during circadian ambulatory BP monitoring in 12 patients with systemic hypertension. Casual BP did not correlate substantially with ECG voltages or with echo measurements of muscle mass. The correlations between whole day, daytime, or nighttime BP averages and ECG voltages were not significant. However, echo LV muscle mass correlated significantly with the averages of whole day, daytime, and nighttime, and 2-hour morning systolic pressures. The correlations between diastolic BP and LV muscle mass were not significant. Therefore serial BP measurements are required to evaluate the relation between BP and LV muscle mass as measured by the M-mode echo. The ECG was of little value in this relation.

Shapiro and Beevers[25] from Birmingham, England, studied electrocardiograms, chest radiographs, and digitized apex echoes in 16 patients with malignant systemic hypertension before and after up to 6 months of antihypertensive treatment and compared them with those of 8 patients with severe benign systemic hypertension. Adequate BP reduction was obtained in 14 with resolution of retinopathy, but 1 patient died and another had poor BP control. Nine had ECG criteria of LV hypertrophy, which did not change with treatment, and 10 had lateral ischemia that resolved in 7. The malignant hypertensive patients were divided into 7 with and 9 without a previous history of hypertension. Both groups had normal echo cavity dimensions, but the former group tended to have hypertrophy (similar to that in benign hypertensive patients) and the latter did not. After adequate reduction of BP, no change in wall and septal thickness occurred (except in 1 patient with poor BP control). At entry, malignant hypertensive patients showed delayed mitral valve opening with significant cavity dimension increase during prolonged isovolumic relaxation, reduced peak rate, and prolonged duration of cavity dimension increase and cavity shape change (inward wall motion) during the upstroke of the apexcardiogram, which showed a tall "a" wave. After reduction of BP, although the delay in mitral valve opening persisted, the timing of A returned toward normal and the dimension change during the upstroke of the apexcardiogram and the relative height of the "a" wave were reduced but remained significantly different from normal. Some patients without a previous history of hypertension may develop a malignant phase without LV hypertrophy on the ECG or echo. They maintain their pump function even with radiologic pulmonary edema, have incoordinate relaxation and contraction, and have abnormal filling. Similar functional abnormalities were found in malignant hypertensive patients with hypertrophy. Treatment to lower BP reduces incoordinate contraction, but impaired diastolic function persists, as in benign hypertension, suggesting that these abnormalities are the result of altered myocardial properties that may occur without hypertrophy.

ECG study

Sparrow and associates[26] from Boston, Massachusetts, observed prospectively for 10 years 1,090 men aged 23–80 years who had baseline BP <140/90 mmHg. The BP was taken at 5- and 10-year follow-up examinations. Multiple linear regression analysis indicated that baseline levels of systolic pressure, age, R-wave amplitude (aV_L), hematocrit, T-wave amplitude (V_5), and S-wave amplitude (V_4, V_5, and V_6) were statistically significant predictors of systolic pressure change. Baseline levels of diastolic pressure, R-wave amplitude (aV_L), and hematocrit were statistically significant predictors of diastolic pressure change. Multiple logistic regression analysis showed that baseline levels of BP, S-wave amplitude (V_1, V_2, and V_3), body mass index, R-wave amplitude (V_4, V_5, and V_6), and T-wave amplitude (V_5) were statistically significant predictors of subsequent hypertension. Whether the identified ECG amplitudes are an indicator of early increases in peripheral resistance or a function of neurohumoral factors, or both, is unknown. This study was followed by an editorial by Tarazi and Gifford[27] from Cleveland, Ohio.

Symposium

A 19 article, 120 page symposium on "Left Ventricular Hypertrophy in Essential Hypertension" appeared in the September 26, 1983, number of *The American Journal of Medicine*.[28]

MANAGEMENT OF MILD HYPERTENSION

Recommendations to treat patients with mild systemic hypertension are based principally on 6 randomized clinical trials conducted in 3 countries between 1964 and 1979. To determine whether the methods and results of these randomized clinical trials justify the current therapeutic policy, Toth and Horwitz[29] from New Haven, Connecticut, performed a clinical epidemiologic analysis of the data focusing on 1) clinical -vs- statistical significance; 2) clinical heterogeneity of patients' baseline state; 3) suitable management of the untreated control patients; and 4) choice of outcome events. This analysis suggested that the results of available studies are better suited to public health decisions (number of cardiovascular deaths prevented nation-wide) than personal health decisions (whether treatment does more good than harm for individual patients), and that current evidence does not justify a uniform policy of treating all asymptomatic patients with mild hypertension.

In contrast to the articles appearing in the January 21 issue of JAMA, Gifford and associates[30] from several USA medical centers developed the argument in favor of the use of drug therapy to reduce diastolic BP when it was consistently >90 mmHg despite a 3–6-month trial of appropriate dietary but nonpharmacologic treatment. Their argument in essence was that it may be more dangerous not to treat than to treat the patient with drugs when dietary and other nonpharmacologic measures do not suffice to lower the diastolic pressure to <90 mmHg.

Another editorial on this subject was written by Ram.[31]

TREATMENT

Sodium restriction

In an investigation carried out by Gillum and associates[32] from Minneapolis, Minnesota, the effects on BP of modest weight reduction and sodium restriction, singly and in combination were examined in 2 studies of obese men with borderline hypertension taking no medication. Weight, 24-hour urinary sodium excretion, and BP change were measured before and after 2 10-week periods of dietary intervention. In the first study of 28 men, an average weight reduction of 5.2 kg with only 18 mmol/24 hour decrease in sodium excretion was associated with a 5.4/2.4 (systolic/diastolic) mmHg average fall in BP. In a second study of 59 men, an average of 3.9 kg weight loss without concomitant change in sodium excretion was associated with a 3.4/1.88 mmHg mean BP decrease, and the combination of a 5.8 kg weight loss with an 80 mmol/24 hour reduction in sodium excretion was associated with a 9.3/6.7 mmHg BP decrease. Thus, even modest weight reduction is associated with a BP decrease independent of changes in sodium intake. Combined modest weight reduction and sodium restriction are associated with substantial decrease in BP and should be combined as the first step in the management of obese patients with, or at high risk for, essential hypertension.

Silman and associates[33] from London, England, compared in a randomized controlled trial the effect of a restricted sodium diet with that of a general health package in 28 patients who had a sustained diastolic BP of 95–104 mmHg and who had no treatment for at least 13 months before the trial. The general health package did not include any specific hypotensive procedures. Changes in BP were measured at predetermined intervals over the course of a year. Within each group both systolic and diastolic BP fell to a highly significant extent after a year, but there was no significant difference between the groups. It would thus seem that the antihypertensive effect of a restricted sodium diet may be related to the increased consultation and monitoring activity of such intervention rather than to the dietary manipulation itself.

Hofman and associates[34] from Rotterdam, The Netherlands, studied the effect of dietary sodium on BP in a double-blind randomized trial with 245 newborn infants assigned to a normal sodium diet and 231 to a low sodium diet during the first 6 months of life. The sodium intake of the normal sodium group was almost 3 times that of the low sodium group. Systolic BP was measured every month from the first week until the 25th week. At 25 weeks, systolic pressure was 2.1 mmHg lower in the low sodium group than in the normal sodium group. The difference between the groups increased significantly during the first 6 months of life. These observations are in agreement with the view that sodium intake is casually related to BP level.

With an index for dietary salt use designed to provide a semiquantitative estimate of salt intake, Holden and associates[35] from New Haven, Connecticut, found that in a sample representative of the 2.1 million adults in Connecticut, the mean BP of those at the 90th percentile or higher of salt intake differed by a quantitative insignificant amount from the mean BP of those at the tenth percentile or lower of salt intake. When the obese (body mass index, 90th percentile or higher) were examined separately, similar results were obtained. These findings indicate that it is unlikely that dietary salt intake has a clinically significant effect on BP in most individuals in a large defined population, but these results do not exclude the possibility of a clinically significant effect in a small subgroup of salt-sensitive individuals. Thus, these authors concluded that it does not appear justifiable or appropriate to undertake large-scale salt restriction in the general population to prevent systemic hypertension.

In an accompanying editorial to the article by Holden and associates, Scribner[36] from Seattle, Washington, disagreed with the implication that sodium restriction was futile in the control of systemic hypertension, arguing that one cannot attain the 10 mEq/day levels achieved by the Kempner diet. Reduction in sodium intake to 50–100 mEq/24 range, however, often prevents the development of systemic hypertension in susceptible persons and makes its treatment much easier and more effective should hypertension develop. Scribner recommends that any person in whom there is a likely propensity for developing hypertension should restrict sodium intake. Included in this group are 1) any patient with chronic renal disease, since hypertension eventually develops in 95% of such patients; 2) any person with 1 or both hypertensive parents; 3) certain racial groups, especially black males, in 50% of whom hypertension develops; and 4) most persons >50 years, since BP tends to increase with age, with the result that >40% of the older population is hypertensive. This trend may be related to the fact that the kidneys' ability to handle a sodium load decreases with age. Scribner quotes the 1976 explanation of Meneely in Battarbee (*The American Journal of Cardiology* 38:768–785, 1976) as to why such studies as that by Holden and associates failed to reveal the true relation between sodium intake and essential hypertension. Meneely and Battarbee termed it "the saturation effect" (Fig. 4-2). What that means is explained to some extent in the figure. The horizontal axis shows the habitual sodium chloride intake of a given population, which can vary from 1 mEq/24 hours to high levels. The vertical axis shows the percent of the population that is hypertensive; that percentage approaches 30% (point B) at the highest levels of habitual sodium intake. This value (point B) may be lower in certain populations and as high as 50% in old or black men. Unfortunately, only points A and B on the curve are

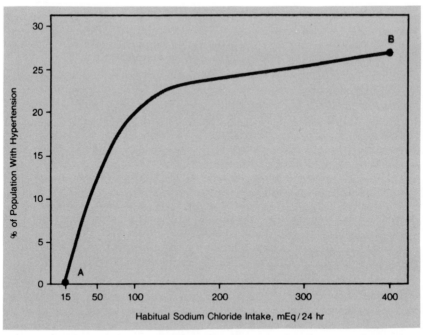

Fig. 4-2. Relation between habitual sodium chloride intake and incidence of hypertension. Only points A and B are documented (see text). Reproduced with permission from Scribner.[36]

known. The evidence now is overwhelming that point A is valid. In other words, among populations worldwide wherein habitual sodium chloride intake is <20 mEq/24 hours, the incidence of hypertension approaches zero and declines in persons >20 years. Point B is known for some population groups and probably varies from 20–50%, depending on genetic and other factors. Unfortunately, no populations have been studied that habitually ingest between 20 and 100 mEq/day sodium chloride so that the shape of the curve really is unknown. The sodium chloride intake among the population studies by Holden and associates ranged from a low of about 100 mEq/24 hours to high levels. Unfortunately, because of the saturation effect, the increase in the percentage of patients with hypertension in this range of salt intake is so small as to be undetectable by the methods employed in large population studies such as this one. The implications of this curve of the saturation effect are both instructive and important. Point A corresponds closely to the set point for the normal regulation of sodium excretion by the kidney. Man from an evolutionary standpoint was designed to survive on low intakes of sodium. Indeed, in certain primitive cultures, such as in the Amazon basin where sodium chloride intake is 1 mEq/24 hours and BP declines with age, the renin levels average 10 times those in our population. Since these people have low BP, the essential role of sodium retention in renal vascular hypertension is apparent.

Why do most modern civilizations consume such huge quantities of salt? The best guess is that early civilizations discovered that sodium chloride in higher concentrations could be used to preserve food and that man slowly adapted his taste for salt to levels of consumption hundreds of times greater than that needed for survival. Point B also is of interest and importance. It can be concluded that man's ability to handle sodium really is amazing; so amazing that as much as 80% of a given population can handle even the highest habitual intakes of salt without danger of essential hypertension developing. Indeed, several studies show no hypertension as a result of salt loading up to 450 mEq/day. Salt loading experiments, however, in normal persons show a linear increase in BP as the intake increases from 450–1,500 mEq/day.

Cooper and associates[37] from Chicago, Illinois, carried out BP screening on a university campus to identify persons with early systemic hypertension or high normal BP. Compared with normotensive control subjects of a similar age, drawn from the same population, persons identified as being at the upper end of the BP distribution had significantly increased levels of sodium-lithium countertransport. This difference persisted when other potential confounding variables, e.g., overweight, sex, ethnicity, sodium excretion, and age, were taken into account. A positive family history was associated with slightly higher levels of sodium-lithium countertransport, although the effect could be explained by higher present levels of BP. These data suggest that abnormalities of cation transport are present early in the course of the development of hypertension. Measurement of transport levels may provide an estimate of risk of hypertension and allow identification of susceptible persons.

Weight reduction

Reisin and associates[38] from New Orleans, Louisiana, measured intravascular volumes and systemic and regional hemodynamic variables before and after weight reduction in 12 patients with obesity and essential hypertension. These findings were compared with those in 9 patients who did not have any weight loss. Reduction of mean arterial pressure significantly correlated with the fall in total body weight. Total circulating and cardiopulmonary blood volumes were significantly reduced, and these changes permitted a decreased venous return and cardiac output. This fall in cardiac output was directly related to a contracted total blood volume and decreased cardiopulmonary blood volume. Patients who did not lose weight showed no changes in any of these hemodynamic measurements. In addition, weight loss was associated with reduced resting circulating levels of plasma norepinephrine, suggesting that diminished adrenergic function may also be related to weight reduction and its associated fall in arterial pressure. The present data provide strong evidence against the concept that the fall in arterial BP with weight reduction resulted from the use of an inappropriate sphygmomanometer cuff, dietary sodium intake, reduced caloric intake, or familiarization with the procedure used to measure arterial BP. In the present study, dietary sodium and choloric intakes were held normal for the 10 days before each hemodynamic study; intraarterial BP was measured directly; and the group of patients with unchanging weight, who were also familiarized with the follow-up and procedure used to measure hemodynamic variables, was studied under similar conditions.

Low-fat diet

Fifty-seven couples living in 2 communities of North Karelia, Eastern Finland, aged 30–50 years, were randomly allocated to 3 groups in a study by Puska and associates[39]. After a 2-week baseline period group I followed a diet low in fat (23% of energy) with a high polyunsaturated/saturated ratio (1.0), group II reduced daily salt intake from 192–77 mmol, and group III (control group) continued the usual diet. After the 6-week intervention period groups I and II reverted to their usual diets. In group I systolic BP declined from 138–130 mmHg and diastolic BP from 89–81 mmHg during the intervention period; the values increased after the switch back to the usual diet. The decrease was greater among hypertensive than among normotensive subjects. In groups II and III the mean BP changed very little during the study.

Cod liver oil

Epidemiologic and experimental data suggest an antiatherothrombotic potential of w-3 polyunsaturated fatty acids. Lorenz and coworkers[40] from Munich, West Germany, supplemented the Western diet that supplies predominately w-6 polyunsaturated fatty acids with 40 ml/day of cod liver oil, which provides about 10 g of w-3 polyunsaturated fatty acids daily, for 25 days in 8 volunteers. The w-3 polyunsaturated fatty acids were incorporated in platelet and erythrocyte membrane phospholipids at the expense of w-6 polyunsaturated fatty acids. Bleeding time increased and platelet count, platelet aggregation upon ADP and collagen and associated thromboxane B_2 formation decreased. The BP and BP response to norepinephrine and angiotensin II decreased without major changes in plasma catecholamines, renin, urinary aldosterone, kallikrein, prostaglandins E_2 and $F_{2\alpha}$, and red cell cation fluxes. Biochemical and functional changes were reversed 4 weeks after cod liver oil was discontinued.

Exercise training

Hagberg and associates[41] from St. Louis, Missouri, studied 25 adolescents (aged 16 ± 1 years) whose BP was persistently above the 95th percentile for their age and sex. They were studied before and after 6 ± 1 months of exercise training and again 9 ± 1 month after the cessation of training. Maximal oxygen consumption (VO_2) increased significantly with training. There was no change in body weight or sum of skinfolds. Both systolic and diastolic BP decreased significantly with training; however, complete BP normalization was not achieved. When the subjects were retested 9 ± 1 months after cessation of training, systolic BP and VO_{2max} had returned to pretraining levels; however, diastolic BP was still below pretraining levels in the subjects who had diastolic hypertension initially. Except in subjects who initially had an elevated cardiac output, no consistent hemodynamic changes were found with training or cessation of training to account for the reductions in BP. The subjects whose resting cardiac outputs were high initially had significantly lower cardiac outputs after training as a result of decreases in both heart rate and stroke volume; however, vascular resistance remained unchanged. Sedentary control subjects with similar BP had no significant change in any of the variables measured over a similar period.

These data indicate that moderate endurance exercise training can lower BP in otherwise healthy hypertensive adolescents as an initial therapeutic intervention.

Calcium supplementation

Epidemiologic and nonhuman animal studies have suggested an inverse relation between calcium intake and BP. Furthermore, calcium intake seems to be inversely related to the incidence of eclampsia in pregnancy. In a randomized clinical trial, Belizan and associates[42] from Guatemala City, Guatemala, and Baltimore, Maryland, allocated young adults to a calcium-supplemented group receiving 1 g/day of elemental calcium (15 men and 15 women) or to a placebo group (14 women and 13 men) for 22 weeks. The calcium-supplemented group had a significant decrease in diastolic BP; this effect was stabilized after 9 weeks in women and 6 weeks in men. The reduction in diastolic BP was 5.6 and 9% from the initial values for women and men, respectively.

Diuretics (hydrochlorothiazide, indapamide)

Vardan and associates[43] from Syracuse, New York, studied 23 patients aged 50–81 years (mean, 66 years) with systolic BP $\geq$160 mmHg and 2 times or more the diastolic BP minus 15. Cardiac output and stroke volume varied widely, with several high values. An elevated systemic vascular resistance, when considered as a function of the cardiac output, was the most prevalent hemodynamic abnormality. After administration of hydrochlorothiazide, 50 mg/day, for 1 month in 20 patients, 18 had a significant fall in BP, systemic vascular resistance, and stroke volume. After 1 year of continuous therapy, the hemodynamics, studied in 14 patients, did not change further. There were no clinical difficulties with carbohydrate intolerance, azotemia, hyperuricemia, or hyopkalemia. No patient had symptoms of orthostatic hypotension or cardiac arrhythmias. Thus, thiazide therapy effectively and safely lowers the BP in most patients with systolic hypertension by reducing systemic vascular resistance.

Indapamide is a new thiazide-like antihypertensive diuretic agent indicated for the treatment of hypertension and edema. The clinical pharmacokinetics and pharmacology of this agent were reported by Caruso and associates[44] from Tuckahoe, New York. Indapamide shows an alteration in vascular reactivity to calcium and other agonists, suggesting the possibility of a direct vascular effect. The drug is recommended in doses of 2.5–5 mg once a day. It is rapidly and completely absorbed from the gastrointestinal tract, resulting in maximal blood levels in approximately 2.3 hours. Coadministration of indapamide with food or antacids does not reduce bioavailability. Linear proportionality of blood concentration with increasing doses is evident following both single and multiple doses. Other pharmacokinetic parameters are not dose related. Indapamide is widely distributed in the body with extensive binding to erythrocytes. Binding to plasma proteins is approximately 76%. Disappearance of indapamide from the blood is biphasic, with a terminal half-life of approximately 16 hours. Renal clearance represents less than 10% of the total systemic clearance of the parent drug, showing the dominant role of hepatic clearance. Studies of patients with renal impairment showed little or no accumulation of indapamide in the blood in comparison to patients with normal renal function. Clinical investigations demonstrate that indapamide has diuretic properties. Free water clearance studies indicate a site of action in the cortical diluting segment of the distal tubules. No adverse effect of indapamide on renal function is evident in normal volunteers, hypertensive patients, or geriatric hypertensive patients, as determined by glomerular filtration rate or effective renal plasma flow. Hemodynamic studies in indapamide in patients with mild to moderate hypertension show a significant ($p < 0.05$) decrease in mean BP (16%) and total peripheral resistance (15%). No other significant hemodynamic effects are evident. These data indicate that indapamide may produce antihypertensive activity through a dual mechanism of action: diuretic and direct vascular. Additionally, the agent appears to be safe even for patients with impaired renal function.

Beta-blocking agents

Cardiac effects of beta-adrenergic blocking drugs represent a balance between depression of myocardial function and relief of pressure load. To determine the relative importance of each, Fouad and associates[45] from Cleveland, Ohio, measured cardiac and hemodynamic indexes by radioisotope technique (technetium-99m-human serum albumin) with essential hypertension treated with either metoprolol (8 patients) or nadolol (13 patients) for 1 month. No significant difference was found between the two groups and the results were pooled. Cardiac output was significantly and equally reduced in the responders and nonresponders (−0.96 -vs- −1.33 liters/min), and EF was not altered significantly in either. The main changes with treatment were observed in the LV volume curves; responders maintained the same ejection velocity despite beta blockade and had a more rapid early ventricular filling rate ($p < 0.05$). In contrast, nonresponders had a reduced velocity of ejection ($p < 0.01$) and a slower rate of ventricular filling ($p < 0.01$), suggesting either altered relaxation rate or decreased LV compliance. Thus, beta-adrenergic blockade can significantly alter ventricular diastolic function, but these effects are overshadowed by BP reduction in responders.

Ruben and associates[46] from Glasgow, Scotland, compared placebo with atenolol in a randomized and double-blind prospective manner in 120 women with mild to moderate pregnancy-associated systemic hypertension. Each of the women became hypertensive during the last trimester of a previously normal pregnancy. Each had been admitted for bed rest. The BP was 140–170 mmHg systolic or 90–110 mmHg diastolic taken after 10 minutes of supine rest or after 5 minutes standing on 2 occasions separated by 24 hours. Atenolol given once daily significantly reduced BP, prevented proteinuria, and reduced the number of hospital admissions. Loss of BP control leading to withdrawal from the study was commoner among the placebo group, whose babies had a high morbidity. Respiratory distress syndrome occurred only in the placebo group. Intrauterine growth retardation, neonatal hypoglycemia, and hyperbilirubinemia occurred with the same frequency in the two groups. Neonatal bradycardia was more common after atenolol, but the systolic BP of the babies was the same in both groups. There was no difference between the groups in maternal symptoms that could have been attributed to beta-blocker therapy. Thus, atenolol is more effective than conventional obstetric management in this form of hypertension and does not adversely affect mother or baby.

Freis and associates[47] of the Veterans Administration Cooperative Study Group on Antihypertensive Agents randomly assigned in a double-blind fashion 365 men with pretreatment diastolic BP of 95–114 mmHg to receive nadolol titrated from 80–240 mg, or bendroflumethiazide 5–10 mg, or the combination. After 12 weeks of treatment, a diastolic BP of <90 mmHg was achieved in 49% who received nadolol, 46% who received bendroflumethiazide, and 85% who received bendroflumethiazide and nadolol. With nadolol, the diastolic BP decreased more in whites than in blacks; with bendroflumethiazide, this racial trend was reversed. Side effects were infrequent; the most common were impotence, lethargy, weakness, and postural dizziness, which occurred more often with bendroflumethiazide than with nadolol. Addition of hydralazine, 25–100 mg twice daily, controlled diastolic BP at a level of <90 mmHg in approximately 60% of those previously uncontrolled. Nadolol, and especially bendroflumethiazide plus nadolol, provided an efficacious once daily treatment for systemic hypertension, and addition of hydralazine was effective in most nonresponders.

A 11 article, 65 page symposium on the usefulness of oxprenolol for control of elevated BP appeared in the November 10, 1983, *American Journal of Cardiology.*[48]

A 15 article, 114 page symposium on the usefulness of labetalol for control of elevated BP appeared in the October 17, 1983, *American Journal of Medicine.*[49]

Calcium channel blockers

Yamakado and associates[50] from Tsu, Japan, treated 16 patients with uncomplicated systemic hypertension with placebo, diltiazem (180 mg/day), and propranolol (60 mg/day) for 1 month each. Each patient performed multistage symptom-limited treadmill exercise tests during each period of administration. There was no significant difference in maximal exercise duration between placebo, diltiazem, and propranolol. Diltiazem significantly decreased both systolic and diastolic BP and heart rate at rest, during submaximal exercise at the same work load, and maximal exercise. Propranolol produced similar changes in systemic BP and heart rate at rest and during exercise. However, the reductions in systolic BP, heart rate, and pressure-rate product with diltiazem during exercise were smaller than those with propranolol at small doses, suggesting that diltiazem in its usual therapeutic dose was almost devoid of beta-blocking activity. Thus, diltiazem benefits hypertensive patients because it reduces systemic BP even during exercise. It is particularly useful when systemic hypertension occurs in association with CAD because of its effects of coronary artery dilation and heart rate reduction.

Hornung and associates[51] from Middlesex, England, examined the action of nifedipine tablets in 17 patients with essential hypertension, focusing particularly on the profile of BP reduction over 24 hours resulting from both twice daily and once daily therapy (dose range, 40–120 mg daily). This new formulation of nifedipine has a more prolonged and lower peak plasma level than an equivalent dose of nifedipine capsules. The patients were fully ambulant and studied by continuous intraarterial recording techniques. The BP responses during isometric and dynamic exercise testing were also observed. Within-patient comparisons of consecutive mean hourly systolic and diastolic BP showed a highly significant effect from twice daily therapy (p < 0.001) for nearly the entire day. Also, significantly lower BP was maintained during isometric and dynamic exercise. Mean hourly heart rates were not significantly altered. The profile of action of the single morning dose was initially similar, but its efficacy diminished from 6 pm to 8 am on the following day. Side effects were not unduly troublesome and did not cause any patient withdrawals. Four patients developed mild ankle edema. Two others had facial flushing. Nifedipine given twice daily in tablet form therefore is an effective antihypertensive drug capable of lowering BP consistently over 24 hours in ambulant patients and during formal exercise testing. Thus, this agent may be useful as initial therapy for systemic hypertension, although the tablets are not as yet widely available.

Nine patients with untreated essential hypertension were studied by McLeay and colleagues[52] from Birmingham, England, in the control state and after 16 weeks of treatment with nifedipine, 10 mg orally every 8 hours. Direct arterial BP monitored continuously over 24 hours showed that nifedipine significantly reduced systolic and diastolic BP throughout the day and night. The variability of BP was not altered by nifedipine therapy. There was no significant change in heart rate after nifedipine therapy. Chronic nifedipine therapy increased forearm blood flow and decreased forearm vascular resistance, consistent with its action as a vasodilator. The absolute BP responses to tilt, hand grip, and cold were reduced but the percent increase in pressure was not altered by therapy. Plasma renin activity was not altered by chronic nifedipine therapy. After chronic nifedipine therapy, there was resetting of the sinoaortic baroreflex and an increase in its sensitivity. Successful control of BP with nifedipine led to a significant reduction in the LV mass index.

Ventura and associates[53] from New Orleans, Louisiana, studied the immediate hemodynamic effects of a new calcium-channel blocking agent, nitrendipine, in 12 patients with mild established essential systemic hypertension. According to the response to mean arterial pressure, patients were classified into responders (decrease ≤10 mmHg, 7 patients) and nonresponders (>10 mmHg, 5 patients). The decrease in arterial pressure in responders was associated with a significant (p < 0.01) decrease in total peripheral resistance and a significant (p < 0.05) increase in heart rate, cardiac index, and LV ejection rate. The plasma norepinephrine level was significantly (p < 0.05) increased in the responders. The response to upright tilt was qualitatively similar to pretreatment values. Thus, nitrendipine lowered arterial pressure as a result of arteriolar dilation associated with a reflexive increase in heart rate and cardiac index. These hemodynamic properties make the drug particularly apt for use in combination with beta-adrenergic blockade for the treatment of arterial hypertension.

Vasodilating agents (endralazine)

A major problem with hydralazine is that its metabolism is subject to genetically determined variations in rate that, in turn, lead to variations in the dosage needed to control BP. Patients who metabolize hydralazine rapidly ("fast acetylators") require significantly higher doses than patients who metabolize it slowly ("slow acetylators"). The BP lowering in slow acetylators is about twice that observed in fast acetylators given the same dose of hydralazine. Slow acetylators are also more likely to develop drug-induced lupus. Endralazine is a new peripheral vasodilator that has been shown to be an effective antihypertensive agent in several animal species. Although chemically related to hydralazine, it is metabolized mainly by the formation of hydrazones with endogenous ketone bodies, acetylation being relatively unimportant. This suggests that acetylator status should not influence the dosage of endralazine needed to achieve good BP control. Holmes and associates[54] in a multicenter clinical study from Basel, Switzerland, Waalwijk, Holland, Helsinki, Finland, and Trondheim, Norway, treated 50 patients with confirmed systemic hypertension with endralazine in addition to the beta blocker, pindolol, to which they had not responded adequately. The BP was lowered from 173/115–143/87 mmHg in the 34 slow acetylators and from 175/111–140/84 mmHg in the 16 fast acetylators. The dosages of both pindolol and endralazine were the same in both groups. Thus, the acetylator phenotype does not affect the therapeutic efficacy or dosage requirement of endralazine.

Alpha-1 blocking agents (trimazosin)

In investigations carried out by Chrysant[55] from Kansas City, Missouri, the acute and chronic autonomic, systemic, and renal hemodynamic effects of trimazosin and placebo were studied in patients with uncomplicated essential hypertension of mild to moderate severity. In these studies, trimazosin effectively reduced arterial pressure through a decrease in peripheral vascular resistance. In the acute studies the cardiac output increased, whereas in the chronic studies it remained unchanged. Acutely, trimazosin selectively increased renal blood flow, which was out of proportion to the increase in cardiac output. No significant effects on autonomic function, metabolic function, or renin and aldosterone release were observed with trimazosin after acute or chronic administration. No tolerance to the action of the drug developed. No significant hemodynamic or metabolic changes were observed when compared with placebo either acutely or chronically. It was concluded that: 1) trimazosin is an effective and safe antihypertensive agent given in single daily doses; 2) it exerts its effects mainly through direct arteriolar dilation and less through autonomic inhibition; 3) its antihypertensive effectiveness is not compromised by the development of tolerance; 4) it exerts a selective beneficial effect on renal circulation that is unrelated to systemic hemodynamic changes; and 5) these properties of trimazosin may make it a desirable drug for the treatment of hypertension complicated by renal failure.

Helgeland[56] from Oslo, Norway, describes a double-blind, parallel, comparative study of trimazosin or propranolol with and without polythiazide in 130 patients with essential hypertension. Both treatment regimens were shown to be effective in achieving statistically significant sustained reduction in BP. Propranolol alone was somewhat more effective, at the doses selected, than trimazosin alone, but the hypertension of nonresponders in each treatment group was effectively controlled by the addition of low doses of polythiazide. Trimazosin had no effect on heart rate, whereas propranolol significantly lowered resting heart rates, which was occasionally troublesome. Side effects were less frequent in the trimazosin-treated group. Trimazosin lowered serum creatinine and blood urea nitrogen, an effect significantly different from that of propranolol. There was also a tendency for serum uric acid to rise in patients receiving propranolol and fall in those receiving trimazosin; polythiazide significantly raised uric acid levels. The effects of trimazosin and propranolol on the lipid profile were small, but the difference between the increase in the HDL cholesterol fraction in trimazosin-treated patients and the decrease in propranolol-treated patients was significant.

Trimazosin and a quinazoline derivative related to prazosin has been extensively examined in >1000 hypertensive patients enrolled in >50 studies evaluated by Taylor and colleagues[57] from Groton, Connecticut, and Sandwich, England. In hypertensive patients, reduction in elevated BP in both supine and standing positions, consequent to a reduction in systemic vascular resistance, persisted in long-term therapy. Progression of hypertension target organ damage did not occur. Improvement in blood lipids with decreased total serum cholesterol was noted in long-term therapy. In long-term studies, 74% of patients responded at a trimazosin dose of ≤300 mg/day; the maximum dose was ≤300 mg/day in 52% of patients and ≤200 mg/day in 36%. Most patients received twice a day therapy. The side-effect profile of trimazosin was comparable to placebo and significantly better than that of either methyldopa or propranolol. Concomitant disease or therapy did not adversely affect the trimazosin safety profile. Hematology, clinical chemistry, and urinary parameters did not indicate deleterious effects. Because of its excellent safety and toleration profile, trimazosin may be particularly suitable in first-line therapy of patients with mild or moderate hypertension.

Terazosin

Drayer and associates[58] from Long Beach and Irvine, California, performed noninvasive BP monitoring in hypertensive patients before and during placebo therapy and before and during therapy with a long-acting peripheral alpha-adrenergic receptor antagonist, terazosin hydrochloride. Placebo therapy did not result in significant changes in casual BP or in averages of whole-day, daytime, or nighttime BPs. Short-term therapy with terazosin did not induce significant changes in casual supine or daytime BPs. However, whole-day BP monitoring disclosed that nighttime BPs were lower during short-term therapy. Moreover, the circadian pattern of BP was shifted downward during terazosin therapy. Long-term therapy with terazosin resulted in significant changes in BP. All BP values were lowered significantly. The differences in the circadian BP pattern between placebo and long-term terazosin therapy showed that in these patients BP was lowered throughout the 24 hours of the day. These results emphasize the usefulness of 24-hour BP monitoring in the evaluation of the effectiveness of long-acting antihypertensive agents.

Captopril

In an investigation by Mookherjee and associates[59] from Syracuse, New York, hemodynamic variables were measured and plasma renin activity

(PRA), angiotensin II (A II), aldosterone, and bradykinin assays performed in 21 hypertensive men without LV dysfunction on regular diet and thiazide diuretics before and 60–90 minutes after 25 mg oral captopril. Heart rate, RV and LV filling pressures, mean cardiac index (CI), and PA resistance remained unchanged. The mean intraarterial pressure (MAP) fell from 140 $\pm$ 5–116 $\pm$ 6 mmHg (p < 0.001) correlating with reduction of systemic vascular resistance (SVR) (r = 0.87; p < 0.001), control PRA (r = 0.59; p < 0.01), and A II levels (r = 0.72; p < 0.005) but not with control bradykinin or its postcaptopril rise (p < 0.01). The decrease in SVR correlated with reduction in plasma A II (r = 0.80; p < 0.001) and aldosterone concentrations (r = 0.53; p < 0.05). Of 4 patients (19%) with precipitous decrease in MAP after captopril, 3 needed volume expansion for circulatory support. It was concluded that: 1) A II reduction by captopril and not bradykinin potentiation explains most of the agent's hemodynamic response in hypertensive circulation; 2) endogenous A II may have a supportive role for SVR and possibly for CI but not for PA resistance; and 3) extra precaution is warranted while captopril is being started in hypertensive patients taking diuretics.

To study the value of low dose captopril (6.25 and 12.5 mg) and a diuretic combination, Thind and colleagues[60] from Louisville, Kentucky, monitored the BP and heart rate of 17 patients with moderate to severe hypertension for 6 hours (in hospital) or 3 hours (office) after a single low dose or larger (25, 50, 100, and 150 mg) of captopril. All patients had preserved renal function and had been taking an oral diuretic (hydrochlorothiazide or furosemide) for at least 4 weeks. The supine and upright acute BP lowering with 6.25 mg was not different from the larger captopril doses; none produced persistent or profound hypotension. There was no deterioration of renal function, new or persistent increase in proteinuria, neutropenia, or agranulocytosis immediately or during 17 weeks follow-up. Low dose captopril (6.25 or 12.5 mg 3 times daily) normalized the supine BP of 35% of these patients. These investigators suggest that in hypertensive patients already taking a diuretic, a lower starting dose of captopril than the recommended 25 mg 3 times a day may be desirable.

Ergotamine

The acute and chronic effects of ergotamine were examined in 4 patients with chronic orthostatic hypotension by Chobanian and colleagues[61] from Boston, Massachusetts. Chronic oral administration of ergotamine tartrate produced significant increases in standing BP and marked clinical improvement without appreciable recumbent hypertension. The BP increases were not associated with significant changes in plasma norepinephrine or plasma renin activity. No major toxicity was observed in doses of 2–6 mg/day over treatment periods of 3–18 months. Hemodynamic studies on the effects of intravenous ergotamine tartrate (0.25–0.50 mg) revealed that the ergotamine-induced increase in BP in the supine position was associated with an increase in total peripheral resistance without a change in cardiac output (CO). During 45–60° upright tilt, ergotamine increased both total peripheral resistance and CO. Forearm plethysmographic studies revealed decreased forearm blood flow and venous volume and increased vascular resistance with ergotamine. The orthostatic hypotensives had more platelet alpha receptors than the control subjects. The increased receptor level was associated with abnormally low circulating levels of norepinephrine and increased pressor responsiveness to infused norepinephrine in 3 of the 4 patients. Chronic ergotamine therapy appeared to reduce platelet alpha receptor number to normal. Thus, the results indicate that ergotamine is of value in certain patients with chronic orthostatic hypotension and that the BP effects are related to vasoconstriction in both aterial and venous beds.

Comparisons

PROPRANOLOL -VS- HYDROCHLOROTHIAZIDE

Freis and associates[62] from Washington, D.C., Miami, Florida, and New York City studied the relation between renin activity and therapeutic response to hydrochlorothiazide or propranolol in 906 patients in 7 Veterans Administration medical centers with diastolic BP of 95–114 mmHg treated with propranolol (40–320 mg twice daily) or hydrochlorothiazide (25–100 mg twice daily). The initial renin profiles were: 102, 56% (n, 300); normal, 33% (n, 174); high, 11% (n, 60). A greater incidence of low and fewer high renin profiles (p < 0.001) were observed in blacks. After furosemide administration (40 mg intravenously), 55% of patients (n, 291) had a low renin response and 45 percent (n, 240) had a normal renin response. No correlation between renin profile and renin response was observed, although low renin response and low renin profile occurred more frequently in older patients. Hydrochlorothiazide administration resulted in a greater decrement in diastolic BP (p < 0.05) in the total group. Irrespective of renin activity, both hydrochlorothiazide and propranolol reduced diastolic BP. When renin profile was considered, no significant variation in response to hydrochlorothiazide therapy was observed, and there was a greater reduction in diastolic BP in the patients with a high renin profile receiving propranolol. In comparing therapeutic response, patients with a low renin profile had a better response to hydrochlorothiazide, and propranolol was more effective in patients with a high renin profile. The anticipated effect of therapy on plasma renin activity was observed. Although these results are consistent with a volume-vasoconstrictor analysis of hypertension, the results of therapy could not have been prejudged from renin profile or responsivity. The slight differences observed do not warrant the expense of renin determinations when a simple determination of therapeutic response is sufficient.

PRAZOSIN -VS- PHENOXYBENZAMINE

Mulvihill-Wilson and associates[63] from Dallas, Texas, investigated the relevance of the selective alpha-1 adrenergic receptor blockade produced by prazosin to its BP lowering efficacy in man. Hemodynamic and neuroendocrine responses to acute and chronic oral administration of prazosin and phenoxybenzamine were compared in a randomized double-blind placebo-controlled crossover study of 11 patients with essential hypertension. In the acute studies, arterial BP decreased to similar levels with prazosin or phenoxybenzamine; however, hemodynamic and neuroendocrine responses differed both before and during sympathetic nervous system activation. Prazosin lowered arterial BP by reducing total peripheral resistance. In contrast, phenoxybenzamine produced a modest reduction in cardiac output with little change in total peripheral resistance, forearm vascular resistance, or forearm blood flow. Additionally, plasma norepinephrine concentration and heart rate rose to significantly higher levels with prazosin than with phenoxybenzamine, a difference that was most evident with lower body negative pressure or dynamic exercise. Baroreceptor control of aterial pressure homeostasis was preserved with both agents, except during marked degrees of cardiovascular stress. With long-term therapy, the circulatory responses adapted to the alpha-adrenergic antagonists, and both drugs produced similar hemodynamic and neuroendocrine profiles. The differences with acute administration may be the result of a more rapid onset of action and a more marked degree of alpha-adrenergic blockade with prazosin than with phenoxybenzamine therapy, rather than to any difference in the alpha-1 and the alpha-2 adrenergic receptor blocking properties. Moreover, these findings suggest that the prejunctional alpha-2 receptor autoinhibitory to sympathetic neuronal norepinephrine release is of no functional significance in patients with essential hypertension.

HYDROCHLOROTHIAZIDE -VS- CLONIDINE

Falkner and associates[64] from Philadelphia, Pennsylvania, performed a study to determine whether the blunted reduction in R-wave amplitude during progressive aerobic exercise observed in adolescents with systemic hypertension could be altered by pharmacologic therapy to reduce BP. Twenty-nine hypertensive adolescents were randomly assigned to treatment with either a diuretic, hydrochlorothiazide, or a centrally acting agent, clonidine. After 16 weeks of therapy, casual BP was significantly reduced in both groups. Repeat exercise stress testing on therapy demonstrated a significant change in R-wave response. In both treatment groups the change in R-wave amplitude during exercise corresponded with the R-wave response pattern observed in normotensive control subjects. These observations indicate that the altered R-wave amplitude response to exercise observed in young hypertensive subjects is reversible and suggest that the altered R-wave response before treatment is related to a higher vascular resistance.

Diuretic-induced hypokalemia

Papademetriou and associates[65] from Washington, D.C., studied 16 patients with diuretic-induced hypokalemia, each of whom underwent 24-hour ambulatory ECG monitoring during and after correction of the hypokalemia. Plasma potassium averaged 2.83 ± 0.08 mEq/liter before and 3.73 ± 0.06 mEq/liter after correction with potassium chloride, triamterene, or both. Premature atrial contractions decreased in 6 patients, increased in 6, and remained unchanged in 4. There was no improvement in ventricular ectopic activity after plasma potassium correction. Ventricular ectopic activity improved in 5 patients, worsened in 10, and remained unchanged in 1. Ventricular tachycardia was not observed in either phase. Plasma magnesium remained normal throughout. The investigators conclude that in patients with uncomplicated hypertension, correction of diuretic-induced hypokalemia does not significantly reduce the occurrence of spontaneous atrial or ventricular ectopic activity.

References

1. VARDAN S, MOORKHERJEE S, WARNER R, SMULYAN H: Systolic hypertension: direct and indirect BP measurements. Arch Intern Med 143:935–938, May 1983.
2. MANNING DM, KUCHIRKA C, KAMINSKI J: Miscuffing: inappropriate blood pressure cuff application. Circulation 68:763–766, Oct 1983.
3. GILLUM RF, PRINEAS RJ, SOPKO G, KOGA Y, KUBICEK W, ROBITAILLE M, BASS J, SINAIKO A: Elevated blood pressure in school children: prevalence, persistence, and hemodynamics: The Minneapolis Children's Blood Pressure Study. Am Heart J 105:316–322, Feb 1983.
4. FOLSOM AR, LUEPKER RV, GILLUM RF, JACOBS DR, PRINEAS RJ, TAYLOR HL, BLACKBURN H: Improvement in hypertension detection and control from 1973–1974 to 1980–1981: The Minnesota Heart Survey experience. JAMA 250:916–921, Aug 19, 1983.
5. PAUL O: Hypertension and its treatment. JAMA 250:939–940, Aug 19, 1983.
6. CHANEY RH, ARNDT S: Predictability of blood pressure response to isometric stress. Am J Cardiol 51:787–790, March 1983.
7. CRIQUI MH, HASKELL WL, HEISS G, TYROLER HA, GREEN P, RUBENSTEIN CJ: Predictors of systolic blood pressure response to treadmill exercise: the lipid research clinics program prevalence study. Circulation 68:225–233, Aug 1983.
8. DLIN RA, HANNE N, SILVERBERG DS, BAR–OR O: Follow-up of normotensive men with exaggerated blood pressure response to exercise. Am Heart J 106:316–320, Aug 1983.
9. FROOM P, BAR–DAVID M, RIBAK J, VAN DYK D, KALLNER B, BENBASSAT J: Predictive value of systolic blood pressure in young men for elevated systolic blood pressure 12–15 years later. Circulation 68:467–469, Sept 1983.
10. MANN S, ALTMAN DG, RAFTERY EB, BANNISTER R: Circadian variation of blood pressure in autonomic failure. Circulation 68:477–483, Sept 1983.
11. MANCIA G, GRASSI G, POMIDOSSI G, GREGORINI L, BERTINERI B, PARATI G, FERRARI A, ZANCHETTI A: Effects of blood pressure measurement by the doctor on patient's blood pressure and heart rate. Lancet 2:695–698, Sept 24, 1983.
12. MESSERLI FH, SUNDGAARD–RIISE K, REISIN E, DRESLINSKI G, DUNN FG, FROHLICH E: Disparate cardiovascular effects of obesity and arterial hypertension. Am J Med 74:808–812, May 1983.
13. PETITTI DB, KLATSKY AL: Malignant hypertension in women aged 15–44 years and its relation to cigarette smoking and oral contraceptives. Am J Cardiol 52:297–298, Aug 1983.
14. NICHOLSON JP, ALDERMAN MH, PICKERING TG, TEICHMAN SL, SOS TA, LARAGH JH: Cigarette smoking and renovascular hypertension. Lancet 2:765–766, Oct 1, 1983.
15. LANG T, DEGOULET P, AIME F, FOURIAUD C, JACQUINET–SALORD MC, LAPRUGNE J, MAIN J, OECONOMOS J, PHALENTE J, PRADES A: Relation between coffee drinking and blood pressure: analysis of 6,321 subjects in the Paris region. Am J Cardiol 52:1238–1242, Dec 1983.
16. IZZO JL, GHOSAL A, KWONG T, FREEMAN RB, JAENIKE JR: Age and prior caffeine use alter the cardiovascular and adrenomedullary responses to oral caffeine. Am J Cardiol 52:769–773, Oct 1983.
17. STRUTHERS AD, REID JL, WHITESMITH R, RODGER JD: Effect of intravenous adrenaline on electrocardiogram, blood pressure, and serum potassium. Br Heart J 49:90–93, Jan 1983.
18. MESSERLI FH, VENTURA HO, GLADE LB, SUNDGAARD–RIISE K, DUNN FG, FROHLICH ED: Essential hypertension in the elderly: hemodynamics, intravascular volume, plasma renin activity, and circulating catecholamine levels. Lancet 2:983–986, Oct 29, 1983.
19. WATT GCM, FOY CJW, HART JT: Comparison of blood pressure, sodium intake, and other variables in offspring with and without a family history of high blood pressure. Lancet 1:1245–1250, June 4, 1983.
20. LIPSITZ LA, NYQUIST P, WEI JY, ROWE JW: Postprandial reduction in blood pressure in the elderly. N Engl J Med 309:81–83, July 14, 1983.
21. CULPEPPER WS, SODT PC, MESSERLI FH, RUSCHHAUPT DG, ARCILLA RA: Cardiac status in juvenile borderline hypertension. Ann Intern Med 98:1–7, Jan 1983.

22. DEVEREUX RB, SAVAGE DD, SACHS I, LARAGH JH: Relation of hemodynamic load to left ventricular hypertrophy and performance in hypertension. Am J Cardiol 51:171–176, Jan 1983.

23. DEVEREUX RB, PICKERING TG, HARSHFIELD GA, KLEINERT HD, DENBY L, CLARK L, PREGIBON D, JASON M, KLEINER B, BORER JS, LARAGH JH: Left ventricular hypertrophy in patients with hypertension: importance of blood pressure response to regularly recurring stress. Circulation 68:470–476, Sept 1983.

24. DRAYER JIM, WEBER MA, DEYOUNG JL: BP as a determinant of cardiac left ventricular muscle mass. Arch Intern Med 143:90–92, Jan 1983.

25. SHAPIRO LM, BEEVERS DG: Malignant hypertension: cardiac structure and function at presentation and during therapy. Br Heart J 49:477–484, May 1983.

26. SPARROW D, THOMAS HE, ROSNER B, WEISS ST: The relationship of the baseline ECG to blood pressure change. JAMA 250:1285–1288, Sept 9, 1983.

27. TARAZI RC, GIFFORD RW: Left ventricular hypertrophy and hypertension. JAMA 250:1319, Sept 9, 1983.

28. MESSERLI FH, SCHLANT RC: Left ventricular hypertrophy in essential hypertension: mechanisms and therapy. Am J Med (Symposium): 1–120, Sept 26, 1983.

29. TOTH PJ, HORWITZ RI: Conflicting clinical trials and the uncertainty of treating mild hypertension. Am J Med 75:482–488, Sept 1983.

30. GIFFORD RW, BORHANI N, KRISHAN I, MOSER M, LEVY RI, SCHOENBERGER JA: The dilemma of "mild" hypertension: another viewpoint of treatment. JAMA 250:3171–3173, Dec 16, 1983.

31. RAM CFS: Should mild hypertension be treated? Ann Intern Med 99:403–405, Sept 1983.

32. GILLUM RF, PRINEAS RJ, JEFFERY RW, JACOBS DR, ELMER PJ, GOMEZ O, BLACKBURN H: Nonpharmacologic therapy of hypertension: the independent effects of weight reduction and sodium restriction in overweight borderline hypertensive patients. Am Heart J 105:128–133, Jan 1983.

33. SILMAN AJ, MITCHELL P, LOCKE C, HUMPHERSON P: Evaluation of the effectiveness of a low sodium diet in the treatment of mild to moderate hypertension. Lancet 1:1179–1182, May 28, 1983.

34. HOFMAN A, HAZEBROEK A, VALKENBURG HA: A randomized trial of sodium intake and blood pressure in newborn infants. JAMA 250:370–373, July 15, 1983.

35. HOLDEN RA, OSTFELD AD, FREEMAN DH, HELLENBRAND KG, D'ATRI DA: Dietary salt intake and blood pressure. JAMA 250:365–369, July 15, 1983.

36. SCRIBNER BH: Salt and hypertension. JAMA 250:388–389, July 15, 1983.

37. COOPER R, LEGRADY D, NANAS S, TREVISAN M, MANSOUR M, HISTAND P, OSTROW D, STAMLER J: Increased sodium–lithium countertransport in college students with elevated blood pressure. JAMA 249:1030–1034, Feb 25, 1983.

38. REISIN E, FROHLICH ED, MESSERLI FH, DRESLINSKI GR, DUNN FG, JONES MM, BATSON HM: Cardiovascular changes after weight reduction in obesity hypertension. Ann Intern Med 98:315–319, Mar 1983.

39. PUSKA P, NISSINEN A, VARTIAINEN E, DOUGHERTY R, MUTANEN M, IACONO JM, KORHONEN HJ, PIETINEN P, LEINO U, MOISIO S, HUTTUNEN J: Controlled, randomised trial of the effect of dietary fat on blood pressure. Lancet 1:1–5, Jan 8, 1983.

40. LORENZ R, SPENGLER U, FISCHER S, DUHM J, WEBER P: Platelet function, thromboxane formation and blood pressure control during supplementation of the western diet with cod liver oil. Circulation 67:504–511, March 1983.

41. HAGBERG JM, GOLDRING D, EHSANI AA, HEATH GW, HERNANDEZ A, SCHECHTMAN K, HOLLOSZY JO: Effect of exercise training on the blood pressure and hemodynamic features of hypertensive adolescents. Am J Cardiol 52:763–768, Oct 1983.

42. BELIZAN JM, VILLAR J, PINEDA O, GONZALEZ AE, SAINZ E, GARRERA G, SIBRIAN R: Reduction of blood pressure with calcium supplementation in young adults. JAMA 249:1161–1165, Mar 4, 1983.

43. VARDAN S, MOOKHERJEE S, WARNER R, SMULYAN H: Systolic hypertension in the elderly: hemodynamic response to long–term thiazide diuretic therapy and its side effects. JAMA 250:2807–2813, Nov 25, 1983.

44. Caruso FS, Szabadi RR, Vukovich RA: Pharmacokinetics and clinical pharmacology of indapamide. Am Heart J 106:212–220, July 1983.

45. Fouad FM, Slominski MJ, Tarazi RC, Gallagher JH: Alterations in left ventricular filling with beta–adrenergic blockade. Am J Cardiol 51:161–164, Jan 1983.

46. Rubin PC, Clark DM, Sumner DJ, Low RA, Butters L, Reynolds B, Steedman D, Reid JL: Placebo–controlled trial of atenolol in treatment of pregnancy–associated hypertension. Lancet 1:431–434, Feb 26, 1983.

47. Veterans Administration Cooperative Study Group On Antihypertensive Agents: Efficacy of nadolol alone and combined with bendroflumethiazide and hydralazine for systemic hypertension. Am J Cardiol 52:1230–1237, Dec 1983.

48. Chobanian AV, Perry HM Jr, Langford HG, Taylor SH: Symposium on the role of oxprenolol in systemic hypertension. Am J Cardiol 52:1D–65D, Nov 10, 1983.

49. Sonnenblick EH: Hypertension and hemodynamics: therapeutic considerations. Am J Med (Symposium): 1–114, Oct 17, 1983.

50. Yamakado T, Oonishi N, Kondo S, Noziri A, Nakano T, Takezawa H: Effects of diltiazem on cardiovascular responses during exercise in systemic hypertension and comparison with propranolol. Am J Cardiol 52:1023–1027, Nov 1983.

51. Hornung RS, Gould BA, Jones RI, Sonecha TN, Raftery EB: Nifedipine tablets for systemic hypertension: a study using continuous ambulatory intraarterial recording. Am J Cardiol 51:1323–1327, May 1983.

52. McLeay RAB, Stallard TJ, Watson RDS, Littler WA: The effect of nifedipine on arterial pressure and reflex cardiac control. Circulation 67:1084–1090, May 1983.

53. Ventura HO, Messerli FH, Oigman W, Dunn FG, Reisin E, Frohlich ED: Immediate hemodynamic effects of a new calcium–channel blocking agent (nitrendipine) in essential hypertension. Am J Cardiol 51:783–786, March 1983.

54. Holmes DG, Bogers WAJL, Wideroe TE, Huunan–Seppala A, Wideroe B: Endralazine, a new peripheral vasodilator: absence of effect of acetylator status on antihypertensive effect. Lancet 1:670–671, March 26, 1983.

55. Chrysant SG: Autonomic, systemic, and renal hemodynamic actions of trimazosin in hypertensive patients. Am Heart J 106:1243–1250, Nov 1983.

56. Helgeland A: Double–blind comparison of trimazosin and propranolol in essential hypertension. Am Heart J 106:1253–1258, Nov 1983.

57. Taylor CR, Leader JP, Singleton W, Munster EW, Falkner FC, O'Neil JA: Profile of trimazosin: an effective and safe antihypertensive agent. Am Heart J 106:1269–1281, Nov 1983.

58. Drayer JIM, Weber MA, DeYoung JL, Brewer DD: Long–term BP monitoring in the evaluation of antihypertensive therapy. Arch Intern Med 143:898–901, May 1983.

59. Mookherjee S, Anderson GH Jr, Eich R, Hill N, Smulyan H, Streeten DHP, Vardan S, Warner R: Acute effects of captopril on cardiopulmonary hemodynamics and renin–angiotensin–aldosterone and bradykinin profile in hypertension. Am Heart J 105:106–112, Jan 1983.

60. Thind GS, Mahapatra RK, Johnson A, Coleman RD: Low–dose captopril titration in patients with moderate–to–severe hypertension treated with diuretics. Circulation 67:1340–1346, June 1983.

61. Chobanian AV, Tifft CP, Faxon DP, Creager MA, Sackel H: Treatment of chronic orthostatic hypotension with ergotamine. Circulation 67:602–609, March 1983.

62. Freis ED, Materson BJ, Flamenbaum W: Comparison of propranolol or hydrochlorothiazide alone for treatment of hypertension: evaluation of the renin–angiotensin system. Am J Med 74:1029–1041, June 1983.

63. Mulvihill–Wilson J, Gaffney FA, Pettinger WA, Blomqvist CG, Anderson S, Graham RM: Hemodynamic and neuroendocrine responses to acute and chronic alpha–adrenergic blockade with prazosin and phenoxybenzamine. Circulation 67:383–393, Feb 1983.

64. Falkner B, Lowenthal DT, Affrime MB, Hamstra B: R–wave amplitude change during aerobic exercise in hypertensive adolescents after treatment. Am J Cardiol 51:459–463, Feb 1983.

65. Papademetriou V, Fletcher R, Khatri IM, Freis ED: Diuretic–induced hypokalemia in uncomplicated systemic hypertension: effect of plasma potassium correction on cardiac arrhythmias. Am J Cardiol 52:1017–1022, Nov 1983.

5

Valvular Heart Disease

MORPHOLOGIC FEATURES OF THE NORMAL AND ABNORMAL
MITRAL VALVE

In this article Roberts[1] from Bethesda, Maryland, reviewed certain anatomic and functional features of the normal and anatomic mitral valve. Of 1,010 personally studied necropsy patients with severe (New York Heart Association functional class III or IV) cardiac dysfunction from primary valvular heart disease, 434 (43%) had MS with or without MR: unassociated with AS or AR or with tricuspid valve stenosis in 189 (44%) patients, and associated with AS in 152 (35%), with pure, meaning no element of stenosis, AR in 65 (15%) patients, and with tricuspid valve stenosis with or without AS in 28 (6%) patients (Table 5-1). The origin of MS was rheumatic in all 434 patients. Of the 1,010 necropsy patients, 165 (16%) had pure MR (papillary muscle dysfunction excluded): unassociated with AS or regurgitation or with tricuspid valve stenosis in 97 (59%) patients and associated with pure aortic regurgitation in 45 (27%) and with AS in 23 (14%) patients. When associated with dysfunction of the aortic valve, pure MR was usually rheumatic in origin, but when unassociated with aortic valve dysfunction it was usually nonrheumatic in origin. Review of operatively excised mitral valves in patients with pure MR unassociated with aortic valve dysfunction disclosed MVP (most likely an inherent congenital defect) as the most common cause of MR. Excluding the patients with MR from CAD (papillary muscle dysfunction), MVP was the cause of MR in 60 (88%) of the other 68 patients, and a rheumatic origin was responsible in only 3 of the 68 patients, all 68 of

TABLE 5-1. *Functional and anatomic classification of valvular heart disease in 1,010 necropsy patients aged ≥15 Years.*

FUNCTIONAL CLASS	PATIENTS (N [%])	ANATOMIC CLASS (N [%])				
		AV	MV	MV-AV	TV-MV	TV-MV-AV
1. AS	292 (29)	256 (87.5)	0	35 (12.1)	0	1 (0.3)
2. MS	189 (19)	0	117 (62)	40 (21)	13 (7)	19 (10)
3. MS + AS	152 (15)	0	0	120 (79)	0	32 (21)
4. AR	119 (12)	107[†] (90)	0	10 (8)	0	2 (2)
5. MR	97 (10)	0	85 (88)	8 (8)	1 (1)	3 (3)
6. MS + AR	65 (6)	0	52 (80)	0	0	13 (20)
7. MR + AR	45 (4)	0	0	39 (87)	0	6 (13)
8. AS + MR	23 (2)	0	0	21 (91)	0	2 (9)
9. Tricuspid stenosis + MS ± AS	28 (3)	0	0	0	4 (14)	24 (86)
Totals	1,010 (100)[‡]	363 (36)	254 (25)	273 (27)	18 (2)	102 (10)

TV = tricuspid valve.
* Excludes patients with mitral regurgitation secondary to CAD (papillary muscle dysfunction), carcinoid heart disease, and HC and those with infective endocarditis limited to 1 or both right-sided cardiac valves. Tricuspid valve regurgitation was present in many patients in most of the 9 functional groups. All patients were in functional class III or IV (New York Heart Association), and more than half had 1 or more cardiac operations.
† In many patients, the aortic valve cusps actually were normal and the regurgitation was the result of disease of the aorta (Marfan and Marfan-like syndromes, syphilis, systemic hypertension, healed aortic dissection).
‡ The hearts in all 1,010 patients were examined and classified by WCR.

whom were >30 years of age. Mitral anular calcium in persons aged >65 years is usually associated with calcific deposits in the aortic valve cusps and in the coronary arteries. Because calcium in each of these 3 sites is common in older individuals residing in the Western world, it is most reasonable to view mitral anular calcium in older individuals as a manifestation of atherosclerosis. Mitral anular calcium appears to be extremely uncommon in persons with total serum cholesterol levels <150 mg/dl. Mitral anular calcium may produce mild MR and, if the deposits are heavy enough, MS.

MITRAL REGURGITATION

Flail leaflet syndrome

The syndrome of a flail mitral leaflet results in acute MR. DePace and associates[2] from Philadelphia, Pennsylvania, performed serial 2-D echo on 29 patients with a flail mitral leaflet. The LV and LA volumes and EF were obtained using a computerized light-pen system. Fifteen patients with the 2-D echo criteria of a flail mitral leaflet were treated medically and followed for a mean of 19 months. Eleven patients did not undergo surgery (group IA). Four patients initially were treated medically, but ultimately required surgery (group IB). On initial examination, there was no difference in volumes and EF between these 2 groups. On follow-up, group IA patients remained in New York Heart Association class I or II. The LV end-diastolic volume increased in the group IA patients from 164 ± 27–203 ± 54 ml (p < 0.01); LV EF tended to increase (from 51 ± 5–56 ± 8, p ≤ 0.06). On follow-up, group IB patients had larger LA and LV volumes than group IA patients. Fourteen patients were initially treated surgically (group II). All but 1 were in New York Heart Association class III or IV. On initial examination LV EF was lower than in group IA patients (51 ± 5 -vs- 43 ± 7; p = 0.05), but there was no difference in LV or LA volumes. On follow-up, a mean of 19 months after surgery, LV EF and LA volumes decreased. We conclude that a subset of patients with a flail mitral leaflet may be followed clinically without deterioration in LV function. Initial LV EF and hemodynamics are reasonably normal. Because increasing LV and LA volumes and changing clinical status are not a function of time, frequent 2-D echo and clinical evaluations are warranted in these patients. After MVR, LV EF decreases without a significant change in LV volume.

Ruptured chordae tendineae

Oliveira and associates[3] from London, England, analyzed 213 patients with MR secondary to rupture of chordae tendineae seen at their hospital between 1970 and 1981. This number represented 12% of patients undergoing mitral valve surgery at their hospital during that period. Of the 213 patients, 159 (75%) had so-called spontaneous or primary chordal rupture (primary group) and the remainder (secondary group) had ruptured chords secondary to rheumatic heart disease (9%) and infective endocarditis on a previously normal valve (9%) and on a rheumatic valve (5%). There were also 5 patients who had ruptured chords secondary to CAD, which I (WCR) find difficult to believe. Additionally, 1 patient was said to have ruptured chords on the basis of acute rheumatic fever, a new observation as far as I (WCR) know.

Oliveira and associates[4] also described results of mitral valve surgery in 183 of the 213 patients with MR secondary to ruptured chordae tendineae. Of the 183 patients, 82 (45%) were treated by mitral valve repair and 101 (55%) by MVR. Mean age at surgery was 57 years. The early mortality was 5%, of whom 5 had undergone MVP and 4, repair. The patients were followed from 0.8–12.2 years (mean, 3.6) and 27 other patients died, 23 of whom had undergone MVP and 4, repair. Cerebral vascular events accounted for 35% of the deaths after MVR and none after mitral valve repair. In 11 patients repair was technically unsatisfactory and MVR was undertaken at the same operation; another 5 patients required late MVR (mean, 1.4 years) for severe MR. Actuarial curves predicted a 6-year survival of 68 ± 6% for all patients after MVR and 88 ± 7% after repair. Thus, actuarial survival curves favor MVR as the procedure of choice for mitral chordal rupture.

Calcium in purely regurgitant valves

Byram and Roberts[5] from Bethesda, Maryland, examined operatively excised purely regurgitant mitral valves in 108 patients aged 21–73 years (mean, 55) (63% men) undergoing isolated MVR for calcific deposits. Of the 108 patients, 19 (18%) had leaflet or chordal calcific deposits or both, but in each the deposits were small and did not appear to alter mitral function. Of the 19 patients with mitral calcium, 6 had had active infective endocarditis and the calcium likely represented healed vegetations; in 6 other patients, the leaflet calcium had extended from the mitral anulus in the setting of MVP. The average total serum cholesterol levels were higher in the patients with than without mitral calcium. Thus, calcium deposits are relatively infrequent in adults with clinically isolated pure MR, and when they occur, the deposits are small and in themselves do not appear to contribute to mitral dysfunction.

Reduced LV afterload and its effect on the resting EF may lead to overestimation of LV function in patients with MR. To evaluate LV function during increased afterload of the heart, Huikuri and associates[6] from Helsinki, Finland, performed an isometric handgrip test during cardiac catheterization in 15 patients with MR (MR group) and in 9 normal subjects (normal group). Twelve months after MVR, the patients were recatheterized, and the value of preoperative stress testing in predicting the change in resting ventricular function after surgery was estimated. Isometric exercise caused an increase in end-systolic wall stress, a measure of ventricular afterload, in both the MR and the control groups ($p < 0.001$). The EF remained unchanged in the control group, but decreased from 0.58 ± 0.08–0.53 ± 0.08 in the MR group ($p < 0.001$). After MVR end-systolic wall stress increased significantly ($p < 0.001$) and the EF decreased from 0.58 ± 0.05–0.51 ± 0.1 ($p < 0.05$). A positive correlation existed between the change in the EF during preoperative stress testing and the change in the resting EF after MVR ($r = 0.65$; $p < 0.01$). In 8 patients whose resting EF was within normal limits (>0.55) preoperatively, the EF was depressed (<0.55) 1 year after surgery. In all but 1 of these patients the isometric exercise revealed the reduced ventricular response to afterload stress preoperatively (decrease of the EF >0.03 during exercise). Therefore the isometric exercise-induced change in LV function appears to predict the influence of MVR on LV function.

Preserving the mitral valve in operations to correct MR

Many patients after MVR for MR are left with depressed EF and elevated LV end-diastolic volume. David and colleagues[7] from Toronto, Canada, evaluated the possible role of the mitral apparatus in LV function after correction of chronic MR. Seventeen patients were divided into 3 groups, 6 had conventional MVR (group I), 6 had MVR with preservation of chordae tendineae and papillary muscles (group II), and 5 had mitral valvuloplasty (group III) (Fig. 5-1). After correction of MR the increase in cardiac index was similar for all 3 groups. The LV end-diastolic volume did not decrease in the group having conventional mitral valve resection, but it did in the groups in which the mitral valve apparatus was preserved. Similarly, LV end-systolic volume increased in the first group and decreased in the second and third groups. The EF decreased in group 1 and did not change in group 2 or 3. The LV end-diastolic pressure increased in group 1 and decreased in groups 2 and 3.

By using a xenograft and leaving the posterior mitral leaflet and papillary muscle chordal apparatus intact LV function was achieved equal to simple anuloplastic repair and better than that seen after conventional mitral valve resection and replacement with a prosthetic device. The number of patients

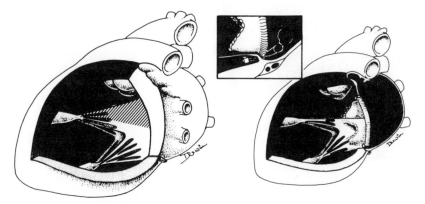

Fig. 5-1. Technique of MVR with preservation of chordae tendineae and papillary muscles. Note that only the central portion of anterior leaflet is excised. Reproduced with permission from David et al.[7]

in each group is small but the changes in LV end-diastolic volume, LV end-systolic volume, EF, and end-diastolic pressure were significant and strongly suggest that continuity between the mitral anulus and LV wall plays an important role in LV function after correction of chronic MR. Most patients in this report had a normal EF before operation.

Reconstructive operations

Between January 1975 and January 1982, 130 patients reported by Lessana and colleagues[8] from Paris, France, underwent mitral valvuloplasty for pure or predominant MR. In general, the mode of reconstruction was modeled after that of Carpentier. The mean age at operation was 30 ± 17 years, 112 patients had rheumatic disease and 59 had another diseased valve that necessitated surgical correction. Three patients died in the first month (2%) and 7 patients required reoperation and 3 of those died. Of the 118 remaining, 116 were in class I or II (Fig. 5-2). Thromboembolic episodes occurred in 4 patients, all of them in AF (Fig. 5-3). Eighty-eight percent of the patients were free of reoperation at 7 years with a rate of reoperation of 1.7 ± 0.7%/patient-year.

Plication of left atrial wall

The giant left atrium associated with mitral valvular disease may be responsible for hemodynamic and respiratory complications after MVR. Kawazoe and associates[9] from Osaka, Japan, described intraoperative management of giant left atrium. They developed a new procedure for paraanular and superior plication combined with conventional right-sided plication and trimming of the LA wall (Fig. 5-4). A total of 40 patients with giant left atrium underwent operation. Ten had the valvular procedure only and 30 had the valvular and plication procedure. The plication procedure resulted in a significant decrease in the incidence of low output syndrome and respiratory failure postoperatively, as well as a marked decrease in mortality. The

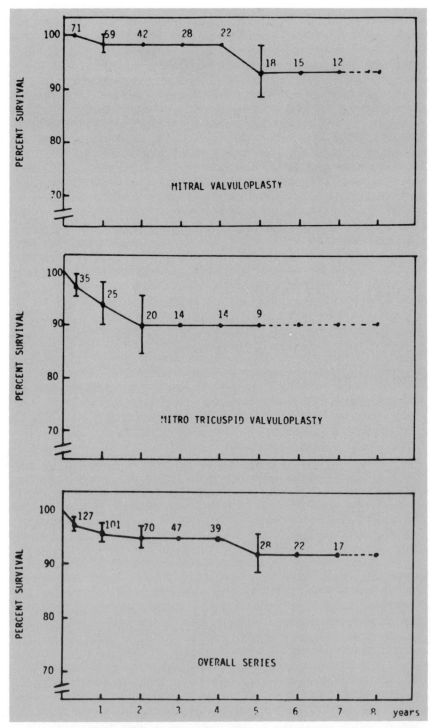

Fig. 5-2. Actuarial survival curve. Hospital mortality rate is included. *Brackets* = 1 SEM. Reproduced with permission from Lessana et al.[8]

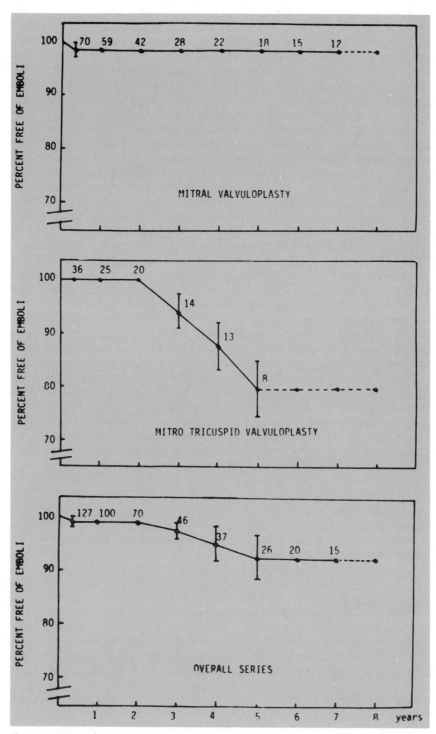

Fig. 5-3. Actuarial curve of thromboembolism-free patients. *Brackets* = 1 SEM. Reproduced with permission from Lessana et al.[8]

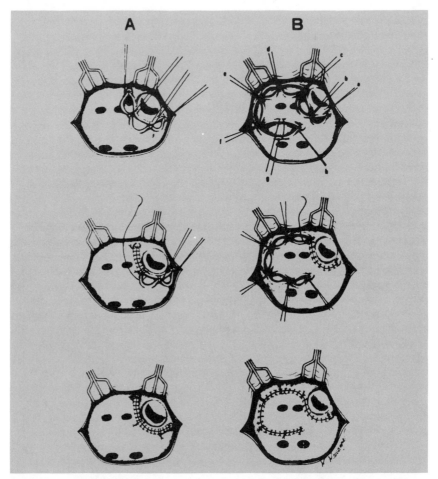

Fig. 5-4. Operative procedure. Drawings on the left *(A)* show paraanular plication. Several stay sutures are placed and continuous over-and-over sutures are used in between. Drawings on the right *(B)* demonstrate superior half plication *(c-h)* continuous with the paraanular plication *(a-c).* Reproduced with permission from Kawazoe et al.[9]

authors concluded that the plication procedure was an effective means of relieving compression of the bronchus and left ventricle in the presence of giant left atrium.

MITRAL VALVE PROLAPSE

In general population

Savage and colleagues[10] from Boston, Massachusetts, obtained epidemiologic information regarding MVP in 2,036 subjects in the original Framingham cohort study (mean age, 70 ± 7 years) and 2,931 of the offspring of the cohort and spouses of the offspring (mean age, 44 ± 10 years) with adequate echoes were evaluated. Echo MVP was detected in 264 (5%) of the total 4,967 subjects. This included 56 (3%) of the 2,036 elderly cohort subjects and 208 (7%) of the 2,931 younger subjects. Females showed a striking decline in prevalence of MVP with age, from 17% for those in their 20s to 1% for those in their 80s. This was in contrast to the similarity of prevalence of MVP (2–4%) in all age decades for men. The strong inverse relation of obesity to prevalence of MVP accounted for much of the difference in prevalence among young and older women and in men of all ages.

To assess the clinical features of the MVP syndrome as found in the general free-living population, 2,931 offspring of the original Framingham cohort (and spouses of the offspring) with adequate echoes were evaluated by Savage and colleagues[11] from Boston, Massachusetts. Chest pain, dyspnea, and syncope were no more common in the 208 subjects with echo MVP than in the remainder of subjects without MVP. Systolic clicks were between 8 (women) and 20 (men) times more common in individuals with than without echo MVP. However, these clicks were found in only 5 (13%) of 38 men and 14 (8%) of 170 women with echo MVP. Systolic murmurs were detected twice as often in those with MVP than in those without MVP. Such murmurs were found in 1 (3%) of 38 men and in 14 (8%) of 170 women with echo-ascertained MVP. Resting and exercise ECG findings were not significantly different in those with and those without echo-ascertained MVP. These data indicate that in the general population, about half of those with systolic clicks have echo MVP, but few individuals with echo MVP have auscultatory findings. Frequency of symptoms and ECG findings are not significantly different in individuals with and without echo MVP in the free-living population.

To compare the frequency of cardiac arrhythmias in free-living individuals with and without echo MVP, 2,840 offspring of the original Framingham cohort (and spouses of the offspring) were evaluated by 1-hour ambulatory ECGs during a clinic visit by Savage and colleagues[12] from Boston, Massachusetts. In 201 of these persons MVP was present. Standard resting 12-lead and exercise ECGs were obtained on nearly all of the subjects. An age-stratified subsample of 179 individuals without echo MVP and 61 individuals with this finding had 24-hour ECG monitoring. Arrhythmias occurred with similar frequency in those with and without echo MVP on the resting 12-lead, exercise, and 1-hour ambulatory ECGs. Nearly half of the subjects with echo MVP had complex (multiform or repetitive VPC) or frequent (>30 in any hour) VPC during 24-hour ECG monitoring. During 24-hour monitoring, 20% of subjects with echo MVP had pairs or runs of VPC and 25% had runs of SVT. Such arrhythmias were less common in those without echo MVP. However, these arrhythmias were so common in those without MVP that the excess of arrhythmias in those with MVP did not reach statistical significance.

Frequency of ruptured chordae

Echo studies were performed on 134 consecutive patients with idiopathic MVP syndrome in an investigation performed by Grenadier and associates[13] from Haifa, Israel. Fifteen patients (11%) had ruptured chordae tendineae on M-mode and in 12 of them the diagnosis was confirmed by 2-D echo. Only 4 patients were referred for surgery as a result of severe MR. At operation, 1 patient had rupture of the anterior mitral chordae and the other 3 had posterior mitral chordal rupture. Eleven patients with chordal rupture had either mild symptoms or were completely asymptomatic. It was concluded that chordal rupture in patients with the MVP syndrome does not always result in severe hemodynamic deterioration and may go undetected unless a high index of suspicion is maintained.

Echo comparisons

One hundred twenty-five consecutive patients with a mid to late systolic click with or without a systolic murmur were evaluated by Abbasi and associates[14] from Long Beach, California, with M-mode, 2-D, and Doppler echo to assess the comparative value of each of these modalities in the detection of MVP. M-mode echo detected 62 of 125 patients (sensitivity, 50%), 2-D echo detected 85 patients (sensitivity, 68%), and Doppler echo detected 90 patients (sensitivity, 72%). When all 3 techniques were combined, 116 of 125 cases were correctly diagnosed (total sensitivity, 93%). Thus, there appears to be value in obtaining 2-D echo and Doppler echo in the evaluation of patients with auscultatory evidence of MVP.

Inheritance

Since its first recognition, the familial occurrence of the MVP syndrome has been extensively recorded. Utilizing echo, auscultation, and phonocardiography, however, few large series of affected families have been reported. Strahan and associates[15] from Baltimore, Maryland, sought evidence of MVP in the families of 12 probands with classic MVP. Seventy parents, sibs, and progeny were included in the analysis: 16 (47%) of 34 of the progeny were affected compared with 3 of 10 of parents; 10 (38%) of 26 sibs were affected.

In individuals ≥ 60 years of age

Kolibash and associates[16] from Columbus, Ohio, reported on 62 patients diagnosed as having MVP, aged 60–81 years. Of the 62 patients, 20 presented with disabling chest pain, 16 with symptoms of arrhythmias, including palpitations and syncope, and 26 with MR and symptoms of CHF. The diagnosis of MVP was made on the basis of a combination of classic auscultatory, echo, and angiographic findings (Figs. 5-5 and 5-6). Thirteen of the 20 patients with chest pain had normal coronary angiograms and 7 had significant CAD. Patients with CAD could not be differentiated by clinical presentation alone. Furthermore, the frequency and types of arrhythmias, the presence of a positive stress test, and hemodynamic findings were similar in all patients in this group whether or not CAD was present. The 16 patients with palpitations had a broad spectrum of rhythm disorders, including both supraventricular and ventricular arrhythmias. Two patients had prehospital "sudden death" and 2 others had systemic emboli. Twenty-one of the 26 patients with MR had valve surgery. Intraoperatively, the valves were described as enlarged, floppy, and with redundant leaflets. Thus, MVP is a cause of symptomatic heart disease in the elderly. It has a predictable pattern of clinical presentation and should be considered in the differential diagnosis

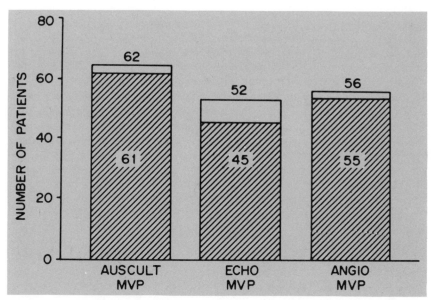

Fig. 5-5. The sensitivity of individual methods used to diagnose MVP. The number of patients with satisfactory examinations is listed at the top of each bar. The number of patients in whom examination indicated MVP is listed in shaded area of the bars. Angio = left ventricular angiography; auscult = auscultatory exam.

of older patients with disabling chest pain and arrhythmias and as the cause of progressive or severe MR.

Sudden death

Chesler and associates[17] from Saint Paul, Minnesota, described clinico-pathologic features of 14 cases of sudden death attributable to arrhythmias associated with MVP. The patients were 14–59 years old; 11 were female and 3 male. Of the 7 with an ECG available, none had prolonged QT intervals, but 2 had repolarization abnormalities. The material was classified according to the degree of prolapse in the pathologic specimen. When obvious prolapse was found, the expected auscultatory findings had been documented. In 3 cases there was minimal MVP. In 1 case with minimal MVP there was a strong family history of sudden death. Endocardial friction lesions were present in 11 cases, including 2 of the 3 with minimal MVP. In 5 cases there was a thrombotic lesion in the angle between the posterior leaflet and the LA wall containing fibrin and platelets.

Cardiovascular regulation

Studies of patients with MVP have suggested autonomic nervous system dysfunction, but a precise definition of mechanisms is lacking. Gaffney and associates[18] from Dallas, Texas, measured supine and standing heart rate, BP, cardiac output, oxygen consumption, plasma catecholamines, and blood volume in 23 symptomatic women with both echo and phonocardiographic signs of MVP and in 17 normal control subjects. An analysis of the results

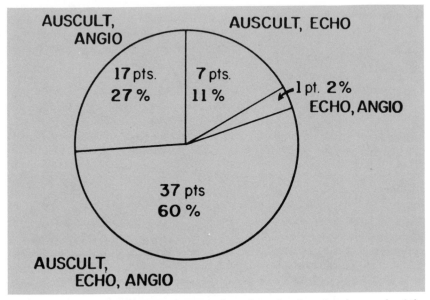

Fig. 5-6. The basis for diagnosis of MVP and number of patients in whom each of the diagnostic methods indicated MVP. Thirty-seven patients (60%) had evidence of MVP by all 3 examinations, whereas diagnosis of MVP in 25 patients (40%) was based on a combination of 2 of the 3 methods that indicated MVP. Angio = left ventricular angiography; auscult = auscultation.

revealed 2 distinct subgroups of patients: those with normal heart rates but increased vasoconstriction (group I: n, 10) and those with orthostatic tachycardia (group II: n, 13). Group II patients had heart rates at rest supine of 97 ± 3 compared with 79 ± 2 in group I patients and 78 ± 8 in control subjects. Estimated total blood volumes were lowest in group I patients, intermediate in group II patients, and highest in control subjects ($p < 0.05$). Other measurements at rest supine were similar in patients and controls. After standing for 5 minutes, patients had a higher mean plasma epinephrine value, diastolic BP (81 ± 2 -vs- 74 ± 3 mmHg; $p < 0.05$), and peripheral resistance (1,878 ± 114 -vs- 1,414 ± 92, dynes/s/cm^{-5}; $p < 0.01$), wider arteriovenous oxygen difference (6.7 ± 0.4 -vs- 5.3 ± 0.5 vol%), and lower stroke volume index (26 ± 2 -vs- 33 ± 2 ml/m^2; $p < 0.01$) than did the control subjects. Cardiac output was normal in group II patients but reduced in group I patients, who demonstrated marked vasoconstriction. No patient had evidence of a "hyperkinetic" circulatory state. A cycle of decreased forward stroke volume, vasoconstriction, and blood volume contraction appears to be present in at least some symptomatic patients with MVP (Fig. 5-7).

Adrenergic stimulation

Boudoulas and associates[19] from Columbus, Ohio, evaluated 16 patients with MVP to determine whether adrenergic stimulation causes symptoms typical of MVP in patients with this abnormality. Isoproterenol infusions

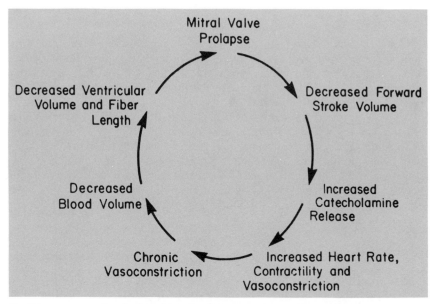

Fig. 5-7. A proposed pathophysiology of orthostatic intolerance in symptomatic patients with MVP. A large myxomatous mitral valve would clearly have a facilitative role, but it is not necessary in order to have MVP or MVP symptoms related to orthostatic intolerance.

(0.5, 1.0, and 2.0 µg/min) resulted in a greater increase in heart rate in the MVP group than in controls. It also reproduced symptoms in a dose-related manner in 14 patients with MVP, but not in control subjects. Thus, symptomatic patients with MVP are hypersensitive to isoproterenol infusion consistent with the concept that some of their symptoms may be catecholamine-related and/or mediated.

Puddu and associates[20] from Montreal, Canada, measured heart rate corrected QT interval (QTc) and plasma catecholamine (CA) and norepinephrine (NE) levels in 15 asymptomatic patients with MVP and in 19 control subjects. The MVP patients showed longer mean QTc and were divided into 2 groups: group A normal QTc (<440 ms) and group B prolonged QTc (≥440 ms). In supine resting conditions CA levels were as follows: group A, 0.420 ± 0.035 ng/ml; group B, 0.619 ± 0.104 ng/ml ($p < 0.05$); both were greater than control values (0.348 ± 0.017 ng/ml; $p < 0.005$). The NE levels were as follows: group A, 0.350 ± 0.031 ng/ml; group B, 0.376 ± 0.052 ng/ml (NS); both were greater than control values (0.242 ± 0.025 ng/ml; $p < 0.05$). When a standing position was assumed, CA and NE levels increased significantly in all groups, and this was most marked in group B compared with control levels (CA, 1.039 ± 0.123 ng/ml -vs- 0.625 ± 0.037 ng/ml; NE, 0.737 ± 0.076 ng/ml -vs- 0.504 ± 0.031 ng/ml) ($p < 0.001$ and $p < 0.05$, respectively). Thus, the longest QTc was observed in patients with MVP who had the highest levels of CA and NE, in both supine and standing positions. It was concluded that these data: 1) account, in part, for the occurrence of severe ventricular arrhythmias in some patients with MVP; and 2) offer a rationale for adrenergic blockade in the subset of patients with MVP and markedly prolonged QTc.

Relation to neurosis

An association has been observed by some between MVP and some neuroses, especially anxiety states, panic disorders, and agoraphobia. Hickey and associates[21] from Sydney, Australia, studied 103 patients with echo-confirmed MVP and tested them with the Eysenck Personality Inventory for neurosis and with the General Health Questionnaire for the presence of neurotic symptoms. The scores for neuroticism and neurotic symptoms were not significantly different from those of patients with other cardiac diseases or from those of patients presenting in primary care. In addition 50 patients with agoraphobia were screened by echo for MVP, but no cases were detected. It appears that some of the earlier evidence for an association between MVP and neurosis may have been based on groups that were incorrectly diagnosed. Thus, this study, at least, demonstrates that MVP and neurosis are independent conditions.

Relation to hypomastia

Mitral valve prolapse has been associated with thoracoskeletal abnormalities, connective-tissue disorders, and coagulopathies. Affected tissues in these disorders are embryologically derived from mesenchymal cell origins. During the sixth week of fetal life, the mitral valve undergoes embryologic differentiation, and the vertebral column and thoracic cage develop their shape and form through chondrification. The breast, which in large part is of mesenchymal origin, undergoes primordial development during the same time. Since both the breast and mitral valve are of mesenchymal origin, Rosenberg and associates[22] from Ann Arbor, Michigan, postulated that an

TABLE 5-2. *Selected anthropometric measurements and prevalence of MVP in 27 patients with hypomastia (group A), 33 controls (group B), and 28 patients with MVP (group C).* Reproduced with permission from Rosenberg et al.[22]

	GROUP A (N = 27)	GROUP B (N = 33)	GROUP C (N = 28)
Age (yr)	32.9 ± 1.5	30.1 ± 1.4	32.7 ± 1.9
Height (cm)	166.4 ± 1.0	165.5 ± 1.4	166.6 ± 1.5
Weight (kg)	53.9 ± 1.0†	60.2 ± 1.7	57.1 ± 1.5
Breast size (cc)	131 ± 6¶	301 ± 15	183 ± 17¶
Hypomastia	27 (100)¶	8 (24)	17 (61)‡
Pectus excavatum	4 (15)	1 (3)	7 (25)
Scoliosis	9 (33)	2 (6)	7 (25)
Straight back	5 (19)	1 (3)	6 (21)
Thoracoskeletal abnormality	11 (40)§	2 (6)	13 (46)¶
Hypomastia, thoracoskeletal abnormality, or both	27 (100)¶	8 (24)	22 (78)¶
Mitral-valve prolapse	13 (48)¶	2 (6)	28 (100)¶

* Values for age, height, weight, and breast size are expressed as means ± S.E.M. All other values are numbers of patients, with percentages given in parentheses.
† P < 0.01 vs. Group B.   ‡ P < 0.005 vs. Group B.
§ P < 0.002 vs. Group B.   ¶ P < 0.001 vs. Group B.

association may exist between breast-size development and MVP. To explore this hypothesis, they studied the prevalence of MVP in patients with primary hypomastia and examined the prevalence of hypomastia in a population with known MVP. The clinical data are summarized in Table 5-2. Of the 27 patients with hypomastia in group A, 13 (48%) had echo evidence of MVP. In contrast, only 2 patients (6%) of the 33 controls in group B had MVP. Conversely, of the 28 patients in group C with MVP confirmed by echo, 17 (61%) had hypomastia compared with 8 (24%) of the controls. Thus, hypomastia is an additional nonauscultatory characteristic associated with MVP. This clinical finding may strengthen a diagnostic impression or arouse suspicion that MVP is present.

MITRAL STENOSIS

Left ventricular function

The status of systolic LV performance in patients with isolated MS remains controversial. Potential alterations in LV architecture and loading conditions may have complex effects on LV ejection performance and muscle function. Gash and associates[23] from Philadelphia, Pennsylvania, measured hemodynamic and angiographic LV EF, velocity of circumferential fiber shortening (Vcf) and stroke work index (SWI), the level of preload (end-diastolic volume index [EDVI]), afterload (end-systolic wall stress [ESS]) and an index of LV contractile function thought to be independent of loading conditions (end-systolic wall stress/end-systolic volume index [ESS/ESVI]) in 9 normal subjects and 16 patients with isolated MS. Although the EF in patients was not statistically different from that in normal subjects, 31% of MS patients had an EF <0.50. The Vcf was lower in MS patients than in normal subjects, as were SWI and EDVI. The ESVI was similar in MS patients and normal patients, whereas stroke volume index was lower in MS patients. Patients with reduced EF had higher ESS than patients with normal performance, yet EDVI was similar in both patient categories. The ESS/ESVI in MS patients was not different from that in normal subjects. Four of 5 MS patients with EF <0.50 and all 6 MS patients with reduced Vcf had a normal ESS/ESVI. Thus, MS patients as a group have reduced EF and reduced preload. The reduction in ejection performance is due to increased afterload without adequate Frank-Starling compensation, but LV muscle function is normal in most MS patients with reduced ejection performance.

Left atrial thrombus

Two-D echo studies were performed by Shrestha and coworkers[24] from Manila, Philippines, in 293 patients with MS who underwent open heart mitral valve surgery during an 18-month period. Of the 293 patients, 33 had LA thrombi by 2-D echo criteria. This diagnosis was confirmed at surgery in 30. A thrombus was not found in 3 patients. In 21 other patients, LA thrombi were present but not detected by 2-D echo. Ten of these 21 had thrombi in the LA body. In 11 patients, thrombi were located in the LA appendage, all of which were missed by 2-D echo. Excluding these 11 left atrial appendage thrombi, the sensitivity of 2-D echo for detecting LA body thrombi was 75%.

Isometric exercise testing

To examine the value of preoperative isometric exercise testing during cardiac catheterization in patients with MS, Huikuri and Takkunen[25] from Oulu, Finland, performed isometric handgrip exercise tests on 28 patients during preoperative diagnostic catheterization. Eighteen patients who subsequently underwent mitral valve surgery were recatheterized and reevaluated clinically 12 months after operation. Preoperatively, the patients were divided into 2 groups: 16 whose mean mitral valve pressure gradient increased >4 mmHg during isometric exercise (group A) and 12 whose pressure gradient decreased or increased <4 mmHg (group B). The EF remained unchanged and the peak systolic pressure/end-systolic volume ratio increased during isometric exercise in group A (p < 0.001). In group B, the EF decreased (p < 0.001) and the peak systolic pressure/end-systolic volume ratio remained unchanged. In the total group, a positive correlation existed between the change in mean mitral valve pressure gradient during isometric exercise and the changes in measures of LV function during exercise. The patients in group A had a significant improvement in both symptoms and in exercise tolerance as determined by symptom-limited bicycle ergometry after surgery. The patients in group B showed minimal or no symptomatic improvement and their exercise tolerance did not improve. The change in mitral valve pressure gradient during isometric exercise appears to reflect the LV response to exercise.

Embolism

Dewar and Weightman[26] from New Castle upon Tyne, England, analyzed 62 patients on chronic anticoagulation, 34 of whom had mitral valve disease and 4 lone AF. All had a history compatible with ≥1 systemic embolus and also 24 patients with mitral valve disease who had no history of systemic embolus. Comparison of the 2 groups disclosed no features that would distinguish those who had emboli from those who did not, other than a higher frequency of men in the emboli group and men of shorter stature. Of the 38 patients with a history of embolism, 9 patients had emboli while still in sinus rhythm. Sixteen (42%) of the 38 had an embolus clinically within 1 year of the onset of AF.

Mitral valvotomy

Kay and associates[27] from London, England, described their experience with open mitral valvotomy in 157 patients operated on from 1968–1980. Preoperatively, all patients were in New York Heart Association functional class 3 or 4. Of the 157 patients, 1 died within 30 days of operation and 1 had a transient cerebral vascular accident. The 157 patients having open mitral valvotomy were among only 222 patients presenting to this group with predominant MS. Of the 124 followed 1–14 years (mean, 7.5 years) 7 died late. Actuarial curves predicted a 90% 10-year survival after open mitral

TABLE 5-3. *Incidence of various events (per 1000 patients/year) at different periods of follow–up. Reproduced with permission from John et al.*[28]

YEARS OF FOLLOW-UP	NO. OF CASES FOLLOWED	MITRAL RESTEN- OSIS	RHEU- MATIC REACTIVITY	MITRAL REGURGI- TATION	SYSTEMIC EMBOLISM	LATE DEATHS
1	3,564	0.0	1.6	4.2	0.3	1.7
5	2,643	4.2	2.2	5.5	0.2	3.4
10	1,473	8.1	1.7	3.5	0.3	3.5
15	670	11.4	1.8	4.7	0.6	3.4
20 or more	186	5.6	1.3	1.9	1.6	3.8

valvotomy. Eight patients (16%) required MVR for restenosis by 10 years. The remaining patients were in functional class 1 or 2.

In India as in other developing countries rheumatic valvular heart disease remains prevalent. The disease strikes the young and most patients rapidly develop MS with significant pulmonary hypertension. John and associates[28] from Vellore, India, reviewed the results of closed mitral valvulotomy performed between 1956 and 1980 in 3,724 consecutive patients: 42% were in New York Heart Association functional class IV (Table 5-3). Hospital mortality was 4% in class IV patients and 4% in class III patients. In the last 5 years of the study, the mortality was 1.5%. After valvotomy, 11 patients (0.3%) developed severe MR necessitating MVR in the immediate postoperative period. A mild degree of postoperative MR was present in 18%. A satisfactory surgical result was achieved in 98% of patients. Restenosis varied in its occurrence from 4.2–11.4 cases per thousand patient-years between the 5th and 15th year of follow-up. Rheumatic activity, embolic phenomena, and MR occurred infrequently. Symptomatic improvement was sustained and actuarial analysis revealed that 78% of patients were alive at the end of 24 years. The presence of moderate calcification and the absence of a loud first heart sound or sharp opening snap did not seem to affect adversely an ultimately good surgical result.

Bonchek[29] from Lancaster, Pennsylvania, in an editorial reviewed results of mitral commissurotomy and pointed out the excellence of the results of this operation, its very low mortality with experienced surgeons, and its continued usefulness in this era of cardiac valve replacement. This is a superb editorial. In an accompanying From-the-Editor column Roberts[30] from Bethesda, Maryland, considered a few other items supporting the view that mitral commissurotomy is being less often performed than it should be.

MITRAL VALVULOPLASTY

Based on concepts originally proposed by Carpentier, Antunes and colleagues[31] from Johannesburg, South Africa, performed mitral anuloplasty on 100 patients operated on from January 1981–March 1982. Fifty-five patients had commissurotomy, 95 patients had chordal resection, 52 patients had chordal shortening, 16 patients had fenestration, and 16 patients had resection of leaflet tissue. Carpentier-Edwards rings were placed in 69 patients. In the first 30 patients there were 4 early and 2 late deaths. In the remaining 70 patients there were no early and 2 late deaths. Three patients in the early group and 3 patients in the later group required a subsequent valve replacement (p < 0.01). The linearized valve failure rate was 12% in the early group and 5% in the later group. Seventy-one percent of the survivors in the first group and 84% of the survivors in the second group had no or only mild residual mitral valve dysfunction. All except 2 patients improved at least one functional class. The relatively low incidence of residual MR was the basis for the authors recommendation of more widespread use of mitral valve reconstruction.

MITRAL ANULAR CALCIUM

To obtain epidemiologic information on mitral anular calcium (MAC), Savage and associates[32] from Framingham, Massachusetts, Bethesda, Maryland, and Boston, Massachusetts, evaluated 2,069 subjects in the original Framingham study cohort (mean age, 70 ± 7 years) and 3,625 of the offspring of cohort and their spouses (mean age, 44 ± 10 years) with adequate echoes. Mitral anular calcium was detected in 162 (2.8%) of the 5,694 subjects: >90% of the subjects with MAC came from the 40% of the study group >59 years of age. Women were more than twice as likely to have such calcium as men. Age in both sexes, systolic BP in men, and obesity in women were significantly and independently associated with MAC. There was a 12-fold excess of AF in subjects with (20 of 162, 12%) compared with those without (53 of 5,532, 1%) MAC.

Nair and associates[33] from Omaha, Nebraska, compared clinical and echo features of 104 patients (53 women and 51 men) with MAC with those of 121 age- and sex-matched control subjects (62 women and 59 men) without MAC. The incidence of CAD, rheumatic heart disease, systemic hypertension, and diabetes mellitus was similar in both groups. Patients with MAC had a greater incidence of cardiomegaly (p < 0.001), cardiac conduction defects (p < 0.001), and aortic outflow tract murmurs (p < 0.005) than did control patients. Patients with MAC and without aortic root calcium had a higher incidence (p < 0.001) of conduction defects than did patients with aortic root calcification without MAC. Control patients with and without aortic root calcification had a similar incidence of conduction defects. A higher incidence of AV block (p < 0.025) and BBB or left anterior hemiblock or intraventricular conduction defect (p < 0.05) was present in anterior MAC than in posterior MAC. In conclusion, patients with MAC have a higher incidence of cardiomegaly, cardiac conduction defects, and aortic outflow tract murmurs than a control group.

To investigate an apparent association of MAC and ECG abnormalities, the relation between location of 2-D echo quantified MAC and conduction disturbances was studied in 140 patients with MAC (MAC group) and in 135 age- and sex-matched patients without MAC (control group) by Takamoto and Popp[34] from Stanford, California. The MAC group was subclassified regarding site and severity of MAC. The site of MAC was defined as type I, near the primary conduction system—MAC located in the medial segment and/or extending to the anterior mitral leaflet—and type II—MAC located at the central and/or lateral segments away from the primary conduction system. The severity of MAC was graded on 2-D echo as mild (localized within 1 segment) and moderate to severe (>1 segment). Seven patients with MAC, and only 1 control subject, had pacemakers in place. Conduction disturbances were present in 44 (31%) of 140 patients with MAC, and in 37 (27%) of 135 control patients (difference not significant). But there were more conduction disturbances in patients with type I MAC (53%) than in those with type II MAC (26%) ($p < 0.01$). Specifically, complete left BBB and intraventricular conduction delay were more prevalent when MAC was near the conduction system. Conduction disturbances also were more prevalent in patients with type I MAC than in the control group: intraventricular conduction delay (12% type I -vs- 4% control; $p < 0.05$) and total conduction disturbances (53 -vs- 28%; $p < 0.01$). These data suggest that moderate to severe degrees of MAC located near the conduction system are associated with conduction disturbances, especially intraventricular conduction delay.

To test the hypothesis that accelerated metastatic calcification in the mitral anulus results from abnormalities in calcium-phosphorus and parathyroid hormone, Nestico and associates[35] from Philadelphia, Pennsylvania, studied 10 patients with end-stage renal disease having echo-proved MAC (group I) and 20 patients without MAC (group II). Serum levels of total calcium, phosphorus, intact and carboxyl terminal parathyroid hormone, serum ionized calcium, and total calcium-phosphorus product were compared for both groups. In addition, other variables, such as sex, supine systolic and diastolic BP, age, duration of hemodialysis, type of renal disease, and diabetes, also were compared in both groups. Although both groups had elevated intact and carboxyl terminal parathyroid hormone levels, group I did not differ significantly from group II. Total serum calcium levels were within normal limits in both groups and were not significantly different. However, the serum ionized calcium level was significantly higher in group I with MAC versus group II without MAC ($p < 0.05$). The serum phosphorus level and calcium phosphorus product were significantly higher in the group with MAC compared with the group without MAC ($p < 0.01$ and $p < 0.001$, respectively). No significant differences were found in the other clinical variables analyzed. It was concluded that MAC in patients with chronic renal failure occurs in the setting of secondary hyperparathyroidism. However, it was found more often in patients with increased ionized calcium and serum phosphorus levels and significantly higher calcium-phosphorus product levels. In chronic renal failure, MAC does not appear to be the result of a degenerative process and high ventricular systolic pressure, as has been previously described.

AORTIC VALVE STENOSIS

Systolic flutter

Chin and associates[36] from Los Angeles, California, postulated that an aortic valve sufficiently pliant to produce systolic flutter on M-mode echo could exclude significant AS, and they reviewed the M-mode echoes of 50 consecutive patients (mean age, 59 years) catheterized for presumed AS; 2-D echo also was performed in 18 patients (36%). In 40 of the 50 patients the aortic valve cusps were easily identified on M-mode echo: 19 of 40 (48%) had systolic flutter with a mean aortic valve gradient of 4 ± 8 mmHg (mean ± SD) and an aortic valve area of 2.8 ± 0.4 cm^2; 21 of 40 (52%) had no systolic flutter with a mean aortic valve gradient of 55 ± 19 mmHg and an aortic valve area of 0.7 ± 0.3 cm^2. In the 10 of 50 patients (20%) in whom aortic valve cusps were not clearly identified, the mean aortic valve gradient was 50 ± 24 mmHg and the aortic valve area 0.8 ± 0.4 cm^2. Systolic flutter was not seen with an aortic valve gradient <30 mmHg or an aortic valve area >1 cm^2. Aortic valve systolic opening by M-mode echo or 2-D echo did not accurately predict the severity of AS. Thus, aortic valve systolic flutter seen on M-mode echo is strong evidence against significant AS, but the absence of systolic flutter does not allow reliable prediction of the severity of AS. The finding of systolic flutter by M-mode echo may be a useful screening test in patients presumed to have AS.

With ruptured mitral chordae

Effron[37] from Stanford, California, identified 10 patients with AS and ruptured mitral chordae tendineae; these patients represented 8% of 125 consecutive surgical cases of ruptured chordae. Six patients presented with acute CHF and 8 patients were in New York Heart Association functional class III or IV. Extensive mitral anular calcium was detected by fluoroscopy in 7 patients. Mean aortic valve index was 0.4 cm^2/M^2 and 9 patients had moderate or worse MR. Only 1 patient had rheumatic alterations involving the mitral valve and 1 had MVP. These data suggest that mitral anular calcium and ventricular hemodynamic alterations that develop in AS may predispose to rupture of mitral chordae tendineae.

Ventricular arrhythmias

Olshausen and associates[38] from Heidelberg, West Germany, investigated the frequency of ventricular arrhythmias in patients with aortic valve disease. Twenty-four-hour ambulatory ECG recordings were obtained in 93 patients without CAD (AS, 38; combined AS and AR, 27; AR only, 28). The arrhythmias were compared with the hemodynamic findings of cardiac catheterization. Of VPC noted in 78 patients (84%), they were rare (<100 VPC/22 hours) in 40 patients (43%), moderately frequent (101–1,000 VPC/22 hours) in 23 patients (25%), and frequent (>1,000 VPC/22 hours) in 15 patients (16%). Multiformity was found in 47 (51%), paired VPC in 32 (34%), and VT in 17 (18%) of the 93 patients studied. The occurrence of ventricular arrhythmia was not related to the type of valve lesion, to the transvalvular gradient in patients with AS, or to the degree of regurgitation in patients with AR. In contrast, the grade of arrhythmia showed a negative correlation with LV EF (AS, r_s = −0.58; AS and AR, r_s = −0.67; AR, r_s = −0.78; all p < 0.001) and a positive correlation with peak systolic LV wall stress (AS, r_s = 0.56; AS and AR, r_s = 0.56; AR, r_s = 0.57; all p < 0.001). The frequency of VPC also showed a negative correlation with LV EF (AS, r_s = −0.63; AS and AR, r_s = −0.65; AR, r_s = −0.71; all p < 0.001). This study indicates that ventricular arrhythmias are present in a large number of patients with aortic valve disease. The severity of arrhythmias is strongly influenced by myocardial performance. Thus, severe arrhythmias are frequently a sign of impaired LV function.

Pulsus alternans

Laskey and associates[39] from Philadelphia, Pennsylvania, studied differences in the mechanics of strong and weak contractions during sustained pulsus alternans in 4 patients with AS. No significant difference was observed between strong (S) and weak (W) beats in M-mode echo end-diastolic minor axis dimension, or end-diastolic meridional wall stress. Peak systolic meridional stress (S, 225×10^3 dynes/cm^2; W, 205×10^3 dynes/cm^2), the time integral of LV meridional systolic stress (S, $5{,}000 \times 10^3$ dynes/cm^2; W, $4{,}500 \times 10^3$ dynes/cm^2) and the area of a stress dimension loop (S, 202×10^3 dynes/cm; W, 165×10^3 dynes/cm) were all greater for strong beats. However, end-systolic meridional stress (S, 100×10^3 dynes/cm^2; W, 115×10^3 dynes/cm^2) and end-systolic minor axis dimension (S, 4.75 cm; W, 5.0 cm) were significantly greater for weak beats. Stress-length relations, derived from resting and postnitroglycerin determinations, revealed higher end-systolic dimensions for weak beats at any level of limiting afterload, suggesting diminished contractile performance of weak beats. Additionally, fractional minor axis shortening for weak beats was diminished at any level of end-systolic stress in comparison with that for strong beats. The results are supportive of theories suggesting alternating contractile performance during pulsus alternans.

Progression

Nestico and associates[40] from Philadelphia, Pennsylvania, analyzed factors related to progression of nonrheumatic AS in 29 adult patients who underwent serial hemodynamic studies over a mean period of 71 months. The AS was congenital in 8 patients and degenerative in 21. The patients were divided into 2 groups on the basis of the change in aortic valve area between the 2 studies. Twelve patients had a ≥25% reduction in aortic valve area (group I) and 17 patients had <25% decrease in aortic valve area (group II). There were no significant differences between the 2 groups in age, interval between studies, cardiac output, LV end-diastolic pressure, LV peak systolic pressure, and origin of AS (congenital or degenerative). Group I patients had significantly larger initial aortic valve areas than did group II patients (1.3 ± 0.9 cm^2 -vs- 0.8 ± 0.4 cm^2; p = 0.02). Also, the initial peak transaortic pressure gradients were lower in group I than in group II (27 ± 19 -vs- 58 ± 38 mmHg; p = 0.01). Group I patients had a significantly greater increase in pressure gradient and a greater reduction in cardiac output than did group II patients (24 ± 21 mmHg in group I -vs- −0.1 ± 24.5 mmHg in group II; p = 0.01; and −1.0 ± 1.3 liters/min in group I -vs- 0.10 ± 1.4 liters/min in group II; p = 0.03). Thus, AS progressed in 41% of a selected group of patients who underwent repeated cardiac catheterization. The progression was not predictable. Although 10 patients (34%) had moderate AR in the second study, it was not related to the origin or rate of progression of AS. Mild AS tends to progress more than severe AS. Congenital AS appears to progress at the same rate as degenerative AS.

Asymmetric septal hypertrophy

Hess and associates[41] from Zurich, Switzerland, evaluated myocardial histologic features and LV dynamics in 24 patients with severe AS, 12 with and 12 without associated asymmetric septal hypertrophy (ASH). In 10 patients with ASH, echo demonstrated a septal posterior wall ratio of 1.5; in the remaining 2 patients, ASH was demonstrated by direct inspection at surgery. Septal myectomy in all 12 of these patients was performed at the time of AVR. The LV end-diastolic and peak systolic pressure, peak pressure gradient, and calculated valvular and angiographic muscle mass did not differ between patients in these 2 groups. Muscle fiber diameter of the anterolateral wall was similar in patients in both groups, but muscle fiber diameter of the septum in patients with associated ASH was significantly smaller than that of the anterolateral wall in patients without associated ASH. No morphologic abnormalities typical of those seen in HC were found in tissue samples from patients in any of the groups. Septal wall thickness decreased significantly from 2.0–1.5 cm and posterior wall thickness from 1.4–1.2 cm by 18 months postoperatively in patients with associated ASH. Similar changes in septal wall and posterior wall thickness had occurred in patients without ASH. In patients with severe AS, ASH appears to be an adaptive mechanism to the long-standing pressure overload rather than a coexistence of HC and aortic valve disease.

Impaired exercise tolerance

To determine the significance of abnormalities of diastolic function in patients with LV hypertrophy, Oldershaw and associates[42] from London, England, performed exercise echo to heart rates of 150 beats/minute in 14 patients who had AVR (for AS in 12 and AR in 2) 5–26 months earlier and in 18 normal subjects. Simultaneous echo, phonocardiograms, and ECGs were recorded. The LV cavity size was determined at end diastole and end systole. The timing of mitral valve opening and closure was measured, and hence LV filling time was derived (expressed either as ms/beat, or s/min when multiplied by heart rate). Isovolumic relaxation was taken as the interval between A_2 and mitral valve opening. Systolic function, assessed from cavity dimensions, peak velocity of circumferential fiber, and Q-A_2 interval was normal in all but 2 patients at rest and on exercise. Isovolumic relaxation was prolonged at rest in the patients to 85 ± 8 ms (normal, 69 ± 9 ms), but LV filling times were normal. With exercise, in normal subjects, isovolumic relaxation remained constant, but filling times dropped strikingly from 380 ± 66 ms/beat or 27 ± 2 s/minute at rest to 115 ± 10 ms/beat or 16 ± 2 s/minute. In patients with LV hypertrophy, isovolumic relaxation dropped on exercise to 41 ± 15 ms. Filling periods were normal at rest, 367 ± 67 ms/beat or 27 ± 3 s/minute, but failed to show the normal drop with exercise, being 240 ± 44 ms/beat or 28 ± 4 s/minute. At heart rates >120/minute, separation between the 2 groups was complete. Thus, striking abnormalities of LV filling can be demonstrated on exercise in patients with LV hypertrophy. They appear to represent loss of mechanisms whereby rapid diastolic filling is achieved in the normal subject.

AORTIC REGURGITATION

Echo findings

To determine whether a LV end-systolic dimension (ESD) >55 mm and LV fractional shortening <25% are risk factors for AVR in patients with AR, Fioretti and associates[43] from Rotterdam, The Netherlands, analyzed the clinical course in M-mode echo in 47 consecutive patients who underwent AVR for isolated symptomatic AR. Group 1 patients (27) had a preoperative ESD <55 mm and group 2 patients had a preoperative ESD >55 mm. One patient in group 1 and 10 patients in group 2 had LV fractional shortening <25%. There were no perioperative or postoperative deaths during an average follow-up of 41 months, ranging from 6–76 months. Five patients had perioperative AMI, 3 in group 1 and 2 in group 2. Since myocardial protection with cold potassium cardioplegia was instituted, no patient had a perioperative AMI. The average preoperative New York Heart Association functional class was 2.3 for group 1 and 2.6 for group 2. Postoperatively, class was 1.2 in group 1 and 1.1 in group 2. Thirty-three patients (20 in group 1 and 13 in group 2) had echoes ≥1 year after AVR. Of these, the LV diastolic dimension decreased from 67–53 mm in group 1 and from 79–55 mm in group 2. The LV ESD also decreased. The LV cross-sectional area and index of LV mass decreased in group 1 from 25–20 cm^2 and in group 2 from 32–20 cm^2. Postoperative ESD and cross-sectional area were not significantly different between the 2 groups. Thus, these investigators concluded that in AR, a preoperative ESD >55 mm does not preclude successful AVR as judged by long-term survival, symptomatic relief, and normalization of LV dimensions assessed by echo.

Surgical correction of chronic AR generally results in a substantial decrease in LV volume and mass. To assess the functional significance of these changes, Carroll and associates[44] from Boston, Massachusetts, examined serial noninvasive tests of LV function in 23 patients after AVR. Three independent tests of LV function were used: 1) the ratio of the LV preejection period (PEP) to the LV ejection time (ET), 2) the echo fractional increase in LV wall thickness (FT), and 3) the mitral E point to septal separation (ESS). Studies were performed before surgery and 0.3 (early), 3–6 (mid), and 9–12 (late) months after surgery. In the early postoperative studies, LV end-diastolic dimension decreased to normal or near normal and the PEP/LV ET ratio increased substantially in 17 patients. Ten of the 17 (group 1) had complete regression of LV hypertrophy and the average values for all 3 indexes of LV function were normal at the time of the late postoperative study (PEP/LV ET, 0.41 ± 0.05; FT, 73 ± 14%; ESS, 6.2 ± 0.9 mm). Seven patients (group 2) with incomplete regression of LV hypertrophy showed borderline to moderately abnormal function indexes at the late study. Six patients had persistent LV enlargement and no postoperative regression of hypertrophy (group 3). These patients did not show the substantial early changes in the function indexes observed in groups 1 and 2; moreover, the indexes remained markedly abnormal at the time of the late postoperative study (PEP/LV ET, 0.52 ± 0.10; FT, 47 ± 13%; ESS, 22.3 ± 7.2 mm). Patients in group 3 had preoperative evidence of abnormal LV function that was more marked than that observed in groups 1 and 2. Thus, the early postoperative changes in LV preload and the subsequent regression of LV hypertrophy are associated with evidence of early LV dysfunction and subsequent improvement. Postoperative LV enlargement and persistent LV hypertrophy are associated with persistent LV dysfunction. These serial data provide a framework for the rational timing and interpretation of postoperative ventricular function tests.

Gaasch and associates[45] from Boston, Massachusetts, evaluated 32 patients who underwent AVR for chronic AR to determine the prognostic value of preoperative echo data. All patients had a preoperative echo and were followed prospectively for 1–6 years after surgery. Postoperatively, 25 patients achieved a normal LV end-diastolic dimension and significant regression of myocardial hypertrophy, but 7 patients had persistent LV enlargement. Patients whose LV hypertrophy and dilation resolved during follow-up had fewer symptoms and used fewer medications than those in whom this did not occur. Survival at 4 years was also better in patients whose hypertrophy and dilatation resolved (96%) than in patients in whom it did not (71%). Preoperatively, a LV dimension at end diastole >3.8 cm/M^2, and end-systolic dimension >2.6 cm/M^2, and end-diastolic radius/wall thickness ratio >3.8 or a product of end-diastolic radius/wall thickness and LV systolic pressure exceeding 600 were predictive of a failure of hypertrophy and dilation to resolve postoperatively. Thus, patients with chronic AR at risk for persistent LV enlargement following aortic valve replacement and diminished survival can be identified by preoperative echo.

Radionuclide studies

Exercise-gated radionuclide ventriculography has been proposed as a method to evaluate cardiac reserve in patients with chronic AR. Characterization of ventricular function, however, in AR is complicated by the dynamic nature of the leak in individual patients and by variations in severity among patients. Steingart and associates[46] from New York City studied 20 patients with isolated chronic AR to assess the effects of exercise on the regurgitant index. The regurgitant index (LV/RV stroke volume counts) estimated the severity of the leak. The regurgitant index at rest was significantly higher in patients with AR than in patients without AR (3.46 ± 1.25 -vs- 1.08 ± 0.16; p < 0.001). In patients with AR, the regurgitant index decreased during exercise to 2.6 ± 0.8 (p < 0.001), whereas it did not change in the control group (1.16 ± 0.21; difference not significant). Also, in patients with AR the greater the regurgitant index at rest, the greater the decrease during exercise (y = 0.56× − 1.08; r = 0.78; p < 0.001). End-diastolic counts and stroke count responses from rest to exercise were highly variable but were explained in part by the decreasing regurgitant index. These data support previous catheterization studies and confirm gated radionuclide ventriculography as a useful tool for monitoring adaptations to exercise in AR.

Huxley and associates[47] from Dallas, Texas, tested the hypothesis that radionuclide ventriculography with exercise allows earlier detection of important LV dysfunction in patients with AR than the other variables. In 16 consecutive asymptomatic or minimally symptomatic patients (8 men and 7 women; mean age, 44 years) with isolated 2–4+ aortic regurgitation, rest and exercise-gated radionuclide ventriculography, M-mode echo, and LV angiography were performed. No other cause of LV dysfunction was apparent in 13 patients; 1 patient had moderate systemic arterial hypertension and 1 had 50% luminal diameter narrowing of the proximal left anterior descending coronary artery. Ten patients did not have an increase in LV EF >0.05 EF units at peak exercise (0.58 ± 0.11–0.50 ± 0.12; mean ± SD) (group 2), whereas 5 had a normal LV EF response to exercise (0.63 ± 0.08–0.69 ± 0.07) (group 1). Eight of the 10 patients with abnormal LV EF responses to exercise had a decrease in LV EF >10% during exercise. The same 8 patients also had an increase in LV end systolic volume index (ESVI) with exercise, whereas the 5 patients with normal LV EF responses to exercise had normal or blunted LV ESVI response to exercise. Only 4 of the 10 patients with exercise-induced LV dysfunction had an angiographic LV ESVI ⩾60 ml/M^2, and only 1 had an echo-determined LV ESD ⩾5.5 cm. Serial follow-up rest and exercise scintigraphic and echo measurements were made in 8 of the patients a mean of 9.4 months after the initial measurements; 3 patients were in group 1 and 5 in group 2. The 5 patients in group 2 again demonstrated abnormal LV function during exercise stress, and 2 of the 3 patients in group 1 then demonstrated an abnormal LV functional response during exercise. Therefore it is concluded that 1) exercise radionuclide ventriculography identifies LV dysfunction earlier than traditionally used assessments; 2) LV dysfunction appears to persist in patients who demonstrate it and develop in others who did not have it originally; and 3) echo dilation of the LV ESD to 5.5 cm appears to be a late and relatively unusual occurrence.

To test the hypothesis that LV performance in AR can be more completely characterized by measurement of LV volumes in addition to EF, Johnson and associates[48] from New York City studied 27 asymptomatic patients (group 1), and 22 symptomatic patients (group 2), and 10 control subjects at rest and during upright bicycle exercise during the first-pass technique and multicrystal scintillation camera. The LV end-diastolic volume was measured by the area-length method. In the control group end-diastolic volume increased 14%, end-systolic volume decreased 22%, and EF increased 22% with exercise. In contrast in group 1 patients with AR, end-diastolic volume was elevated at rest and during exercise. The 18% decrease in end-diastolic volume during exercise was significantly different from the control response (p < 0.01). End-systolic volume was also elevated at rest and during exercise, but the 30% decrease during exercise was a response not significantly different from the control. Although mean EF increased 15% in these patients, EF at peak exercise was significantly lower than that in the controls. In group 2 patients with AR, resting EF was reduced, the EF response to exercise was abnormal, and end-diastolic and end-systolic volume responses to exercise were significantly different from those in group 1: end-diastolic volume did not change and end-systolic volume increased. In contrast to the fairly uniform volume responses among all group 1 patients, there were 2 subgroups based on volume changes within group 2: 7 of 22 had a decrease in end-diastolic volume and end-systolic volume during exercise and 8 of 22 showed an increase in end-diastolic and end-systolic volume during exercise.

In conclusion, LV volumes at rest and exercise give more information about LV functional reserve in symptomatic patients with AR than do EF responses alone and may be useful in separating symptomatic patients who show a normal end-systolic volume response to exercise from those in whom worsening failure develops during exercise.

Boucher and associates[49] from Boston, Massachusetts, measured serial radionuclide LV EF during graded supine exercise in 35 asymptomatic or minimally symptomatic patients with severe AR and in 16 control subjects. Simultaneous pulmonary gas exchange analysis permitted determination of the anaerobic threshold, which is the point during exercise at which lactic acid begins to accumulate in the blood. The EF and oxygen uptake were measured at rest, anaerobic threshold, and peak exercise. The mean EF (± 1 SD) in control patients increased from 0.65 ± 0.06 at rest to 0.73 ± 0.05 at anaerobic threshold ($p < 0.01$). No further change in EF occurred between anaerobic threshold and peak exercise (0.73 ± 0.09). Peak oxygen uptake in control patients was 20 ± 4 m/kg/minute. Patients with AR were classified into 2 groups based on a peak oxygen uptake 16 ml/kg/minute (group I: n, 26) and 16 ml/kg/minute (group II: n, 9). In group I the mean oxygen uptake at the anaerobic threshold and peak exercise was similar to or greater than that in control patients, whereas in group II patients it was less than in control patients. In group I, the mean rest EF (0.62 ± 0.07) was similar to that in control patients; there was no change at the anaerobic threshold (0.61 ± 0.10), and then it decreased at peak exercise (0.57 ± 0.12; $p < 0.05$). In group II, the mean rest EF (0.44 ± 0.12) was below that in control patients ($p < 0.01$); there was a decrease at the anaerobic threshold (0.35 ± 0.10; $p < 0.01$), and then it decreased further at peak exercise (0.30 ± 0.09; $p < 0.05$). The anaerobic threshold and peak oxygen uptake reflect rest and exercise LV EF in AR and may provide an additional approach of assessing cardiac performance in these patients. Exercise-induced changes in LV EF should be based on the changes occurring before the anaerobic threshold, because changes between anaerobic threshold and peak exercise are of uncertain diagnostic value.

With ascending aortic aneurysm

The selection of an appropriate surgical technique for repair of aneurysm of the ascending thoracic aorta with associated AR is unsettled. Grey and associates[50] from Houston, Texas, analyzed 140 patients who underwent repair. Anuloaortic ectasia was the most common indication followed by acute and chronic dissection. Eighty-nine patients (64%) underwent composite replacement with coronary reimplantation, and 51 (36% had separate graft and valve repair or primary repair of the aneurysm). Cardiopulmonary bypass methods, times, and postoperative complications were comparable between the 2 groups. Hospital mortality for the whole series was 8% (11 of 140) with 6% in patients having conduit replacement and 14% in patients having separate supracoronary graft and valve repair. In patients with anuloaortic ectasia, use of separate graft and valve had a greater mortality ($p = 0.005$), and in patients with atherosclerotic aneurysm use of conduit repair had greater mortality ($p = 0.05$). No patient has required reoperation for conduit malfunction or has required repair of aneurysm or paravalvular leak below a supracoronary graft.

CONGENITALLY BICUSPID AORTIC VALVE

Bicuspid aortic valve is one of the most common congenital cardiac anomalies, occurring in 0.4–2% of all births. Because its complications, namely, stenosis, pure regurgitation, with or without infective endocarditis, and infective endocarditis, early identification of this valvular anomaly is important. Brandenburg and associates[51] from Rochester, Minnesota, reviewed preoperative 2-D echoes of all patients <50 years of age in whom the aortic valve had been directly inspected by the surgeon or the pathologist or both. From June 1977 to June 1981, 283 patients aged ≤50 years had aortic valve surgery at the Mayo Clinic: 115 (aged 1–50 years [mean, 32]) had 2-D echo preoperatively (Table 5-4). The echo was reviewed blindly, and the aortic valve structure was categorized as bicuspid, tricuspid, or indeterminate. On the basis of combined surgical and pathologic inspection, 50 aortic valves were congenitally bicuspid, 60 were tricuspid, 4 were unicommissural, and 1 was quadricuspid. By 2-D echo, the number of cusps was indeterminate in 29 patients (25%). When these patients were excluded, the sensitivity,

TABLE 5-4. *Two–dimensional echo in aortic valve disease: diagnosis in 115 patients.*

AORTIC VALVE STRUCTURE	PATIENTS	
	N	%
Bicuspid	31	27
Tricuspid	55	48
Indeterminate	29	25
Calcified valve	14	...
Inadequate visualization	15	...

TABLE 5-5. *Correlation between surgical pathologic diagnosis and 2-D echo diagnosis in 84 patients.*

AORTIC VALVE STRUCTURE BY 2-D ECHO	SURGICAL-PATHOLOGIC DIAGNOSIS OF AORTIC VALVE CUSP NUMBER	
	BICUSPID	TRICUSPID
Bicuspid	28	2
Tricuspid	8	47
Diagnostic accuracy for		
Bicuspid valve	93%	
Tricuspid valve	85%	
Sensitivity	78%	
Specificity	96%	

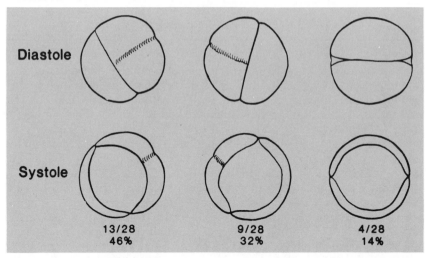

Fig. 5-8. Diagram of parasternal short axis scan shows commissural orientation in 28 patients with bicuspid aortic valves correctly diagnosed by 2-D echo. Orientation of commissures was indeterminate in 2 patients. The most common pattern (left pair) demonstrated posterior commissure at the 4 or 5 o'clock position and anterior commissure at the 9 or 10 o'clock position, with raphe (when visualized) at the 1 or 2 o'clock position. This pattern resulted in a larger anterior and slightly smaller posterior cusp. In the next most common pattern (middle pair), anterior commissure was at the 1 or 2 o'clock position and posterior commissure usually at the 6 o'clock position, with raphe (when visualized) at the 9 or 10 o'clock position. This pattern usually resulted in a larger right than left cusp. Least frequently visualized (right pair) were commissures at the 3 and 9 o'clock positions (no raphe) resulting in equal sized anterior and posterior cusps.

specificity, and diagnostic accuracy of 2-D echo for bicuspid aortic valve were 78, 96, and 93%, respectively (Table 5-5; Fig. 5-8). Thus, with adequate 2-D images, echo is a sensitive and highly specific technique for the diagnosis of bicuspid aortic valve.

THE MARFAN SYNDROME

Come and associates[52] from Boston, Massachusetts, and Baltimore, Maryland, compared echo abnormalities of the mitral valve and aortic root with auscultatory findings and with assessment of aortic root size by chest roentgenography in 61 patients with the Marfan syndrome. Echo was more sensitive than physical examination in detecting valvular and aortic root abnormalities. Although physical examination revealed findings of mitral valve disease and/or AR in 52% of patients (mitral valve disease in 44% and AR in 23%), echo detected abnormalities of the mitral valve and/or aortic root in 82% of patients (MVP in 57% and aortic root enlargement in 69%). Prevalence of MVP was approximately equal in male and female patients, whereas aortic root enlargement was more frequent in males (83%) than in females (50%). Aortic root enlargement detected by echo was frequently not apparent on chest x-ray. Indeed, 5 patients with markedly increased aortic root diameters (ranging from 6.0–7.9 cm) had no evident enlargement of the aortic root on routine chest x-ray. The authors caution that mitral valve disease may not be detected on occasion by echo in patients with LV dilation. Additionally, anteroposterior LA compression by the enlarged aorta may cause the LA size to be underestimated in patients with dialated aortic roots.

The prevalence, age of onset, and natural history of mitral valve dysfunction in the Marfan syndrome are uncertain. Therefore, Pyeritz and Wappel[53] from Baltimore, Maryland, reviewed all patients in their clinic who met strict diagnostic criteria for the Marfan syndrome and who had clinical and echo examinations before age 22 years. Of the 166 patients (84 males aged 12 ± 0.6 years and 82 females aged 11 ± 0.6 years), 52% had auscultatory and 68% had echo evidence of mitral valve dysfunction, generally MVP. Prevalence did not differ between the sexes. Follow-up in 115 patients averaged 5 examinations over a mean of 4 years; 17% were followed for more than 6 years. Criteria for progression of mitral valve dysfunction were: 1) on auscultation, the appearance of new systolic clicks or apical systolic murmurs, a murmur of MR increased by 2 grades, or appearance of CHF not due to AR; and 2) on echo, the new appearance of MVP or abnormally increased LA dimension. Nearly half the patients met ≥1 criterion and 25% had both auscultatory and echo evidence of progressive mitral valve dysfunction. Twice as many females had worse mitral valve function with time. Eight of the 166 patients either died as a result of mitral valve dysfunction or required MVR. Severe MR developed in an additional 15 patients. Rupture of chordae tendineae was uncommon. Antibiotic prophylaxis was routine, and no cases of infective endocarditis of the mitral valve occurred. These results suggest that mitral valve dysfunction is extremely common in young patients with Marfan syndrome and usually presents as MVP. Serious MR develops in 1 of every 8 patients by the third decade. Thus, the prevalence and natural history of MVP in the Marfan syndrome appear distinct from MVP associated with other conditions, including idiopathic or familial MVP.

TRICUSPID VALVE DISEASE

Nanna and associates[54] from Los Angeles, California, reviewed the M-mode and 2-D echoes of 100 consecutive patients with rheumatic heart disease. All patients were subsequently studied by cardiac catheterization and angiography. In 4 patients, cardiac catheterization revealed tricuspid stenosis (TS) (average mean diastolic gradient, 6 mmHg) which was confirmed during cardiac surgery. M-mode echo showed a diminished EF slope in 12 patients, including the 4 patients with TS. Seven of the 8 patients without TS had significant pulmonary hypertension. Four patients were diagnosed as having TS by 2-D echo on the basis of diastolic doming and restricted leaflet motion of the tricuspid valve; these 4 patients with TS were also diagnosed by cardiac catheterization. These investigators concluded that 2-D echo was useful in the diagnosis of TS.

In a 5-year period 2-D echo detected 327 patients with rheumatic mitral valve disease studied by Daniels and associates[55] from Philadelphia, Pennsylvania. Of these patients, 23 (6%) had tricuspid valve involvement. Two-D echo criteria of rheumatic tricuspid valve disease included thickened leaflets with restriction in motion, diastolic doming, and encroachment of the leaflet tips on the ventricular inlet. These criteria provided a sensitivity of 100%, a specificity of 90%, a predictive accuracy of 21%, and a negative predictive value of 100% in diagnosing hemodynamically significant TS. Hemodynamic variables in patients with rheumatic tricuspid valve disease (group I) were compared with those in patients with no rheumatic tricuspid disease (group II). The only significant difference was mean RA pressure (15 ± 7 mmHg -vs- 11 ± 5 mmHg; p < 0.02). Both groups were classified into patients with (A) and without (B) significant TR. There was no significant difference in any hemodynamic variable when group IA was compared with group IIA. In addition, there was no difference in any hemodynamic variable when patients with functional TR (group IIA) were compared with those with rheumatic mitral valvular disease without TR (group IIB). Two-D echo and cardiac catheterization provide complementary diagnostic information in these patients.

Brown and Anderson[56] from Lancaster, England, studied the tricuspid valve of 40 subjects using 2-D echo: 40 normal subjects, 31 with MVP, 22 with clinically probable tricuspid valve prolapse (TVP), and 20 with chronic CHF, and 30 with miscellaneous cardiac conditions, but no features of right-sided cardiac disease. Using multiple views, it was possible to record all 3 leaflets in 75% of the patients and anterior and septal leaflets in 95%. In 13 patients TVP was recognized: 6 with associated MVP and 7 without. The TVP involved all 3 leaflets in 1 patient, both anterior and septal leaflets in 6 patients, anterior and posterior leaflets in 3, septal leaflet alone in 2 patients, and anterior leaflet alone in 1. Thus, 2-D echo allows definition of individual tricuspid valve leaflets, and prolapse of any or all leaflets can be diagnosed. Tricuspid valve prolapse is commonly associated with MVP.

Tei and associates[57] from Los Angeles, California, examined the tricuspid valve by 2-D echo in 14 patients with TVP and in 16 normal subjects. Individual leaflets were identified anatomically and for frequency of prolapse. Maximal and minimal anular sizes were measured. Multiple tomograms of the tricuspid anulus were recorded at 30° intervals around the tricuspid anulus with the transducer placed at the RV apex. Anuli were reconstructed from the 6 planes and corrected for body surface area. Three leaflets of the tricuspid valve could be anatomically identified in all patients. Prolapse of all 3 leaflets was observed in 6 patients, 2 leaflets in 5, and 1 in 3. Frequency of individual leaflet prolapse was 93% for the septal cusp, 86% for the anterior, and 43% for the posterior. Maximal anular circumference and area in TVP were 7.9 ± 0.6 and 8.9 ± 1.3 cm^2/M^2, respectively—significantly larger than values in normal subjects (6.4 ± 0.5 cm/M^2 and 6.1 ± 0.9 cm^2/M^2, respectively) (p < 0.001). Percent reductions in circumference and area in TVP were 14 ± 3 and 25 ± 5%, respectively—significantly smaller values than in normal subjects (19 ± 4 and 33 ± 4%, respectively). Contrast echo detected TR in 7 of 14 patients with TVP. The severity of TR appeared to be minimal in 6 of the 7 patients and was not associated with an increase in anular size. Thus, TVP is associated with anular dilation irrespective of associated TR.

Contrast echo and inferior vena cava ultrasonography are useful techniques in diagnosing TR but are not helpful in estimating its severity. Using a computerized light-pen method for tracing the RA border during systole and diastole in the apical 4-chamber view, DePace and associates[58] from Philadelphia, Pennsylvania, calculated single-plane volume determinations in 10 normal subjects (group I), 18 patients with AF and no TR (group II), 14 patients with MS and mild TR (group IIIa), and 8 patients with MS and severe TR (group IIIb). The TR was quantitated as absent, mild, or severe by contrast right ventriculography. The RA end-systolic volume was 36 ± 13 ml in group I patients, 59 ± 17 ml in group II patients, 77 ± 55 ml in group IIIa patients, and 155 ± 57 ml in group IIIb patients (all groups -vs- group I, p < 0.001). The mean RA emptying volume, which equals RA end-systolic volume—RA end-diastolic volume, was 15 ± 5 for group I, 18 ± 3 for group II, 30 ± 8 for group IIIa, and 71 ± 25 for group IIIb. All 8 patients with severe TR but none of the 14 patients with mild TR had an RA emptying volume >40 ml (p < 0.001). In addition, all 28 patients in groups I and II but only 4 of 14 patients in group III had an RA emptying volume <26 ml (p < 0.01). The mean RA pressure measured at cardiac catheterization correlated with RA emptying volume (r = 0.71; p < 0.001). Thus, RA emptying volume is useful for separating severe from mild TR in patients with MS.

To determine whether TR can be diagnosed by direct imaging of RA regurgitant flow using contrast echo, Meltzer and associates[59] from Tel Hashomer, Israel, performed echo in 35 patients using peripheral intravenous injections of 5% dextrose solution. Fifteen patients had TR judged by v-wave synchronous contrast appearance on the inferior vena cava echo (a previously validated method for diagnosing TR), 5 of whom had clinically obvious TR. Twenty patients had no TR on inferior vena cava contrast echo, 9 of whom were normal volunteers. On subsequent blind review, 13 of the 15 patients with TR were correctly identified on the basis of the regurgitant contrast flow just posterior to the tricuspid valve. Of the 20 without TR, 19 were correctly identified and there was 1 false positive res' .t. Using different criteria for the diagnosis (insisting on imaging of flow across the tricuspid valve in systole), another blinded observer correctly diagnosed only 8 of the 15 patients as having TR, but had no false positive results. To avoid false positive results, it is important to realize that there are 2 regions where retrograde flow can normally be seen in the right atrium: briefly at the onset of systole coincident with tricuspid valve closure, and in the posterior right atrium, as distinct from the anterior RA area just behind the tricuspid valve where T . is diagnosed in this study. It was concluded that direct imaging of regurgitant flow in the right atrium just posterior to the tricuspid valve is an accurate method for diagnosing or excluding TR and is ideally complementary to inferior vena cava contrast echo in making this diagnosis.

To determine the critical anular dilation required for functional TR and the role of systolic anular shortening in the severity of TR, Ubago and associates[60] from Santander, Spain, performed right ventriculography in 67 patients. These patients were classified into group I, control (n, 12), and group II, patients with rheumatic valvular disease (n, 55). Group II patients were subclassified as follows: IIa, without TR (n, 19); IIb, with mild TR (n, 22); and IIc, with moderate to severe TR (n, 14). The angiographic maximal early systolic and minimal end-systolic diameters were measured (Fig. 5-9). The shortening of the tricuspid anulus was expressed as percent reduction of the maximal diameter. The average maximal diameter (mm/M^2) was: group I, 21 ± 2; group IIa, 24 ± 2; group IIb, 31 ± 4; and group IIc, 37 ± 4. The av-

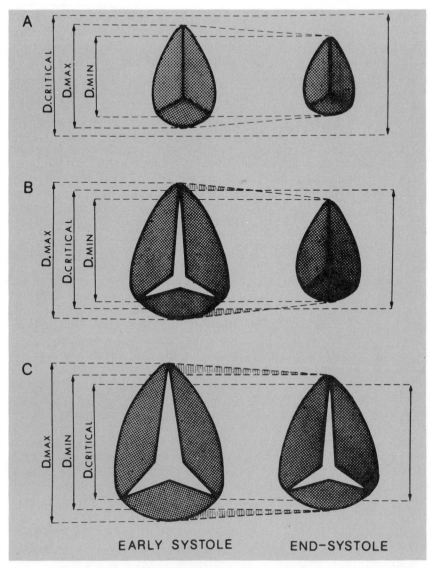

EARLY SYSTOLE   END-SYSTOLE

Fig. 5-9. Diagram of the tricuspid valve in patients with rheumatic heart disease. Panel A, patients without TR (group IIa). Both maximal early systolic diameter (D. MAX) and minimal end–systolic diameter (D. MIN) are below the critical diameter. Cusp apposition is present throughout systole. Panel B, patients with mild TR (group IIb). D. MAX is larger and D. MIN is smaller than the critical diameter (D. CRITICAL). No cusp apposition during early and mid–systole occurs. Panel C, patients with moderate to severe TR (group IIc). D. MAX and D. MIN are above the critical diameter. No cusp apposition occurs. The shaded areas represent the systolic period during which TR is present.

erage minimal diameter (mm/M^2) was: group I, 15 ± 2; group IIa, 18 ± 2; group IIb, 23 ± 2; and group IIc, 31 ± 3. The average percent shortening was: group I, 30 ± 7%; group IIa, 25 ± 7%; group IIb, 26 ± 5%; and group IIc, 15 ± 3%. The rheumatic patients had a larger maximal diameter than did those in the control group. Anular shortening was reduced only in the group with moderate to severe TR and preserved in the other groups, including those with mild TR. The critical diameter was determined to be between the maximal diameter in the rheumatic patients without TR and the minimal diameter in the patients with moderate to severe TR, or 27 mm/M^2. Thus this easily measured parameter can determine the presence and significance of functional TR, adding objectivity to the angiographic diagnosis of TR.

Equilibrium gated RNA was performed by Handler and associates[61] from Chicago, Illinois, in 2 control groups (15 patients with no organic heart disease and 24 patients with organic heart disease but without right-or left-sided valvular regurgitation) and in 9 patients with clinical TR. The regurgitant index, or ratio of LV to RV stroke counts, was significantly lower in patients with TR than in either control group (range and mean ± SEM, 0.4–1.0, 0.7 ± 0.1 -vs- 1.0–1.5, 1.3 ± 0.1 and 1.0–2.9, 1.5 ± 0.1, respectively; p < 0.001). Time activity variation over the liver was used to compute a hepatic expansion fraction that was significantly higher in patients with TR than in either control group (1.4–11.4, 5.8 ± 1.0% -vs- 0.6–3.4, 1.9 ± 0.3% and 1.0–5.1, 2.3 ± 0.2%, respectively; p < 0.001). Fourier analysis of time activity variation in each pixel was used to generate amplitude and phase images. Only pixels with values for amplitude at least 7% of the maximum in the image were retained in the f display. All patients with TR had >100 pixels over the liver were automatically retained by the computer These pixels were of phase comparable to that of the right atrium and proxi mately 180° out of phase with the right ventricle. In contrast, no patient with no organic heart disease and only 1 of 24 patients with organic heart disease had any pixels retained by the computer. Thus, patients with TR were characterized on equilibrium gated angiography by an abnormally low regurgitant index (7 of 9 patients), reflecting increased RV stroke volume, increased hepatic expansion fraction (7 of 9 patients), and increased amplitude of count variation over the liver in phase with the right atrium (9 of 9 patients).

ACUTE RHEUMATIC FEVER

Acute rheumatic fever (ARF) and rheumatic heart disease have declined greatly in North America and in western Europe during the past 50 years. The precise incidence of ARF in metropolitan areas of the USA at the present time remains unknown. Land and Bisno[62] from Memphis, Tennessee, surveyed the incidence of ARF in the county including Memphis, Tennessee, during the 5-year period 1977–1981. Only 41 patients met the modified Jones criteria, of whom 16 had conditions that were diagnosed in Memphis but they resided elsewhere. The overall ARF incidence in these county residents was 0.64/100,000 population each year. The highest rate, 3.7, was in blacks aged 5–17 years residing in the inner city, whereas white children in the suburban and rural areas had a rate of only 0.5. Current strategies for prevention and diagnosis of ARF must take into account the extraordinarily low level to which the incidence of ARF has fallen in certain surburban USA populations.

Stollerman[63] from Boston, Massachusetts, in an editorial pointed out that ARF still ranks as a major health problem in large segments of the populations of Asia, Africa, and South America. In fact, the industrialization of some native or aboriginal third world populations has resulted in an alarming prevalence of ARF, estimated to be increasing in some areas of South Africa. These estimates actually exceed ARF incidence rates of 61/100,000/year calculated for Manhattan school children in 1964, a time when the incidence of ARF was already declining rapidly in the USA. In commenting on the article by Land and Bisno[66], Stollerman raised several questions: How is this virtual disappearance of a major disease in such a short time to be explained in the face of continued, frequent isolation of group A streptococci from school children's throats? Is the diagnosis so precise and the antibiotic therapy all that effective? Has host resistance been greatly improved? Is our housing, even in our poorest urban areas, that spacious and decongested? Or have most of the virulent, rheumatogenic group A streptococci of the past become attenuated and the few that remain virulent retreated to the darkest recesses of our inner cities? If, indeed, the group A streptococci that are now extant in the affluent societies of the world are no longer of sufficient virulence to be rheumatogenic, can we change our strategies of the past 3 decades for treatment of streptococcal sore throat? Must we still use antibiotic therapy according to the same stringent regimens that were recommended a few decades ago? If ARF is no longer expected as a complication of the kind of streptococcal pharyngitis we now encounter, must it be treated at all? Will rheumatogenic streptococcal pharyngitis become a traveler's disease? These are questions with which expert committees of the American Heart Association are now struggling in their deliberations over whether or not to alter their long-standing recommendations on the primary prevention of ARF.

Although the incidence of ARF in North America and western Europe has plummeted during this century, group A Streptococcus has clearly not disappeared from the environment. Holmberg and Faich[64] from Providence, Rhode Island, in a comprehensive survey of physicians, laboratories, and hospital records in Rhode Island showed that >157,000 throat cultures in a population of 930,000 people were performed in 1980. Eighty-seven percent of primary care physicians prescribed antibiotic therapy before culture results were known, and almost 40% continued antibiotic therapy for 10 days regardless of culture results. The throat culture positivity rate for β-hemolytic Streptococcus was 17% statewide in 1980. Only 3 definite and 7 possible cases of ARF were identified by hospital chart reviews and a physician survey covering the 5 years 1976–1980. Current throat culture practices probably have little influence on treatment of streptococcal pharyngitis and control of ARF in the state.

In an accompanying editorial, Bisno[65] from Memphis, Tennessee, wrote: "Presuming that the conclusions of the study by Holmberg and Faich are valid, ie, that current throat culture practices probably have little influence on treatment of streptococcal pharyngitis and control of ARF . . . , and may be generalized to other parts of the USA, what options are available nationally? One might simply bow to the inevitable and dispense with the throat culture. Such a maneuver would leave physicians dependent on "clinical judgment" or on clinical algorithms to diagnose strep throat. This is, de facto, the strategy currently employed by many Rhode Island physicians, and it probably leads to considerable overtreatment. One might deemphasize any treatment of uncomplicated strep throat in private patients, given the extraordinarily low risk of ARF in Rhode Island. This course is probably unacceptable to most primary care practitioners because of the uncertainty as to what extent antibiotic therapy has contributed to the disappearance of rheumatic fever. Finally, we may recognize that, in the current milieu, the aim of a throat culture is more to prevent extraneous antibiotic treatment than to prevent the rare case of ARF. If so, we would need to redouble our efforts to educate physicians in the proper use of this tool (in the mode of pediatricians and more recent medical graduates in Rhode Island) and to ensure universal availability of inexpensive, timely streptococcal screening cultures. Can this be accomplished in a setting wherein interest in streptococcology may be waning pari passu with the decline of ARF? Only time will tell."

INFECTIVE ENDOCARDITIS

Surgery -vs- medicine

Croft and associates[66] from Cape Town, South Africa, and Dallas, Texas, analyzed 108 patients with infective endocarditis involving native valves studied from 1972–1980. Of the 108 patients, 23 (group A) underwent valve replacement during the active stage of the infective process because of progressive CHF (12 patients), persistent severe hypotension (3 patients), uncontrolled infection for over 21 days (11 patients), aortic root abscess (2 patients), and pericarditis (1 patient). The other 85 patients (group B) with active native valve infective endocarditis were treated medically and matched for severity of illness. Two patients (9%) in group A and 43 patients (51%) in group B died during the hospital admission ($p < 0.001$). Any difference in long-term cumulative survival rate between the 2 groups was largely due to the beneficial impact of surgical management on the hospital mortality. Of 23 patients in group A, 11 (48%) had an entirely uncomplicated postoperative course. Long-term mortality rates in those with aortic valve endocarditis treated medically (79%) were significantly higher than in those with mitral valve involvement (47%) (<0.05) (Fig. 5-10). Patients with aortic valve involvement treated surgically had a better hospital ($p < 0.005$) and long-term ($p < 0.0005$) survival rate than those treated medically. Two groups at risk for postoperative complications were identified; 3 of 11 patients (27%) with uncontrolled infection had an early postoperative recurrence, and 4 of 7 patients (57%) with an aortic root abscess had postoperative prosthetic paravalvular regurgitation. Surgery therefore effects a substantial reduction in hospital mortality in patients with complicated active infective endocarditis (9 -vs- 51%), but patients with preoperative prolonged periods of uncontrolled infection or with aortic root abscess are liable to postoperative complications.

Nakamura and associates[67] from Tokyo, Japan, studied clinical and echo features of 8 patients with infective pulmonary valve endocarditis. In 2 patients, the vegetation was limited to the pulmonary valve and in the other 6

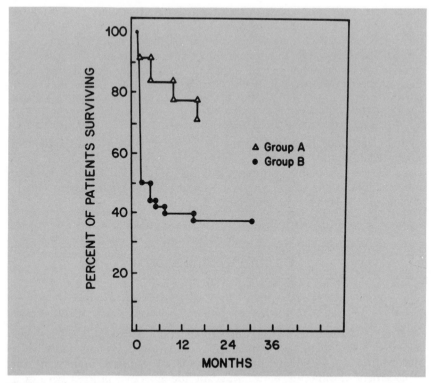

Fig. 5-10. Plot of the cumulative hospital and long–term survival rate of all patients in groups A and B. Plots are extended until the last death in each group. The overall survival rate for patients in group A is significantly better than that for patients in group B (p = 0.0004).

it also involved mitral or aortic valves. No patient was addicted to narcotics. Seven of the 8 patients had underlying congenital heart disease. In 6 patients, the responsible organism was alpha Streptococcus. The investigators found 2-D echo using a wide angle sector scanner was more useful than M-mode echo for evaluating patients with pulmonary valve endocarditis.

Usefulness of echo

M-mode and 2-D echo commonly are used to confirm the presence of vegetations in active infective endocarditis (IE). Two-D echo has been demonstrated to be more sensitive in detecting vegetations than M-mode echo. Wong and associates[68] from Los Angeles, Long Beach, and Irvine, California, examined by both M-mode and 2-D echo 34 patients with active IE. Vegetations were identified in 16 patients (47%) by M-mode and in 27 patients (87%) by 2-D echo. Vegetations identified by 2-D echo were categorized as small (<5 mm), medium (5–9 mm), or large (≥10 mm). Large vegetations were caused by several organisms, had a high frequency of surgery (44 -vs- 0%), and had no increased incidence of stroke or death. The larger the vegetation, the more often it was detected by M-mode echo. Aortic valve vegetations were associated with a high incidence of CHF (67 -vs- 14%) and stroke (44 -vs- 9%).

Mitral valve aneurysm

Five patients with clinical and echo pathologic findings documenting mitral valve aneurysm were described by Reid and associates[69] from Los Angeles, California. Two-D echo features in these patients were helpful in making the correct diagnosis by demonstrating a bulge of the mitral valve leaflet toward the left atrium persisting throughout the cardiac cycle. All 5 of these patients had clinical evidence of both AR and MR. Four patients had AVR for severe AR and CHF resulting from endocarditis on their aortic valve and 1 patient died shortly after hospital admission from severe CHF before surgery could be performed. Aortic valves in all 4 patients undergoing surgery had vegetations with extensive destruction of the valve leaflets. The remaining 4 patients died following cardiac surgery. Three patients died within 10 days of surgery and the 4th died suddenly 18 months after replacement of his aortic valve. The data obtained suggest that the probable mechanism of formation of mitral valve aneurysm is destruction of the aortic valve resulting in a regurgitant jet that strikes the anterior leaf of the mitral valve creating a secondary site of infection that leads to the development of an aneurysm. Perforation of these aneurysms occurred in 3 of these patients, resulting in MR and severe LV failure.

CARDIAC CATHETERIZATION BEFORE CARDIAC VALVE SURGERY

Several articles have been summarized in the past 2 years concerning the need for cardiac catheterization before valve replacement. The article by Sutton and associates in the *New England Journal of Medicine* in 1981 strongly suggested that catheterization was not necessary before most cardiac valve operations, but a large percent of the patients studied never had catheterization to know whether the noninvasive or purely clinical assessments were correct. In this article Hall and associates[70] from Newcastle upon Tyne, England, studied prospectively 106 consecutive patients with valvular heart disease in whom valve surgery was considered on clinical grounds to assess how frequently and accurately the need for valve surgery and the operation required could be specified on noninvasive grounds alone; history and physical examination, ECG, chest X-ray, and M-mode echo. Two-D echo also was performed in 65 patients. On the basis of this noninvasive assessment alone, the patients were assigned to group A if a definite surgical recommendation, including the operation required, could be made, or group B if catheterization was judged necessary before such a recommendation could be made. After they had been assigned to group A or B, all patients were catheterized. There were 62 patients in group A; subsequent catheterization and surgical findings confirmed that the surgical recommendation based on the noninvasive findings was correct in all patients. In 16 of these patients the surgeon was requested to operate on a specified valve or valves and also asked to inspect another valve or valves about which there was some doubt. In only 6 patients did the subsequent catheter resolve this doubt before operation. The remaining 44 patients were placed in group B. The most frequent reason for catheterization was doubt about severity of the valve lesion (24 patients). Such doubt was significantly more frequent in aortic or combined aortic and mitral valve than in mitral valve disease alone. Nine of the 24 patients had echoes that were interpreted as showing that valve disease was mild, and in all 9 subsequent catheterization proved this correct; This experience suggests that catheterization was unnecessary in these patients. The other 20 patients in group B were catheterized because of diagnostic doubt introduced by coexistent severe respiratory disease (8 patients), to assess the extent of suspected severe lesions in asymptomatic patients (4 patients), or to assess suspected associated nonvalvular lesions (8 patients), such as poor LV function or abnormal aortic anatomy. Therefore catheterization was not needed to establish the severity of valve disease or the valve operation required in 71 (67%) of the patients studied (all group A and the 9 patients with definite echo evidence of mild disease in group B), since noninvasive assessment did this with complete accuracy. I (WCR) continue to believe that cardiac catheterization, with relatively few exceptions, should be performed before sending a patient to a cardiac valve operation.

CARDIAC VALVE REPLACEMENT

Warfarin plus dipyridamole or warfarin plus aspirin after valve replacement

Despite the use of oral anticoagulation in patients with prosthetic heart valves, persistent thromboembolism warrants a search for improved methods of prevention. Chesebro and associates[71] from Rochester, Minnesota,

TABLE 5-6. *Thromboembolism and bleeding: actuarial analysis of events.**

YEAR	WARFARIN + ASA (N = 170)		WARFARIN + DIP (N = 181)		WARFARIN ONLY (N = 183)	
	N†	%	N†	%	N†	%
Percent Survivors Free of Thromboembolism						
1	149	98	164	99	166	97
2	85	96	110	99	135	97
3	20	96	28	99	81	97
Percent Survivors Free of Bleeding						
1	141	89‡	160	97	170	98
2	80	86‡	103	96	134	95
3	16	86‡	23	96	80	95
Percent Survivors Free of Thromboembolism and Bleeding						
1	138	87‡	158	95	165	95
2	76	84‡	103	95	129	91
3	15	84‡	23	95	77	91

* Deaths without event are withdrawn alive.
† Number still under observation without event.
‡ $p < 0.01$ compared with each of the other 2 groups.
ASA = acetylsalicylic acid; DIP = dipyridamole.

randomized patients receiving ≥1 mechanical prosthetic heart valve to therapy with warfarin plus dipyridamol (400 mg/day) or warfarin plus aspirin (500 mg/day) on the basis of location and type of valve and surgeon, and followed up with a concurrent, nonrandomized control group taking warfarin alone. In 534 patients followed 1,319 patient-years, excessive bleeding (necessitating blood transfusion or hospitalization) was noted in the warfarin plus aspirin group (23 of 170 [14%], or 6.0/100 patient-years) compared with warfarin plus dipyridamole (7 of 181 [4%], or 1.6/100 patient-years, p < 0.001), or warfarin alone (9 of 183 [5%], or 1.8/100 patient-years, p < 0.001) (Table 5-6). A trend was evident toward a reduction in thromboembolism in the warfarin plus dipyridamole group (2 of 181 [1%], or 0.5/100 patient-years) compared with warfarin plus aspirin (7 of 170 [4%], or 1.8/100 patient-years), or warfarin alone (6 of 183 [4%], or 1.2/100 patient-years). Adequacy of anticoagulation (based on 12,720 prothrombin time determinations) was similar in all 3 groups with 65% of prothrombin times in the therapeutic range (1.5 ≤ prothrombin time/control ≤ 2.5), 30% too low, and 5% too high. Warfarin plus aspirin therapy resulted in excessive bleeding and is contraindicated. Longer follow-up study is needed to determine whether further separation of the incidence of thromboembolism can be detected.

Hemodynamics after mitral valve replacement

Horstkotte and colleagues[72] from Dusseldorf, West Germany, compared the hemodynamic features of several different prosthetic heart valves that have equal tissue diameter (29 mm or comparable) in 75 patients with isolated MVR. These patients were catheterized approximately 1 year after operation while at rest and during bicycle exercise. There were 19 patients with the Bjork-Shiley (BS) standard prosthesis, 5 with a Hall-Kaster (HK), 7 with the Ionescu-Shiley (IS), 12 with Lillehei-Kaster (LK), 12 with a Starr-Edwards (SE) silastic ball, and 20 with a St. Jude (SJ). The PA and LA pressures were reduced significantly in all the groups postoperatively; however, PA and LA pressure was somewhat lower after BS and SJ

TABLE 5-7. *Comparison of hemodynamic data of valve prostheses. Reproduced with permission from Horstkotte et al.[72]*

	BS (N, 19)	HK (N, 5)	IS (N, 7)	LK (N, 12)	SE (N, 12)	SJ (N, 20)
External diameter (mm)	29	29	29	28.5	30	29
Total area (cm^2)	6.61	6.61	6.61	6.38	7.07	6.61
GOA (cm^2)	4.52	4.52	5.07	3.80	2.85	4.41
dp (mm Hg)	4.5 ± 1.6	5.2 ± 3.3	5.3 ± 1.6	7.1 ± 1.3	6.3 ± 2.0	2.3 ± 0.6
Q (cm^2)	2.2 ± 0.5	1.9 ± 0.5	1.9 ± 0.8	1.7 ± 0.3	1.8 ± 0.4	3.1 ± 0.8
Eff./GOA	0.49	0.42	0.38	0.45	0.62	0.70
Eff./total GOA	0.33	0.28	0.29	0.27	0.25	0.46

Data from patients at rest.
GOA = geometric orifice area of the prosthesis (area within the valve housing); dp = diastolic pressure difference area; Q = effective orifice area calculated by Gorlin formula; Eff./GOA = effective area to GOA ratio; Eff./total GOA = effective area to total prosthetic valve orifice area ratio.

implantation than the comparable pressures in other groups (Table 5-7). Average diastolic pressure gradients in patients at rest were 2.3 ± 0.6 mm after the SJ, 4.5 ± 1.6 after the BS, 5.2 ± 3.3 after the HK, 5.3 ± 1.6 after the IS, 7.1 ± 1.3 after the LK, and 6.3 ± 2.0 after the SE implantation. Effective valve orifice areas were calculated to be 3.1 ± 0.8 cm² in the SJ group and 2.2 ± 0.5 cm² in the BS group and even smaller in the other groups. Total volume regurgitation was not significantly different among the valve types examined by left ventricular angiography. The SJ prosthesis appeared to perform best in terms of lowest pressure gradients and largest effective orifice areas.

Starr-Edwards prosthesis

The Starr-Edwards (SE) noncloth covered silicone ball prosthesis (model 6120) has been widely used for MVR for >15 years. Miller and associates[73] from Stanford, California, investigated its performance characteristics at the 10–15 year follow-up (Fig. 5-11). Their study included 509 patients. Twenty-two percent of hospital deaths and 27% of late deaths were valve related. Overall 46 ± 2% of patients had a valve-related complication by 5 years, 62 ± 3% by 10 years, and 75 ± 4% at 14 years. No cases of mechanical failure of the valve were identified; however, 16% of the valve failures were due to valvular occlusion (thrombotic or tissue ingrowth), which was associated with a 79% mortality. Thromboembolism occurred at a linearized rate (%/patient-year) of 5.7. At 5 years 62 ± 2% of patients were free of thromboembolism and at 10 years, 55 ± 3% were free of thromboembolism. The risk of

Fig. 5-11. Composite function incorporating all valve–related morbidity and mortality. Includes all cases of valve failure plus complications which did *not* result in death or reoperation. Priority was given to valve failure over other complications in the compilation of this function. The instantaneous hazard was nonconstant (23% ± 2%/patient–year for the first postoperative year -vs- 6.2% ± 0.5%/patient-year thereafter [p < 0.05]). *ACH* = anticoagulant-related hemorrhage. *PVE* = prosthetic valve endocarditis. Reproduced with permission from Miller et al.[73]

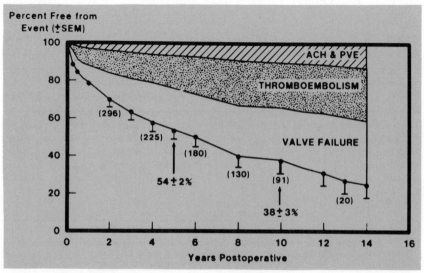

thromboembolism was significantly higher for the first year, but thereafter the probability of thromboembolism did not change significantly. The risk of anticoagulant hemorrhage was statistically constant through the entire postoperative follow-up. Total valve-related morbidity and mortality occurred at a linearized annual rate of 8.5% per patient-year. Only 38 ± 3% of patients were free of a serious valve-related complication 10 years postoperatively.

The 2320 SE aortic valve has a composite seat with metallic studs that protrude through the cloth. Warnes and associates[74] from Bethesda, Maryland, described certain clinical and morphologic findings in 6 patients who had this prosthesis in situ for 50–144 months (mean, 92). Considerable disruption of the cloth covering both struts and base and varying degrees of wear of the metallic studs that line the luminal side of the prosthetic ring occurred in each. Excessive stud wear resulted in severe disruption of the cloth lining the interior of the prosthetic ring. Cloth disruption may be associated with hemolytic anemia, embolic consequences, or both. Of 6 patients, 4 had severe hemolytic anemia, 4 had neurologic events compatible with emboli, and 1 died suddenly. Stud wear as observed in the 2320 series SE prosthesis also may occur in the models 2310 and 2400 prostheses, which have the same composite seat.

Rosenzweig and Nanda[75] from Rochester, New York, studied real-time 2-D echo of impaction of the SE mitral valve prosthesis with the LV wall in 8 patients (septum in 7, posterior wall in 1). One patient with echo evidence of posterior wall impaction died; necropsy revealed grooving of the LV posterior wall by the cage. Four of 7 patients with ventricular septal impaction developed ventricular arrhythmias in the in-hospital postoperative period, which were persistent and difficult to control in 2 patients, but were not fatal. None of the 22 patients without ventricular wall impaction had ventricular arrhythmias. Two-D echo appears to be useful in detecting LV wall impaction by mitral prosthesis.

Björk-Shiley prosthesis

Verdel and colleagues[76] from Utrecht, The Netherlands, developed a method in which cineradiography is used for the assessment of the opening angle of implanted Björk-Shiley prosthetic valves. The method is based on the fact that the ring and the disc, which are known to be circular, appear to be elliptical on x-ray films. The spatial position of the valve can be retrieved from the characteristics of these ellipses when vector analysis is applied. The method's accuracy does not depend on the position of the patient with respect to the direction of the x-ray beam. The accuracy of the method was demonstrated with the use of a phantom valve. The difference between the measured and the opening angle was −0.7°. Results were reproducible in patients to within −0.1°. In 18 patients with normally functioning valves, it could be demonstrated with frame-by-frame analysis that the valves opened very rapidly up to about 60°. Closing patterns varied. In 1 of the patients with valvular thrombosis insufficient valvular opening could be demonstrated by the method before the patient's complaints drew attention to the valvular dysfunction.

Olin and colleagues[77] from Stockholm, Sweden, addressed the problem of AVR in the small aortic root. A special technique for inserting large Björk-

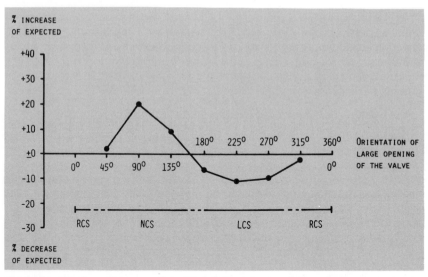

Fig. 5-12. Effective orifice area of the Björk-Shiley valve in relation to orientation of major opening of the prosthesis. *RCS* = right coronary sinus; *NCS* = noncoronary sinus; *LCS* = left coronary sinus. Reproduced with permission from Olin et al.[77]

Shiley valves without using outflow patches or anuloplastic procedures was developed. The method included allowing the right portion of the aortic incision to end about 0.5 cm above the noncoronary sinus, the use of simple interrupted sutures, placement of the prosthetic sewing ring on top of the anulus of the noncoronary sinus, thereby tilting the valve slightly in the outflow tract, and routine orientation of the major opening of the valve toward the anulus of the noncoronary sinus. This orientation resulted in the largest effective orifice area at postoperative catheterization. No man received a valve <23 mm and no woman was given a valve <21 mm. The convex/concave model was used in 71% of the patients. In this consecutive group of 250 patients, there were no operative deaths and all patients left the hospital in good condition. The combination of adequate myocardial protection, relatively short aortic cross-clamping, and the use of a large properly oriented Björk-Shiley valve resulted in perfect operative survival in this experience and is indeed an impressive performance. The authors have also provided information on operative technique and the orientation of this popular prosthetic device (Fig. 5-12). Other methods are available to relieve LV outflow tract stenosis in small aortic roots satisfactorily. These include placing various prosthetic devices in a supraanular position, tilting the device, or using the St. Jude prosthesis. Anuloplastic procedures may or may not add an incremental risk to AVR. The authors have shown that their technique has resulted in no mortality and have suggested that in each patient, an adequate sized prosthesis could be placed.

St. Jude medical prosthesis

To determine whether the flow characteristics of aortic and mitral St. Jude Medical prosthesis could be defined noninvasively, Weinstein and colleagues[78] from St. Louis, Missouri, analyzed Doppler transprosthetic flow velocity spectra in 23 relatively asymptomatic patients. Results were interpreted in the framework of M-mode and 2-D echo data and were compared with Doppler transvalvular flow velocity spectra from native valves of healthy subjects. Although the morphologic characteristics of Doppler spectra were similar, peak and mean transprosthetic mitral flow velocities were higher than values obtained across native valves. Calculated pressure half-times were not different and calculated transprosthetic mitral gradients were small. Similarly, the morphologic characteristics of aortic Doppler flow spectra in St. Jude and native valves were analogous. However, prosthetic valves exhibited higher peak and mean velocities and slightly prolonged time to peak flow. M-mode and 2-D studies did not show useful quantitative measures of prosthetic function and did not demonstrate evidence of paravalvular leaks, which were detected in 4 cases by Doppler techniques. Thus, Doppler echo provides quantitative information about transprosthetic flow characteristics in patients with implanted St. Jude prostheses and is useful in identifying patients with prosthetic dysfunction.

Porcine bioprostheses

Thompson and associates[79] from Pittsburgh, Pennsylvania, evaluated 10 patients with porcine heterograft valves not receiving anticoagulant agents to determine the effect of the valve on red blood cell survival and on platelet activation and consumption as measured by 1) quantification of the coagulation mechanism, 2) platelet function studies, and 3) chromium-51 platelet survival time. There was no evidence of significant intravascular hemolysis as determined by the reticulocyte count, serum iron and iron binding capacity, serum bilirubin level, or lactic dehydrogenase activity. The coagulation profile and the platelet function studies were normal. No statistically significant difference was found in the platelet survival time in the 10 patients with porcine heterograft valves (half-life, 3.2 ± 0.8 days) and the 11 normal control subjects (half-life, 3.6 ± 0.6 days) (p > 0.2). The finding of a normal platelet survival time in patients with porcine heterograft valves is consistent with clinical experience, indicating that this device is associated with a low incidence of systemic embolization, approximating 3% per year.

Lader and associates[80] from New York City described 2 patients who developed severe and medically refractory hemolytic anemia within several weeks of AVR with a porcine bioprosthesis. Additional valve replacement was necessary in both cases. Careful evaluation of the removed aortic prosthesis demonstrated perforation of the bioprosthetic cusps in both cases. Thus, perforation of a bioprosthetic cusp may lead to important hemolytic anemia, and this possibility should be considered in patients developing this abnormality following AVR.

To determine the clinical value of echo evaluation of porcine bioprosthetic valves, Alam and associates[81] from Detroit, Michigan, analyzed echoes in all patients who had porcine bioprosthetic valve replacement from 1978–1982. The study included 309 normal and 59 dysfunctioning bioprosthetic valves. Valve dysfunction resulted from spontaneous cusp degeneration in 39 (34 valve regurgitations, 5 stenoses), infective endocarditis in 12, paravalvular regurgitation in 5, regurgitation of redundant cusps, mitral valve thrombi, and aortic stent stenosis in 3 others. Echo findings were correlated with gross surgical pathologic or autopsy findings in 45 of the 59 dysfunctioning valves. Echo abnormalities were demonstrated in 41 of 59 (69%) dysfunctioning valves. A systolic mitral or diastolic aortic valve flutter was diagnostic of a regurgitant valve caused by a torn or unsupported cusp margin and was observed in 28 (82%) of 34 regurgitant valves with no false positive studies. Echo cusp thickness of ≥3 mm correctly identified all regurgitant and stenotic valves with gross anatomic evidence of localized or generalized cusp thickening or calcific deposits. Echo valve abnormalities were observed in only 4 of 12 patients with infective endocarditis and in 1 of 5 with paravalvular regurgitation. Thus, echo provides important information regarding the function of porcine bioprosthetic valves and is of value in the decision to replace these valves, especially when dysfunction is due to spontaneous cuspal degeneration. Echo is neither sensitive nor specific in patients with infective endocarditis and paravalvular regurgitation.

Effron and Popp[82] from Stanford, California, used 2-D echo to evaluate 80 patients with Hancock porcine heterograft valves. Abnormalities in these valves were subsequently characterized by type of valvular abnormality: group I, dysfunction due to primary tissue failure (41 valves); group II, dysfunction due to paravalvular leak without infection (5 valves); group III, infective endocarditis with or without hemodynamic dysfunction (28 valves); and group IV, control cases without dysfunction or infection (21 valves). Increased size of the heterograft leaflet image was observed in 46% of instances with primary heterograft failure and in 62% of those with leaflet vegetations due to endocarditis. Prolapse of leaflet echoes to below the level of the bioprosthetic sewing ring occurred in 76% of instances with torn leaflets and in 46% of valves with vegetations on intact leaflets. The only echo sign helping to distinguish infection from degeneration was extension of leaflet echoes beyond the level of stents, which was observed in 4 of 16 cases with leaflet vegetations. Thus, 2-D echo identifies some valves with leaflet degeneration or infection, but it does not allow a precise separation of these 2 clinical problems.

A high resolution method of spectral analysis of the class generally called "maximum entropy method," was used by Faole and coworkers[83] from Boston, Massachusetts, in a study of aortic porcine valve closing sounds in 37 patients. Spectra from 27 normal xenografts, implanted from 2 weeks to 61 months previously were characterized by a dominant frequency peak, F_1 at 89 Hz, with a lower amplitude peak, F_2 at 154 Hz. Eight of 9 patients with aortic porcine valve dysfunction were proved surgically to have leaflet degeneration or infection and had either F_1 139 Hz and/or F_2 195 Hz, significantly higher than normal. In 2 patients with paravalvar leak but no leaflet abnormality, F_1 and F_2 were in the normal range. Estimation of F_1 and F_2 was highly reproducible and was unaffected by duration of implant up to 5 years. Spectral analysis of aortic porcine valve closing sounds by the maximum entropy method may be useful for detection of intrinsic xenograft dysfunction.

To ascertain relations among site, incidence, and mechanisms of clinically evident failure of porcine bioprosthetic heart valves, Schoen and associates[84] from Boston, Massachusetts, reviewed the frequency of failure of 1,110 valves in 1,001 adult operative survivors from January 1972 to January 1982 and correlated the findings with morphologic features of 22 consecutive dysfunctional valves. There were 373 mitral, 519 aortic, and 109 double replacements, yielding for study 482 mitral and 628 aortic valves at risk. Infective endocarditis occurred in 1.9% (8 mitral, 7 aortic, and 4 double). Twenty-three valves (13 mitral and 10 aortic) with documented primary dysfunction were explanted, a mean of 55 months (range, 9–94) after surgery. The primary dysfunction rate for the 333 valves implanted for ≥5 years was 6.8% (11 of 161) for mitral and 4.1% (7 of 172) for aortic valves. Valves implanted for ≥5 years had a failure rate of 0.7%. The actuarially determined freedom from primary valve failure was 98 ± 1% for mitral and 98 ± 1% for aortic valves at 5 years and 79 ± 7% for mitral and 91 ± 4% for aortic valves at 10 years. Recovered valves (12 mitral and 10 aortic) with detailed morphologic analysis were functioning for a mean duration of 52 months (range, 12–87). Causes of failure included calcification-related tears in 7 (4 mitral and 3 aortic; mean, 66 months), tear without calcium deposits in 4 (4 mitral; mean, 44 months), cuspal stiffening without tear but with calcium deposits in 2 (1 mitral and 1 aortic; mean, 80 months) and thrombosis in 1 (aortic). Late primary dysfunction was most frequently a result of degenerative processes, especially calcification, often with secondary tears, but cuspal tears in the absence of calcium deposits and thrombosis predominated at shorter intervals.

Many reports have described degenerative changes in porcine bioprostheses implanted in either the mitral or aortic valve positions. None, however, have described morphologic alterations in bioprostheses in both positions in the same patient. The latter situation, of course, allows one bioprosthesis to serve as a control for the other. Warnes and associates[85] from Bethesda, Maryland, Orlando, Florida, San Jose, California, and Columbia, South Carolina, reexamined porcine bioprostheses implanted in both the mitral and aortic valve positions simultaneously in 5 patients, aged 20–61 years (mean, 45), 18–107 months (mean, 51) later. In 4 patients, the degenerative changes were distinctly more severe in the bioprostheses in the mitral than in the aortic valve position. The reasons for the more extensive degeneration of the bioprostheses in the mitral position are unclear, but at least these factors need consideration: 1) the closing pressure on the bioprosthesis in the mitral position is higher than on the bioprosthesis in the aortic position; 2) the pressure difference across the closed bioprosthesis in the mitral position is far higher than that across the closed bioprosthesis in the aortic position; and 3) the presence of a bioprosthesis composed of a semilunar valve in the AV valve position may prevent equal distribution of the LV systolic pressure on each of the cusps, whereas the aortic diastolic pressure is probably equally distributed on each of the 3 aortic valve cusps. Thus, it is not enough to know whether a patient has a mechanical valve or a tissue valve, but also it is important to know into which valve position the tissue valve is to be inserted.

Bovine parietal pericardial bioprosthesis

Szkopiec and associates[86] from Phoenix, Arizona, reported phonocardiographic findings in 19 patients with normally functioning Ionescu-Shiley prostheses in the mitral or aortic valve position. Opening clicks were recorded in all 8 patients with mitral prostheses at a mean second heart sound (A_2) to opening click interval of 94 ms. In 9 subjects, apical systolic murmurs were found. All 11 patients with the prosthesis in the aortic position had systolic ejection murmurs. Opening clicks were observed in 8 patients with a mean Q wave to opening click interval of 125 ms; closing clicks were found in 9 of 11. No diastolic murmurs occurred in this group. These acoustic characteristics serve as a reference source for the noninvasive evaluation of the bovine pericardial prosthesis.

Using M-mode and 2-D echo, Szkopiec and associates[87] from Phoenix, Arizona, characterized ultrasonic features of the Ionescu-Shiley valve. A 23 mm prosthesis was placed in a saline-filled chamber and subjected to pulsatile flow. Production of a linear tear at the base of a cusp resulted in coarse fluttering in the open position, and there was a reduction in the anterior cusp slope. Partial detachment of a cusp from its stent produced high amplitude low frequency fluttering during ejection. Alteration of transducer position eliminated the abnormal echoes. Fourteen patients with aortic and 11 with mitral prostheses were studied. There was a close approximation of echo-determined values for the bare stent internal diameter, cusp excursion, and valve orifice diameter compared with the manufacturer's specifications. Random punctiform echoes were noted when the cusps opened. Cusp echoes were superimposed on stent echoes in 21% of patients, and a third cusp was detected in 29%. Good quality 2-D echo was recorded in the vast majority of subjects. Cusp echoes were smooth and had a consistent motion in both the short and longitudinal axes. Multiple transducer positions were required to delineate prosthetic components with optimal clarity. It is concluded that 1) M-mode and 2-D echo is useful in assessing Ionescu-Shiley valve function, 2) in vitro valve tears or detachment produces characteristic cusp fluttering, 3) careful attention to transducer positions is necessary to record high quality valve images, and 4) these findings represent a data base for the longitudinal follow-up study of patients with the Ionescu-Shiley valve.

The Ionescu-Shiley bovine pericardial valve was evaluated in the USA by Gonzalez-Lavin and coworkers[88] from Palo Alto, California. Between 1977 and 1982, 168 patients underwent AVR with the Ionescu-Shiley device. There was 100% follow-up of the 156 patients discharged from the hospital. Thirteen died during follow-up, 5 with infective endocarditis, 1 of AMI, and 1 with CHF. The 4 other deaths were of noncardiac origin. Patients were not placed on anticoagulants. Thromboembolism occurred in 4 patients (1.3/100 patient-years). Bioprosthetic failure resulting from structural deterioration occurred only once and was due to calcification (0.3/100 patient-years). Disruption, tear, or perforation of the cusps was not encountered. The actuarial freedom from valve failure at 5 years was 96 ± 4%. The authors maintained that clinical performance in the surviving patients has been good. Of the 79 survivors who received a 17, 19, or 21 mm valve, all are in New York Heart Association class I or II.

Aortic valve homograft

Qureshi and associates[89] from Harefield, England, described results of MVR using unstented antibiotic sterilized aortic homografts in 379 patients followed 52–138 months (mean, 102 months). The most common cause of the valvular disease was rheumatic (321 patients). There were 37 early deaths (10%) and 97 late deaths (28%). The actuarial survival of operative survivors was 83 months at 3 years, 75% at 5 years, and 55% at 9 years.

Technical valve failure occurred in 6 patients (1.6%), infective endocarditis in 19 (5%), and degeneration of the valve in 43 (13%). The cumulative probability of freedom from valve degeneration was 97% at 5 years and 48% at 10 years. There were no early embolic episodes, but late embolism occurred in 5 patients (1.5%). Valve failure was described as valvular dysfunction necessitating reoperation or causing death regardless of ideology. Thus, this homograft valve produced results similar to those with porcine bioprostheses with perhaps a marginally slower rate of degeneration. In children the use of unstinted homografts offers the advantage of the slowest rate of degeneration of tissue valves currently available.

Porcine bioprosthesis -vs- Björk-Shiley prosthesis for mitral regurgitation

Marshall and colleagues[90] from Birmingham, Alabama, evaluated survival and the incidence of thromboembolism in 357 patients receiving a Björk-Shiley and 96 patients receiving a porcine bioprosthesis in the mitral position (Fig. 5-13). The median duration of follow-up was 46 months in the Björk-Shiley group and 32 months in the porcine bioprosthesis group. At 5 years, survival was 70% for the Björk-Shiley group and 68% for the bioprosthesis group (p, NS). The percentage of patients free of thromboembolic episodes was 77% for the Björk-Shiley and 78% for the porcine bioprosthesis. All patients in the Björk-Shiley group and 14 in the bioprosthesis group received long-term anticoagulant therapy. The presence of AF LA enlargement, preoperative thromboembolic episodes, and LA thrombus had no affect on

Fig. 5-13. Actuarial incidence of event–free survival following primary MVR. Reproduced with permission from Marshall et al.[90]

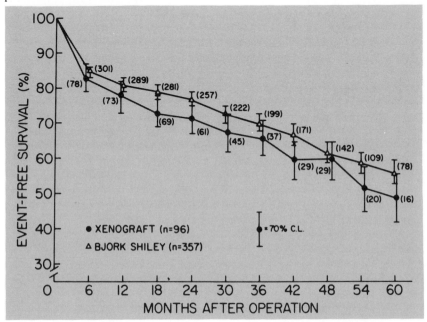

the incidence of thromboembolic complication with either prosthesis. Additionally when patients with AF and LA enlargement were compared with those with normal sinus rhythm and small left atria, there was no difference in the incidence of thromboembolism. The major advantage of the porcine bioprosthesis over the Björk-Shiley prosthesis is its use in patients in whom long-term anticoagulation is contraindicated. The choice of a prosthesis or necessity of anticoagulation need not be influenced by LA size, cardiac rhythm, the presence of preoperative embolus or the presence of LA thrombus.

Combined aortic valve replacement and aortocoronary bypass grafting

Nunley and associates[91] from Portland, Oregon, provided 10-year follow-up of patients having concurrent CABG and AVR. There were 197 patients operated on between 1969 and 1981. Operative mortality between the period 1969–1975 was 16% compared with 5% for the years 1976–1981 (p < 0.02). The incidence of perioperative AMI declined over the same period from 14–2% (p < 0.1). Functional class and LV end-diastolic pressure significantly influenced mortality, whereas age, sex, duration of symptoms, cardiac index, wall motion abnormality, type of valve lesion, and completeness of revascularization did not. Actuarial analysis shows a survival rate during the 10-year follow-up equal to that of patients undergoing isolated AVR (Fig. 5-14). Patients with combined AVR and CAD obtained by CABG a prognostic curve apparently determined by their valvular disease alone (Fig. 5-15). Long-term survival as it relates to the operative time frame demonstrates improved survival in the more recently operated group (p = 0.053).

Fig. 5-14. Relative survival for 197 patients having AVR with CABG and 595 patients undergoing AVR alone during 1970–1981. Relative survival is the ratio of the observed survival of the group in question to that of an age– and sex–matched group from the normal population. The increase in AVR-CABG relative survival in the sixth and tenth years indicates a slightly better than normal survival. Reproduced with permission from Nunley et al.[91]

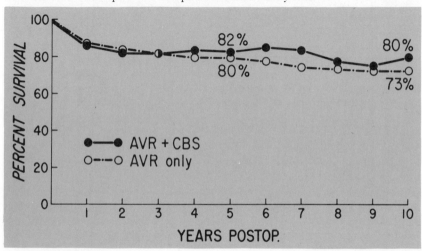

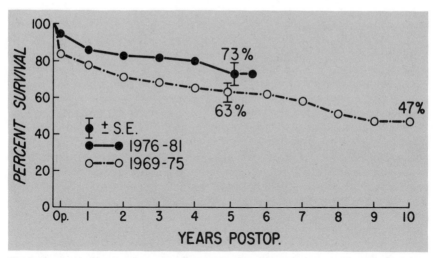

Fig. 5-15. Survival by time frame of operation for 96 patients having AVR with CABG bypass in 1969–1975 and 101 patients undergoing AVR with CAGB in 1976–1981. This difference approaches significance at 5 years (p = 0.053). Reproduced with permission from Nunley et al.[91]

Of 500 consecutive patients undergoing AVR and CAB reported by Lytle and associates[92] from Cleveland, Ohio, in the years from 1967–1981, 29 (6%) died in the hospital. Current operative mortality for 1978–1981 was 3%. Univariate and multivariate analyses were used to identify determinants of early and late risk. Female sex, AR, and advanced age increased in-hospital mortality, whereas use of cardioplegia decreased it. At follow-up of 471 patients who survived hosptialization for 1–135 months (mean, 41) after surgery, 96 late deaths were documented. At 2, 5, and 10 years after surgery, survival rates were 87, 80 and 55%, and event-free survival rates were 80, 65, and 39%, respectively. The late survival rate was unfavorably influenced by the presence of moderately or severely impaired LV function and 2-vessel CAD; the rate was enhanced for patients aged 50–59 years old and was not influenced by the method of myocardial protection. The event-free survival rate decreased with the presence of moderately or severely impaired LV function and was enhanced for patients with New York Heart Association class I or II symptoms before surgery. Patients with bioprostheses who did not receive anticoagulants had higher survival and event-free survival rates than did either patients with bioprostheses who received anticoagulants or patients with mechanical valves, whether they received anticoagulants or not.

Tricuspid valve replacement

Thorburn and associates[93] from Sydney, Australia, described observations in 71 patients having tricuspid valve replacement. The operative mortality rate was 10% and the actuarial survival rate was 73% at 5 years and 47% at 10 years (Fig. 5-16). Survival was unaffected by the number of valves replaced or the type used (27 Starr-Edwards, 32 Björk-Shiley, 8 Lillehei-Kaster, and 4 porcine xenografts). Complications were common: 3

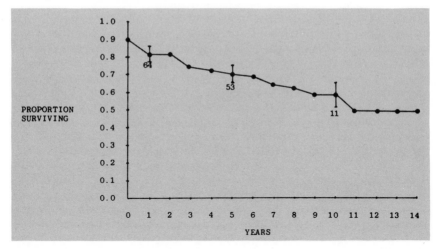

Fig. 5-16. Actuarial survival curve with 95% confidence limits for all patients (n, 71) undergoing tricuspid valve replacement.

deaths were related to anticoagulation and 1 was due to a systemic embolus. Six patients required permanent pacing. There was a very high incidence of thrombosis of the prosthetic tricuspid valve. Twenty percent of the tilting disc valves thrombosed, compared with 4% of the Starr-Edwards valves (p < 0.05). Symptoms of thrombosis were usually insidious, and its diagnosis was often delayed. There was a continuing risk of this complication, and presentation occurred up to 12 years after the original operation. Thrombolytic therapy with streptokinase was successful in 1 of 2 patients. Replacement of the thrombosed prosthetic valves was carried out without mortality in 8 patients.

Prosthetic valve regurgitation—its relation to heart rate and cardiac output

No well-controlled study previously had evaluated the influence of such factors as cardiac output or heart rate on backflow through prosthetic heart valves. Dellsperger and associates[94] from Shrevesport, Louisiana, studied 4 prosthetic aortic valves (size, 27 mm)—St. Jude Medical, Björk-Shiley spherical disc, Björk-Shiley convexo concave, and Starr-Edwards model 1260—in the aortic chamber of a pulse duplication system at heart rates of 50, 80, 110, and 140 beats/minute, cardiac output of 2, 4, 6, and 8 liters/minute, and mean aortic pressure of 100 mmHg. Regurgitation was calculated in percentage and found to vary directly with heart rate and inversely with cardiac output. The range of values obtained was 5.5% for the Starr-Edwards model 1260 valve at 110 beats/minute and 8 liters/minute to 37.5% for the Björk-Shiley convexo concave valve at 140 beats/minute and 2 liters/minute. Regurgitation ranged from 3.4 ml/stroke for the Starr-Edwards model 1260 valve at 140 beats/minute and 2 liters/minute to 17.3 ml/stroke for the Björk-Shiley spherical disc valve at 50 beats/minute and 2 liters/minute. Regurgitation associated with prosthetic heart valves may present a problem clinically, particularly under conditions of low cardiac output and tachycardia.

Reoperation for malfunctioning prosthetic cardiac valve

Husebye and associates[95] from Rochester, Minnesota, reported on risk factors associated with 552 patients undergoing reoperation for repair or replacement of a prosthetic heart valve. Operative mortality for the first reoperation (530 patients) was 6% for the aortic position and 20% for the mitral position. Overall operative mortality (for both positions) was 14% for second reoperation (69 patients) and 7% for third reoperation (14 patients). In addition to valve position, operative mortality for first reoperation appeared to be related to functional class and urgency of operation. The first reoperation mortality for mitral valve patients in New York Heart Association class II was 4%, class III, 9%, and class IV, 41%. In the aortic position reoperative mortality was 2% for class I, 2% for class II, 6% for class III, and 21% for class IV. The mortality for elective mitral valve reoperation was 0, for urgent reoperation, 23%, and for emergency procedures, 55%. Elective aortic valve reoperation carried a 1% mortality, urgent procedures, 8%, and emergency procedures, 38%. These data appeared to suggest that when significant prosthetic valve dysfunction is first noted reoperation should be undertaken to minimize operative risk. The 5-year survival rate for these patients was 73%, and this is compared with 8% in patients at the same institution undergoing initial AVR or MVR. The 2 survival rates are not comparable, since the reoperative study spans a 19-year experience as opposed to a 5-year follow-up in patients with initial valve replacement and the percentage of class IV patients undergoing reoperation was twice that of such patients undergoing initial valve replacement. The authors recommend that when significant prosthetic valve dysfunction is first noted operation should be undertaken to both minimize the operative risk and perhaps improve long-term survival.

Complications

Karchmer and associates[96] from Boston, Massachusetts, Richmond, Virginia, and Birmingham, Alabama, studied 75 episodes of prosthetic valve endocarditis (PVE) from *Staphylococcus epidermidis* retrospectively. Methicillin-resistant isolates caused 53 (87%) of 61 infections occurring within 1 year of valve replacement, but only 2 of 9 after 1 year. Resistance to methicillin was heterogeneic and extended to the cephalosporins. Of 55 isolates, 43 (78%) were susceptible to gentamicin and all to vancomycin and rifampin. In 55 patients PVE was complicated by tissue invasion or valve dysfunction. Among these 55 patients, 30 of the 32 who were cured needed surgery. Methicillin-resistant *S. epidermidis* causing PVE was cured in 21 of 26 patients treated with vancomycin and 10 of 20 treated with beta-lactam antibiotic therapy (p = 0.055). Cure rates of patients treated with vancomycin but not beta-lactam antibiotics were increased by the addition of rifampin or gentamicin to therapy. Vancomycin plus rifampin, or an aminoglycoside, should be used to treat PVE from methicillin-resistant *S. epidermidis*. Surgical intervention is important in treating complications of PVE.

Detection and quantitation of circulating immune complex (CIC) levels have been suggested as aids in diagnosis and assessment of therapeutic efficacy in active infective endocarditis (IE). In patients with acute bacteremic infections, however, CIC determinations have been of limited use in distinguishing valvular from nonvalvular infection. Conversely, in patients with active IE and a long duration of antecedent symptoms, CIC levels tend to be high (>101–200 $\mu g/ml^2$) and to differentiate patients with IE from those with bacteremias of other origin. Often associated with a subacute clinical onset is PVE, which would seem to be an ideal syndrome for measurement of CIC levels. Using the Raji cell radioimmunoassay, Hooper and associates[97] from Boston, Massachusetts, Los Angeles, California, and LaJolla, California, determined CIC levels in 36 patients with prosthetic valves during 38 episodes of fever. Fever resulted from PVE in 27 instances and from other causes in 11. Peak initial CIC levels higher than 100 $\mu g/ml$ occurred more frequently in the group with PVE, whereas peak initial CIC values less than 30 $\mu g/ml$ were more frequent in the control group. Levels of CIC decreased substantially with completion of antibiotic therapy in 28 (78%) of the patients with PVE. Late CIC elevations were associated with drug-related rashes and replacement of persistently infected prostheses. These data suggest that the predictive value of measurement of CIC levels in patients with fever and prosthetic valves is excluding PVE in patients with CIC levels persisting below 30 $\mu g/ml$.

Schoen and associates[98] from Houston, Texas, reviewed records of 378 patients who died after cardiac valve replacement and underwent autopsy at 1 hospital in Houston, Texas. The patients died from 1962–1979. Patients were divided according to postoperative interval at death: within 30 days (early) or 30 days to 10 years (late). Early deaths (279 patients) were due almost exclusively to cardiovascular abnormalities or operative complications (94%) (Fig. 5-17). Only 6% of early deaths were caused by prosthesis-associated complications. In contrast, late deaths (99 patients) were valve related in 47% of cases, including complete thrombotic occlusion or systemic thromboembolism (21%), prosthetic valve endocarditis (14%), valve dehiscence (6%), anticoagulation-related hemorrhage (3%), and mechanical degeneration (2%). Nine percent of late deaths were unrelated to cardiovascular disease. Thus, although early deaths primarily reflected the severity of

Fig. 5-17. Early and late causes of death after cardiac valve replacement, 1962–1979. Reproduced with permission from Schoen et al.[98]

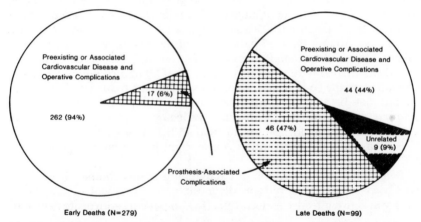

Early Deaths (N=279)   Late Deaths (N=99)

preexisting or associated cardiovascular disease, prosthesis-associated complications were an important cause of late death after cardiac valve replacement.

Physical, psychologic, social, and economic outcomes after cardiac valve replacement

Jenkins and associates[99] from Galveston, Texas, and Boston and Worcester, Massachusetts, studied before and 6 months after valve replacement 89 patients at 4 teaching hospitals. More than 60 indicators of the quality of life were assessed. Most persons showed improvement in physical function, emotional states, and social activity. Of those with exertional angina or dyspnea before surgery, about two-thirds were completely relieved at 6 months after surgery. There was a substantial reduction in number (from 31–7) of persons with 5 or more days of disability per month due to cardiac symptoms. The majority remained the same in their usual level of physical activity, most psychologic traits and attitudes, and social support networks. Most previously employed persons returned to work. Improvements in the conditions of patients who had had valve surgery closely paralleled those of patients who had undergone CABG in the same hospitals.

References

---

1. ROBERTS WC: Morphologic features of the normal and abnormal mitral valve. Am J Cardiol 51:1005–1028, March 1983.

2. DEPACE NL, MINTZ GS, REN JF, KOTLER MN, MATTLEMAN S, VICTOR MF, ROSS J, MINTZ PS: Natural history of the flail mitral leaflet syndrome: a serial 2–dimensional echocardiographic study. Am J Cardiol 52:789–795, Oct 1983.

3. OLIVEIRA DBG, DAWKINS KD, KAY PH, PANETH M: Chordal rupture, II: comparison between repair and replacement. Br Heart J 50:318–324, Oct 1983.

4. OLIVEIRA DBG, DAWKINS KD, KAY PH, PANETH M: Chordal rupture, I: aetiology and natural history. Br Heart J 50:312–317, Oct 1983.

5. BYRAM MT, ROBERTS WC: Frequency and extent of calcific deposits in purely regurgitant mitral valves: analysis of 108 operatively excised valves. Am J Cardiol 52:1059–1061, Nov 1983.

6. HUIKURI HV, IKAHEIMO MJ, LINNALUOTO MMK, TAKKUNEN JT: Left ventricular response to isometric exercise and its value in predicting the change in ventricular function after mitral valve replacement for mitral regurgitation. Am J Cardiol 51:1110–1115, Apr 1983.

7. DAVID TE, UDEN DE, STRAUSS HD: The importance of the mitral apparatus in left ventricular function after correction of mitral regurgitation. Circulation 68 (suppl II), II-76–II-82, Sept 1983.

8. LESSANA A, VIET TT, ADES F, KARA SM, AMEUR A, RUFFENACH A, GUERIN F, HERREMAN F, DEGEORGES M: Mitral reconstructive operations: a series of 130 consecutive cases. J Thorac Cardiovasc Surg 86:553–561, Oct 1983.

9. KAWAZOE K, BEPPU S, TAKAHARA Y, NAKAJIMA N, TANAKA K, ICHIHASI K, FUJITA T, MANABE H: Surgical treatment of giant left atrium combined with mitral valvular disease: plication procedure for reduction of compression to the left ventricle, bronchus, and pulmonary parenchyma. J Thorac Cardiovasc Surg 85:885–892, June 1983.

10. SAVAGE DD, GARRISON RJ, DEVEREUX RB, CASTELLI WP, ANDERSON SJ, LEVY D, MCNAMARA PM, STOKES J III, KANNEL WB, FEINLEIB M: Mitral valve prolapse in the general population, I. epidemiologic features: The Framingham Study. Am Heart J 106:571–576, Sept 1983.

11. SAVAGE DD, DEVEREUX RB, GARRISON RJ, CASTELLI WP, ANDERSON SJ, LEVY D, THOMAS HE, KANNEL

WB, FEINLEIB M: Mitral valve prolapse in the general population, II. clinical features: The Framingham Study. Am Heart J 106:577–581, Sept 1983.

12. SAVAGE DD, LEVY D, GARRISON RJ, CASTELLI WP, KLIGFIELD P, DEVEREUX RB, ANDERSON SJ, KANNEL WB, FEINLEIB M: Mitral valve prolapse in the general population, III. dysrhythmias: The Framingham Study. Am Heart J 106:582–586, Sept 1983.

13. GRENADIER EH, ALPAN G, KEIDAR S, PALANT A: The prevalence of ruptured chordae tendineae in the mitral valve prolapse syndrome. Am Heart J 105:603–610, Apr 1983.

14. ABBASI AS, DeCRISTOFARO D, ANABTAWI J, IRWIN L: Mitral valve prolapse: comparative value of M–mode, 2–dimensional and Doppler echocardiography. J Am Coll Cardiol 2:1219–1223, Dec 1983.

15. STRAHAN NV, MURPHY EA, FORTUIN NJ, COME PC, HUMPHRIES JO: Inheritance of the mitral valve prolapse syndrome: discussion of a 3–dimensional penetrance model. Am J Med 74:967–972, June 1983.

16. KOLIBASH AJ, BUSH CA, FONTANA MB, RYAN JM, KILMAN J, WOOLEY CF: Mitral valve prolapse syndrome: analysis of 62 patients aged 60 years and older. Am J Cardiol 52:534–539, Sept 1983.

17. CHESLER E, KING RA, EDWARDS JE: The myxomatous mitral valve and sudden death. Circulation 67:632–639, March 1983.

18. GAFFNEY FA, BASTIAN BC, LANE LB, TAYLOR WF, HORTON J, SCHUTTE JE, GRAHAM RM, PETTINGER W, BLOMQVIST CG, MOORE WE: Abnormal cardiovascular regulation in the mitral valve prolapse syndrome. Am J Cardiol 52:316–320. Aug 1983.

19. BOUDOULAS H, REYNOLDS JC, MAZZAFERRI E, WOOLEY CF: Mitral valve prolapse syndrome: the effect of adrenergic stimulation. J Am Coll Cardiol 2:638–644, Oct 1983.

20. PUDDU PE, PASTERNAC A, TUBAU JF, KROL R, FARLEY L, DE CHAMPLAIN J: QT interval prolongation and increased plasma catecholamine levels in patients with mitral valve prolapse. Am Heart J 105:422–428, March 1983.

21. HICKEY AJ, ANDREWS G, WILCKEN DEL: Independence of mitral valve prolapse and neurosis. Br Heart J 50:333–336, Oct 1983.

22. ROSENBERG CA, DERMAN GH, GRABB WC, BUDA AJ: Hypomastia and mitral valve prolapse: evidence of a linked embryologic and mesenchymal dysplasia. N Engl J Med 309:1230–1232, Nov 17, 1983.

23. GASH AK, CARABELLO BA, CEPIN D, SPANN JF: Left ventricular ejection performance and systolic muscle function in patients with mitral stenosis. Circulation 67:148–154, Jan 1983.

24. SHRESTHA NK, MORENO FL, NARCISO FV, TORRES L, CALLEJA HB, PALILEO MR, ESMELE LW, CABALLERO AC, LEANO RL: Two–dimensional echocardiographic diagnosis of left atrial thrombus in rheumatic heart disease: a clinicopathologic study. Circulation 67:341–347, Feb 1983.

25. HUIKURI HV, TAKKUNEN JT: Value of isometric exercise testing during cardiac catheterization in mitral stenosis. Am J Cardiol 52:540–543, Sept 1983.

26. DEWAR, WEIGHTMAN: A study of embolism in mitral valve disease and atrial fibrillation. Br Heart J 49:133–140, Feb 1983.

27. KAY PH, BELCHER P, DAWKINS K, LENNOX SC: Open mitral valvotomy: 14 year's experience. Br Heart J 50:4–7, July 1983.

28. JOHN S, BASHI VV, JAIRAJ PS, MURALIDHARAN S, RAVIKUMAR E, RAJARAJESWARI T, KRISHNASWAI S, SUKUMAR IP, SUNDAR RAO PSS: Closed mitral valvotomy: early results and long–term follow–up of 3,724 consecutive patients. Circulation 68:891–896, Nov 1983.

29. BONCHEK LI: Current status of mitral commissurotomy: indications, techniques, and results. Am J Cardiol 52:411–415, Aug 1983.

30. ROBERTS WC: Mitral commissurotomy: still a good operation. Am J Cardiol 52:A9–A10, Aug 1983.

31. ANTUNES MJ, COLSEN PR, KINSLEY RH: Mitral valvuloplasty: a learning curve. Circulation 68 (suppl II): II-70–II-75, Sept 1983.

32. SAVAGE DD, GARRISON RJ, CASTELLI WP, McNAMARA PM, ANDERSON SJ, KANNEL WB, FEINLEIB M: Prevalence of submitral (anular) calcium and its correlates in a general population–based sample (The Framingham Study). Am J Cardiol 51:1375–1378, May 1983.

33. NAIR CK, ARONOW WS, SKETCH MH, MOHIUDDIN SM, PAGANO T, ESTERBROOKS DJ, HEE TT:

Clinical and echocardiographic characteristics of patients with mitral anular calcification: comparison with age– and sex–matched control subjects. Am J Cardiol 51:992–995, March 1983.

34. TAKAMOTO T, POPP RL: Conduction disturbances related to the site and severity of mitral anular calcification: a 2–dimensional echocardiographic and electrocardiographic correlative study. Am J Cardiol 51:1644–1649, June 1983.

35. NESTICO PF, DEPACE NL, KOTLER MN, ROSE LI, BREZIN JH, SWARTZ C, MINTZ GS, SCHWARTZ AB: Calcium phosphorus metabolism in dialysis patients with and without mitral anular calcium: analysis of 30 patients. Am J Cardiol 51:497–500, Feb 1983.

36. CHIN ML, BERNSTEIN RF, CHILD JS, KRIVOKAPICH J: Aortic valve systolic flutter as a screening test for severe aortic stenosis. Am J Cardiol 51:981–985, March 1983.

37. EFFRON MK: Aortic stenosis and rupture of mitral chordae tendineae. J Am Coll Cardiol 1:1018–1023, Apr 1983.

38. OLSHAUSEN KV, SCHWARZ F, APFELBACH J, ROHRIG N, KRAMER B, KUBLER W: Determinants of the incidence and severity of ventricular arrhythmias in aortic valve disease. Am J Cardiol 51:1103–1109, Apr 1983.

39. LASKEY WK, SUTTON MS, UNTEREKER WJ, MARTIN JL, HIRSHFELD JW, REICHEK N: Mechanics of pulsus alternans in aortic valve stenosis. Am J Cardiol 52:809–812, Oct 1983.

40. NESTICO PF, DEPACE NL, KIMBIRIS D, HAKKI A, KHANDERIA B, ISKANDRIAN AS, SEGAL B: Progression of isolated aortic stenosis: analysis of 29 patients having more than 1 cardiac catheterization. Am J Cardiol 52:1054–1058, Nov 1983.

41. HESS OM, SCHNEIDER J, TURINA M, CARROLL JD, ROTHLIN M, KRAYENBUEHL HP: Asymmetric septal hypertrophy in patients with aortic stenosis: an adaptive mechanism or a coexistence of hypertrophic cardiomyopathy? J Am Coll Cardiol 1:783–789, March 1983.

42. OLDERSHAW PJ, DAWKINS KD, WARD DE, GIBSON DG: Diastolic mechanisms of impaired exercise tolerance in aortic valve disease. Br Heart J 49:568–573, June 1983.

43. FIORETTI P, ROELANDT J, BOS RJ, MELTZER RS, VAN HOOGENHUIJZE E, SERRUYS PW, NAUTA J, HUGENHOLTZ PG: Echocardiography in chronic aortic insufficiency: is valve replacement too late when left ventricular end–systolic dimension reaches 55 mm? Circulation 67:216–221, Jan 1983.

44. CARROLL JD, GAASCH WH, ZILE MR, LEVINE HJ: Serial changes in left ventricular function after correction of chronic aortic regurgitation: dependence on early changes in preload and subsequent regression of hypertrophy. Am J Cardiol 51:476–482, Feb 1983.

45. GAASCH WH, CARROLL JD, LEVINE HJ, CRISCITIELLO MG: Chronic aortic regurgitation: prognostic value of left ventricular end–systolic dimension and end–diastolic radius/thickness ratio. J Am Coll Cardiol 1:775–782, March 1983.

46. STEINGART RM, YEE C, WEINSTEIN L, SCHEUER J: Radionuclide ventriculographic study of adaptations to exercise in aortic regurgitation. Am J Cardiol 51:483–488, Feb 1983.

47. HUXLEY RL, GAFFNEY A, CORBETT JR, FIRTH BG, PESHOCK R, NICOD P, RELLAS JS, CURRY G, LEWIS SE, WILLERSON JT: Early detection of left ventricular dysfunction in chronic aortic regurgitation as assessed by contrast angiography, echocardiography, and rest and exercise scintigraphy. Am J Cardiol 51:1542–1550, May 1983.

48. JOHNSON LL, POWERS ER, TZALL WR, FEDER J, SCIACCA RR, CANNON PJ: Left ventricular volume and ejection fraction response to exercise in aortic regurgitation. Am J Cardiol 51:1379–1385, May 1983.

49. BOUCHER CA, KANAREK DJ, OKADA RD, HUTTER AM, STRAUSS HW, POHOST GM: Exercise testing in aortic regurgitation: comparison of radionuclide left ventricular ejection fraction with exercise performance at the anaerobic threshold and peak exercise. Am J Cardiol 52:801–808, Oct 1983.

50. GREY DP, OTT DA, COOLEY DA: Surgical treatment of aneurysm of the ascending aorta with aortic insufficiency. J Thorac Cardiovasc Surg 86:864–877, Dec 1983.

51. BRANDENBURG RO, TAJIK AJ, EDWARDS WD, REEDER GS, SHUB C, SEWARD JB: Accuracy of 2–dimensional echocardiographic diagnosis of congenitally bicuspid aortic valve: echocardiographic–anatomic correlation in 115 patients. Am J Cardiol 51:1469–1473, May 1983.

52. COME PC, FORTUIN NJ, WHITE RI, MCKUSICK VA: Echocardiographic assessment of cardiovascular abnormalities in the Marfan syndrome. Am J Med 74:465–474, March 1983.

53. Pyeritz RE, Wappel MA: Mitral valve dysfunction in the Marfan syndrome: clinical and echocardiographic study of prevalence and natural history. Am J Med 74:797–807, May 1983.

54. Nanna M, Chandraratna PA, Reid C, Nimalasuriya A, Rahimtoola SH, Butler M: Value of 2–dimensional echocardiography in detecting tricuspid stenosis. Circulation 67:221–224, Jan 1983.

55. Daniels SJ, Mintz GS, Kotler MN: Rheumatic tricuspid valve disease: 2–dimensional echocardiographic, hemodynamic, and angiographic correlations. Am J Cardiol 51:492–496, Feb 1983.

56. Brown AK, Anderson V: Two–dimensional echocardiography and the tricuspid valve: leaflet definition and prolapse. Br Heart J 49:495–500, May 1983.

57. Tei C, Shah PM, Cherian G, Trim PA, Wong M, Ormiston JA: Echocardiographic evaluation of normal and prolapsed tricuspid valve leaflets. Am J Cardiol 52:796–800, Oct 1983.

58. DePace NL, Ren JF, Kotler MN, Mintz GS, Kimbiris D, Kalman P: Two–dimensional echocardiographic determination of right atrial emptying volume: a noninvasive index in quantifying the degree of tricuspid regurgitation. Am J Cardiol 52:525–529, Sept 1983.

59. Meltzer RS, Vered Z, Benjamin P, Hegesh J, Visser CA, Neufeld HN: Diagnosing tricuspid regurgitation by direct imaging of the regurgitant flow in the right atrium using contrast echocardiography. Am J Cardiol 52:1050–1053, Nov 1983.

60. Ubago JL, Figueroa A, Ochoteco A, Colman T, Duran RM, Duran CG: Analysis of the amount of tricuspid valve anular dilatation required to produce functional tricuspid regurgitation. Am J Cardiol 52:155–158, July 1983.

61. Handler B, Pavel DG, Pietras R, Swiryn S, Byrom E, Lam W, Rosen KM: Equilibrium radionuclide gated angiography in patients with tricuspid regurgitation. Am J Cardiol 51:305–310, Jan 1983.

62. Land MA, Bisno AL: Acute rheumatic fever: a vanishing disease in suburbia. JAMA 249:895–898, Feb 18, 1983.

63. Stollerman GH: Global strategies for the control of rheumatic fever. JAMA 249:931, Feb 18 1983.

64. Holmberg SD, Faich GA: Streptococcal pharyngitis and acute rheumatic fever in Rhode Island. JAMA 250:2307–2312, Nov 4, 1983.

65. Bisno AL: Treating the patient with sore throat: theory vs practice. JAMA 250:2351, Nov 4, 1983.

66. Croft CH, Woodward W, Elliott A, Commerford PJ, Barnard CN, Beck W: Analysis of surgical versus medical therapy in active complicated native valve infective endocarditis. Am J Cardiol 51:1650–1655, June 1983.

67. Nakamura K, Satomi G, Sakai T, Ando M, Hashimoto A, Koyanagi H, Hirosawa K, Takao A: Clinical and echocardiographic features of pulmonary valve endocarditis. Circulation 67:198–204, Jan 1983.

68. Wong D, Chandraratna AN, Wishnow RM, Dusitnanond V, Nimalasuriya A: Clinical implications of large vegetations in infectious endocarditis. Arch Intern Med 143:1874–1877, Oct 1983.

69. Reid CL, Chandraratna AN, Harrison E, Kawanishi DT, Chandrasoma P, Nimalasuriya A, Rahimtoola SH: Mitral valve aneurysm: clinical features, echocardiographic–pathologic correlations. J Am Coll Cardiol 2:460–464, Sept 1983.

70. Hall RJ, Kadushi OA, Evemy K: Need for cardiac catheterisation in assessment of patients for valve surgery. Br Heart J 49:268–275, March 1983.

71. Chesebro JH, Fuster V, Elveback LR, McGoon DC, Pluth JR, Puga FJ, Wallace RB, Danielson GK, Orszulak TA, Piehler JM, Schaff HV: Trial of combined warfarin plus dipyridamole or aspirin therapy in prosthetic heart valve replacement: danger of aspirin compared with dipyridamole. Am J Cardiol 51:1537–1541, May 1983.

72. Horstkotte D, Haerten K, Seipel L, Korfer R, Budde T, Bircks W, Loogen F: Central hemodynamics at rest and during exercise after mitral valve replacement with different prostheses. Circulation 68 (suppl II): II-161–II-168, Sept 1983.

73. Miller DC, Oyer PE, Stinson EB, Reita BA, Jamieson SW, Baumgartner WA, Mitchell RS, Shumway NE: Ten to 15 year reassessment of the performance characteristics of the

Starr–Edwards model 6120 mitral valve prosthesis. J Thorac Cardiovas Surg 85:1–20, Jan 1983.

74. WARNES CA, McINTOSH CL, ROBERTS WC: Wear of the metallic studs on the composite seat of the 2320 Starr–Edwards aortic valve and its clinical consequences. Am J Cardiol 52:1062–1065, Nov 1983.

75. ROSENZWEIG MS, NANDA NC: Two–dimensional echocardiographic detection of left ventricular wall impaction by mitral prosthesis. Am Heart J 106:1069–1076, Nov 1983.

76. VERDEL G, HEETHAAR RM, JAMBROES G, VAN DER WERF T: Assessment of the opening angle of implanted Björk–Shiley prosthetic valves. Circulation 68:355–359, Aug 1983.

77. OLIN CL, BOMFIM V, HALVAZULIS V, HOLMGREN AG, LAMKE BJ; Optimal insertion technique for the Björk–Shiley valve in the narrow aortic ostium. Ann Thorac Surg 36:567–576, Nov 1983.

78. WEINSTEIN IR, MARBARGER JP, PEREZ JE: Ultrasonic assessment of the St. Jude prosthetic valve: M–mode, 2–dimensional and Doppler echocardiography. Circulation 68:897–905, Nov 1983.

79. THOMPSON ME, LEWIS JH, PORKOLAB FL, HASIBA U, SPERO JA, WILSON J, SNYDER M: Indexes of intravascular hemolysis, quantification of coagulation factors, and platelet survival in patients with porcine heterograft valves. Am J Cardiol 51:489–491, Feb 1983.

80. LADER E, KRONZON I, TREHAN N, COLVIN S, NEWMAN W, ROSEFF I: Severe Hemolytic anemia in patients with a porcine aortic valve prosthesis. J Am Coll Cardiol 1:1174–1176, Apr 1983.

81. ALAM M, LAKIER JB, PICKARD SD, GOLDSTEIN S: Echocardiographic evaluation of porcine bioprosthetic valves: experience with 309 normal and 59 dysfunctioning valves. Am J Cardiol 52:309–315, Aug 1983.

82. EFFRON MK, POPP RL: Two–dimensional echocardiographic assessment of bioprosthetic valve dysfunction and infective endocarditis. J Am Coll Cardiol 2:597–606, Oct 1983.

83. FOALE RA, JOO TH, McCLELLAN JH, METZINGER RW, GRANT GL, MYERS GS, LEES RS: Detection of aortic porcine valve dysfunction by maximum entropy spectral analysis. Circulation 68:42–49, July 1983.

84. SCHOEN FJ, COLLINS JJ, COHN LH: Long–term failure rate and morphologic correlations in porcine bioprosthetic heart valves. Am J Cardiol 51:957–964, March 1983.

85. WARNES CA, SCOTT ML, SILVER GM, SMITH CW, FERRANS VJ, ROBERTS WC: Comparison of late degenerative changes in porcine bioprostheses in the mitral and aortic valve position in the same patient. Am J Cardiol 51:965–968, March 1983.

86. SZKOPIEC RL, DESSER KB, BENCHIMOL A, SHEASBY C: Phonocardiographic findings in patients with normally functioning Ionescu–Shiley prostheses. Am J Cardiol 51:969–972, March 1983.

87. SZKOPIEC RL, TORSTVEIT J, DESSER KB, SAVAJIYANI RD, BENCHIMOL A, SOLOMON DK: M–mode and 2–dimensional echocardiographic characteristics of the Ionescu–Shiley valve in the mitral and aortic positions. Am J Cardiol 51:973–980, March 1983.

88. GONZALEZ-LAVIN L, CHI S, BLAIR TC, JUNG JY, GABAZ AG, McFADDEN PM, LEWIS B, DAUGHTERS G: Five–year experience with the Ionescu–Shiley bovine pericardial valve in the aortic position. Ann Thorac Surg 36:270–280, Sept 1983.

89. QURESHI SA, HALIM MA, CAMPALANI G, COE YJ, TOWERS MK, YACOUB MH: Late results of mitral valve replacement using unstented antibiotic sterilised aortic homografts. Br Heart J 50:564–569, Dec 1983.

90. MARSHALL WG, KOUCHOUKOS NT, KARP RB, WILLIAMS JB: Late results after mitral valve replacement with the Björk-Shiley and porcine prostheses. J Thorac Cardiovasc Surg 85:902–910, June 1983.

91. NUNLEY DL, GRUNKEMEIER GL, STARR A: Aortic valve replacement with coronary bypass grafting: significant determinants of 10–year survival. J Thorac Cardiovasc Surg 85:705–711, May 1983.

92. LYTLE BW, COSGROVE DM, LOOP FD, TAYLOR PC, GILL CC, GOLDING LAR, GOORMASTIC M, GROVES LK: Replacement of aortic valve combined with myocardial revascularization: determinants of early and late risk for 500 patients, 1967–1981. Circulation 68:1149–1162, Dec 1983.

93. THORBURN CW, MORGAN JJ, SHANAHAN MX, CHANG VP: Long–term results of tricuspid valve

replacement and the problem of prosthetic valve thrombosis. Am J Cardiol **51:1128–1132**, April 1983.

94. DELLSPERGER KC, WIETING DW, BAEHR DA, BARD RJ, BRUGGER JP, HARRISON EC: Regurgitation of prosthetic heart valves: dependence on heart rate and cardiac output. Am J Cardiol **51:321–328**, Jan 1983.

95. HUSEBYE DG, PLUTH JR, PIEHLER JM, SCHAFF HV, ORSZULAK TA, PUGA FJ, DANIELSON GK: Reoperation on prosthetic heart valves: an analysis of risk factors in 552 patients. J Thorac Cardiovasc Surg **86:543–552**, Oct 1983.

96. KARCHMER AW, ARCHER GL, DISMUKES WE: *Staphylococcus epidermidis* causing prosthetic valve endocarditis: microbiologic and clinical observations as guides to therapy. Ann Intern Med **98:447–455**, Apr 1983.

97. HOOPER DC, BAYER AS, KARCHMER AW, THEOFILOPOULOS AN, SWARTZ MN: Circulating immune complexes in prosthetic valve endocarditis. Arch Intern Med **143:2081–2084**, Nov 1983.

98. SCHOEN FJ, TITUS JL, LAWRIE GM: Autopsy-determined causes of death after cardiac valve replacement. JAMA **249:899–902**, Feb 18, 1983.

99. JENKINS CD, STANTON BA, SAVAGEAU JS, OCKENE IS, DENLINGER P, KLEIN MD: Physical, psychologic, social, and economic outcomes after cardiac valve surgery. Arch Intern Med **143:2107–2113**, Nov 1983.

6

Myocardial Heart Disease

IDIOPATHIC DILATED CARDIOMYOPATHY

Quantitative morphologic findings of myocardium

Schwarz and associates[1] from Heidelberg, West Germany, assessed the relation between quantitative morphologic findings and LV contractile function in patients with idiopathic dilated cardiomyopathy (IDC). The LV endomyocardial biopsy catheter specimens were obtained from 73 patients during diagnostic cardiac catheterization. All patients had normal coronary arteriograms but abnormal ECGs. Twenty-six patients had normal LV function (EF ≥ 55%), and 47 patients had contractile dysfunction (EF ≤ 54%). Myocardial fiber diameter, volume fraction of interstitial fibrosis, and intracellular volume fraction of myofibrils were determined by light microscopic morphometry. Results of light microscopic morphometry were confirmed by electron microscopic morphometry in 12 patients. The coefficient of variation (analysis of several biopsies from the same patient) was 6% for determination of fiber diameter, 43% for interstitial fibrosis, and 3% for volume fraction of myofibrils. Fiber diameter (r = −0.32; p < 0.01) and fibrosis (r = −0.47; p < 0.001) showed a negative correlation, the volume fraction of myofibrils (r = 0.55; p < 0.001) and calculated myofibrillar mass per 100 g of myocardium (r = 0.64; p < 0.001) a positive correlation with the EF. Thus, sampling error is low for determination of fiber diameter and myofibrils but high for evaluation of fibrosis, and a reduction in the volume fraction of myofibrils and an increase in fibrosis are morphologic correlates of LV dysfunction in patients with IDC.

Ventricular tachycardia

To evaluate the significance of VT in IDC, Huang and associates[2] from Chicago, Illinois, studied 35 consecutive patients (Figs. 6-1 and 6-2, Table 6-1). All patients had right- and left-sided heart catheterization, left ventriculography, and coronary cineangiography. Long-term ambulatory ECGs (Holter) were obtained in all patients at diagnosis. There were 24 men and 11 women, aged 22–72 years (51 ± 12, mean ± SD). Frequent (>30/hour) VPC were observed in 29 patients (83%): complex VPC (Lown grades 3, 4, and 5) in 93% and simple VPC in 7%. Twenty-one patients (60%) had nonsustained VT consisting of 3–46 beats (8 ± 5) with rates from 75–210 beats/minute. No difference between patients with and without VT was observed with regard to the presenting symptoms, functional classification, ECG findings, heart size on chest radiograph, and the hemodynamic measurements, including cardiac index, LV end-diastolic pressure, and EF. Patients with VT were older (p < 0.05). Follow-up observation from 4–74 months (34 ± 17) showed that 2 patients died suddenly (1 with and 1 without previous VT), a third patient died from intractable CHF, and the fourth, from sepsis. It is concluded that the incidence of ventricular arrhythmias in IDC is high, VT is frequent and tends to occur in the nonsustained form, and (3) there is no correlation between VT and the clinical and hemodynamic findings. In patients with IDC VT does not appear to predict prognosis during a relatively short follow-up period.

Fig. 6-1. ECG findings in patients with IDC. The numbers inside each bar represent number of patients with different ECG findings in the VT and the non-VT group. Left BBB or intraventricular conduction delay (IVCD) was the most common finding (54%). There were no significant differences in ECG findings in 2 groups. 1° AVB = first degree AV block; IACD = intraarterial conduction defect; LAD = left axis deviation; LAHB = left anterior hemiblock; LVH = left ventricular hypertrophy; RVH = right ventricular hypertrophy.

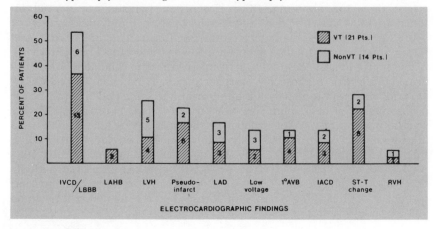

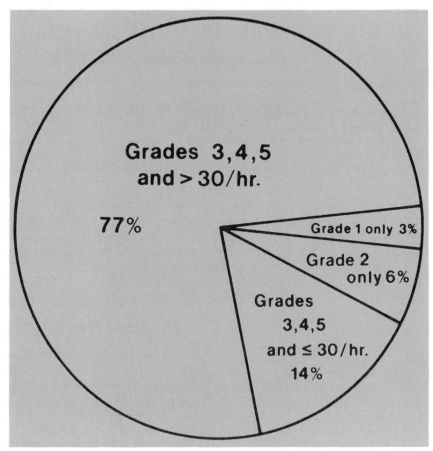

Fig. 6-2. The prevalence of ventricular arrhythmias by modified Lown's grades in 35 patients with IDC.

Regression of myocardial cellular hypertrophy with vasodilator therapy

Unverferth and associates[3] from Columbus, Ohio, evaluated 49 patients with IDC to determine the hemodynamic and morphologic effects of vasodilator therapy. Hydralazine (225 mg/day; H), isosorbide dinitrate (160 mg/day; I), and combination H plus I therapy were compared with placebo (P) at baseline and after 3 months of continuous therapy. Thirty-three randomly assigned patients completed the study. Hemodynamic parameters included the echo percent change of LV diameter (% ΔD), the systolic time intervals ratio of preejection period to LV ejection time (PEP/LV ET), the pulmonary capillary wedge pressure, mean pulmonary artery pressure, cardiac index, systemic vascular resistance, and pulmonary vascular resistance. An endomyocardial biopsy was performed at baseline and after 3 months; the myocardial cell diameter of 50 cells per biopsy was measured. During the 3-month study, 5 patients died; there was not a significant

TABLE 6-1. *Holter monitoring findings in 35 patients.*

	N	%
Atrial fibrillation	7	20
Atrial premature beats (>30/h)	15	54
Supraventricular tachycardia	7	25
Ventricular premature beats (>30/h)	29	83
Simple (uniform)	2	7
Complex (grades 3, 4, and 5)	27	93
VT	21	60

difference among the groups in the number of deaths. The % ΔD and PEP/LV ET did not change in the P or I groups but did improve significantly from baseline in the H and H plus I groups. The pulmonary capillary wedge and mean pulmonary artery pressures and the pulmonary vascular resistance did not change in the P or H groups but did decrease significantly in the I and H plus I groups. The P and I groups did not have improvement in systemic vascular resistance or cardiac index, whereas the H group had a decrease in systemic vascular resistance and an increase in cardiac index from 2.5 ± 0.4–3.1 ± 0.4 liters/min/M^2 (p < 0.05). The H plus I group also had a decrease in systemic vascular resistance; the cardiac index increased from 2.3 ± 0.4–3.1 ± 0.4 liters/min/M^2 (p < 0.01). Myocardial cell diameter did not change in the P or I group. Cell diameter of the H group decreased from 25.4 ± 3.1 μm at baseline to 23.1 ± 3.8 μm (p < 0.05) after 3 months of continuous therapy. The H plus I group decreased its cell diameter from 23.9 ± 3.7–22.2 ± 2.2 μm (p < 0.05). Compared with P and H, patients treated with I alone or H plus I had a significant reduction of preload. In contrast to P and I, H alone and H plus I elicited improvement in parameters of inotropy and afterload, and this improvement was accompanied by a reduction in cell diameter. Chronic therapy of heart failure with H and H plus I effects a persistent augmentation of cardiac function and improvement of myocardial cellular morphology.

Coronary dilatory capacity

Opherk and associates[4] from Heidelberg, West Germany, measured hemodynamic function and overall coronary blood flow (argon technique) in 16 patients with IDC and in 12 patients without detectable heart disease (controls) referred for precordial pain. In patients with IDC, coronary blood flow was normal at rest (78 ± 17 ml/100 g · min -vs- 78 ± 9 in control subjects). During maximal inducible coronary vasodilation (dipyridamole, 0.5 mg/kg), coronary blood flow was significantly reduced (142 ± 38 ml/100 g · min -vs- 301 ± 64 in control subjects; p < 0.001). Consequently, obtainable minimal coronary resistance was increased in IDC (0.54 ± 0.20 mmHg/ml/100 g · min -vs- 0.23 ± 0.04 in control subjects; p < 0.001). In patients with IDC, LV end-diastolic pressure was significantly increased (19 ± 11 mmHg -vs- 6 ± 3 in control subjects; p < 0.005), and the LV EF was diminished (36 ± 11% -vs- 72 ± 3% in control subjects; p < 0.001). In patients with IDC, LV end-diastolic pressure correlated significantly with the obtained minimal coronary resistance after application of dipyridamole (4 = 0.85; p < 0.001). The LV catheter biopsy specimens revealed no alterations in myocardial microvasculature. Thus, coronary dilatory capacity is impaired in patients with IDC, due partially to an increase in extravascular component of coronary resistance.

Mechanism of mitral regurgitation

Boltwood and coworkers[5] from Los Angeles, California, sought to evaluate the mechanism of MR in IDC. Quantitative 2-D echo was performed in 27 patients, 18 with IDC (9 with and 9 without MR on physical examination) and 9 without underlying heart disease. The MR and no MR patients were clinically comparable. Spatial reconstructions from multiple apical cross sections were used to estimate the mitral leaflet area needed to occlude the orifice for a given midsystolic coaptation configuration (LEAF) and mitral anular area index, LV volume, and LA volume. Similarly, reconstruction from parasternal short-axis views were used to estimate central chordae tendineae length and angulation. From selective parasternal views, papillary muscle length and contraction and the tethering length from its base to the anular plane were measured. The MR group was characterized by markedly enlarged occlusional leaflet area, striking mitral anular dilation, and LA enlargement. Chordal length and angulation, papillary muscle length, contraction, tethering length, and LV volume were not significantly different in the MR -vs- the no MR group. Noncoaptation of the mitral leaflets at their free margins was not observed in any MR patient with the use of stepwise linear regression. LEAF was determined chiefly by anular size, with LV size having little additional influence. Thus, IDC is associated with enlargement of the mitral anulus, which is more pronounced in those patients with MR. Based on the quantitative estimates of occlusional leaflet area, the investigators postulated that mitral leaflet tissue can stretch somewhat to accommodate dilation of the mitral complex, but as the requirement for occlusional leaflet area increases less tissue is available for coaptation. Thus, although coaptation continues to occur, the valvular seal becomes ineffective once a critical LEAF is reached. The chief determinant of LEAF is the mitral anular size, whereas LV size is a less important factor.

Usefulness of pulsed Doppler echo

The ability of pulsed Doppler echo to identify patients with LV systolic dysfunction was evaluated in 12 patients with IDC by Gardin and associates[6] from Orange, California. A range-gated, spectrum analyzer-based Doppler velocimeter was used to record blood flow velocity in the ascending aorta and pulmonary trunk. Doppler blood flow velocity data in the IDC patients were compared with data from 20 normal subjects. Measurements from the ascending aorta revealed that peak aortic flow velocity discriminated between IDC patients (mean, 47 cm/s; range, 35–62) and normal subjects (mean, 92 cm/s; range, 72–120) with no overlap in data (p < 0.001). Aortic flow velocity integral also was able to separate the patients with IDC (mean, 7 cm; range, 4–9) from normal subjects (mean, 16 cm; range 13–23) with no overlap in data (p < 0.001). Although mean values for average aortic acceleration and aortic ejection time also were significantly different (both p

< 0.005), there was some overlap between the 2 groups. The PA blood flow demonstrated significantly increased average acceleration and decreased ejection time (both p < 0.05), but no difference in average deceleration or peak flow velocity in IDC patients compared with normal persons was observed. Compared with PA flow measurements, aortic Doppler flow velocity measurements allowed better separation of IDC and normal groups. In addition, aortic peak flow velocity appeared to correlate well (r = 0.83) with M-mode echo measurement of LV percent fractional shortening; both parameters were equally useful in discriminating patients with normal LV function from those with global dysfunction. Thus, pulsed Doppler echo appears to be a useful addition to M-mode and 2-D echo in the quantitative noninvasive assessment of LV systolic function.

Left ventricular myocardial dopamine

The adrenergic nervous system is chronically activated in patients with chronic CHF. One consequence of this is depletion of the normally high levels of myocardial norepinephrine. Pierpont and associates[7] from Minneapolis, Minnesota, reported myocardial norepinephrine and dopamine concentrations from the LV walls of 3 patients undergoing cardiac transplantation for severe refractory CHF. The dopamine/norepinephrine ratios were high in all 3 patients (29, 58, and 26%). This finding supports data from nonhuman animal studies suggesting a change in the rate-limiting step of myocardial norepinephrine synthesis in CHF. Conversion of tyrosine to dopa by tyrosine hydroxylase is replaced as the rate-limiting step by inability to hydroxylate dopamine to norepinephrine. Thus, dopamine accumulates but norepinephrine is depleted.

Amrinone therapy

Leier and associates[8] from Columbus, Ohio, administered amrinone, 100 mg orally every 8 hours, to 13 patients with moderate to severe CHF for 1 month on an outpatient basis to determine the beneficial and undesirable effects of this new cardioactive agent in this setting. The patients received conventional CHF medications during the study. Ten patients who received conventional CHF medications alone served as a control group. Changes in functional classification were not significantly different between the 2 treatment groups. Amrinone augmented exercise capacity 37% above baseline compared with a 12% improvement for the control group. Noninvasive indexes of resting LV function (echo and systolic time intervals) did not change significantly for either group, nor was there a significant change in the exercise EF. All patients treated with amrinone had ≥1 symptom-related or laboratory-detected adverse effect. An increase in the frequency of VPC was noted at rest in 4 and with exercise in 6 patients (salvos of nonsustained VT in 2). Six subjects treated with amrinone had gastrointestinal symptoms and 8 developed a viral-like illness. Other adverse effects noted in the amrinone-treated group included near syncope, headaches, marked anxiety, chest pain, palpitations, maculopapular rash, hypokalemia, and elevation of serum transaminase levels. The control patients had significantly fewer adverse effects. Although individual patients with CHF may benefit from long-term amrinone therapy, the low benefit to risk of adverse effect ratio does not warrant widespread application of this drug in the outpatient management of CHF and requires caution when prescribing.

HYPERTROPHIC CARDIOMYOPATHY

Relation of ECG abnormalities to patterns of LV hypertrophy determined by 2-D echo

Maron and associates[9] from Bethesda, Maryland, assessed by wide-angle 2-D echo the distribution of LV hypertrophy in 153 patients with HC and compared the findings with the scalar ECG in the same patients. The most common ECG alterations were ST segment changes and T-wave inversion (61%), LV hypertrophy (47%), abnormal Q waves (25%), and LA enlargement (24%). The LV hypertrophy on the ECG was significantly more common in patients with the most extensive distribution of LV hypertrophy on 2-D echo involving substantial portions of both the ventricular septum and LV free wall (type III; 51 of 69, 74%) than in those with more limited distribution of LV hypertrophy (21 of 84, 25%; p < 0.001). Most patients with HC and normal ECGs (13 of 23) had localized (type I) hypertrophy, but only 4 had the extensive type III pattern of hypertrophy. Abnormal Q waves were significantly more common in those patients without hypertrophy of the anterior, basal septum (type IV; 15 of 27, 56%) than in those with basal septal hypertrophy (23 of 126, 18%; p < 0.001); abnormal Q waves were uncommon in extensive type III distribution of hypertrophy (13 of 69, 19%). Thus, although no single ECG abnormality is characteristic of HC, 2-D echo clarifies the significance of certain ECG patterns: 1) LV hypertrophy on the ECG, although present in only about half of the study group, was a relatively sensitive (74%) marker for extensive (type III) LV hypertrophy; 2) abnormal Q waves cannot be explained by ventricular septal hypertrophy alone; and 3) a normal ECG was most commonly a manifestation of localized LV hypertrophy.

Ventricular arrhythmia induction in the operating room

To evaluate vulnerability to ventricular arrhythmia induction, Anderson and associates[10] from Stanford, California, performed programmed electrical stimulation in the operating room in 17 consecutive patients undergoing myotomymyectomy for obstructive HC. A control group of 5 patients undergoing CABG with normal LV function and no previous AMI also were tested. Of the 17 patients with HC, 14 had inducible sustained VT or VF, 1 had inducible unsustained VT, and the remaining 2 had <6 VPC/minute. In contrast, none of the 5 control patients had an inducible sustained ventricular arrhythmia, 1 had inducible unsustained VT, and the remaining 4 had <3 VPC. The difference between the 2 groups with respect to induction of a sustained ventricular arrhythmia, unsustained VT, or <6 VPC was significant (p < 0.001). Thus, patients with severe obstructive HC are unusually vulnerable to ventricular arrhythmia induction.

Myocardial fiber diameter and regional distribution in the ventricular wall of normal adult hearts, hypertensive hearts, and hearts with HC

• Hoshino and coworkers[11] from Kyoto, Japan, measured myocardial fiber diameters to determine their distribution throughout the ventricular wall in normal adult hearts, hypertensive hearts, and hearts with HC. In normal adult hearts and hypertensive hearts, the diameter decreased from the inner to the outer third of the LV free wall and from the LV side to the RV side of the septum. In HC, these regional differences were preserved in the LV free wall but not in the septum. The diameter was greatest in the middle third of the septum where myocardial fiber disarray was widely distributed. The diameters of the fibers in the RV side of the septum were significantly larger than those of the fibers in the LV side of the septum in HC. This finding, in contrast to that in normal adult or hypertensive hearts, was considered to be related to the inward convex curvature of the LV chamber. Although there was no significant difference in the diameter of the myocardial fibers in the LV free wall between hypertensive hearts and hearts with HC, the diameters of those in the RV free wall, in the RV side of the septum, and in the middle third of the septum were significantly larger in HC than in hypertensive hearts. These investigators concluded that there is a transmural variation in myocardial fiber diameter in the LV free wall and the ventricular septum, and such transmural variation in HC is different from that in hypertensive hearts.

Number and size of myocytes and amount of interstitial space in the ventricular septum and in the LV free wall

The wall thickness of the myocardium depends on 3 variables: the number of muscle layers, the mean size of myocytes, and the percent area of interstitial space. To clarify the pathogenesis of asymmetric septal hypertrophy (ASH) in HC, Fujiwara and associates[12] from Kyoto, Japan, measured these 3 variables and wall thickness in the ventricular septum (VS) and in the LV posterior wall. The VS/LV ratio of wall thickness was correlated with the VS/LV ratios of the 3 variables in the hearts of 10 patients in HC with ASH and in 37 control patients without ASH (25 with no cardiac disease and 12 with systemic hypertension). The VS/LV ratios (mean ± SD) in hearts with HC were 1.6 ± 0.2 for wall thickness, 1.8 ± 0.3 for the number of transmural muscle layers, 0.9 ± 0.1 for mean size of myocytes, and 1.1 ± 0.1 for percent area of transmural interstitial space. The VS/LV ratios in control hearts were 1.0 ± 0.1 for wall thickness, 1.0 ± 0.1 for number of transmural muscle layers, 1.0 ± 0.1 for mean size of myocytes, and 1.0 ± 0.1 for percent area of interstitial space. The VS/LV ratios of wall thickness and transmural muscle layers correlated well. In hearts with ASH in HC, the number of muscle layers was greater in the VS (630 ± 80) and smaller in the LV free wall (360 ± 70) than in the control hearts (500 ± 60 and 480 ± 50, respectively). Thus, the pathogenetic factor of ASH in HC is an increased VS/LV ratio of the number of muscle layers, and the degree of ASH is determined by the combined abnormalities in the numbers of transmural muscle layers in the VS and the LV free wall.

Significance of LV outflow tract cross-sectional area

The morphologic determinants of subaortic obstruction in patients with HC are not completely understood. To define the relation between LV outflow tract orifice size and presence or absence of subaortic obstruction, Spirito and Maron[13] from Bethesda, Maryland studied 65 patients with HC and 16 normal controls by quantitative 2-D echo. The LV outflow tract area was measured at the onset of systole in the short-axis view in the stop-frame mode. The LV outflow tract area was significantly smaller in patients with HC and subaortic obstruction than in patients without obstruction. Of 21 patients with obstruction, 20 had a LV outflow tract area <4.0 cm², whereas 28 of 30 patients without obstruction had a LV outflow tract area ≥4.0 cm². The outflow tract area in patients with provocable obstruction was intermediate between the areas of patients with and without obstruction. The LV outflow tract area was significantly smaller in patients with HC than in normal subjects. These investigators concluded that the cross-sectional outflow tract area is closely related to the presence or absence of subaortic obstruction in patients with HC. Thus, the size of the outflow tract at the level of the mitral valve appears to be of major pathophysiologic significance in producing obstruction.

Mitral regurgitation (Doppler echo)

Kinoshita and associates[14] from Osaka, Japan, investigated by 2-D Doppler echo 28 patients with MR and HC: 14 had systolic anterior motion (SAM) of the anterior mitral leaflet and 14 did not. The Doppler technique detected MR in all 14 with SAM and in 7 of the 14 without SAM. Doppler signals of MR started immediately after the first heart sound. The MR flow was often distributed from the entire mitral orifice over the entire or the posterior half of the left atrium in the patients with SAM. In the cases without SAM, the MR was usually localized near the mitral orifice. These features are different from those observed in patients with MR of rheumatic origin or from MVP. The Doppler technique in these patients was as good as left ventriculography in detecting MR. The early systolic component of the murmur of HC is considered to result primarily from concomitant MR.

Morphologic expression of genetic transmission

To determine the degree to which LV morphology is similar in related patients with HC, 40 index cases with this disease and 66 of their affected first degree relatives were studied by Ciro and associates[15] from Bethesda, Maryland, with 2-D echo. A diverse variety of patterns of distribution of LV hypertrophy were identified. In 48% of patients, hypertrophy involved both the ventricular septum and anterolateral LV free wall: 20% of the patients showed hypertrophy involving LV regions other than the basal anterior ventricular septum; therefore HC could not be diagnosed from M-mode echo, and 2-D echo was required. In the remaining patients, hypertrophy either was confined to the anterior portion of the ventricular septum or involved the entire septum but not the free wall. The LV morphology was compared in pairs of first-degree relatives. Only 41 of 105 pairs of first degree relatives showed phenotypically similar hearts with the same pattern of LV hypertrophy. Morphologic similarity was most common in patients who had diffuse distribution of hypertrophy involving the septum and free wall. Further analysis of LV morphology was performed by assessing whether hypertrophy was present in each of the 10 segments of LV wall. Using this method, only 32 of 105 pairs of relatives were found to have a similar or identical morphologic LV appearance. Thus, almost all patterns of distribution of LV hypertrophy may represent expressions of genetically transmitted HC. Furthermore, the morphologic LV appearance is particularly variable and markedly dissimilar in most closely related individuals with the genetically transmitted form of HC. This marked morphologic variability in closely related patients suggests that in screening families for HC, both M-mode and 2-D echo should be used.

Relation to asymmetric septal hypertrophy in families

Emanuel and associates[16] from London, England, studied 19 families in whom HC and/or isolated asymmetric septal hypertrophy (ASH) occurred in successive generations. All 19 propositi had HC proved by cardiac catheterization and angiocardiography, operation, or necropsy. These 19 families consisted of the 19 propositi and their 39 siblings, 38 parents, and 23 children. Of these 119, 114 were examined or, if dead before the study, there was sufficient evidence from necropsy or operation reports to establish the diagnosis. In 5 (4 parents and 1 sibling) who had died before the study there was insufficient evidence to establish the presence or absence of heart disease. These 19 families were selected from >100 cases of familial cardiomyopathy with a minimum follow-up of 5 years. The main points leading to selection were the presence of the disease in 2 successive generations and the availability of the first degree relatives for examination. The families were divided into 2 groups: Subset I of 12 families in which 1 of the parents as well as the propositus had all the clinical manifestations of HC; and subset II of 7 families in which the propositus had proved HC and 1 of the parents had isolated ASH with no other manifestation of cardiovascular disease. Differentiation was made between relatives with clinical, radiologic, ECG, and echo signs of HC, and those in whom the only abnormality was in the ventricular septum and detected solely by echo. The term "isolated ASH" was applied to the latter if the ventricular septal/LV posterior wall ratio was ≥1/3. In subset I there were 12 propositi and 22 siblings. Nineteen of these 34 were found to have HC and one had isolated ASH; thus there were 20 affected. In subset II, there were the 7 propositi with 17 siblings. Eleven of these 24 had HC and 1 had isolated ASH; thus 12 were affected. Applying Smith's method of analysis, the expected number affected if the condition was inherited as a dominant characteristic was 20/1 in subset I and 13/4 in subset II. These figures did not differ significantly from those actually found, that is, 24 and 12, respectively. The conclusions are that in familial HC isolated ASH is part of the clinical spectrum and has the same genetic implications as HC. Thus, parents with clinical HC can produce offspring with either isolated ASH or clinical HC. Conversely, parents with isolated ASH can produce children with either anomaly. In all circumstances other than HC, ASH does not appear to be an inherited characteristic.

Relation of systolic anterior motion of anterior mitral leaflet to site of outflow pressure gradient

Nagata and associates[17] from Osaka, Japan, determined the mechanism of systolic anterior motion (SAM) of the anterior mitral leaflet and the localization of the LV outflow pressure gradient in 15 patients with obstructive HC by the combined use of real time 2-D echo and intracardiac manometry. The SAM was classified into 2 types based on 2-D echo findings. In type I, the echo sources of SAM were the anterially shifted mitral chordae and, in part, the papillary muscles. The intraventricular pressure gradient occurred at the level of the tip of the papillary muscle. The suprapapillary part of the outflow tract and the inflow part had a low pressure, but the apical portion had a high pressure. In the second type, the echo sources of SAM were the anterior and posterior mitral leaflets, which were oriented in such a way as to obstruct the LV outflow tract. The pressure gradient occurred at the level of the anterior and posterior mitral leaflets. The inflow tract and outflow tract just below the tips of the mitral leaflets had a high pressure in contrast to the type I SAM. The authors concluded the inappropriate and maloriented papillary muscles played an essential role in causing both types of SAM and LV outflow obstruction. The direction of the access of the papillary muscle was changed in late systole, moving its tip away from the ventricular septum and resulting in a simultaneous reduction in SAM.

Systolic anterior motion of the posterior mitral leaflet

Dynamic obstruction to LV outflow in patients with HC usually occurs when the anterior mitral leaflet moves forward in systole and approaches or contacts the ventricular septum. Maron and colleagues[18] from Bethesda, Maryland, identified by M-mode and 2-D echo 21 patients with HC who presented a unique pattern of mitral valve motion characterized by abnormal mitral valve coaptation and systolic anterior motion (SAM) of the posterior mitral leaflet. This abnormality was most reliably identified with 2-D echo in LV views obtained from the apex. At end diastole, the anterior and posterior mitral leaflets did not appear to coapt at their distal free margins. Rather, in mitral valve closure, the anterior mitral leaflet contacted the basal portion of the posterior mitral leaflet. Subsequently, during systole, the "residual" distal portion of posterior mitral leaflet approached or contacted the ventricular septum. Morphologic observations in 9 other patients with HC suggested that SAM of the posterior mitral leaflet is due to elongation of the middle scallop of its leaflet, which probably comes into apposition with the ventricular septum during systole by passing through the space created by the normal pattern of chordal attachments onto the anterior mitral leaflet. Of the 16 patients who underwent cardiac catheterization, 9 had basal subaortic gradients of 20–85 mmHg, which were apparently due to moderate or marked SAM of the posterior mitral leaflet. Ventricular septal myotomy-myectomies were performed in 2 patients and resulted in markedly diminished SAM of the posterior mitral leaflet in each and abolition of subaortic gradient in the 1 patient who underwent postoperative cardiac catheterization. Thus, in patients with HC, SAM of the posterior mitral leaflet 1) identifiable in about 10% of patients, according to a consecutively studied series; 2) constitutes a previously undescribed mechanism for dynamic subaortic obstruction; and 3) is due to a malformation of the posterior mitral leaflet.

Ventricular septal and free wall dynamics

Kaul and associates[19] from Los Angeles, California, used 2-D echo to evaluate ventricular, septal, and free wall alterations in 8 normal subjects and 8 patients with HC. Comparisons between normal individuals and those with HC demonstrated: 1) the lower and midseptal alterations did not appear different between the 2 groups; 2) the lower septum seemed to move more than the corresponding free wall; and 3) the upper septum moved and thickened less than the rest of the septum in both groups but was less mobile in patients with HC ($p < 0.05$). Thus, these observations indicate that the ventricular septum in HC is not akinetic.

Rest and exercise LV function

In a study carried out by Manyari and associates[20] from London, Canada, LV EF at rest and during exercise was measured in 19 HC patients without CHF by means of RNA. The results were compared with those in 20 normal subjects. Based on hemodynamic data, patients with HC were divided into 3 groups: in group I, no demonstrable LV outflow obstruction, 5 patients had a LV EF increase from 68% ± 9 (mean ± SD) at rest to 74% ± 9 during exercise ($p < 0.05$); in group II, latent obstruction, 6 patients had a LV EF at rest (75% ± 8) and at peak exercise (79% ± 7) that was not statistically different ($p > 0.05$); in group III obstruction present at rest, 8 patients had a LV EF at rest of 83% ± 9 that decreased significantly during exercise (76% ± 8; $p < 0.01$). In normal subjects resting LV EF was 66% ± 8; it increased to 76% ± 7 ($p < 0.001$). Exercise duration and exercise heart rate times BP product were lower in groups II and III. Thus, there are significant differences in LV systolic function both at rest and during exercise between major hemodynamic subgroups of HC based on presence or absence of LV outflow obstruction.

Verapamil's effect in children

Spicer and associates[21] from Ann Arbor, Michigan, studied the acute affects of verapamil in 9 patients aged 7 months to 19 years with HC. Diagnosis was made by echo in each. All patients were symptomatic; 7 had resting or provocable LV outflow tract gradients of 18–139 mmHg. Verapamil (0.1 mg/kg) was given as an intravenous bolus followed by an infusion of 0.007 mg/kg/minute. At rest, verapamil increased cardiac index from 3.3 ± 0.9–3.7 ± 0.9 liters/min/M^2 and decreased LV end-diastolic pressure from 19.3 ± 8.1–14.5 ± 6.9 mmHg. In addition, during supine bicycle exercise, verapamil resulted in increased total work performed, maximal cardiac index during exercise, decreased maximal exercise LV end-diastolic pressure from 21.9 ± 10.1–19.3 ± 10.4 and in LV outflow tract gradient from 31.2 ± 10.5–1.75 ± 1.7 mmHg. These studies indicate an excellent prompt result in terms of hemodynamic improvement with intravenous verapamil. No serious side effects were noted, although P-R interval increased in all patients.

Children with serious conduction system disease or the combination of LV end-diastolic pressure >20 mmHg and LV outflow tract obstruction >50 mmHg were excluded because of serious side effects in adults with this combination.

Atrial systole and LV filling and effect of verapamil

Many patients with HC have impaired LV rapid diastolic filling. To quantitate the contribution of atrial systole to LV filling, Bonow and associates[22] from Bethesda, Maryland, used RNA to study 30 normal volunteers and 42 patients with HC before and after oral administration of verapamil (320–560 mg/day). The LV time activity curves were constructed by combined forward and reverse gating from the R wave, and the onset of atrial systole was determined by the P-R interval. The percent of LV stroke volume filled during rapid diastolic filling and atrial systole then was computed. Peak LV filling rate during rapid diastolic filling was expressed in end-diastolic volume (EDV)/second. Peak rate of rapid diastolic filling was not different in normal patients and those with HC (3.3 ± 0.6 -vs- 3.3 ± 1.1 EDV/s) and was within the normal range in 34 patients with HC (81%). However, the contribution to LV filling volume by rapid diastolic filling was diminished in patients with HC (83 ± 7% normal, 67 ± 17% HC; p < 0.001) and the contribution of atrial systole was increased (16 ± 8% normal, 31 ± 18% HC; p < 0.001). The LV filling volume during atrial systole was above the upper normal limit of 31% in 17 patients (40%), including 13 patients with a normal peak filling rate. After verapamil, peak filling rate increased (to 4.2 ± 1.2 EDV/s; p < 0.001), percent LV filling during rapid diastolic filling increased (to 83 ± 7%; p < 0.001), and percent LV filling during atrial systole decreased (to 16 ± 9%; p < 0.001). Percent LV filling volume during atrial systole was abnormal after verapamil in only 3 patients (7%). Hence, although the peak rate of rapid diastolic filling may be normal in patients with HC, the contribution to LV filling by rapid diastolic filling is reduced and that of atrial systole is thereby increased. Increased rate and magnitude of rapid diastolic filling during verapamil is associated with decrease and normalization of the contribution of atrial systole to LV filling. These data suggest that many patients with HC are at risk of hemodynamic decompensation with the onset of atrial fibrillation or other tachyarrhythmias and loss of the atrial contribution to LV filling. This risk may be reduced during verapamil therapy.

Effects of verapamil on LV function

To investigate the effects of verapamil on LV systolic and diastolic function in patients with HC, Bonow and colleagues[23] from Bethesda, Maryland, studied 14 patients at catheterization with a nonimaging scintillation probe before and after serial intravenous infusions of low, medium, and high dose verapamil (total dose, 0.17–0.72 mg/kg). Percent change in radionuclide stroke counts after verapamil correlated well with percent change in thermodilution stroke volume, and changes in diastolic and systolic counts were used to access relative changes in LV volumes after verapamil. Verapamil produced dose-related increases in end-diastolic counts, end-systolic counts, and stroke counts. This was associated with a decrease in EF (83% control, 73% verapamil) and in the 10 patients with LV outflow tract gradients, a reduction in gradient (62 mmHg control, to 32 mmHg verapamil). The end-systolic pressure-volume relation was shifted downward and rightward in all patients, suggesting a negative inotropic effect. In 10 patients, LV pressure-volume loops were constructed with simultaneous micromanometer pressure recordings and the radionuclide time activity curve. In 5 patients, verapamil shifted the diastolic pressure-volume curve downward and rightward, demonstrating improved pressure-volume relations despite the negative inotropic effect, and also increased the peak rate of rapid diastolic filling. In the other 5 patients, the diastolic pressure-volume relation was unaltered by verapamil, and increased end-diastolic volume occurred at higher end-diastolic pressures; in these patients, the peak rate of LV diastolic filling was not changed by verapamil. The negative inotropic effects of intravenous verapamil are potentially beneficial in patients with HC by decreasing LV contractile function and increasing LV volume. Verapamil also enhances LV diastolic filling and improves diastolic pressure-volume relations in some patients despite its negative inotropic effect.

To determine the hemodynamic effect of verapamil at rest and during exercise, Hanrath and associates[24] from Hamburg, West Germany, studied 18 patients with HC before and after 7 weeks of treatment with oral verapamil (maximal dose, 720 mg/day). At rest and at peak exercise, verapamil produced a significant increase in LV systolic performance in terms of stroke volume index (rest, from 43 ± 11–53 ± 11 ml/M^2; $p < 0.001$; exercise, from 46 ± 11–51 ± 10 ml/M^2; $p < 0.01$), whereas heart rate decreased (rest, from 81 ± 14–70 ± 11 min^{-1}; $p < 0.001$; exercise, from 150 ± 21–141 ± 18 min^{-1}; $p < 0.01$). Cardiac index at rest and during exercise remained unchanged. Systolic vascular resistance did not change at rest, but decreased significantly during exercise (974 ± 243–874 ± 174 dynes/s/cm^{-5}; $p < 0.05$). After verapamil administration, PA pressures did not change at rest, but decreased significantly during exercise. This was probably due to a shift in the LV pressure-volume relation. The improvement in LV hemodynamics was associated with a significant increase in exercise capacity. The findings of this study indicate that in patients with HC, hemodynamic improvement at rest and during exercise can be achieved by chronic administration of verapamil.

TenCate and coworkers[25] from Rotterdam, The Netherlands, studied the effects of short-term administration of verapamil on LV isovolumetric relaxation and early and late diastolic filling dynamics in 10 patients with HC by a combined hemodynamic-ultrasonic technique. The LV pressures recorded with high fidelity macromanometers were determined simultaneously with M mode echo. After 10 mg of verapamil was given intravenously at the rate of 2 mg/minute, LV contractility and systolic pressure dropped significantly. The LV dP decreased from 1,947–1,489 mmHg/s, maximal velocity of the contractile element at zero load decreased from 50–42 liters/s, peak velocity contraction of the contractile element decreased from 37–29 liters/s, and LV systolic pressure decreased from 149–127 mmHg. The LV negative dP/dt increased from 1,770–1,477 mmHg/s, and the time constant of isovolumetric pressure decay was prolonged from 48–64 ms. The LV end-diastolic pressure rose from 21–23 mmHg. The time constant of isovolumetric pressure decay was calculated in 3 different ways, but none of these

measurements was influenced by verapamil. Time of isovolumetric relaxation, duration of rapid ventricular filling, and peak rate of LV lengthening
were not significantly influenced by verapamil and remained highly abnormal. In contrast, peak rate of LV posterior wall thinning declined further
after verapamil from 2.9–2.4 liters/s. The constructed pressure-dimension
loops did not show any change after verapamil. Plasma levels of verapamil in
8 of the 10 patients were in the therapeutic range; heart rate did not change.
The data of these investigators indicate that abnormal relaxation and
disturbed LV filling dynamics persisted after short-term administration of
verapamil. Further studies in well-defined subgroups of patients after long-
term oral treatment with verapamil are needed to establish the merits of
medical treatment of HC.

Follow-up of 10–21 years after partial septal myectomy

Beahrs and associates[26] from Rochester, Minnesota, reviewed the outcome in 36 consecutive patients who survived partial septal myectomy for HC
operated on between 1960 and 1972. All patients were followed until death
or until June 1981 (mean, 13.4 years). Of the 26 survivors, 17 had been more
than mildly symptomatic preoperatively, but only 1 remained so postoperatively. The operation was effective in relieving the obstruction (peak systolic
pressure gradient reduced from 79–8 mmHg [p < 0.001]) and MR was
relieved. No survivors' symptoms worsened, but 10 died late—4 suddenly, 5
from CHF, and 1 from a malignancy (Fig. 6-3). The 10-year survival rate was
77% (Fig. 6-4). No correlation with outcome was found with respect to age,
surgical approach, preoperative functional class, pressure gradient, LV end-
diastolic pressure, or presence of AF, but AF occurring late postoperatively

Fig. 6-3. Mortality (cardiac and noncardiac) and survivorship in 36 patients surviving septal
myectomy. Follow–up is 7–19 years (mean, 11.7).

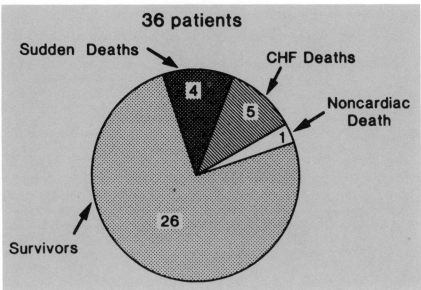

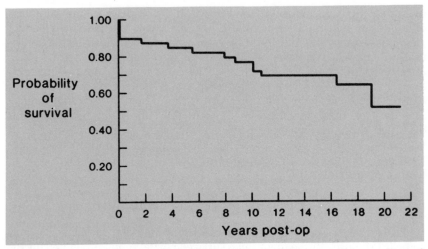

Fig. 6-4. Survivorship after septal myectomy for HC, including operative mortality and postoperative deaths (excluding 1 noncardiac death).

(12 patients) was associated with an increased frequency of late death (7 of 10 late deaths) or continuing New York Heart Association functional class III status. Early or late postoperative complete heart block occurred in 1 patient each. Thus, these results suggest a favorable effect of operation and support continued surgical intervention for appropriate patients.

CARDIAC AMYLOIDOSIS

Analysis of 54 necropsy patients with cardiac dysfunction

Roberts and Waller[27] from Bethesda, Maryland, described clinical and morphologic findings in 54 necropsy patients (32 men [59%]) aged 21–97 years (mean, 64) with cardiac amyloid deposits extensive enough to cause fatal cardiac dysfunction. Chronic CHF was present in 46 (85%). The duration of CHF, known in 39 patients, ranged from 1–108 months (mean, 18) and lasted ≤12 months in 25 patients (64%). All 8 patients without CHF died suddenly and unexpectedly. Systemic arterial pressures were recorded in the last 3 months of life in 43 patients: the peak indirect systolic pressure was ≤130 mmHg and the diastolic pressure <90 mmHg in all. The ECGs, recorded in the last 6 months of life in 40 patients, were abnormal in each: low voltage in 35 (63%); "myocardial infarction pattern" in 33 (83%); abnormal QRS axis in 29 (73%); arrhythmias in 29 (73%); first, second, or third degree heart block in 28 (45%); and complete BBB in 7 (18%) (Table 6-2). In 30 patients, the QRS amplitude in all 12 leads was measured: in the 15 men it ranged from 60–197 mm (mean, 99) (10 mm = 1 mV) and in the 15 women from 58–199 mm (mean, 109) (Table 6-3). Diagnosis of amyloidosis was established by biopsy of noncardiac organs or tissues during life in only

TABLE 6-2. *Cardiac amyloid causing cardiac dysfunction: ECG observations in 40 patients.**

ABNORMALITY [NO. (%)]	NO. OF PATIENTS (%)
1. Low voltage (QRS ≤ 15 mm in I + II + III)	25 (63)
2. Myocardial infarct pattern	33 (83)
Anterior = 26 (79)	
Posterior = 2 (6)	
Both = 5 (15)	
3. Abnormal QRS axis	29 (73)
Right (+111 to +210°) = 6 (21)	
Left (−30 to −90°) = 23 (79)	
4. Arrhythmias	29 (73)
Atrial fibrillation = 9 (31)	
Atrial or junctional tachycardia = 10 (34)	
Ventricular premature complexes = 21 (72)	
5. Heart block	18 (45)
P-R interval > 0.20 = 9 (50)	
2° AV block = 4 (22)	
3° AV block = 5 (28)	
6. Complete bundle branch block (QRS ≥ 0.12)	7 (18)
Right = 5	
Left = 2	

18 (33%) patients. During life the condition simulated HC in 5 patients, constrictive pericardial disease in 3, and CAD (because of angina pectoris) in 4. At necropsy, the hearts ranged in weight from 300–900 g (mean, 554), and all but 1 had a "rubbery," noncompliant consistency. In addition to their presence in myocardial interstitium (53 patients) and in intramural coronary arteries (54 patients) amyloid deposits were present grossly in mural endocardium in all 54 patients and in valvular endocardium in 46 (85%). The cardiac ventricles were not dilated in 43 patients (80%), but both atria were dilated in all 54 patients. Intracardiac thrombi were present in 14 patients (26%). Cardiac amyloidosis must be considered in any elderly patient with chronic CHF unassociated with chest pain when BP is normal and the ECG discloses low voltage and a pattern of "healed myocardial infarction."

Sensitivity of technetium-99m pyrophosphate for diagnosis

To determine the value of technetium-99m pyrophosphate myocardial scintigraphy in diagnosis of amyloid heart disease, Falk and associates[28] from Boston, Massachusetts, prospectively studied 20 consecutive patients with biopsy proved primary amyloidosis. Eleven patients had echo abnormalities compatible with cardiac amyloid, 9 of whom had CHF. Diffuse myocardial pyrophosphate uptake was of equal or greater intensity than that of the ribs in 9 of the 11 patients with echoes suggestive of amyloid, but in only 2 of the 9 with normal echoes, despite abnormal ECGs (p < 0.01). Increased wall

TABLE 6-3. *ECG QRS voltage (mm) in each of 12 leads in 15 men and 15 women with cardiac amyloidosis causing fatal cardiac dysfunction.*

CASE	NECROPSY NUMBER	AGE (YR) AT DEATH	INTERVAL (DAYS) ECG TO DEATH	LEADS I	II	III
		Men				
1	A63-125	32	88	6	10	6
2	Vt. MCV A75-174	35	56	4	4	3
3	A65-159	38	10	2	4	6
4	A70-254	38	2	2	2	5
5	A79-25	45	2	5	4	8
6	A81-6	46	13	5	5	5
7	NNMC 80A-15	49	107	6	3	4
8	A60-19	54	0	4	4	1
9	A56-81	55	23	2	3	2
10	A61-190	55	2	2	4	5
11	GT 74A-259	62	9	2	3	3
12	A65-232	65	103	7	20	12
13	A69-187	68	5	5	5	7
14	A67-241	68	35	9	5	6
15	A66-151	69	59	4	3	5
Mean		52	34	4.3	5.3	5.2
		Women				
1	A65-25	21	58	5	5	5
2	A68-23	48	50	4	3	3
3	GT 80A-262	50	91	4	3	3
4	A68-277	53	15	3	2	3
5	HU A77-19	54	51	5	2	8
6	Wil., D. WMC A79-24	55	8	1	8	9
7	SH A81-47	61	0	2	6	6
8	GT 71A-67	67	76	8	8	8
9	GT 81A-90	70	42	3	4	2
10	GT 71A-435	72	70	5	14	12
11	SH A79-76	75	30	7	10	7
12	GT 79A-127	78	49	3	5	4
13	WHC A82-120	82	6	5	8	12
14	GT 79A-195	89	160	3	5	1
15	Sibley A80-99	93	3	10	6	12
Mean		65	47	4.5	5.9	6.3
Total (mean)		58	41	4.4	5.6	5.8

thickness measured by M-mode ECG correlated with myocardial pyrophosphate uptake ($r = 0.68$; $p < 0.01$). None of 10 control patients with nonamyloid, nonischemic heart disease had a strongly positive myocardial pyrophosphate uptake. Thus, myocardial technetium-99m pyrophosphate scanning is a sensitive and specific test for the diagnosis of cardiac amyloidosis in patients with CHF of obscure origin. It does not appear to be of value for the early detection of cardiac involvement in patients with known primary amyloidosis without echo abnormalities.

TABLE 6-3. *ECG QRS voltage (mm) in each of 12 leads in 15 men and 15 women with cardiac amyloidosis causing fatal cardiac dysfunction. (Continued)*

| | | | LEADS | | | | | | TOTAL QRS | HEART |
R	L	F	V_1	V_2	V_3	V_4	V_5	V_6	12-LEAD	WEIGHT (G)
					Men					
8	4	7	11	23	16	14	11	9	125	700
4	3	4	5	9	9	11	13	8	77	750
2	5	6	5	19	11	6	9	7	82	410
1	3	3	4	18	16	16	9	5	84	600
2	6	6	12	27	21	22	30	15	158	780
4	4	3	2	10	17	19	19	13	106	545
3	6	3	14	20	15	12	9	4	99	850
4	3	3	10	10	3	10	8	5	65	550
2	1	3	5	9	11	11	7	4	60	480
3	4	5	3	15	14	12	12	6	85	535
2	2	3	1	6	23	21	11	2	79	470
11	3	15	8	15	24	32	27	23	197	560
3	6	6	13	16	11	9	8	6	95	550
7	7	3	11	7	13	15	12	6	101	420
3	5	4	7	10	11	8	5	4	69	450
3.9	4.1	4.9	7.4	14.3	14.3	14.5	12.7	7.8	99	570
					Women					
5	5	3	11	28	30	16	10	12	135	530
3	3	3	5	7	9	8	9	8	65	450
2	3	3	11	24	20	18	11	14	116	460
1	3	3	6	10	10	10	4	3	58	370
2	7	6	7	15	15	4	7	6	84	420
4	5	9	14	21	17	9	9	5	110	430
5	3	6	6	19	21	16	9	8	107	385
7	6	7	7	19	18	17	14	8	127	650
3	1	3	3	11	14	9	8	7	68	485
9	6	12	3	4	12	24	12	8	121	480
6	12	5	16	18	17	17	15	15	145	510
4	2	3	4	9	16	17	21	9	97	520
4	7	10	8	18	34	41	25	27	199	900
4	2	3	3	9	14	18	20	9	91	440
5	10	10	9	10	11	14	14	6	117	380
4.3	5.0	5.7	7.5	14.8	17.2	15.8	12.5	9.7	109	494
4.1	4.6	5.3	7.5	14.5	15.8	15.2	12.6	8.7	104	532

CARDIAC HEMOSIDEROSIS—EFFECTS OF IRON REMOVAL

The echo features of idiopathic hemochromatosis (IH) were studied by Candell-Riera and associates[29] from Barcelona, Spain, in 22 patients. The results were compared with a control group of 22 patients without heart disease. Statistically significant increases in LV mass, end-diastolic and end-systolic diameters of the LV, and in LA dimension were observed in patients with IH; significant changes of systolic function indexes (decrease in fractional shortening and EF and increase in distance of the E point to the septum) were seen as well. These echo abnormalities were mainly seen in patients with abnormal ECGs. In 11 patients with IH, iron removal therapy was carried out by means of periodic phlebotomies. In patients with impaired LV function at the beginning of therapy, comparison between measurements of the initial echo and posttreatment echo showed significant improvement in LV diameters, fractional shortening, EF, distance from the E point to the septum, LV mass, and LA dimension.

ENDOMYOCARDIAL DISEASE WITH OR WITHOUT EOSINOPHILIA

Two-D echo assessment

Cardiac manifestations in the idiopathic hypereosinophilic syndrome include MR and peripheral emboli. To determine the anatomic basis of these abnormalities, Gottdiener and associates[30] from Bethesda, Maryland, performed real-time, wide-angle, and 2-D echo in 21 patients with hypereosinophilic syndrome. Nine patients had MR and each had localized thickening of the posterobasal LV wall behind the posterior mitral leaflet, and absent (7 patients) or diminished motion (2 patients) of the posterior leaflet. Anatomic observations at operation or necropsy in 4 patients with MR demonstrated that the echo abnormalities resulted from posterior mitral leaflet thickening and adherence of the leaflet to the underlying mural endocardium of the posterobasal wall. On 2-D echo, each of the 6 patients with peripheral emboli had either apical LV echo-dense targets consistent with thrombus or thickening of the LV posterobasal wall, and these findings were validated at necropsy or operation in 3 patients. Therefore, in patients with the hypereosinophilic syndrome, 2-D echo is useful in identifying the probable etiology of 2 important cardiac manifestations.

Heart disease characterized by endomyocardial fibrosis is the major cause of morbidity and mortality in the idiopathic hypereosinophilic syndrome. Harley and associates[31] from Bethesda, Maryland, from their series of 50 patients with idiopathic hypereosinophilia, defined the noncardiovascular characteristics that distinguish patients at risk of developing endomyocardial fibrosis from those who remained free of heart disease (Fig. 6-5). These groups did not differ with respect to the extent of eosinophilia or the duration of disease. Patients with clinically overt heart disease were more likely ($p <$ 0.05) to be male, HLA-Bw44 positive, and to have splenomegaly, thrombocytopenia, elevated serum levels of vitamin B_{12}, hypogranular or vacuolated eosinophils, and abnormal early myeloid precursors in the peripheral blood. These idiopathic hypereosinophilic patients with heart disease also were more likely to have fibrosis and decreased megakaryocytes in the bone marrow. In contrast, those who remained free of heart disease tended to be female and have angioedema, hypergammaglobulinemia, elevated serum levels of immunoglobulin E, and circulating immune complexes. Therefore in the idiopathic hypereosinophilic syndrome, male patients with a myeloproliferative type disorder and the HLA-Bw44 haplotype were at a much

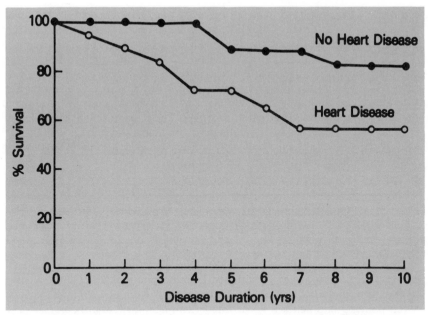

Fig. 6-5. The survival of patients with overt heart disease (○) compared with that in patients who remain free of heart disease (●).

increased risk for the development of endomyocardial fibrosis. However, those patients with a hypersensitivity-like illness and angioedema who were female did not develop heart disease. Appreciation of this relative degree of risk for the major complication of the idiopathic hypereosinophilic syndrome should prove useful in the early identification and appropriate treatment of patients in whom endomyocardial fibrosis might develop.

Surgical therapy

The surgical treatment of endocardial fibrosis has not been utilized with any frequency. Moraes and colleagues[32] from Recife and Sao Paulo, Brazil, collected 30 patients (26 females) with endomyocardial fibrosis who had endocardial decortication and AV valve replacement in the years 1977–1981. Their ages ranged from 14–48 years (mean, 32). Thirteen patients had biventricular disease. A RV endocardial decortication was performed in 27 patients, of whom 14 had isolated right-sided and 13 biventricular involvement. The right atrium was always dilated and thickened. This was opened and the tricuspid orifice exposed. There were 7 patients in whom an organized thrombus in the area of the atrial appendage was removed. The tricuspid valve was preserved in 4 patients but was resected in the remaining 23. The RV endocardial scar was entirely removed, care being taken to preserve the adjacent myocardium. In 16 patients with either biventricular disease or left-sided disease, LV endocardial decortication was performed by the same guidelines as used for right-sided disease. However, the LV approach varied according to LA size. Only 6 patients had a dilated left atrium and good exposure was obtained by a large atriotomy in them. In the remainder, the procedure was performed either by an incision in the atrial septum or by a left ventriculotomy. In only 2 patients was the mitral valve preserved; it was replaced by tissue valves in the other 14. There were 6 deaths during the postoperative period (20%). The main postoperative complication was AV dissociation in 5 patients. Twenty-four survivors were followed 3–53 months and 23 improved clinically. The mean cardiothoracic ratio decreased and the size of the RV cavity increased postoperatively and the LV configuration returned to normal. There were 5 late deaths. The authors suggest that because systolic performance of the heart is usually only slightly depressed and the surgical procedure is easily performed, operation ought to be done fairly soon in the course.

MYOCARDITIS—DIAGNOSIS AND CLASSIFICATION BY ENDOMYOCARDIAL BIOPSY

Fenoglio and associates[33] from New York City diagnosed myocarditis by endomyocardial biopsy in 34 patients with unexplained CHF. On the basis of both clinical and histologic findings, the patients were divided into 3 groups. Seven patients had acute myocarditis (mean age, 20 years; mean EF, 22%) characterized by an interstitial inflammatory infiltrate and extensive, acute cell damage. Five of these patients died after a mean duration of illness of 8 weeks. Eighteen patients had rapidly progressive myocarditis (mean age, 35 years; mean EF, 19%) characterized by patchy acute and healing cell damage and fibrosis; 17 of them died after a mean duration of illness of 23 months. Nine patients had chronic myocarditis (mean age, 31 years; mean EF, 31%) characterized by focal inflammation and cell damage. All 9 were alive after a mean follow-up period of 39 months. In 4 of these 9, clinical and hemodynamic improvement occurred after 1 month of immunosuppressive therapy. This study suggests that a clinically useful classification of myocarditis can be accomplished by endomyocardial biopsy. James[34] commented on this article in an accompanying editorial.

ARRHYTHMOGENIC RV DYSPLASIA

Arrhythmogenic RV dysplasia (ARVD) is a recently described entity characterized by RV myopathic changes and VT of RV origin. The presence or extent of LV dysfunction in ARVD is not known. Manyari and coworkers[35] from Calgary, Canada, assessed RV and LV function and size in 6 patients with ARVD by echo and RNA in patients at rest and during exercise. All patients had recurrent VT of left BBB morphology, and RV origin of the VT was confirmed by endocardial mapping in 4 patients. The results were compared with those of 10 normal subjects and 5 patients with WPW syndrome taking amiodarone. The latter was a control group, since the investigators did not withhold amiodarone therapy in 4 patients with ARVD. Mean RV Ef in patients with ARVD was 25% at rest and 26% during exercise. In normal subjects, RV EF was 51% at rest and 59% during exercise. The RV/LV end-diastolic diameter was 0.60 in patients with ARVD and 0.37 in normal subjects. The RV/LV end-diastolic volume ratio was 2.4 in patients with ARVD and 1.2 in normal subjects. Measured in patients at rest, a subnormal LV EF was present in 2 patients with ARVD, but an abnormal LV EF was present in all 6 patients during exercise. Mean LV EF in patients with ARVD was 57% at rest and 55% during exercise. In normal subjects, LV EF was 61% at rest and 72% during exercise. New LV wall motion abnormalities were seen during exercise in all but 1 patient with ARVD. At rest and exercise, LV and RV EF in patients with WPW syndrome were similar to those of normal subjects. The investigators concluded that RV dysfunction predominates in patients with ARVD, but latent LV dysfunction is present more often than is commonly recognized.

DOXORUBICIN CARDIOMYOPATHY

Clinical and morphologic cardiac findings

Isner and associates[36] from Bethesda, Maryland, evaluated the relation between clinical evidence of and histologic signs of anthracycline cardiotoxicity by reviewing the clinical and morphologic findings in 64 patients studied at necropsy, all of whom had received doxorubicin or daunorubicin chemotherapy during life. Of the 64 patients, 20 (31%) had docuumented clinical toxicity consisting of impaired LV systolic performance; in 7 (35%) of these 20 patients, histologic signs of toxicity were absent. In the remaining 13 patients with clinical toxicity, histologic signs of toxicity ranged from mild to severe. Of the 44 (69%) patients without clinical signs of drug toxicity, 21 (48%) had no histologic sign of cardiotoxicity; in 23 (52%) of the patients without clinical toxicity, however, morphologic signs of cardiotoxicity were nevertheless present, mild in most patients, but extensive in 4. Signs of extensive histologic toxicity (19 [30%] of 64 patients) were associated with large doses (>450 mg/M^2) of the drug, mediastinal irradiation, and age >70 years. This study suggests that attempts to monitor cardiotoxicity by serial evaluation of cardiac histology in patients undergoing anthracycline chemotherapy may be seriously limited by the fact that clinical evidence of toxicity may be present without histologic signs of toxicity; likewise, histologic signs of anthracycline toxicity may be present without clinical evidence of toxicity.

Radionuclide assessment

Although previous studies have demonstrated that sequential RNA allows identification of patients at risk for development of CHF and prediction of the appropriate time for safe discontinuation of doxorubicin, these studies were based predominantly on patients with normal baseline LV performance. A report by Choi and colleagues[37] from New Haven, Connecticut, addresses the use of doxorubicin in patients with abnormal LV EF ($<55\%$) prior to drug administration. Of 337 patients referred for evaluation of LV performance prior to doxorubicin therapy during a 36-month period, 45 (13%) had abnormal baseline LV performance determined by first-pass RNA. Sixteen patients had antecedent cardiovascular disease, and 16 patients had received thoracic radiation, whereas only 4 patients had both. The LV EF in each of these subgroups was comparable. In 7 of 16 patients who only had a baseline determination of LV function, doxorubicin was not administered because of a significant concern for the potential risk of doxorubicin cardiotoxicity. In the group of 29 patients followed sequentially 3–15 months (mean, 6 months), there was no significant difference between baseline and final LV EF (48 ± 5 -vs- 47 ± 9%). Only in the 12 patients who received ≥350 mg/M² cumulative dose was there a small but significant decrease in LV EF (48 ± 4 -vs- 43 ± 8%; p < 0.05). Only 1 patient developed CHF. This study demonstrates that doxorubicin can be administered safely to patients with abnormal baseline LV performance using serial radionuclide studies as a means of monitoring therapy.

McKillop and associates[38] from Stanford, California, examined radionuclide-determined LV EF at rest and during graded exercise in 37 patients receiving doxorubicin (Adriamycin) therapy in whom the risk of developing CHF was precisely defined by endomyocardial biopsy and right heart catheterization. Echo and phonocardiographic measurements of LV function were also determined. An abnormal LV EF at rest (≤45%) had a sensitivity of 53% and a specificity of 75% for detecting patients at moderate or high risk of developing CHF. The addition of exercise LV EF increased the sensitivity of detection of moderate or high risk patients to 89% but lowered the specificity to 41%. Exercise LV EF improved the sensitivity of detection of high risk patients from 58–100%. Echo fractional shortening and systolic time intervals yielded lower sensitivities than rest or exercise LV EF. As a single test, exercise LV EF possesses the sensitivity for use of a single value as a definitive test. Single rest LV EF determinations, although more specific than exercise LV EF, do not possess the sensitivity for use as screening or definitive tests.

RADIATION CARDIOMYOPATHY—DETECTION BY RA

Burns and associates[39] from Toronto, Canada, studied 21 asymptomatic adults by rest and exercise gated RNA 7–20 years after their having received 2,000–7,600 rads to the mediastinum for Hodgkin's disease. Twelve patients (57%) had abnormal LV (<53% at rest and/or >5% decrease at peak exercise) and/or RV (<27% at rest and/or >5% decrease at peak exercise) EF. Thus, rest and exercise RNA is a sensitive method for assessing systolic ventricular function and reveals a high prevalence of cardiac ventricular disease that can be linked to the previous radiotherapy.

ASSOCIATION WITH A CONDITION AFFECTING PRIMARILY A NONCARDIAC STRUCTURE

Sickle cell anemia

Covitz and associates[40] from Augusta, Georgia, studied cardiac performance by RNA at rest and during exercise in 22 adolescents with sickle cell anemia (SCA) and the results were compared with those in 12 control subjects. At rest, cardiac contractility was normal; cardiac output and end-diastolic volume were increased. At maximal exercise, heart rate, cardiac output response, and work capacity were reduced; the reduction was related to the degree of anemia. The LV end-diastolic volume decreased with exercise most markedly in patients with ischemic exercise ECGs. An abnormal EF response to exercise occurred in 4 patients; ECG signs of ischemia developed in all 4, and wall motion abnormalities in 2. Those patients who had ECG signs of ischemia had a significantly lower heart rate, EF, and cardiac output response to exercise, and a lower hematocrit level than subjects with normal results on exercise ECG. The increase in cardiac output was not sufficient to maintain a normal level of exercise. The decrease in end-diastolic volume suggests that diastolic function was abnormal during exercise. Cardiac dysfunction was manifested by an abnormal EF response, wall motion abnormalities, and incomplete LV filling during exercise.

Although ventricular dysfunction is suspected of underlying CHF in SCA, ejection indexes of LV pump performance have been found to be normal. The increased preload and decreased afterload of SCA increases the ejection phase indexes and might obscure true LV dysfunction. Denenberg and associates[41] from Philadelphia, Pennsylvania, compared the preload and afterload independent end-systolic stress-volume index in 11 patients with SCA and in 11 normal volunteers. End-systolic pressure and echo LV dimensions were determined during rest, leg raise, hand-grip, and amyl nitrite inhalation. Systemic vascular resistance (afterload) was decreased to $1,033 \pm 314$ dynes/s/cm^{-5} (mean $\pm$ SD) in SCA from $1,701 \pm 314$ dynes/s/cm^{-5} in normal subjects. End-diastolic volume index (preload) was increased to 102 ± 24 ml/M^2 in SCA from 66 ± 10 ml/M^2 in normal subjects. Cardiac index was increased to 4.7 ± 1.1 liters/min/M^2 in SCA from 2.8 ± 0.8 liters/min/M^2 in normal subjects. The EFs were similar: 0.59 ± 0.09 in SCA -vs- 0.62 ± 0.07 in normal subjects. However, in patients with SCA, the ratio of resting end-systolic stress-volume index was decreased (1.5 ± 0.5 in SCA -vs- 2.8 ± 0.6 in normal subjects) and the slope of the end-systolic stress -vs- end-systolic volume index relation was decreased (2.7 ± 1.3 in SCA -vs- 4.4 ± 1.8 in normal subjects), suggesting LV dysfunction in those patients. Thus, LV muscle contractile performance is depressed in SCA. Increased preload and decreased afterload compensate for the LV dysfunction and maintain a normal EF and high cardiac output.

Manno and associates[42] from Philadelphia, Pennsylvania, evaluated LV and RV function at rest and during exercise during radionuclide ventriculography in 10 patients, aged 19–53 years, with SCA. Seven patients were in New York Heart Association functional class I and 3 were in class II. The resting LV EF was normal in 9 patients and the resting RV EF was normal in 4. The LV dilation and high cardiac output were observed in 6 patients at rest. The LV EF during exercise was normal in all 10 patients, whereas only 2 patients had normal RV EF at rest and during exercise. The LV EF was lower in patients with SCA at rest ($54 \pm 4\%$ -vs- $61 \pm 6\%$; p < 0.001) and exercise ($66 \pm 4\%$ -vs- $74 \pm 6\%$; p < 0.001) than in 42 age-matched normal subjects. Rest thallium-201 images from 9 patients showed abnormal RV uptake in 8 and normal LV uptake in 8. Thus, in adult patients with SCA, LV function was normal during exercise in all patients and at rest in all but 1 patient. The LV EF, however, was lower than that in age-matched normal subjects. The RV function was abnormal in most patients at rest and during exercise. The RV thallium-201 uptake suggested pressure or volume overload (or both), most likely due to pulmonary vaso-occlusive complications of the disease.

References

1. SCHWARZ E, MALL G, ZEBE H, BLICKLE J, DERKS H, MANTHEY J, KUBLER W: Quantitative morphologic findings of the myocardium in idiopathic dilated cardiomyopathy. Am J Cardiol 51:501–506, Feb 1983.

2. HUANG SK, MESSER JV, DENES P: Significance of ventricular tachycardia in idiopathic dilated cardiomyopathy: observations in 35 patients. Am J Cardiol 51:507–512, Feb 1983

3. UNVERFERTH DV, MEHEGAN JP, MAGORIEN RD, UNVERFERTH BJ, LEIER CV: Regression of myocardial cellular hypertrophy with vasodilator therapy in chronic congestive heart failure associated with idiopathic dilated cardiomyopathy. Am J Cardiol 51:1392–1398, May 1983.

4. OPHERK D, SCHWARZ F, MALL G, MANTHEY J, BALLER D, KUBLER W: Coronary dilatory capacity in idiopathic dilated cardiomyopathy: analysis of 16 patients. Am J Cardiol 51:1657–1662, June 1983.

5. BOLTWOOD CM, TEI C, WONG M, SHAH PM, TRIM PA: Quantitative echocardiography of the mitral complex in dilated cardiomyopathy: the mechanism of functional mitral regurgitation. Circulation 68:498–508, Sept 1983.

6. GARDIN JM, ISERI LT, ELKAYAM U, TOBIS J, CHILDS W, BURN CS, HENRY WL: Evaluation of dilated cardiomyopathy by pulsed Doppler echocardiography. Am Heart J 106:1057–1065, Nov 1983.

7. PIERPONT GL, FRANCIS GS, DEMASTER EG, LEVINE TB, BOLMAN RM, COHN JN: Elevated left ventricular myocardial dopamine in preterminal idiopathic dilated cardiomyopathy. Am J Cardiol 52:1033–1035, Nov 1983.

8. LEIER CV, DALPIAZ K, HUSS P, HERMILLER JB, MAGORIEN RD, BASHORE TM, UNVERFERTH DV: Amrinone therapy for congestive heart failure in outpatients with idiopathic dilated cardiomyopathy. Am J Cardiol 52:304–308, Aug 1983.

9. MARON BJ, WOLFSON JK, CIRO E, SPIRITO P: Relation of electrocardiographic abnormalities and patterns of left ventricular hypertrophy identified by 2-dimensional echocardiography in patients with hypertrophic cardiomyopathy. Am J Cardiol 51:189–194, Jan 1983.

10. ANDERSON KP, STINSON EB, DERBY GC, OYER PE, MASON JW: Vulnerability of patients with obstructive hypertrophic cardiomyopathy to ventricular arrhythmia induction in the operating room: analysis of 17 patients. Am J Cardiol 51:811–816, March 1983.

11. HOSHINO T, FUJIWARA H, KAWAI C, HAMASHIMA Y: Myocardial fiber diameter and regional distribution in the ventricular wall of normal adult hearts, hypertensive hearts and hearts with hypertrophic cardiomyopathy. Circulation 67:1109–1116, May 1983.

12. FUJIWARA H, HOSHINO T, YAMANA K, FUJIWARA T, FURUTA M, HAMASHIMA Y, KAWAI C: Number and size of myocytes and amount of interstitial space in the ventricular septum and in the left ventricular free wall in hypertrophic cardiomyopathy. Am J Cardiol 52:818–823, Oct 1983.

13. SPIRITO P, MARON BJ: Significance of left ventricular outflow tract cross-sectional area in hypertrophic cardiomyopathy: a two-dimensional echocardiographic assessment. Circulation 67:1100–1108, May 1983.

14. KINOSHITA N, NIMURA Y, OKAMOTO M, MIYATAKE K, NAGATA S, SAKAKIBARA H: Mitral regurgitation in hypertrophic cardiomyopathy: non-invasive study by 2-dimensional Doppler echocardiography. Br Heart J 49:564–573, June 1983.

15. CIRO E, NICHOLS PF III, MARON BJ: Heterogeneous morphologic expression of genetically transmitted hypertrophic cardiomyopathy. Two-dimensional echocardiographic analysis. Circulation 67:1227–1233, June 1983.

16. EMANUEL R, MARCOMICHELAKIS J, WITHERS R, O'BRIEN K: Asymmetric septal hypertrophy and hypertrophic cardiomyopathy. Br Heart Journal 49:309–316, Apr 1983.

17. NAGATA S, NIMURA Y, BEPPU S, PARK YD, SAKAKIBARA H: Mechanism of systolic anterior motion of mitral valve and site of intraventricular pressure gradient in hypertrophic obstructive cardiomyopathy. Br Heart J 49:234–243, Mar 1983.

18. MARON BJ, HARDING AM, SPIRITO P, ROBERTS WC, WALLER BF: Systolic anterior motion of the posterior mitral leaflet: a previously unrecognized cause of dynamic subaortic obstruction in patients with hypertrophic cardiomyopathy. Circulation 68:282–293, Aug 1983.

19. KAUL S, TEI C, SHAH PM: Interventricular septal and free wall dynamics in hypertrophic cardiomyopathy. J Am Coll Cardiol 1:1024–1030, Apr 1983.

20. MANYARI DE, PAULSEN W, BOUGHNER DR, PURVES P, KOSTUK WJ: Resting and exercise left ventricular function in patients with hypertrophic cardiomyopathy. Am Heart J 105:980–987, June 1983.

21. SPICER RL, ROCCHINI AP, CROWELL DC, VASILIEDES AJ, ROSENTHAL A: Hemodynamic effects of verapamil in children and adolescents with hypertrophic cardiomyopathy. Circulation 67:413–420, Feb 1983.

22. BONOW RO, FREDERICK TM, BACHARACH SL, GREEN MV, GOOSE PW, MARON BJ, ROSING DR: Atrial systole and left ventricular filling in hypertrophic cardiomyopathy: effect of verapamil. Am J Cardiol 51:1386–1391, May 1983.

23. BONOW RO, OSTROW HG, ROSING DR, CANON RO III, LIPSON LC, MARON BJ, KENT KM, BACHARACH SL, GREEN MV: Effects of verapamil on left ventricular systolic and diastolic function in patients with hypertrophic cardiomyopathy: pressure-volume analysis with a nonimaging scintillation probe. Circulation 68:1062–1073, Nov 1983.

24. HANRATH P, SCHLUTER M, SONNTAG E, DIEMERT J, BLEIFELD W: Influence of verapamil therapy on left ventricular performance at rest and during exercise in hypertrophic cardiomyopathy. Am J Cardiol 52:544–548, Sept 1983.

25. TENCATE FJ, SERRUYS PW, MEY S, ROELANDT J: Effects of short-term administration of verapamil in left ventricular relaxation and filling dynamics measured by a combined hemodynamic-ultrasonic technique in patients with hypertrophic cardiomyopathy. Circulation 68:1274–1279, Dec 1983.

26. BEAHRS MM, TAJIK AJ, SEWARD JB, GIULIANI ER, McGOON DC: Hypertrophic obstructive cardiomyopathy: ten- to 21-Year follow-up after partial septal myectomy. Am J Cardiol 51:1160–1166, Apr 1983.

27. ROBERTS WC, WALLER BF: Cardiac amyloidosis causing cardiac dysfunction: analysis of 54 necropsy patients. Am J Cardiol 52:137–146, July 1983

28. FALK RH, LEE VW, RUBINOW A, HOOD WB, COHEN AS: Sensitivity of technetium-99m-pyrophosphate scintigraphy in diagnosing cardiac amyloidosis. Am J Cardiol 51:826–830, March 1983.

29. CANDELL-RIERA J, LU L, SERES L, GONZALEZ JB, BATLLE J, PERMANYER-MIRALDA G, DELCASTILLO G, SOLER-SOLER J: Cardiac hemochromatosis: beneficial effects of iron removal therapy. An echocardiographic study. Am J Cardiol 52:824–829, Oct 1983.

30. GOTTDIENER JS, MARON BJ, SCHOOLEY RT, HARLEY JB, ROBERTS WC, FAUCI AS: Two-dimensional echocardiographic assessment of the idiopathic hypereosinophilic syndrome. Anatomic basis of mitral regurgitation and peripheral embolization. Circulation 67:572–578, March 1983.

31. HARLEY JB, FAUCI AS, GRALNICK HR: Noncardiovascular findings associated with heart disease in the idiopathic hypereosinophilic syndrome. Am J Cardiol 52:321–324, Aug 1983.

32. MORAES CR, BUFFOLO E, LIMA R, VICTOR E, LIRA V, ESCOBAR M, RODRIGUES J, SARAIVA L, ANDRADE JC: Surgical treatment of endomyocardial fibrosis. J Thorac Cardiovasc Surg 85:738–745, May 1983

33. FENOGLIO JJ, URSELL PC, KELLOGG CE, DRUSIN RE, WEISS MB: Diagnosis and classification of myocarditis by endomyocardial biopsy. N Engl J Med 308:12–18, Jan 6, 1983.

34. JAMES TN: Myocarditis and cardiomyopathy. N Engl J Med 308:39–41, Jan 6, 1983.

35. MANYARI DE, KLEIN GJ, GULAMHUSEIN S, KOSTUK WJ, BOUGHNER D, GUIRAUDON GM, WYSE GL, MITCHELL LB: Arrhythmogenic right ventricular dysplasia: a generalized cardiomyopathy? Circulation 68:251–257, Aug 1983.

36. ISNER JM, FERRANS VJ, COHEN SR, WITKIND BG, VIRMANI R, GOTTDIENER JS, BECK JR, ROBERTS WC: Clinical and morphologic cardiac findings after anthracycline chemotherapy. Am J Cardiol 51:1167–1174, Apr 1983.

37. Choi BW, Berger HJ, Schwartz PE, Alexander J, Wackers FJ, Gottschald A, Zaret BL: Serial radionuclide assessment of doxorubicin cardiotoxicity in cancer patients with abnormal baseline resting left ventricular performance. Am Heart J 106:638–643, Oct 1983.

38. McKillop JH, Bristow MR, Goris ML, Billingham ME, Bockemuehl K: Sensitivity and specificity of radionuclide ejection fractions in doxorubicin cardiotoxocity. Am Heart J 106:1148–1156, Nov 1983.

39. Burns RJ, Bar-Shlomo BZ, Druck MN, Herman JG, Gilbert BW, Perrault DJ, McLaughlin PR: Detection of radiation cardiomyopathy by gated radionuclide angiography. Am J Med 74:297–302, Feb 1983.

40. Covitz W, Eubig C, Balfour IC, Jerath R, Alpert BS, Strong WB, Durant RH, Hadden BG: Exercise-induced cardiac dysfunction in sickle cell anemia: a radionuclide study. Am J Cardiol 51:570–575, Feb 1983.

41. Denenberg BS, Criner G, Jones R, Spann JF: Cardiac function in sickle cell anemia. Am J Cardiol 51:1674–1678, June 1983.

42. Manno BV, Burka ER, Hakki A, Manno CS, Iskandrian AS, Noone AM: Biventricular function in sickle-cell anemia: radionuclide angiographic and thallium-201 scintigraphic evaluation. Am J Cardiol 52:584–587, Sept 1983.

7

Congenital Heart Disease

ATRIAL SEPTAL DEFECT, SECUNDUM TYPE

It is well recognized that patients with secundum ASD often have MR. Utilizing 2-D echo, Nagata and associates[1] from Osaka, Japan, sought the presence of mitral valve lesions in 120 patients with secundum ASD. The 57 men and 63 women patients ranged in age from 15–74 years (mean, 40). Cardiac catheterization was performed in 37 of the 120 patients and 36 of them had operative closure of the ASD. The most frequent observation was a dislocation of the anterior and posterior mitral leaflets at the coaptation zone. One mitral leaflet was dislocated to the LA side in its closed position. The grade of severity of the mitral lesion was assessed by measuring the distance of the dislocation between the anterior and posterior leaflets at the area of coaptation. Mitral valve lesions were seen in 7 of 18 patients aged 15–24 years and in 56 of the 102 patients aged 25–74 years. Sixty patients had the abnormality only in the anterior mitral leaflet and the other 3 in both leaflets. Among 25 healthy control subjects, dislocation of both mitral leaflets occurred in only one subject. The dislocation in all patients was near the posteromedial commissure. In 41 of the 63 patients the lesion extended to the central part of the anterior leaflet and it was further toward the anterolateral commissure in 15 patients. Both the presence and severity of the dislocation mitral lesion was higher in the older compared with the younger patients. In 18 of the 37 patients who had left ventriculography MR was observed, and the worse the dislocation, the greater the MR. In about half of the patients, the mitral lesion disappeared after closure of the ASD.

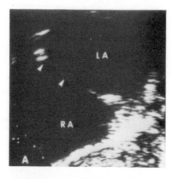
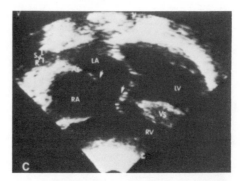
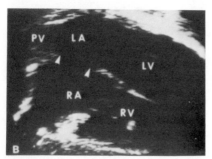
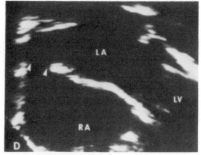

Fig. 7-1. Two-dimensional ECG images (still frame photographs) of various types of ASD, as viewed from the subcostal approach. A and B, Two examples of ostium secundum. C, Ostium primum defect. D, Sinus venosus defect. Arrowheads demarcate the defect in A, B and D; arrows indicate defect in C. 1 = inferior; L = left; R = right; S = superior; VS = ventricular septum; LA = left atrium; LV = left ventricle; RA = right atrium; RV = right ventricle; PV = pulmonary vein. Reproduced with permission from Shub et al.[2]

Shub and associates[2] from Rochester, Minnesota, reviewed the diagnostic sensitivity of subcostal echo imaging of ASD in 154 patients aged 2 months to 74 years (mean, 31 years). Echoes successfully visualized 93 of 105 secundum ASD, all 32 primum defects, and 7 of 16 sinus venosus defects. Echo contrast studies in 69 of 71 patients revealed abnormal findings, most often a bidirectional atrial shunt. Contrast studies revealed defects in 3 of 5 patients with secundum defects and 5 patients with sinus venosus defects in whom imaging alone was negative. Doppler studies in 7 patients with secundum defects were positive in each instance, showing a typical diastolic flow disturbance in the RA in the region of the atrial septum. This study provides important sensitivity data regarding echo diagnosis of ASD. Figure 7-1 shows the typical findings in patients with the 3 types of ASD studied. With the use of contrast, the authors were able to increase sensitivity to 93%. Sinus venosus defects remain the most difficult to visualize, with recent sensitivity of 55%. The question of false positives was not brought up by these authors.

COMPLETE ATRIOVENTRICULAR CANAL

A major goal of corrective surgery for complete AV canal is to leave the patient with a competent mitral valve. In an effort to improve results in this regard, Kawashima and coworkers[3] from Osaka, Japan, used a vertical Dacron patch with horizontal wings of Dacron or parietal pericardium in 10 patients undergoing repair of this defect since 1975. The basic surgical technique described by Rastelli is employed and the vertical patch of Dacron used to close the interventricular and interatrial communications. The wings of Dacron or parietal pericardium were sutured to the AV valve leaflets to enlarge the leaflet area of the mitral and tricuspid valves. There was one hospital death from tricuspid stenosis. Postoperative catheterization studies were performed in 7 of 9 survivors between 2 and 10 months (mean, 4.4) after operation: MR was absent in 4, trivial in 3; TR was absent in 2, mild in 4, and moderate in 1. Postoperative improvement in MR was observed in each of 5 patients. Of 2 patients without MR preoperatively, trivial MR was present postoperatively in 1, none in the other. The magnitude of postoperative TR was related to higher PA pressure postoperatively. The authors believe that use of this method will reduce the magnitude of residual MR after operation. This technique should be kept in mind as a method of increasing the ratio of leaflet/orifice area and may be particularly useful in selected patients who have deficient leaflet tissue.

Silverman and associates[4] from Chicago, Illinois, reviewed their experience with 21 consecutive patients <1 year of age with complete AV canal. Severe MR (3–4+) was present in 4 patients and trace to 2+ in 17. Eleven had concomitant closure of a PDA and 2, repair of coarctation. There was 1 hospital death. Postoperative (4–41 months) cardiac catheterization studies in 10 patients showed significant reduction and PA pressure and flow. All were symptomatically improved and 4 have undergone subsequent total correction. The authors believe PA banding is a rational alternative to complete repair and offer this to infants <1 year of age as the initial mode of surgical treatment. These results are not different from those for primary corrective repair, as reported from Boston, Birmingham, and Nashville during the current era. Return to a uniform policy of 2-stage surgical management for infants with complete AV canal seems inappropriate, but in selected patients who have anatomic and functional incremental risk factors for increased hospital mortality after primary repair, PA banding may be useful.

VENTRICULAR SEPTAL DEFECT

Nakazawa and associates[5] from Tokyo, Japan, studied 17 infants and young children with VSD. Hydralazine (0.3 mg/kg intraveneously) was used to study the effect on shunt flow and vascular resistance. Systemic vascular resistance (SVR) decreased in all but 2 patients, and the magnitude of reduction correlated with control of SVR. Systemic blood flow (Qs) increased from 3.7 ± 0.7–5.0 ± 0.8 liters/min/M^2 (p < 0.05). Pulmonary blood flow (Qp) did not change significantly, but Qp/Qs ratio was reduced from 3.6 ± 0.4–2.4 ± 0.2 (p < 0.05) in patients with a control SVR $\geq$20 units/M^2 but Qp/Qs was unchanged in patients with a lower SVR. After hydralazine, the Qp/Qs ratio, expressed as a percent of the control value, was inversely correlated with control SVR (r = −6.1; p = 0.02) in patients with elevated SVR. Thus, controlling SVR is important for predicting the hemodynamic effects of afterload reduction in infants and children with large VSD. The drug may be beneficial in patients with high SVR, but since Qp does not change, the long-term effect of this reduction may be minimal. Afterload reduction should be tried in the catheterization laboratory before chronic therapy is begun.

PATENT DUCTUS ARTERIOSUS

Alverson and associates[6] from Albuquerque, New Mexico, estimated descending aortic blood flow using a range-gated pulsed Doppler velocity meter and a suprasternal approach in 18 preterm infants with PDA. Ages ranged from 26–34 weeks and birth weight from 750–2,100 g. Ascending aortic flow (Qao) averaged 343 ml/min/kg in infants with PDA, a value well above the normal of 232 ± 9 ml/min/kg. After PDA closure with surgery or indomethacin, Qao decreased to 250 ml/min/kg. These studies indicate that changes in LV output can be estimated with this method, and LV output is extremely high in preterm infants with PDA. These methods could aid considerably in monitoring LV output in any critically ill child with cardiopulmonary compromise.

Gersony and associates[7] from New York City reported a national collaborative study regarding the incidence and therapy for PDA. Among 3,559 infants with birth weight less than 1,750 g, 421 developed a clinically significant PDA and entered a randomized trial to evaluate indomethacin in the management. Indomethacin given with usual medical therapy at the time of diagnosis resulted in ductal closure in 79% -vs- 35% with palcebo (p < 0.001). Indomethacin as backup to usual medical treatment resulted in similar closure rates. To assess overall effects, 3 management strategies were compared: indomethacin with initial medical therapy, indomethacin only if usual therapy failed, and surgery alone as the only backup to failure of medical therapy. Mortality did not differ among the 3 strategies, but a lower incidence of bleeding in those to whom indomethacin was given with initial therapy and lower rates of pneumothorax and retrolental fibroplasia in those to whom no indomethacin was administered with surgery as the only backup indicated that indomethacin used only when medical treatment failed appeared to be the preferable approach. This national collaborative study has resulted in a number of important aspects of diagnosis and management of PDA being clarified. Indomethacin is now used commonly on a national scale in patients with a symptomatic ductus. There does appear to be a significant decrease in the effectiveness of indomethacin in the smallest and youngest premature infants, and patients who fail to respond probably have either rapid clearance of the indomethacin or an increased volume of distribution. These latter patients may require 3 doses of indomethacin given over a relatively rapid time interval (24–36 hours) to achieve effective constriction. One major problem with continuing indomethacin therapy in infants whose ductus initially constricts but then reopens is the prolongation of ventilator time and delay of final effective closure by surgery. Thus, if indomethacin is not effective in achieving enough ductal constriction for ventilator weaning on a rapid basis, consideration for early surgery should be given.

Controversy continues over the use of medical -vs- surgical therapy for closure of the PDA in premature infants. Mavroudis and coworkers[8] from Louisville, Kentucky, reviewed their experience with surgical closure in 86 neonates 452–2,400 g (mean, 1,135), 42 were <1,000 g. Although no deaths occurred at operation, overall mortality was 17% and necrotizing enterocolitis or intestinal perforation occurred in 10%. This experience was compared with a previous institutional analysis of the use of indomethacin in 82 neonates. Ductal closure was achieved in 54 and serious gastrointestinal complications occurred in 21. Overall mortality in this group was 40%. The authors concluded that surgical therapy was preferable and can be safely accomplished in the neonatal nursery.

PULMONIC STENOSIS

Lima and associates[9] from Tucson, Arizona, and Sao Paulo, Brazil, compared Doppler estimations of transpulmonary gradients in 16 children with pulmonary valve stenosis (PS) within 12 hours of catheterization. Both a pulsed Doppler and a continuous-wave Doppler system were evaluated. Patient ages were 1 month to 16 years and catheterization gradients ranged from 15–180 mmHg. Imaging was performed from a precordial parasternal short-axis view. Maximal velocity was found and recorded by changing the position of the sample volume until the highest frequency audible signals were identified and the highest maximal systolic velocity recorded. In 3 patients were velocities quantifiable without ambiguity using the pulsed Doppler system. The correlation between Doppler predicted transvalvular gradients and catheterization gradient was excellent.

Lock and coworkers[10] from Minneapolis, Minnesota, performed balloon dilation angioplasty (BDA) in 7 children with either stenosis or hypoplasia of both right and left main PAs. Angioplasty was possible in 5 of 7 patients aged 1.5–16 years. The BDA was successful in decreasing gradient in all 5: RV pressure fell from 104 ± 42–80 mmHG, gradient across the obstruction fell from 61 ± 51–32 ± 22 mmHg, and diameter of narrowed artery increased from 3.7 ± 1.2–6.8 ± 1.1 mm. In addition, quantitative lung scans showed an increase in percentage of pulmonary flow to the dilated lungs from 41 ± 16–52 ± 22%. No morbidity was observed in these patients. Follow-up angiograms 2–12 months later in 3 patients showed persistence of the dilated diameters, and perfusion scans in 2 patients showed a further small increase in the proportion of flow to the lung with the dilated artery.

PULMONIC VALVE ATRESIA WITH INTACT VENTRICULAR SEPTUM

Continued controversy surrounds the initial surgical approach to the infant with pulmonary atresia and intact ventricular septum. Lewis and associates[11] from Los Angeles, California, reviewed the records of 27 infants (23 < 1 week of age) treated between 1970 and 1982. The size of the RV cavity was estimated using an RV index calculated from angiographic measurements of the sum of the TV anulus and RV inflow and outflow tracts and normalized to the diameter of the descending thoracic aorta. This ratio was 13.5 ± 1.4 in 20 control subjects and 7.3 ± 2.6 in the study group (p < 0.001). Pulmonary valvotomy plus a Blalock-Taussig shunt was performed in

10 infants with 1 death, and postoperative cardiac catheterization studies showed an increase in RV index from 8.0–12.5 in the 5 survivors. In contrast, patients who underwent a shunt alone had no change in RV cavity size. The authors concluded that pulmonary valvotomy usually must be combined with a systemic-pulmonary shunt. In a few patients, however, an RV index >11 appears to be sufficient to sustain adequate pulmonary blood flow after valvotomy alone. In these patients, prostaglandin E_1 infusion should be continued for 3–5 days postoperatively to maintain adequate pulmonary blood flow during the initial recovery period. The author's method of quantitating RV cavity size may prove useful in selecting the initial surgical approach to these patients and also in following future RV growth. It remains to be demonstrated that these small right ventricles will increase in size and permit complete circulatory support by a 2-ventricular system.

Bass and coworkers[12] from Minneapolis, Minnesota, studied 6 patients aged 11 months to 10 years with hypoplastic right heart and atrial right-to-left shunts. Five patients had pulmonary atresia and 1 patient had TF with tricuspid stenosis. At catheterization, RA pressure, aortic pressure, systemic saturation, and right-to-left shunt were determined before and after balloon occlusion of the ASD. Five patients tolerated complete occlusion without significant changes in atrial or aortic pressures and with improvements in systemic saturation. All 5 underwent surgical closure of ASD without evidence of postoperative systemic venous hypertension. Attempted occlusion in the sixth patient caused profound systemic venous hypoxia and surgical occlusion was not attempted. This method should be used in all patients before surgical ASD closure in situations in which RV hypoplasia is a potential problem and right-to-left atrial shunting is present.

PULMONIC VALVE ATRESIA WITH VENTRICULAR SEPTAL DEFECT

Patients with TF and congenital pulmonary atresia often have hypoplasia of the branch PAs and arborization anomalies. Shimazaki and associates[13] from Osaka, Japan, reviewed their results with total correction in 18 patients in an attempt to provide information regarding the adequacy of the size of the main right and left PAs. The RV-PA continuity was established with a transanular patch in 4 patients (no deaths) and with a valved extracardiac conduit in 14 (5 deaths). An average cross-sectional area of the right and left PAs (PA area) was calculated from preoperative angiograms and compared with the cross-sectional area of the normal right PA (N-rPA). The ratio PA area/N-rPA area ranged from 0.03–1.05 and averaged 0.54. Three patients who died from postrepair suprasystemic RV pressure had a ratio equal to <0.20. Fifteen patients had a ratio >0.20 and 1 of them died from pulmonary edema related to a persistent large aortopulmonary collateral artery and another died from pulmonary vascular obstructive disease. The authors concluded that a PA area/N-rPA area ratio >0.20 is essential to accomplish a corrective repair.

Enlargement of severely hypoplastic PAs has been demonstrated after systemic-PA shunting or palliative outflow tract patching, leaving the VSD open, in some patients with TF with pulmonary atresia. The ultimate goal of such procedures is to provide a PA size and distribution compatible with successful complete repair. Freedom and coworkers[14] from Toronto, Canada, evaluated their results with pericardial outflow patch reconstruction in 15 patients operated between 1977 and 1981. An extensive aortopulmonary collateral circulation was present in 7 patients and 8 had undergone a previous systemic-PA shunt. There was 1 hospital death. Postoperative cardiac catheterization studies, performed in 11 patients 2 weeks to 3 years later, disclosed that none had a normal caliber and distribution of each PA considered adequate for corrective repair. Severe proximal stenosis of the left PA was present in 7 patients, right PA stenosis in 1, and bilateral stenoses in 2. Thus, no patient had normal PAs achieved by palliative RV outflow tract construction. This is an excellent article that points out problems with enlarging hypoplastic PAs associated with TF and pulmonary atresia. Although no patient was ultimately suitable for correction, some patients achieved satisfactory PAs from either systemic-to-PA shunting or palliative transanular patching. Therefore attempts to produce suitable PAs in these patients are justified although satisfactory results may be disappointing.

TETRALOGY OF FALLOT

Kirklin and coworkers[15] from Birmingham, Alabama, reviewed their experience with 1,103 operations performed for all types of TF from 1967–1982. Repair was accomplished in 836 patients with 88 hospital deaths (11%). Incremental risk factors for hospital death included PA problems, major associated cardiac anomalies, small size, and >1 previous operation. In patients with pulmonary stenosis, hospital mortality has decreased with time but the incremental of a high hematocrit and of transanular patching has persisted. In the current era, risk of repair in patients with pulmonary stenosis is estimated to be 2% at 5 years and at 12 months to be 4% without and 8% with transanular patching. Hospital mortality for repair when pulmonary atresia is present and a valved extracardiac conduit is used was lowest (5%) between 5.5 and 16 years of age. No deaths occurred among 53 patients with pulmonary stenosis receiving a primary classic or modified Blalock-Taussig shunt, and 6 deaths (12%) occurred in 51 patients with pulmonary atresia similarly treated.

Pulmonary regurgitation (PR) is present in all patients having a transanular patch, and in many without this, as part of the repair of TF. Shaher and associates[16] from Albany, New York, described 10 patients among 147 undergoing repair of TF from 1962–1981 who required late reconstruction of the RV outflow tract. Average age at repair was 9 years, and the interval between this and subsequent reconstruction ranged from 3–10 years (average, 5.3). Each of 5 group I patients had a transanular patch as part of the initial repair and at restudy each had severe PR, decreased RV contractility, and an outflow tract aneurysm. Severe right PA stenosis was present in 2 and severe TR, in 4. Secondary repair included resection of outflow aneurysm and placement of a porcine valved RV-PA conduit in each and tricuspid valve anuloplasty in 2. There was 1 hospital death. Initial repair in each of 5 group II patients did not include a transanular patch, and 2 of these had congenital absence of the left PA. Severe PR was present in 4, pulmonary stenosis in 1, outflow aneurysm in 3, and severe RV dysfunction and TR in 2. One had a large residual VSD and 1, severe AR. The pulmonary valve was replaced with a homograft valve in 3 early patients, a porcine valve in 2, and in 1 of these a tricuspid anuloplasty and AVR also was done. There were no deaths in this group. Hemodynamic studies after secondary repair were performed in 7 of 9 survivors and were considered good or excellent in 5 and unsatisfactory in 2 who had significant gradients across their homograft valve. Thus, severe PR after repair of TF may not be well tolerated, especially when it coexists with other residual defects.

Bove and colleagues[17] from Syracuse, New York, evaluated 20 patients 3–15 years (mean, 9) after complete repair of TF. Age at operation ranged from 2–14 years (mean, 7). In each patient, catheterization studies after repair showed a resting peak RV systolic pressure ≤60 mmHg, resting RV-PA peak systolic gradient ≤30 mmHg, and no TR. Group I (8 patients) had no clinical PR, whereas group II (12 patients) had moderate to severe PR. A transanular patch had been used in 6 of the latter patients. Age at operation, duration of follow-up, RV pressure, RV-PA gradient were similar in each group. No patient had a residual shunt and all were New York Heart Association class I. Twenty-four-hour Holter monitoring showed serious ventricular arrhythmias in 38% of group I and 50% of group II (p, NS), and older age at operation was the only incremental risk factor identified. The RV/LV end-diastolic echo dimension was greater in patients with PR (p < 0.01). Radionuclide ventriculography showed significant reduction of both RV and LV EF in group II patients. The authors concluded that patients with significant PR following repair of TF have impaired ventricular function late after operation. Serial prospective assessment of RV function may provide guidelines for future pulmonary valve replacement to preserve RV function.

In an effort to determine the short-term variations of $P_{RV/LV}$ after repair of TF, Bertranou and associates[18] from Paris, France, studied 50 consecutive patients comparing this ratio measured in the operating room immediately after repair with that measured during the third postoperative week. The ratio fell in 64% of patients, remained unchanged in 6%, and increased in 30%. Mean $P_{RV/LV}$ immediately after repair was 0.52 ± 0.12 and at 3 weeks it was 0.47 ± 0.16 (p, 0.04). This was similar whether or not a transanular patch was used at repair. The authors confirm the usefulness of $P_{RV/LV}$ measured in the operating room immediately after repair and indicate that on the average it will fall by 10% 3 weeks later.

Deanfield and associates[19] from London, England, analyzed clinical and necropsy data in 6 patients who died suddenly 1–9 years after repair of TF. All patients had right BBB and 2 patients had multiform VPCs on routine ECG. Two patients had stress tests and neither developed arrhythmia. Catheterization in 4 patients revealed elevated (50–100 mmHg) systolic RV pressure. There were no residual shunts or PA hypertension. One patient died during strenuous physical exercise. Necropsy performed in 3 patients disclosed no evidence of histologic damage of the AV node, AV bundle, or left bundle branch. There was extensive fibrosis of the RV myocardium at the ventriculotomy site in 3, septum in 1, and outflow tract in 1. These data give further evidence that heart block is an unlikely cause for late sudden death in TF patients. Ventricular arrhythmia remains the most likely cause and a poor hemodynamic result with resultant elevated RV pressure and volume may contribute in some but not all patients. Prevention of severe hypoxia before surgical repair, adequate myocardial protection during repair, and reoperation for significant residual defects are important in an attempt to reduce the incidence of this tragic consequence. Postoperative patients should have ambulatory monitoring and exercise stress testing on a periodic basis after repair. If symptoms are in the least way indicative of arrhythmia, then prolonged monitoring and detailed electrophysiologic evaluation should be performed.

Garson and associates[20] from Houston, Texas, performed electrophysiologic studies in 27 patients who had undergone repair of TF 7 months to 21 years (mean, 2) previously. Syncope in 4 patients was not related to ventricular arrhythmia on rest ECG, 24 hour ECG, or exercise testing, but was associated with nonsustained in 2 or sustained in 2 inducible VT. Two of these 4 had RV pressure ≥70 mmHg, 1 had RV dysfunction and TR, and 1 had a septal aneurysm. The 9 patients with inducible VT had a greater prevalence of more complex ventricular arrhythmia on 24-hour ECG, long His-to-ventricle interval, RV pressure >70 mmHg, and decreased RV EF compared with the 15 without. These data indicate that 4 postoperative TF patients with syncope had inducible VT. In addition, all patients at risk for syncope could not be identified by routine or 24-hour ECG or treadmill testing. Hemodynamic abnormalities were present in patients with syncope and inducible VT. These authors also found, however, that VT was inducible in 23 patients who had a "routine" catheterization and electrophysiologic study with no history to suggest ventricular arrhythmia. Whether or not these patients are at risk for significant ventricular arrhythmia and sudden death is still unclear. These authors recommend routine postoperative hemodynamic catheterization for all postoperative TF patients and periodic 24-hour ECG into adulthood. In addition, treatment is recommended for patients with syncope and inducible VT, patients with elevated RV systolic pressure or reduced RV EF with more than infrequent uniform VPC on 24-hour ECG, and any patient with VT on 24-hour ECG.

COMPLETE TRANSPOSITION OF THE GREAT ARTERIES

Ventricular function postoperatively

Parrish and associates[21] from Nashville, Tennessee, performed RNA at rest and with supine bicycle exercise in 11 patients with complete TGA after the Mustard intraatrial repair and 2 patients with TGA after Rastelli's ventricular repair. Studies were performed 3 months to 14 years after the repair and comparisons were made with 15 normal and 5 patients with congenitally corrected TGA (CCTGA). Mean ages (years) at repair were 1.5 for Mustard and 10 for Rastelli procedures and at study they were 9 for Mustard and 10 for Rastelli; mean for CCTGA is 14 years and normal is 11 years. Residual abnormalities in patients after Mustard repair were mild systemic venous obstruction in 5 patients, small VSD in 2, and mild pulmonary venous obstruction in 1. For the CCTGA group, 2 had VSD plus pulmonary stenosis (PS), 1 had complete AV block with ventricular pacemaker, and 1 had undergone surgery for VSD plus PS 3 years before the study. There were no significant differences among groups in exercise capacity, heart rate, or BP response to exercise. Systemic ventricular EF was normal at

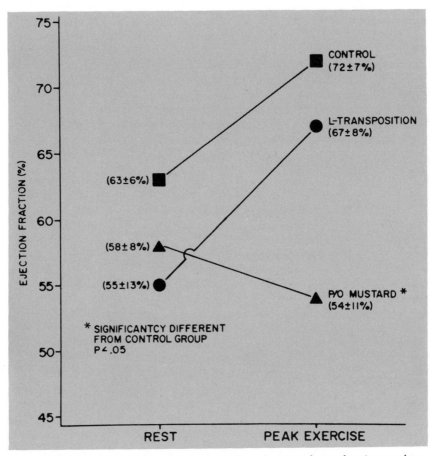

Fig. 7-2. The mean LV EF at rest and peak exercise for each group. The numbers in parentheses indicate the mean EF (±SD). Reproduced with permission from Parrish et al.[21]

rest but failed to increase normally with exercise in 6 of the Mustard patients, 2 of the Rastelli patients, and all of the CCTGA patients. In addition, pulmonary ventricular EF failed to increase normally in 10 Mustard patients, 2 Rastelli patients and 2 CCTGA patients. No correlation was found between exercise response and residual defects, age at repair, or duration of intraoperative arrest time in TGA patients. An abnormal RV EF response to exercise in patients studied many years after Mustard repair of TGA has been reported previously from the Toronto group (*Circulation* 65:1052–1059, 1982). The present study showed in addition an abnormal LV EF response in both Mustard and Rastelli patients (Fig. 7-2). These data suggest that factors other than the inability of the right ventricle to provide normal systemic ventricular pump function are operative in these patients. Preoperative hypoxemia and intraoperative myocardial ischemia with inadequate myocardial protection are possible causes for the postoperative ventricular functional abnormalities. Further longitudinal data on RV and LV function are needed in TGA patients without residual defects, who were operated upon early in infancy, who never had severe hypoxemia, and who had newer methods of intraoperative myocardial protection. These latter patients will form the data base for comparison of postoperative RV and LV function with TGA patients after arterial switch.

Redundant tricuspid leaflet tissue

Riggs and coworkers[22] from Chicago, Illinois, studied 6 infants and children with TGA, VSD, and subvalvular pulmonary stenosis. In each patient pulmonary stenosis resulted from redundant tricuspid valve tissue that protruded through the VSD into the LV outflow tract. Patients with normally related great arteries may have a similar pouch but unless this pouch protrudes into the LV outflow tract, systolic obstruction usually is not present. This angiographic and echo study is important in terms of preoperative evaluation of patients with TGA and VSD. At surgery with the heart arrested, the obstructive nature of the pouch may not be manifested and thus postoperative obstruction could be a major problem. With 4-chamber angiographic or echo data, the diagnosis should be clear and data available preoperatively for the surgeon.

Left ventricular geometry

VanDoesburg and associates[23] from Boston, Massachusetts, studied LV geometry in 19 neonates with TGA using subziphoid echo. Repeat echo and catheterization were performed preoperatively in 16 of 19 patients at 3–10 months of age and postoperatively in 5 of 19 at 6–22 months of age. Echo geometry was compared with 30 subjects aged 1 day to 6.5 months with no clinical evidence of cardiopulmonary disease. The LV geometry was classified as type I: round LV with bowing of the septum into the RV; type II: flattened septum; and type III: septum bowing into LV. The minor axis ratio (MAR) determined at end diastole and end systole was used as a quantitative index of these geometric types. In normal patients, type I end-systolic geometry was present in 29 of 30 with MAR ranging from 0.72–1.21 (mean, 0.91 ± 0.13). Neonates with TGA showed type II geometry in 13 of 19, with mean systolic MAR of 0.58. In preoperative TGA patients, type III geometry was found in 15 of 16, with a mean systolic MAR of 0.32. Significant pulmonary venous obstruction was found in 2 of 5 postoperative patients associated with a reversion to type II or type I geometry with an increase in MAR in both patients. The end-systolic ratio shows significant correlation ($r = 0.58$; $p < 0.01$) with the peak systolic LV/RV pressure ratio. These data demonstrate changes in LV geometry as a function of alterations in LV pressures in patients with TGA. Assessment of MAR in the same patient with time will be useful. A marked change in ventricular geometry or MAR toward a more spherical LV suggests the possibility of a significant increase in LV pressure.

Prostaglandin E_2

Beitzke and Suppan[24] from Graz, Austria, reported the use of prostaglandin E_2 (PGE_2) intravenous infusions before atrial septostomy in 15 infants with TGA and severe hypoxemia. Twelve patients had simple TGA and 3 had small VSD. The infusion resulted in an increase in PA oxygen from 22 ± 3–37

± 5 torr within 1–2 hours. Only 1 patient did not respond to treatment. After balloon septostomy PGE_2 was discontinued but had to be reinstituted within 24 hours in 2 of 15 patients whose PA oxygen decreased to ≤25 torr. Two patients developed prolonged patency of the ductus with CHF requiring ductal ligation at the age of 5 days in 1. These authors present objective data regarding the benefits of this therapy before catheterization. It appears to be useful in nearly all patients with TGA and probably fails only in those patients whose ductus has already closed or in whom the foramen ovale is extremely small. What to do with the rare patient who continues to be hypoxic following septostomy continues to be a problem. Prolonged hypoxemia is a possible contributing factor to myocardial hypoxia at times of stress with resultant increased myocardial oxygen demand and the potential for irreversible myocardial injury. It seems reasonable to try to get the systemic oxygen saturation to ≥60% at rest before hospital discharge.

Mustard operation

Since a variety of surgical options are currently available to treat patients with complete TGA, it becomes important to document the early and late results of each specific procedure. Park and coworkers[25] from Pittsburgh, Pennsylvania, reviewed the pre- and postoperative catheterization studies of 82 survivors who underwent the Mustard operation for TGA between 1964 and 1980. Their ages range from 0.3–14 years (mean, 3): 46 had TGA, intact septum, and 36 had either a VSD or pulmonary stenosis (PS) or both. A Blalock-Hanlon atrial septectomy had been performed in 20 patients, PA banding in 7, and a Blalock-Taussig shunt in 4. In 74 (90%), parietal pericardium was used to construct the baffle and other materials in the remaining 8 patients. Postoperative catheterization studies were performed 20 days to 10 years after operation (mean, 2.5 years): 11 patients (13%) had significant systemic venous obstruction, 5 (6%) had severe pulmonary venous obstruction. Important baffle leakage was present in 2 patients and TR was present in 2 of 58 patients who did not -vs- 6 of 24 patients who did have surgical closure of a VSD. This was severe and surgically treated in 2. Some degree of LV outflow obstruction was present before operation in 31 (38%) and was surgically treated in 12. Six patients who had localized obstruction had a good result but the others had little or no relief. Mild to moderate gradients regressed spontaneously in most patients after the Mustard procedure. Baffle dysfunction after the Mustard operation is probably multifactorial and dependent upon the precise surgical technique employed, baffle material, patch enlargement of the pulmonary venous atrium, and age at operation. Generally, younger age has been associated with a higher incidence of venous obstructive complications. In the series, the mean age at operation was 3.2 years, considerably older than a modern day experience with a primary repair. The low incidence of late TR in those without an associated VSD is noteworthy.

Senning operation

Penkoske and associates[26] from Boston, Massachusetts, reviewed their experience (1978–1982) with VSD closure and Senning operation in 46 infants 12 days to 12 months of age. Hospital mortality was similar for 32 patients <6 months of age to that for 14 patients 6–12 months of age, and the overall early mortality was 15%. Eight patients had LV outflow tract obstruction of varying etiology. There were 2 late deaths over the follow-up period (4%). Postoperative cardiac catheterization studies were done in 17 patients within 1 year of operation: 6 (13%) had mild TR and 3 patients (7%) underwent successful TV replacement for severe TR. Three patients (7%) had an important residual VSD and 2 survived secondary closure. Pulmonary venous obstruction was found in 3 patients, 2 of whom survived reoperation. Secondary cardiac procedures were required in 23% of hospital survivors. Six (13%) had temporary and 4 (9%) had permanent complete heart block; 2 of the latter died and the other 2 received a permanent pacemaker. The authors believe this study provides baseline data for the Senning operation with VSD closure in this defect. Comparable studies after VSD closure and an arterial switch operation should permit useful comparison.

Satomi and associates[27] from Tokyo, Japan, studied 16 patients with echo following Senning's procedure for TGA. Three patients had pulmonary venous channel stenosis detected by echo and confirmed at catheterization. The newly created pulmonary venous channel was assessed with a short-axis view at the base of the heart (Fig. 7-3), and LV shape was assessed by short-axis view at the level of the papillary muscles. A ratio of minor axis LV diameters >0.55 was associated with LV pressure of >60 mmHg. In addition, pulmonary venous stenosis was associated with an echo-derived channel measurement of 3, 5, and 6 mm compared with ≥10 mm in patients without stenosis. This is a very useful method for assessing pulmonary venous stenosis and LV hypertension in postoperative TGA patients.

Postoperative arrhythmias are present after the Mustard operation for patients with TGA and over the years modifications in the surgical technique have reduced their incidence. Few reports have carefully documented the incidence of arrhythmias following the Senning operation. Martin and coworkers[28] from St. Louis, Missouri, studied the cardiac rhythm of 29 patients with TGA who underwent the Senning operation between 1979 and 1982. Their ages ranged from 3–23 months (mean, 9). There were 3 early deaths (10%) and 24-hour Holter monitoring 7 days to 30 months (mean, 11 months) was done in 23 patients: 8 (35%) had normal sinus rhythm for the entire recording period, 7 (30%) had occasional atrial or VPC; 4 (17%) had normal sinus rhythm for >50% of the recording period with episodes of junctional escape during sinus arrest or slowing and/or periods of accelerated junctional rhythm with sinus node suppression; 3 (13%) had a nonsinus mechanism during >50% of the recording period and this was junctional in each; 1 had SVT. Each patient was asymptomatic despite the rhythm disturbance and in this group there have been no late deaths or need for permanent pacemakers.

Arterial switch repair

Repair of TGA-VSD by VSD closure and venous switching has less good early and late results than venous switching for simple TGA. This, the presence of a prepared left ventricle and the attractiveness of leaving the left as the systemic ventricle, has led to a variety of arterial switch operations. Pacifico and colleagues[29] from Birmingham, Alabama, reported their experience with 6 patients 2–18 months of age with TGA and large VSD. An arterial

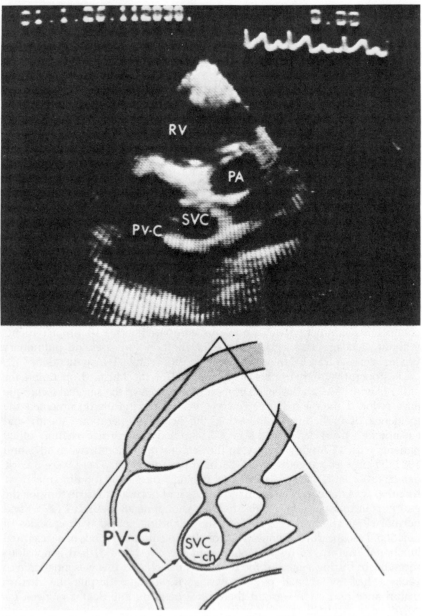

Fig. 7-3. *Top,* Two-dimensional echo of the first view. *Bottom,* Schematic illustration showing how to measure the diameter of the pulmonary venous channel (PV-C). PA = pulmonary artery; RV = right ventricle; SVC = superior vena cava. Reproduced with permission from Satomi et al.[27]

switch operation using the method described by Lecompte, with translocation of the coronary ostia, was successfully accomplished in each. Catheterization studies in 4 patients 0.25–7.5 months later showed normal ventricular function, a competent aortic valve in 2, trivial and mild AR in 1 each. The method used is best suited for those with "normal" coronary artery anatomy and when the aorta is directly anterior to the pulmonary trunk. This small experience lends additional support to the use of anatomic correction for patients with TGA and large VSD.

Dynamic LV outflow tract obstruction is relatively common in patients with TGA and may result in significant LV-PA gradients. Yacoub and colleagues[30] from Harefield, England, reviewed their experience with 14 patients who survived anatomic correction. Preoperatively, they had LV-PA gradients from 20–120 mmHg (mean, 40); 10 having an intact ventricular septum and 4 an associated VSD. No organic obstruction was observed at operation and no attempt at surgical widening was made. Postoperative echo showed a normal LV outflow tract in each and catheterization studies in 10 patients, 6–26 months later, showed no gradient from the LV to the aorta. The authors concluded that the arterial switch operation resulted in immediate resolution of dynamic LV outflow obstruction, demonstrating that this form of obstruction preoperatively is due to the reversed roles of each ventricle.

Transmitral approach to relief of outflow obstruction

Wilcox and coworkers[31] from Chapel Hill, North Carolina, reported their experience with resection of LV outflow tract obstruction in 3 patients by exposing the area through the mitral valve, as suggested by Oelert and Borst. Each operation was successful and postrepair systolic LV pressure varied between 35 and 45 mmHg. The authors described in detail the area "safe" for resection as viewed by the surgeon and they believe this method provides excellent exposure to permit effective relief of LV outflow obstruction.

CONGENITALLY CORRECTED TRANSPOSITION OF THE GREAT ARTERIES

Sutherland and associates[32] from London, England, studied 49 patients with AV discordance using cross-sectional echo. The atrial arrangement was consistently predicted by echo analysis of the patterns of pulmonary and systemic venous drainage. The ventricular arrangement was consistently predicted by direct identification of ventricular morphology. In the 47 patients with 2 AV valves, ventricular morphology was determined by the pattern of implantation of chordae to the ventricular myocardium. An inlet valve showing chordae implanting into the septum correctly identified a morphologic RV in 47 patients and an inlet valve with chordae implanting into the free wall of the ventricle correctly identified a morphologic LV in 47 patients. The reversal of the normal pattern of implantation of AV valve septal leaflets into the AV junction is diagnostic of AV discordance with intact ventricular septum. This finding, however, cannot be used in patients with a large perimembranous VSD in which there is a common level of attachment of AV valve septal leaflets. This article should be studied in detail by physicians dealing with patients with complex congenital heart disease.

These authors present convincing evidence for correctly identifying AV discordance and its spectrum of associated lesions, even in the most complex hearts using a segmental, sequential analysis and cross-sectional echo examinations.

Huhta and associates[33] from Rochester, Minnesota, reviewed data on 107 patients with congenitally corrected TGA: 77% had VSD, 53% had pulmonary stenosis, 34% had tricuspid insufficiency, and 23% had dextrocardia. Complete AV block was found in 23: at birth in 4, and developing unrelated to surgery in 19 at ages 4 months to 53 years (mean, 18 years). Pacemaker was implanted in 9, 4 with the onset of block and 5 an average of 11 years later. One patient without a pacemaker died suddenly at age 28 years, 4 years after the onset of block and with a resting rate of 40 beats/minute. The risk of natural onset complete AV block was increased in patients with intact ventricular septum. A VSD closure without surgical AV block did not confer an increased risk of late onset complete AV block in excess of that expected without surgery. The risk of natural onset AV block occurred at a rate of approximately 2% a year. In the absence of symptoms and a heart rate >50 beats/minute, pacemaker therapy is probably not needed. Patients with heart rates lower than this at rest probably need more extensive evaluation, including ambulatory ECG monitoring and stress testing.

Morphologic abnormalities of the specialized conduction tissue are present in patients with corrected TGA. Surgically induced complete heart block has been reported in 15–67% of patients undergoing closure of an associated VSD, and also may be produced by local resection of subpulmonary stenosis. Doty and coworkers[34] from Iowa City, Iowa, reviewed surgical implications of conduction tissue abnormalities in this defect. Applying the technique described in DeLeval, they closed a large VSD by placing a prosthetic patch on the morphologic RV side of the septum in 5 patients, working through the right AV valve. In 2 patients the VSD was closed by direct suture. In 3 patients with severe pulmonary stenosis, a unique and innovative posteriorly placed spiral patch was used to widen the subpulmonary area, pulmonary valve anulus, and pulmonary trunk. An extracardiac conduit was used to relieve pulmonary stenosis in 1 and valvotomy and subanular posterior resection in another. Complete heart block was present in 1 patient preoperatively and developed in 1 patient who had direct VSD suture closure. All patients survived operation and 1 sudden death occurred 3.5 months later from probable complete heart block.

LEFT VENTRICULAR OUTFLOW OBSTRUCTION

Lima and associates[35] from Tucson, Arizona, and Sao Paulo, Brazil, studied 16 children aged 6 months to 17 years with valvular AS (n, 12) or with discrete subaortic stenosis (n, 4) and compared Doppler estimates of pressure gradients with catheterization gradients. Continuous-wave Doppler guided by echo imaging was used and gradient was estimated with the equation: gradient $= 4 \times$ (maximal velocity)^2. There was an excellent correlation between severity of obstruction estimated by the 2 methods with r $= 0.94$ (SEE $\pm$ 7.5 mmHg). Catheterization gradients ranged from 20–155 mmHg and Doppler gradients from 14–100 mmHg. These results indicate a reasonably good correlation of Doppler and catheterization gradients.

AORTIC VALVE ATRESIA

Aortic valve atresia (AVA) is a complex and relatively common congenital cardiac defect that untreated is fatal during infancy. Lang and Norwood[36] from Boston, Massachusetts, reported their results of postoperative cardiac catheterization studies in 10 hospital survivors after initial palliative surgery. Thirty-five patients underwent palliative operations for AVA between 1979 and 1982, with 13 hospital survivors (37%). Of the 10 patients restudied, systemic blood flow from the right ventricle to the descending thoracic aorta was established in 4 (group 1) by placing a conduit proximally connected to the RV free wall or pulmonary trunk, banding the pulmonary trunk and closing the PDA. A Blalock-Taussig shunt was made in 1. Conduit obstruction developed in 2 and pulmonary vascular resistance remained excessively elevated in the remaining 2. In the remaining 6 patients (group 2), systemic blood flow was established by direct anastomosis of the pulmonary trunk to the ascending aorta and aortic arch, and pulmonary blood flow provided by a central or Blalock-Taussig shunt. The ASD was enlarged in each. Catheterization studies 2 weeks to 16 months after surgery (median, 6 months) showed systemic arterial oxygen between 65 and 80%, and each of the 6 group 2 patients were candidates for physiologic correction. This was accomplished in 3 of them, with 2 survivors.

TRICUSPID VALVE ATRESIA

The Fontan operation, first performed in 1968, has undergone a continual evolution both in regard to the precise technique employed and the specific indication for its use. This procedure and its modifications are currently widely employed for patients with tricuspid atresia (TA) and other complex cardiac defects. Complete analysis of early and late results is sorely needed. Fontan and coworkers[37] from Bordeaux, France, and Leiden, The Netherlands, analyzed their experience with 100 consecutive patients with TA who received this procedure between 1968 and 1981. Previous palliative procedures had been performed in 71 patients, a systemic-PA shunt in 63 and a Glenn shunt in 17. A variety of surgical methods was used to effect RV exclusion, and an aortic homograft valve was employed in each of 27 patients with ventriculoarterial discordant connection and in 14 of 73 patients with a concordant connection. Hospital mortality was 12% overall, and in 82 patients between 4 and 16 years of age it was 7% compared with 33% in the group of 18 patients either <4 or >16 years at operation (p < 0.001). There were 6 late deaths, each occurring during the first postoperative year, and actuarial survival at 14 years was 80%. Fourteen patients required reoperation, 1 day to 5 years, to repair residual shunt in 6, an obstructed conduit in 2, and late subaortic stenosis in 1. Two Glenn shunts were unsuccessfully performed early postoperatively because of RA hypertension. Follow-up cardiac catheterization studies were made in 54 patients 2 weeks to 1 year postoperatively. In patients with ventriculoarterial concordance who had a RA-RV homograft valve, mean pressure in the right atrium was significantly lower than the others. No RA-PA gradients were found. Those with concordance and a RA-RV homograft valve had arterial type PA pressure curves and an increase in systolic PA pressure that was not observed in other groups. At follow-up, 94% of patients were New York Heart Association class I or II. The highest proportion (88%) of class I survivors was in the group with concordance and an RA-RV homograft valve. Late exercise capacity was studied in 30 patients and was >70% of normal in 15. The best results were obtained in 10 patients with an RA-PA and in 2 patients with an RA-RV homograft valve. Seven studied patients with a coexistant Glenn shunt had the lowest exercise capacity. The authors believe the strict selection criteria, previously published, are necessary to obtain good early and late results after the Fontan operation. Young age at operation is an incremental risk factor. Evaluation of functional status, exercise capacity, and catheterization data tend to demonstrate that a homograft valve is a valuable adjunct to the operative technique. This article is a complete and thorough analysis of a large series of patients receiving the Fontan operation and should be studied by all interested in congenital heart surgery.

Bull and associates[38] from London, England, compared the hemodynamics postoperatively of 18 patients who underwent an atrial-pulmonary connection with those of 17 patients with an atrial-ventricular connection incorporating a subpulmonary ventricular chamber (SPVC) as part of a Fontan procedure for treatment of TA or other univentricular hearts. Early postoperatively the mean PA pressure was not greater than mean RA pressure in any patient regardless of the connection used. In 2 patients with recatheterization 12–30 months postoperatively, the mean RA pressure was lower than the mean PA pressure and SPVC growth was documented. In 11 other patients with late recatheterization, the SPVC pressure at rest was either similar to or marginally higher than the mean PA pressure. These investigators attempted to determine differences between short- and long-term results for the Fontan operation in patients with or without a SPVC. Early postoperative data indicated that there was little contribution of RV contraction to forward pulmonary flow. Data in a small number of patients ≥1 year after operation indicate that significant contributions of RV contraction to forward pulmonary flow can develop with a SPVC. Thus, any afterload resistance to the right atrium by anastomotic stenoses, conduit gradients, gradients across the SPVC or pulmonary valve, increased pulmonary vascular resistance, or raised LA pressure due to mitral or LV dysfunction will cause marked increases in systemic venous pressure so that systemic capillary leakage is common. Use of an SPVC connection, particularly when there is a sinus portion of the right ventricle and not simply an infundibular portion, appears to have significant potential for late improvement in the ability of the combined RA-RV chamber to provide more effective pulmonary flow at a lower systemic venous pressure.

The original operation described by Fontan for physiologic correction of TA included a cavopulmonary anastomosis (Glenn shunt) and a homograft valve between the right atrium and pulmonary trunk and at the entrance of the inferior vena cava. More recently, a simultaneous Glenn shunt has been excluded from the operative procedure and the need for valves within the circuit questioned. DeLeon and associates[39] from Chicago, Illinois, reported their experience with 27 patients, 3–22 years of age, who underwent the Fontan repair. Seventeen had TA and 10 other complex lesions. Twelve patients had an established Glenn shunt, in 3 it was constructed simultaneous with and in 1 following the Fontan operation. There was 1 early death (4%) and 2 late deaths (7%) within 6 months of operation. The 9 patients with TA and an established Glenn shunt had a shorter hospital stay (average, 10 days) and were without pleural or pericardial effusions, whereas the 7 similar patients without a Glenn shunt had an average hospital stay of 18 days and significant effusions were present in 3. Postoperative effusions did not occur in 3 of the patients with complex defects who had an established Glenn shunt compared with significant effusions in 5 of the remaining 7 without this. One patient with a complex defect required takedown of the Fontan 2 days later and another required a Glenn shunt at 4 days. The presence of the Glenn shunt was considered lifesaving for 2 patients who had major tricuspid patch disruption and for 1 of these who later developed complete occlusion of the valved conduit 2 months later. The patients own pulmonary valve or a porcine valved heterograft was included in the RA-PA connection in each of the 27 patients. The Glenn shunts were evaluated after 4 months to 13 years (average, 9 years) in 14 patients and 10 had homogeneous perfusion of the right lung, 4 had preferential flow to the middle and lower lobes and 1 had a pulmonary arterial venous fistula. Twenty-three patients were followed from 8 months to 5 years after the Fontan operation (average, 26 months): 20 were asymptomatic, 2 limited because of myocardial dysfunction, and 1 with a Glenn shunt was cyanotic because of the pulmonary arterial venous fistula. The authors believe an established Glenn shunt improves the result of the Fontan operation in patients who are less than ideal candidates. They also believe the Glenn shunt should be considered for younger patients with complex lesions who are in need of increased pulmonary blood flow and who are future candidates for the Fontan operation.

EBSTEIN'S ANOMALY

Shiina and associates[40] from Rochester, Minnesota, studied 25 patients with Ebstein's anomaly (aged 7 days to 71 years) who subsequently had cardiac surgery. An apical 4-chamber view (Fig. 7-4) with measurements of various aspects of RA and RV size and leaflet anatomy was used to assess patients (Fig. 7-5). Echo findings of anterior leaflet tethering with restriction of motion as well as a small functional RV were the strongest indicators for valve replacement requirement at surgery. Plication/anuloplasty was performed in 17 patients who differed from patients needing valve excision in that the anterior tricuspid leaflet was elongated, was not tethered, and showed a large excursion. These investigators have extensive experience with Ebstein's anomaly. The use of these quantitative aspects of the echo examination should be useful to measure severity of the disease and to determine with some accuracy which patients are likely to require valve excision at the time of surgery (Fig. 7-6).

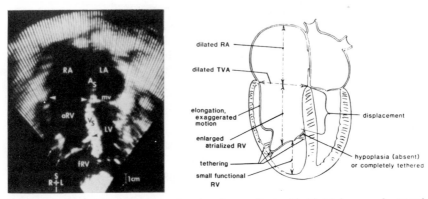

Fig. 7-4. *Left,* Typical 4-chamber echo view in a patient with Ebstein's anomaly. Septal tricuspid leaflet was markedly displaced downward into the right ventricle (black arrowhead) and thus divided the right ventricle into 2 components: an atrialized right ventricle (aRV) and a functional right ventricle (fRV). LV = left ventricle; LA = left atrium; RA = right atrium; VS = ventricular septum; AS = atrial septum; mv = mitral valve; S = superior; L = left; I = inferior; R = right. *Right,* Schematic representation of abnormalities. TVA = tricuspid valve anulus (white arrowheads). Reproduced with permission from Shiina et al.[40]

Fig. 7-5. Schema illustrating measurement of displacement of septal leaflet and intracardiac dimensions. RA = right atrium; LA = left atrium; TVa = tricuspid valve anulus; aRV = atrialized right ventricle; fRV = functional right ventricle; RV = whole right ventricle; dSTL = displacement of septal tricuspid leaflet; LV = left ventricle; S = superior; L = left; I = inferior; R = right. Reproduced with permission from Shiina et al.[40]

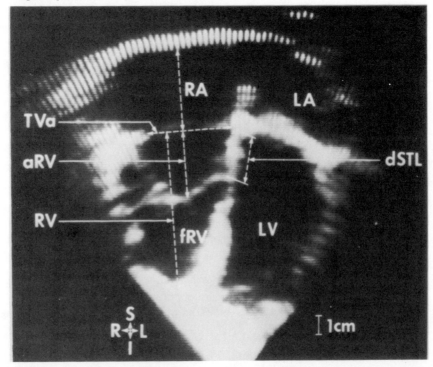

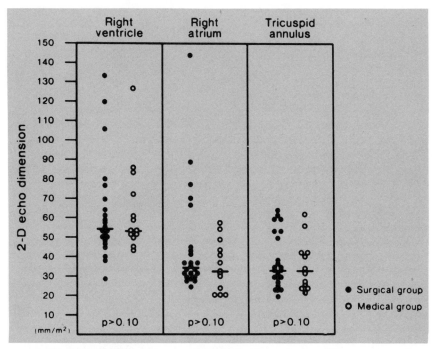

Fig. 7-6. Comparison of dimensions of right ventricle, right atrium, and tricuspid anulus in surgical and medical groups. Note that there is no significant difference between the 2 groups, but a right atrium of more than 60 mm/m² was seen only in patients who underwent surgery. Reproduced with permission from Shiina et al.[40]

AORTIC ISTHMIC COARCTATION

Echo diagnosis

Duncan and associates[41] from Toronto, Canada, used 2-D echo to study 51 neonates in whom "coarctation" of the aorta had been diagnosed clinically. In 40 patients, studies showed coarctation or arch interruption that was later confirmed at angiography, surgery, or necropsy. Of the remaining 11 studies, 1 gave a false positive result, 1 was technically poor, 3 had echo evidence of only mild arch narrowing, and 6 were negative. There were 2 false negative studies; 4 studies were true negatives. Many additional anomalies were correctly identified by echo, although some, such as PDA and small VSD, were frequently missed. Twelve patients underwent surgery without preoperative catheterization. Thus, 2-D echo is very useful in confirming the diagnosis of neonatal aortic coarctation and sometimes obviates the need for invasive catheterization.

Smallhorn and associates[42] from London, England, studied 48 neonates and infants with coarctation of the aorta. By combining information on the peripheral pulses, isthmic size, and the presence of a discrete shelf in the aorta, it was retrospectively possible to predict correctly the presence of coarctation in 45 cases. Imaging of a posterior shelf in the ductal region was possible in 38 of 47 patients. In 9 of 40 patients with preductal coarctation, the shelf was not visible, but isthmic narrowing was found in 7 of 9. One patient with a normal thoracic echo had an abdominal coarctation. The standard long axis suprasternal cut of the aorta may not visualize the posterior shelf, but rotation of the transducer into a ductal cut visualizes most coarctations. These authors have demonstrated the ability successfully to diagnose coarctation in most symptomatic infants. Pitfalls in diagnosis include failure of rotation of the transducer into the ductal cut, failure to rule out discrete coarctation in instances of isthmic hypoplasia in association with a wide open ductus, and confusing the site of entry of a ductus into the anterior aortic wall as the posterior shelf of a coarctation. It is obvious that experience is required in these examinations before sending infants to surgery on the basis of echo data alone. It does appear, however, that by combining clinical, echo, and Doppler data that diagnosis of coarctation and associated defects can be made successfully in most infants.

Hemodynamic, angiographic, and morphologic studies

Although many studies of juxtaductal coarctation of the aorta have been reported, none has correlated clinical, hemodynamic, angiographic, anatomic, and operative findings. Glancy and associates[43] from Bethesda, Maryland, studied 84 such patients (62 male and 22 female; age range, 1–49 years [mean, 17]) (Fig. 7-7). All had murmurs, 76 had absent, diminished, or delayed femoral pulsations, 50 had cuff systolic BPs in the arm >140 mmHg, and 30 had diastolic pressures >90 mmHg (Table 7-1). The average pressure gradients (mmHg) by direct measurements above and below the coarctation in 35 patients were peak systolic, 45; mean, 17; and diastolic, 5 (Table 7-2). Rib notching, visible in chest roentgenograms in 43 patients, correlated

Fig. 7-7.   Ages of the 84 patients with juxtaductal aortic coarctation.

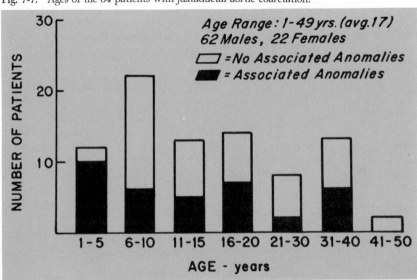

TABLE 7-1. *Physical findings in aortic coarctation.*

| | ASSOCIATED ANOMALIES | |
	ABSENT (48)	PRESENT (36)
Systolic murmur	100%	100%
Diastolic or continuous murmur	27%	67%
Palpable thrill	21%	58%
Systolic ejection click	29%	33%
Absent, diminished, or delayed femoral pulse	94%	86%
Palpable collateral pulsations	35%	39%
Prominent arterial pulses in the neck	46%	22%
Retinal arterial narrowing	44%	18%
Systolic blood pressure (mmHg)		
Range	110–227	108–215
Average	156	145
>140 mmHg	69%	47%
Diastolic blood pressure (mmHg)		
Range	62–123	30–115
Average	91	80
>90 mmHg	44%	25%
Height <11th percentile*	3/20	8/16
Weight <11th percentile*	2/20	10/16

* Children under 13 years of age.

directly with age and inversely with the diameter of the coarctation. Moderate or marked cardiomegaly by radiograph was present in only 1 of 48 patients with isolated coarctation and in 17 of 36 with associated cardiovascular malformations (Table 7-3). The ECGs were abnormal in more than two-thirds of patients with associated anomalies, but were normal in more than three-fourths of those with isolated coarctation. In 70 excised, serially sectioned coarctations the aortic lumens were completely occluded in 4 patients, up to 0.5 mm in internal diameter in 22 patients, from 0.6–2 mm in 26 patients, from 2.1–5 mm in 14, and >5 mm in 4, and correlated directly with lumens measured angiographically. The most significant anatomic factor causing the coarctation was invagination of the medial from the posterior aortic wall, but intimal proliferation (jet lesion) at and immediately distal to the invagination contributed to the narrowing. Three (each with associated anomalies) of 70 patients died early after coarctation repair. Systolic or diastolic BPs decreased early postoperatively in 58 (87%) of 67 surviving patients, and both pressures decreased in 42 (63%). Late postoperatively (mean follow-up, 4.7 years), the systolic BP remained elevated in 25% of patients.

Angioplasty

Sperling and associates[44] from Irvine and Orange, California, performed successful dilation of congenital coarctation of the aorta using the Gruntzig technique in 2 patients, a 3-week-old boy and an 11-month-old girl. The systolic gradients across the narrowings were lowered from 50–8 mmHg and

TABLE 7-2. *Hemodynamic findings in aortic coarctation.*

	ASSOCIATED ANOMALIES	
	ABSENT (12)	PRESENT (23)
Gradient Across Coarctation (mmHg)		
Peak systolic		
Range	39–100	13–90
Average	55	41
Mean		
Range	13–36	5–34
Average	21	16
End diastolic		
Range	1–11	0–15
Average	6	5
Brachial artery–femoral artery	(9 patients)	(12 patients)
Pulse lag (second)		
Range	0.09–0.20	0.06–0.15
Average	0.14	0.09

from 23–8 mmHg. Although the femoral pulses later disappeared in the younger patient, surgery was avoided. The second patient's gradient remained minimal for 8 months and no surgery has been performed.

Lock and associates[45] from Minneapolis, Minnesota, attempted balloon dilation angioplasty 9 times in 8 infants and children with aortic coarctation. In 3 infants with VSD or ASD, angioplasty was attempted preoperatively. Although the gradient fell ≥40%, there was no late gradient evidence of improvement. Angioplasty was performed in 4 infants and children who had previously undergone surgery: (anastomosis, bypass graft, and subclavian flap). Angioplasty was successful in all with an increase in diameter at the coarctation site (4.7 ± 2.6–7.7 ± 4.0 mm; $p < 0.05$) and a decrease in the gradient measured 24 hours after dilation (42 ± 16–12 ± 11 mmHg; $p <$

TABLE 7-3. *Roentgenographic findings in aortic coarctation.*

	ASSOCIATED ANOMALIES	
	ABSENT (48)	PRESENT (36)
Coarctation seen on barium swallow	66%	53%
Rib notching	65%	33%
Aortic lumen completely closed	2/2	2/2
Diameter of aortic lumen <0.5 mm	13/15	5/7
Diameter of aortic lumen 0.6–2.0 mm	8/15	4/11
Diameter of aortic lumen >2.0 mm	4/12	0/6
Heart size		
Normal	63%	6%
Slightly enlarged	35%	47%
Moderately or markedly enlarged	2%	47%

0.05). In 1 patient with hypoplasia of a thoracic aorta and similar lesions of the brachiocephalic arteries, a preliminary attempt to dilate a severely narrowed subclavian artery was unsuccessful. Postdilation angiograms demonstrated small intimal tears in 3 of 5 successful dilations. Follow-up (1–6 months) demonstrated continued gradient relief in 4 of 5 children. These authors have pioneered work with angioplasty in infants and children with congenital cardiac defects. Their data indicate that a short-term fall in gradient across a coarctation site is an unreliable indicator of the success of angioplasty. In addition, dilation, when successful, appears to be in most cases associated with an intimal tear. Thus, the potential for late morbidity and mortality from this procedure is real and these patients will require close clinical and probable angiographic follow-up for a prolonged period.

Kan and coworkers[46] from Baltimore, Maryland, performed percutaneous transluminal angioplasty to treat coarctation restenosis in 7 patients aged 10 months to 17 years. Initial repair had been performed 10 months to 17 years previously. End-to-end anatomosis had been performed in 3 patients, bypass graft in 2, patch angioplasty in 1, and repair of interrupted aortic arch with suture line stenosis was present in 1 patient. Angioplasty reduced systolic gradients from a mean of 58–13 mmHg immediately after the procedure. Follow-up from 1–14 months has indicated sustained relief of restenosis. One patient died 6 hours after an uncomplicated angioplasty, and necropsy revealed no anatomic features to explain the death. The area of stenosis showed small intimal tears without disruption of the media. These data suggest that coarctation restenosis can be treated in some patients by balloon angioplasty. Further data are needed in this situation to indicate which patients are candidates for this procedure and what the risk of the procedure is. Of particular importance will be the risk of late aneurysm formation at the site of intimal tears.

Operative repair

Controversy persists regarding the optimal timing for repair of coarctation of the aorta. Bergdahl and associates[47] from Stockholm, Sweden, assessed the influence of age at operation on long-term results in 3 groups of patients of whom 19 were operated between 5 and 15 years of age, 19, between 16 and 31, and 20, between 35 and 62. There were 4 early deaths and surviving patients were followed for a mean period of 28, 29, and 15 years, respectively. There were 12 late deaths, 9 of which were related to cardiovascular complications. The incidence of late systemic hypertension and cardiovascular symptoms was related to older age at operation. Twenty-nine patients had postoperative cardiac catheterization studies and a gradient of ≥ 20 mmHg was present in 2. Aortic valve disease was present in 37–58% of each group. The authors concluded that coarctation of the aorta should be repaired before school age to prevent systemic hypertension but that patients must have careful follow-up to detect aortic valve disease.

Todd and associates[48] from Liverpool, England, studied 16 patients, 2–9 years after subclavian flap aortoplasty (SFA) for coarctation of the aorta in infancy. There were no major symptoms in the left arm. Parents noted that the left arm was cooler than the right in 4, noticeably smaller in 2, and both colder and thinner in 1. Each patient had diminished or absent pulses in the left arm and the systolic pressure difference between each limb varied from

10–60 mmHg (mean, 37). Anthropometric studies showed the left arm to be shorter than the right in each patient. This was compared with normal right-handed boys, demonstrating significant shortening of the left upper arm only with no difference for the left forearm or hand. The authors concluded that the good results after SFA are not compromised by the effects of ligating the left subclavian artery in infancy.

Fripp and colleagues[49] from Hershey, Pennsylvania, studied the BP response to exercise of 8 children 4.6 ± 0.9 years of age who underwent SFA repair at a mean age of 4.6 months. Doppler systolic pressures were measured in the arm and leg during treadmill exercise using a standard Bruce protocol. Twelve normal volunteer children (aged 5 ± 1 year) were used for control. Mean resting systolic BP in the upper limb was 121 ± 10 mmHg in the patient group and 107 ± 14 mmHg in the control group (p > 0.05). With exercise, this increased similarly in each group. The mean upper to lower limb systolic gradient did not change significantly with dynamic exercise in either group. The authors concluded that SFA is an effective form of treatment for infants with coarctation of the aorta and can be expected to result in a low incidence of *subclinical* residual obstruction.

Waldman and coworkers[50] from San Diego, California, reviewed their experience with 31 patients operated on during the first year of life, 26 being ≤3 months of age. The technique of repair was resection and end-to-end anastomosis in 14, SFA in 6, patch aortoplasty in 5, and various other procedures in 6. Hospital mortality was 3%. The efficacy of repair was evaluated by Doppler arm-to-leg pressure measurements at rest and with stress preoperatively and serially after repair. Preoperatively, arm-to-leg gradients at rest were present in 12 of 18 infants (mean, 77 mmHg), which increased with stress to a median of 92 mmHg. During the first 20 days after repair, most infants had gradients >10 mmHg either at rest or with stress, a finding that was not present in normal control patients. Serial later studies demonstrated gradual resolution of most gradients found early postoperatively. Late data obtained an average of 29 months after operation in 21 patients showed gradients of <10 mmHg at rest in 19 of 21 children and with stress in 15. There was no difference in any of these measurements according to the type of repair employed. The authors concluded that stress testing was useful to unmask gradients not present in the resting state and that most patients have insignificant stress gradients after a variety of operations used to repair coarctation. They believe the optimal method of surgical therapy should depend upon the specific anatomy present.

ECHOCARDIOGRAPHY

As basis for surgery

Stark and associates[51] from London, England, operated on 70 children for congenital heart disease without catheterization. Diagnosis was established by clinical x-ray, ECG, and echo examinations. The following lesions were repaired: coarctation (28 patients), total anomalous pulmonary venous drainage (6 patients), AS (17 patients), mitral and tricuspid valve lesions (4 patients), TGA (3 patients), infective endocarditis (3 patients), truncus (2 patients), and others (13 patients). Three diagnostic errors occurred and in 4 patients the diagnosis was incomplete. No child died as a consequence of diagnostic error and 1 inappropriate operation was carried out (abdominal coarctation of the aorta). Echo should be used to visualize every cardiac structure and every major intrathoracic vessel. In situations in which there is a question of the diagnosis, angiographic studies should be performed. In addition, further comprehensive reports, such as this one detailing the possible diagnostic errors that can occur, will be important to continue to evaluate which anomalies can be safely operated upon without catheterization.

In double orifice mitral valve

Warnes and Somerville[52] from London, England, studied 11 patients aged 10 months to 20 years with double orifice mitral valve. Ten patients had an ostium primum ASD, and 1 had a single atrium. Diagnosis was made by a 2-D echo. This rare additional anomaly in endocardial cushion defects can cause considerable difficulty at surgery and shortly thereafter. It occurs in 3–5% of patients with ostium primum ASD or common atrium. It also occurs rarely with complete AV canal. Radical repair of the double orifice MV was unsuccessful in this series, and these authors suggest that the best surgical results are obtained when the valve is sufficiently competent to be left untouched or when minor repair of a cleft in one orifice results in satisfactory function. This anomaly should be looked for carefully before operation in these patients.

In pulmonary atresia with VSD and in truncus arteriosus

Vargas Barron and associates[53] from Tucson, Arizona, evaluated M-mode and 2-D echo in 13 patients with pulmonary atresia with VSD and in 6 patients with truncus arteriosus to identify echo features distinguishing these 2 abnormalities. M-mode features compatible with the diagnosis of pulmonary atresia with VSD were a small but identifiable space anterior to the aorta and/or immobile pulmonic valve echoes opening during diastole rather than systole. By 2-D echo, the proximal and distal segments of the RV outflow tract could be imaged and the length of the atretic segment estimated. In truncus arteriosus, no RV outflow tract could be identified by 2-D or M-mode echo, and the origin of the PA from the truncus could be imaged directly in 4 patients with type I (main PA arises directly from truncus) and in 1 patient with type II (both PA branches arise separately from truncus) truncus. Abnormalities of the truncal valve also were present and were imaged by 2-D echo in 3 of 5 patients. This study identified specific echo criteria for rapidly diagnosing truncus arteriosus and pulmonary atresia with VSD and for differentiation between these 2 conditions, which may present with overlapping clinical features.

In double chamber right ventricle

Matina and associates[54] from Montreal, Canada, studied 14 patients with doubled chambered right ventricle (DCRV) with 2-D echo. Diagnosis was confirmed at catheterization or necropsy. Diagnosis was based on visualization in the subziphoid short-axis view of an anomalous muscle bundle at the lower margin of the RV infundibulum. A common associated lesion is VSD, found in 13 of 14 patients. Both TF and pulmonary stenosis are easily distinguished with echo. These investigators clearly showed echo criteria for diagnosing DCRV. Doppler studies are needed in this group to determine if estimations of gradients are accurate in this type of PS associated with VSD.

In VSD associated with coarctation of the aorta

Smallhorn and associates[55] from London, England, studied 18 neonatal infants with coarctation of the aorta and large VSD. Twelve patients had a perimembranous defect with varying degrees of extension into the inlet, trabecular, or outlet septum and 10 of 12 had associated aortic override with normal position of the outlet septum. Three patients had malalignment defects with associated LV outflow tract narrowing. Two had a doubly committed subarterial defect with malalignment of the point of continuity between aortic and pulmonary valves on the crest of the trabecular septum. Abnormal insertion of the tricuspid valve that partly obscured the VSD was observed in 10 cases. These authors showed that in most patients with

Fig. 7-8. Parasternal short-axis stop-frame images of the left ventricle in a normal child at end diastole, midsystole, and end systole. The typical rounded configuration of the interventricular septum is demonstrated throughout the cardiac cycle. LV = left ventricle; RV = right ventricle. Reproduced with permission from King et al.[59]

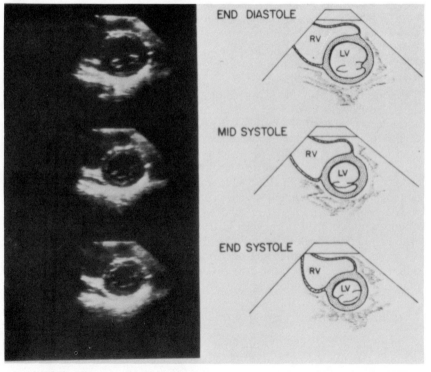

coarctation and VSD, the morphology of the VSD and ventricular outflow tracts is such that LV ejection is directed more toward the pulmonary artery than the aorta. Most patients with coarctation and VSD have interventricular anatomy that might be expected to reduce the amount of LV blood reaching the aortic isthmus and contribute to development of coarctation in utero.

For diameter of right pulmonary artery

Lappen and associates[56] from Chicago, Illinois, determined right PA diameter in 50 normal infants using suprasternal echo. An excellent correlation between right PA diameter and body surface area was observed. Right PA diameter was less than the third percentile in 16 of 37 patients with TF, but exceeded the 97th percentile in 17 of 30 with ASD and 8 of 12 with pulmonary regurgitation. Excellent agreement between angiographic and echo measurements of right PA was found. These measurements are of particular importance in patients with decreased pulmonary blood flow in whom operations are performed in an attempt to increase PA size.

Fig. 7-9. Parasternal short-axis stop-frame images of the left ventricle from a patient with RV systolic hypertension. The interventricular septum becomes progressively flattened from end diastole to end systole. RV = right ventricle; LV = left ventricle. Reproduced with permission from King et al.[59]

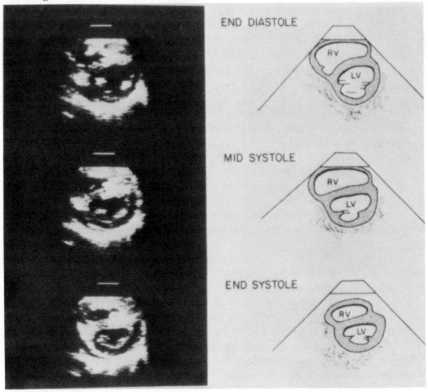

In anomalous left coronary artery

Infants having anomalous origin of the left coronary artery (LCA) from the PA may at times be difficult to distinguish clinically from those having dilated cardiomyopathy (DC). Five children having anomalous LCA and 15 having DC were evaluated by Caldwell and associates[57] from Indianapolis, Indiana, with 2-D echo and angiography. The LCA was demonstrated by 2-D echo to arise normally in all children having DC. The LCA aortic ostium was not recorded in any child with anomalous LCA; however, the LCA was recorded in 3 patients. The 2-D echo recorded the LCA originating from the pulmonary trunk in 2 of 3 infants. A prominent right coronary artery was seen in all patients with anomalous LCA. Thus, 2-D echo is helpful in distinguishing patients having anomalous LCA from those with DC.

For mitral valve area

Riggs and coworkers[58] from Chicago, Illinois, measured mitral valve area (MVA) with echo in 50 normal subjects, 15 patients with congenital MS, and

Fig. 7-10.   Parasternal short-axis stop-frame images of the left ventricle from a patient with suprasystemic RV pressures. The interventricular septum is flattened at end diastole, and at end systole reverses its curvature to become convex toward the left ventricle. RV = right ventricle; LV = left ventricle. Reproduced with permission from King et al.[59]

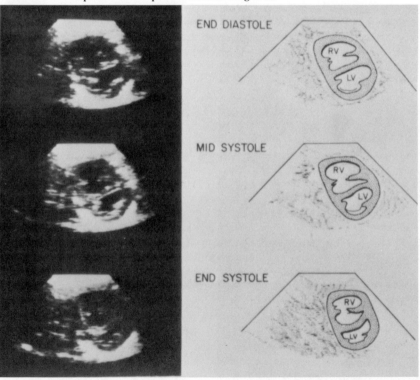

7 patients with tricuspid atresia. Mitral area was measured near the tips of the mitral leaflets and MVA was correlated with body surface area (BSA) and the regression equation obtained: MVA = 4.83 × BSA − 0.07. Patients with MS had MVA <3rd percentile. In 8 patients, there was an excellent correlation between MVA calculated with the Gorlin from catheterization data. All patients with tricuspid atresia had a large MVA (>99 percentile). These investigations indicate that noninvasive MVA can be accurately and reproducibly achieved with echo. This is helpful in assessment on a diagnostic basis and for follow-up.

For septal configuration

King and coworkers[59] from Boston, Massachusetts, examined ventricular septal position and motion in 20 normal children compared with 29 children aged 2 weeks to 20 years with RV hypertension due to a variety of congenital or acquired abnormalities. Echo was used to measure the septal radius of curvature (r) normalized for the ideal (circular) radius for the LV cavity (r_i) in the parasternal short-axis view (Fig. 7-8). With increasing levels of RV systolic hypertension, there is flattening of the septum (Fig. 7-9) and subsequently reversal of the normal curvature with suprasystemic RV pressure (Fig. 7-10). The reciprocal of r/r_i at end systole was <0.5 for patients with RV pressure, >50% of systemic pressure, and the average value for this group was 0.19 at end systole -vs- 0.85 for normal patients. This use of septal configuration with quantitation of the degree of septal flattening as an estimate of RV systolic pressure may prove useful in estimating significant RV and PA hypertension. More data need to be collected in a large number of patients to assess clearly the specificity, sensitivity, and predictive accuracy with various congenital and acquired cardiac abnormalities.

MISCELLANEOUS TOPICS IN PEDIATRIC CARDIOLOGY

Ventricular and pulmonary artery volumes with absent pulmonary valve

Hiraishi and associates[60] from Los Angeles, California, and Birmingham, Alabama, determined RV and LV volumes and right PA volumes in 19 patients with absent pulmonary valve syndrome. Patients were divided into 4 groups: 4 newborn infants who responded to medical management; 7 newborn infants who died; 4 infants aged 1–10 months; and 4 children aged 2–8 years. The RV end-diastolic volume was significantly greater, as was the right PA volume in newborn infants who died. Right PA compliance was greater than normal in all groups but more than 2 times normal in newborn infants who died. Increased right PA compliance and pulmonary regurgitation in patients with absent pulmonary valve syndrome contribute to bronchial obstruction and right-sided CHF and are the causes of high morbidity and mortality in these patients. Many studies have indicated that the primary problem in the sickest patients is bronchial obstruction due to the aneurysmally dilated PAs. Patients with only moderate PA dilation generally can be handled medically and are good candidates for repair after infancy. If medical management fails in the sick newborn, surgery should be attempted to reduce the size of the right PA and eliminate the hemodynamic abnormalities.

Ventricular response to exercise in VSD or ASD

In patients with VSD or ASD, the ventricle, which is chronically volume overloaded, might not appropriately respond to increased demand for an augmentation in cardiac output and thereby might limit total cardiac function. Peter and associates[61] from Durham, North Carolina, simultaneously measured RV and LV response to exercise in 10 normal individuals, 10 patients with VSD, and 10 patients with ASD. The normal subjects increased both RV EF and LV EF, RV and LV end-diastolic volume, and RV and LV stroke volume to achieve higher cardiac output during exercise. Patients with VSD did not increase RV EF, but increased RV end-diastolic volume and RV stroke volume; LV end-diastolic volume did not increase in these patients but LV EF, LV stroke volume, and forward LV output achieved during exercise were comparable to the response observed in healthy subjects. In the patients with ASD, no rest-to-exercise change occurred in either RV EF, RV end-diastolic volume, or RV stroke volume. In addition, LV end-diastolic volume failed to increase, and, despite an increase in LV EF, LV stroke volume remained unchanged from rest to exercise. It was concluded that 1) cardiac output is augmented principally by the heart rate increase in these patients; and 2) RV function is the major determinant of total cardiac output during exercise in patients with cardiac septal defects and left-to-right shunt.

Digital angiography

Levin and coworkers[62] from New York City compared digital subtraction angiography (DSA) with conventional cut film angiography or cineangiography in 42 patients aged 2 months to 18 years. There were 29 diagnoses, including regurgitant and obstructive lesions, shunt lesions, and a group of miscellaneous anomalies. For right-sided injections distant from the anomalies, the dose of contrast was 60–100% of the dose during standard angiography. With injections close to the anomaly, contrast dose was 28–42% of the conventional dose. Radiation dose was markedly reduced with DSA and only 5 of 92 studies were suboptimal for diagnosis. Digital subtraction angiography has been used both as a minimally invasive technique with intravenous contrast that can be used for outpatients as well as for selective angiography during routine catheterization to reduce radiation and contrast dose. Intravenous studies in children are primarily helpful for aortic or PA lesions, such as coarctation of the aorta or PA branch stenosis. Most other congenital cardiac lesions can be imaged equally well noninvasively with echo. Thus, the potential for this modality in outpatient studies for diagnosis of congenital heart disease is probably minimal. In contrast, use of this modality in the catheterization laboratory may prove extremely useful for contrast enhancement and for reduction of radiation exposure. Unfortunately, there are no biplane DSA units at the present time. Thus, multiple injections would be needed to evaluate children with congenital heart disease. This drawback negates to some extent the potential for the use of decreased amounts of contrast.

Coronary arteriography

Takahasha and coworkers[63] from Los Angeles, California, performed selective coronary arteriography in 34 patients, 7 months to 18 years of age. Indications for study included Kawasaki disease with clinical or echo suggestion of coronary aneurysms, patients with congenital heart disease and angina or ECG changes of ischemia, and patients with congenital heart disease and suspected coronary anomalies. Catheters were shaped for left and right coronary injections according to the patient's size and aortic root dimensions. There was no mortality, but 1 patient had VF and 1 had transient bradycardia and hypotension without sequelae. The need for coronary arteriography in children is rare, but with the increasing prevalence of patients with Kawasaki disease, the number of studies performed will probably increase. Most patients with this illness do not need coronary arteriography, and it should be reserved for those with suspected ischemia or infarction in whom bypass surgery or changes in medical management are contemplated. In addition, patients with complex congenital heart disease with suspected coronary anomalies or the need for detailed coronary anatomy before right ventriculotomy is performed also are candidates for coronary arteriography. Finally, patients with cardiac tumor may benefit from coronary arteriography if surgical removal is contemplated. These studies should be performed only by groups who have considerable experience both with infants and children and with coronary arteriography and anatomy. It represents a real opportunity for collaboration between cardiologists, pediatric cardiologists, and cardiovascular radiologists.

Neonatal pulmonary hypertension

St. John Sutton and Meyer[64] from Cincinnati, Ohio, assessed regional and global LV function in 23 neonates with persistent PA hypertension using computer-assisted analysis of LV echoes and compared results with 50 normal neonates. The LV end-diastolic dimension was normal, but end-systolic dimension was increased and fractional shortening and peak VCF were mildly decreased, suggesting impaired systolic performance. In addition, the peak rate of increase in LV diameter on early diastole was decreased and the durations of rapid filling and isovolumic relaxation were prolonged, suggesting abnormal diastolic LV properties. Seven neonates with persistent PA hypertension died and 3 of 7 examined at necropsy all had LV hypertrophy with 2 of 3 showing extensive subendocardial hemorrhage and infarction affecting RV and LV papillary muscles. These authors present intriguing data regarding LV dysfunction in infants with persistent PA hypertension. This situation occurs in neonates with many different etiologic factors, and whether the LV dysfunction is primary or whether it is secondary to a combination of hypoxemia and acidemia is unclear. There was no correlation between severity of LV dysfunction and clinical outcome.

Psychologic development after cardiac operation

Welles and associates[65] from London, England, determined IQ scores from cognitive, memory, perceptual, quantitative, and verbal tests in 31 patients 5 years following operations performed with total circulatory arrest between 1972 and 1976. These patients were compared with three control groups: 19 patients with similar defects operated upon using moderate hypothermia and continuous cardiopulmonary bypass; 16 children who were the siblings of the total circulatory arrest patients; and 14 children who were the siblings of the cardiopulmonary bypass patients. The hypothermic temperatures reached were closely clustered around 15°C in the arrest group and 28°C in the bypass group. Circulatory arrest times ranged from 22–71 minutes. The mean IQ score of the arrest group was significantly lower than that of their siblings (91 -vs- 106), but the score for bypass patients was not different from that of their siblings (102 -vs- 96). The difference between patient and sibling in verbal, quantitative, and general cognitive scores in the arrest group was associated with duration of arrest. These data question the "safe" period of total circulatory arrest of 60 minutes. There are some difficulties with the data, including the lack of an appropriate control group and the fact that the siblings of the patients in the total arrest group had a higher IQ than those in the cardiopulmonary bypass group. Further studies are needed in regard to long-term psychologic development in similar patient groups. The technique of total circulatory arrest to provide an adequate intracardiac repair frequently is required in infants with complex congenital defects. The authors agree that the use of total circulatory arrest in selective patients is not abrogated by these studies but suggest that continued attempts to minimize total circulatory arrest times are needed.

MISCELLANEOUS TOPICS IN PEDIATRIC CARDIAC SURGERY

Coronary artery fistula

Urrutia-S and coworkers[66] from Houston, Texas, in 25 years treated 58 patients with coronary artery fistulas. A single fistula was present in 49 patients, multiple fistulas in 9. The fistula arose from the right coronary artery in 44%, LAD in 29%, and LC in 22%. They drained into the right ventricle in 33%, PA, 31%, right atrium, 22%, left ventricle, 10%, left atrium, 1%. Preoperative symptoms were present in 29 of 37 patients with no associated cardiac lesions and in 17 of 19 patients with associated cardiac lesions, the commonest being CAD. Surgical closure of the fistula was accomplished in 56 patients without mortality. Each patient >25 years of age was symptomatic. The authors therefore recommended surgical treatment at diagnosis. Direct closure of the drainage site of the fistula using cardiopulmonary bypass methods was recommended.

Cor triatriatum

Cor triatriatum is a rare anomaly in which the left atrium is divided into a dorsal chamber receiving the pulmonary veins and a ventral chamber containing the LA appendage and leading to the mitral valve. A communication of varying size is present in the fibromuscular diaphragm between these 2 chambers and either 1 may or may not connect via an interatrial communication to the right atrium. Oglietti and associates[67] from Houston, Texas, reviewed their experience with 25 patients who underwent surgical correction from 1959–1980. They ranged in age from 4 months to 38 years. Five patients (20%) had isolated cor triatriatum and 20 patients had other associated cardiac defects, including anomalous pulmonary venous return in 24%, persistent left superior vena cava in 32%, ASD in 60%, single ventricle in 8%, and complete atrioventricular canal in 8%. There were 21 hospital survivors (mortality, 16%) and the 4 patients who died were infants with major associated cardiac anomalies. The dividing membrane was resected via the left atrium in 40%, right atrium in 48%, and both atria in 12%. The authors favor a surgical approach through the right atrium and atrial septum.

Branch pulmonary artery from ascending aorta

Origin of either the right or left PA from the ascending aorta is rare. A PDA is the most common associated anomaly when the right PA is involved, and TF is most frequently associated with aortic origin of the left PA. Penkoske and coworkers[68] from Boston, Massachusetts, reported 3 patients who underwent surgical repair between 2 and 8 weeks of age. This was accomplished by detaching the anomalous PA from the aorta and anastomosing it to the pulmonary trunk in the normal anatomic position. Each patient survived and although PA pressure was systemic preoperatively, it was almost normal 24 hours later. The authors indicated that the untreated course of these patients is dismal and that operation should be performed as early as possible to prevent the development of irreversible pulmonary vascular obstructive disease.

Total anomalous pulmonary venous connection

Mazzucco and colleagues[69] from Padova, Italy, reviewed their experience with 20 patients who underwent repair of total anomalous pulmonary venous connection (TAPVC) at 1 day to 12 months of age (9 < 1 month). Each of 4 patients with associated intracardiac defects died. There were 2 deaths among 16 with isolated TAPVC, both repaired during the first month of life and having infradiaphragmatic drainage with severe pulmonary venous obstruction. Analysis of this group shows a possible (p = 0.17) incremental effect due to young age and pulmonary venous obstruction. There were no late deaths and no late complications among the 14 survivors followed 7 months to 10 years (mean, 44 months). The authors recommended an aggressive surgical approach regardless of age, degree of PA hypertension, and type of anatomic connection. Those with associated malformations are at significantly greater risk.

Interrupted aortic arch

Kron and coworkers[70] from Charlottesville, Virginia, reported their experience treating 9 patients <8 days of age for interrupted aortic arch and associated VSD. Each presented with severe CHF and acidosis. The partial repair was accomplished by division of the carotid or proximal subclavian artery and connecting this end-to-side to the descending thoracic aorta in 7 patients. In 2, the subclavian artery arising distal to the interruption was divided and anastomosed end-to-side to the left common carotid artery. Banding of the PA also was done in 5 patients. There were 4 hospital deaths. Five survivors have been followed between 4 months and 7 years and an anastomotic gradient ≤10 mmHg was present in 3, 40 mmHg in 1, and 55 mmHg in 1. Anastomotic growth was demonstrated in the 3 patients followed between 4 and 7 years after operation. Operations were performed between 1972 and 1982. The author's current approach to the management of these ill neonates includes initial prostaglandin E_1 infusion and patient stabilization, aortic arch reconstruction with endogenous arch vessels, and selective PA banding for those with large VSD.

Double outlet right ventricle

Double outlet right ventricle (DORV) is an uncommon anomaly that is usually amenable to corrective surgery. Luber and associates[71] from Boston, Massachusetts, reported their early and late results after repair of DORV in 57 patients operated between 1973 and 1981. Eighteen patients (32%) were <1 year of age. Pulmonary stenosis was present in 35 and a valved extracardiac conduit was used in the repair of 15. Subaortic stenosis was present in 6. There were 7 hospital deaths (12%), 3 occurring among 5 patients with associated AV valve abnormalities. A tunnel repair connecting the VSD with the aorta was accomplished in 46 patients with 5 early deaths (11%) and connecting the VSD with the PA plus venous switch in 7 patients with 1 death. Three patients (0 deaths) had VSD and PA closure and LV-PA conduit, and 1 nonsurvivor with severe subaortic stenosis had connection of the proximal PA to the aorta, LV-PA conduit, and venous switch. Young age was not related to hospital mortality. There were no late deaths among the 50 survivors who were followed between 2 months and 9 years (mean, 3.6 years). Postoperative cardiac catheterization studies in 28 patients and 12 of 14 with significant abnormalities underwent successful reoperation (rate, 24%) for residual VSD in 5, AV valve regurgitation in 3, subaortic or subpulmonic obstruction in 3, and AR in 1. The authors concluded that surgical risk is related to the anatomic complexity of the malformation and the rather high incidence of residual hemodynamic abnormalities underscores the need for close long-term follow-up.

Blalock-Taussig anastomosis

Pulsed Doppler echo has been used to detect continuous turbulent flow in the right PA after Blalock-Taussig (B-T) shunts. Since continuous turbulent flow could also arise from PDA (frequently present in the neonate), continuous turbulent flow in the right PA is not specific for B-T shunt function. Stevenson and associates[72] from Seattle, Washington, evaluated 35 B-T shunts from suprasternal or high parasternal approach for flow in the right PA, and in the B-T shunts themselves. From precordial approach, Doppler evaluations of the main PA were also made in search of flow characteristics of PDA. Doppler detection of flow within the B-T shunts indicated shunt patency, and that continuous turbulent flow in the right PA was not due to only PDA. Shunts were proved patent in 31 patients, occluded in 4. Twelve patients also had PDA. By Doppler, the right PA had continuous turbulent flow in 30 of 31 patients in whom the right PA was found. From the suprasternal or high parasternal approach, the right B-T shunts were detected by marked continuous turbulent flow directed away from the transducer, between the aortic and superior vena caval flow signals. Left B-T shunts had similar directional continuous turbulent flow. Prosthetic shunts were identified by the dense shunt material. Twenty-four of 31 functional shunts were identified, and all contained continuous turbulent flow. Three left-sided shunts were missed. All 4 occluded shunts were identified by Doppler and had no lumen flow within. The B-T shunts were not confused with PDA in any patient. Doppler echo provided correct diagnosis (detection plus patency or occlusion) in 80% of all B-T shunts and in 91% of prosthetic shunts. Pulsed Doppler has reliable accuracy in evaluation of B-T shunts per se, and in differentiation from PDA. Doppler echo is also very useful when no murmur is heard or when a murmur can be attributed to shunt, PDA, or both.

Guyton and coworkers[73] from Atlanta, Georgia, reviewed their experience with 64 patients with varying congenital cardiac anomalies who underwent a classic B-T shunt. Thirty-one patients were <2 months of age at operation. There were 2 hospital deaths (3%) and no early shunt closures. Heparin was administered intraoperatively and continued for 2 days in 41 patients. Reexploration for bleeding was required in 5 (12%) of these 41 and in 1 (4%) of 23 who did not receive heparin postoperatively (p < 0.05). There were 3 late cardiac deaths in patients with complex heart disease. A life-table analysis showed 87% of the shunts functioning at 1 year and 78% at 2 years. Younger age at operation did not influence late patency. Postoperative pulmonary arteriograms were reviewed in 42 patients and showed mild tenting at the site of the shunt in 4, severe kinking in 2. Branch PA diameter was compared with the diameter of the descending aorta at the diaphragm and showed equal bilateral growth that was more rapid in those with initially small pulmonary arteries. The authors concluded that the B-T shunt can be performed with low risk and provides good palliation and PA growth even when performed in small infants. Effective palliation persists in 80% of patients 1 year postoperatively.

Limb vascular effects of subclavian artery division

Lodge and coworkers[74] from San Diego, California, evaluated the acute and chronic effects of division of the subclavian artery in 28 patients, 23 undergoing a Blalock-Taussig shunt, 4 a subclavian flap angioplasty to repair coarctation, and 1 for aberrant left subclavian artery. Age at operation varied between 1 day and 4 years (median, 2 months). Bilateral systolic brachial artery pressure was measured by Doppler preoperatively and at various intervals during the first postoperative year. Brachial artery pressure on the operated side/control side was 0.99 preoperatively, 0.39 between 4 and 48 hours after operation, 0.62 at 3 weeks, and 0.70 thereafter (p < 0.001 at each interval). Exercise significantly increased brachial artery pressure in both operated and nonoperated limbs similarly (mean change, 25–30 mmHg). No significant differences were present in patients who had no -vs- ≥2 subclavian artery branches ligated.

Pulmonary artery banding

Various surgical protocols are currently employed to provide optimal PA constriction during banding. Some patients do require postoperative band adjustment, and thus Muraoka and associates[75] from Shizuoka, Japan, reported their experience with a new technique of adjustable PA banding employed in 6 patients. A heavy monofilament ligature enclosed in a Goretex sleeve was placed about the PA and a tourniquet formed by enclosure within a polyvinyl tube. Intraoperative PA banding was accomplished while measuring systemic and PA pressures, heart rate, systemic PA oxygen, and the degree of constriction by intraoperative 2-D echo. After appropriate constriction, hemoclips were placed at the distal end of the polyvinyl tube to secure the tourniquet and this end was buried within the anterior chest wall. Each patient survived the banding procedure, and postoperative adjustment using local anesthesia was performed in 4, loosening the band in 2 shortly after operation and tightening the band in 2 at 3 and 4 months after surgery. This was effectively accomplished in each. The authors believe this technique of PA banding allows simple later adjustment and may optimize early and late results.

Pericardial patch for aortic root enlargement

Many surgeons have avoided the use of autogenous parietal pericardium as a patch material in the systemic circulation, fearing aneurysm formation. The impervious nature of parietal pericardium, however, makes it an attractive patch material. Piehler and coworkers[76] from Rochester, Minnesota, reviewed their experience with 96 patients operated from 1965–1981 who received autogenous parietal pericardial patch enlargement during AVR. The patch was used to enlarge the supravalvular aorta in 81 and to enlarge the aortic anulus (including subvalvar and supravalvular areas) in 15. Follow-up data were available in 92 patients (96%) 6 months to 15 years after surgery (mean, 5.4 years). None of the 92 hospital survivors had clinical evidence of sudden patch failure or patch aneurysm detected by chest x ray. More direct information was available in 48 patients, 24 at reoperation, 6 at necropsy, 16 with 2-D echo, and 2 with aortic root angiography. No instance of patch aneurysm was observed and in each patient the patches were nicely incorporated into adjacent tissues.

Fontan operation for complex defects with common atrium

The Fontan operation, originally described and employed for patients with classic tricuspid atresia, has been extended to other forms of single ventricle and other types of complex heart disease associated with low pulmonary artery pressure. Di Carlo and associates[77] from Amsterdam, The Netherlands, described their experience with this type of operation in 4 patients with complex cardiac malformations, including a common atrium. Three had a complete form of AV canal defect with double outlet right ventricle and 1 had left AV valve atresia. A common atrium was present in each and 3 had pulmonary and systemic venous anomalies. Complex atrial baffles were placed to divert pulmonary venous return through the AV valve and into the ventricle, and the right atrium was connected to the PA via a valved conduit. There was 1 hospital survivor and each of the 3 patients with venous anomalies died. The authors suggest that complex rerouting of blood within the atria may result in an increased hospital mortality when combined with the Fontan-type operation. Experience at the University of Alabama in Birmingham and also at the Mayo Clinic has shown an increased risk for the Fontan-type operation for cardiac anomalies other than tricuspid atresia. Since there is no theoretical reason that completely explains this, these experiences support the idea that the pathways created within the atrium and connecting the atrium to the PA must be completely unobstructive. Further experience and technical improvement may neutralize this difference in hospital mortality.

Valved extracardiac conduits

Stewart and associates[78] from Rochester, New York, evaluated late results of 18 children who received a RV-PA Hancock valved extracardiac conduit between 1974 and 1977 as part of repair of a variety of congenital cardiac defects. Their ages range from 18 months to 18 years (mean, 7 years). Two patients with TGA, VSD, and pulmonary stenosis died within 12 months of repair from chronic CHF. Fifteen long-term survivors were followed between 6 and 9 years and were New York Heart Association functional class I. Routine cardiac catheterization studies were performed at a mean of 16 months and again at a mean of 6 years after repair. The mean RV-PA gradient was 25 mmHg at 16 months, but 2 patients had a gradient >50 mmHg. The mean gradient at the late study was 43 mmHg and 7 patients had a gradient ≥50 mmHg. Each of 5 patients survived reoperation for conduit replacement. The principal site of obstruction in each of the conduits was in the region of the valve and was due to either thickened peel formation and/or degenerated rigid leaflets. Conduit compression was not observed.

Daskalopoulos and coworkers[79] from Rochester, Minnesota, described an uncommon complication from use of valved extracardiac conduits in 3 children 2–8 years of age. Two died within 24 hours of operation and 1, 4 months later, from coronary artery compression by the metallic stent of a Hancock in 1, Carpentier-Edwards in 1, and Ionescu-Shiley in 1. In a fourth patient, coronary artery compression by the conduit was diagnosed intraoperatively during the presence of low cardiac output, which was successfully managed by repositioning the conduit. Careful intraoperative assessment of coronary anatomy must be undertaken at the time of any procedure requiring a valved extracardiac conduit.

Extracardiac conduits are most commonly placed between RV and PA to repair a variety of congenital cardiac malformations. Successful placement of a valved extracardiac conduit from the left atrium to the left ventricle was reported by Lansing and coworkers[80] from Louisville, Kentucky. They described the case of a 15-year-old girl who at the age of 10 had a small Starr-Edwards ball valve prosthesis placed for congenital MS. She had severe CHF from a gradient across this prosthesis and underwent successful placement of a porcine valved conduit from the body of the left atrium to the left ventricle. The conduit has functioned nicely and demonstrates the feasibility of using extracardiac conduits in this position.

References

1. NAGATA S, NIMURA Y, SAKAIBARA H, BEPPU S, PARK YD, KAWAZOE K, FUJITA T: Mitral valve lesion associated with secundum atrial septal defect: analysis by real time two dimensional echocardiography. Br Heart J 49:51–58, Jan 1983.

2. SHUB C, DIMOPOULOS IN, SEWARD JB, CALLAHAN JA, TANCREDI RG, SCHATTENBERG TT, REEDER GS, HAGLER DJ, TAGIK AJ: Sensitivity of 2-dimensional Echocardiography in the direct visualization atrial septal defect utilizing the subcoastal approach: experience with 154 patients. J Am Coll Cardiol 2:127–135, July 1983.

3. KAWASHIMA Y, MATSUDA H, HIROSE H, NAKANO S, SHIMAZAKI Y, MIYAMOTO K: Surgical treatment of complete atrioventricular canal defect with an endocardial cushion prosthesis. Circulation 68 (suppl II):139–143, Sept 1983.

4. SILVERMAN N, LEVITSKY S, FISHER E, DUBROW I, HASTREITER A, SCAGLIOTTI D: Efficacy of pulmonary artery banding in infants with complete atrioventricular canal. Circulation 68 (suppl II):148–153, Sept 1983.

5. NAKAZAWA M, TAKAO A, CHON Y, SHIMIZU T, KANAYA M, MOMMA K: Significance of systemic vascular resistance in determining the hemodynamic effects of hydralazine on large ventricular septal defects. Circulation 68:420–424, Aug 1983.

6. ALVERSON DC, ELDRIDGE MW, JOHNSON JD, BURSTEIN R, PAPILE L, DILLON P, YABEK S, BERMAN W: The effect of patent ductus arteriosus on left ventricular output in premature infants. J Pediatr 102:754–757, May 1983.

7. GERSONY WM, PECKHAM J, ELLISON RC, MIETTIEN OS, NADAS AS: Effects of indomethacin in premature infants with patent ductus arteriosus: results of a national collaborative study. J Pediatr 102:895–906, June 1983.

8. MAVROUDIS C, COOK LN, FLEISCHAKER JW, NAGARAJ HS, SHOTT RJ, HOWE R, GRAY LA JR: Management of patent ductus arteriosus in the premature infant: indomethacin versus ligation. Ann Thorac Surg 35:561–566, Nov 1983.

9. LIMA CO, SAHN DJ, VALDEZ-CRUZ LM, GOLDBERG SJ, BARRON JV, ALLEN HD, GRENADIER E: Non-invasive prediction of transvalvular pressure gradient in patients with pulmonary stenosis by quantitative 2-dimensional echocardiographic Doppler studies. Circulation 67:866–871, April 1983.

10. LOCK JE, CASTANEDA-ZUNIGA WR, FUHRMAN BP, BASS JL: Balloon dilation angioplasty of hypoplastic and stenotic pulmonary arteries. Circulation 67:962–967, May 1983.

11. LEWIS AB, WELLS W, LINDESMITH GG: Evaluation and surgical treatment of pulmonary atresia and intact ventricular septum in infancy. Circulation 67:1318–1323, June 1983.

12. BASS JL, FUHRMAN BP, LOCK JE: Balloon Occlusion of atrial septal defect to assess right ventricular capability in hypoplastic right heart syndrome. Circulation 68:1081–1086, Nov 1983.

13. SHIMAZAKI Y, KAWAXHIMA Y, HIROSE H, NAKANO S, MATSUDA H, KITAMURA S, MORIMOTO S: Operative results with pseudotruncus arteriosus. Ann Thorac Surg 35:294–299, March 1983.

14. FREEDOM RM, PONGIGLIONE G, WILLIAMS WG, TRUSLER GA, ROWE RD: Palliative right ventricular outflow tract construction for patients with pulmonary atresia, ventricular septal defect, and hypoplastic pulmonary arteries. J Thorac Cardiovasc Surg 86:24–36, July 1983.

15. KIRKLIN JW, BLACKSTONE EH, KIRKLIN JK, PACIFICO AD, ARAMENDI J, BARGERON LM JR: Surgical results and protocols in the spectrum of tetralogy of Fallot. Ann Surg 198:251–265, Sept 1983.

16. SHAHER RM, FOSTER E, FARINA M, SPOONER E, SHEIKH F, ALLEY R: Right heart reconstruction following repair of tetralogy of Fallot. Ann Thorac Surg 35:421–426, April 1983.

17. BOVE EL, BYRUM CJ, THOMAS FD, KAVEY REW, SONDHEIMER HM, BLACKMAN MS, PARKER FB JR: The influence of pulmonary insufficiency on ventricular function following repair of tetralogy of Fallot. J Thorac Cardiovasc Surg 85:691–696, May 1983.

18. BERTRANOU EG, THIBERT M, AIGUEPERSE J: Short-term variations of the right ventricular/left ventricular pressure ratio following repair of tetralogy of Fallot. Ann Thorac Surg 35:427–429, April 1983.

19. DEANFIELD JE, HOAGUE S, PHIL M, ANDERSON RA, McKENNA WJ, ALLWORK SP, HALLIDIE-SMITH KA: Late sudden death after repair of tetralogy of Fallot: a clinicopathologic study. Circulation 67:626–631, March 1983.

20. GARSON A, PORTER CJ, GILLETTE PC, McNAMARA DG: Induction of ventricular tachycardia during electrophysiologic study after repair of tetralogy of Fallot. J Am Coll Cardiol 1:1493–1502, June 1983.

21. PARRISH MD, GRAHAM TP JR, BENDER HW, JONES JP, PATTON J, PARTAIN CL: Radionuclide angiographic evaluation of right and left ventricular function during exercise after repair of transposition of the great arteries: comparison with normal subjects and patients with congenitally corrected transposition. Circulation 67:178–183, Jan 1983.

22. RIGGS TW, MUSTER AJ, AZIZ KU, PAUL MH, ILBAW IM, IDRISS FS: 2–dimensional echocardiographic and angiocardiographic diagnosis of subpulmonary stenosis due to tricuspid valve pouch in complete transposition of the great arteries. J Am Coll Cardiol 1:484–491, Feb 1983.

23. VanDOESBURG NH, BIERMANN FZ, WILLIAMS RG: Left ventricular geometry in infants with D-transposition of the great arteries and intact interventricular septum. Circulation 68:733–739, Oct 1983.

24. BEITZKE A, SUPPAN CH: Use of prostaglandin E_2 in management of transposition of great arteries before balloon atrial septostomy. Br Heart J 49:341–344, Apr 1983.

25. PARK SC, NECHES WH, MATHEWS RA, FRICKER FJ, BEERMAN LB, FISCHER DR, LENOX CC, ZUBERBUHLER JR: Hemodynamic function after the Mustard operation for transposition of the great arteries. Am J Cardiol 51:1514–1519, May 1983.

26. PENKOSKE PA, WESTERMAN GR, MARX GR, RABINOVITCH M, FREED MD, NORWOOD WI, CASTANEDA AR: Transposition of the great arteries and ventricular septal defect: results with the Senning operation and closure of the ventricular septal defect in infants. Ann Thorac Surg 36:281–288, Sept 1983.

27. SATOMI G, NAKAMURA K, TAKAO A, IMAI Y: Two dimensional echocardiographic detection of pulmonary venous channel stenosis after Senning's operation. Circulation 68:545–549, Sept 1983.

28. MARTIN TC, SMITH L, HERNANDEZ A, WELSON CS: Dysrhythmias following the Senning operation for dextro-transposition of the great arteries. J Thorac Cardiovasc Surg 85:928–932, June 1983.

29. PACIFICO AD, STEWART RW, BARGERON LM JR: Repair of transposition of the great arteries with ventricular septal defect by an arterial switch operation. Circulation 68 (suppl II):49–55, Sept 1983.

30. YACOUB MH, ARENSMAN FW, KECK E, RADLEY-SMITH R: Fate of dynamic left ventricular outflow tract obstruction after anatomic correction of transposition of the great arteries. Circulation 68 (suppl II):56–62, Sept 1983.

31. WILCOX BR, HENRY GW, ANDERSON RH: The transmitral approach to left ventricular outflow tract obstruction. Ann Thorac Surg 35:288–293, March 1983.

32. SUTHERLAND GR, SMALLHORN JF, ANDERSON RH, RIGBY ML, HUNTER S: Atrial ventricular discordance: cross sectional echocardiographic-morphological correlative. Br Heart J 50:8–20, July 1983.

33. HUHTA JC, MALONEY JD, RITTER DG, ILSTRUP DM, FELDT RH: Complete atrioventricular block in patients with atrioventricular discordance. Circulation 67:1374–1377, June 1983.

34. DOTY DB, TRUESDELL SC, MARVIN WJ: Techniques to avoid injury of the conduction tissue during the surgical treatment of corrected transposition. Circulation 68 (suppl II):63–69, Sept 1983.

35. LIMA CO, SAHN DJ, VALDES-CRUZ LM, ALLEN HD, GOLDBERG SG, GRENADIER E, BARRON JV: Prediction of the severity of LV outflow tract obstruction by quantitative 2–D echo Doppler studies. Circulation 68:348–354, Aug 1983.

36. LANG P, NORWOOD WI: Hemodynamic assessment after palliative surgery for hypoplastic left heart syndrome. Circulation 68:104–108, July 1983.

37. FONTAN F, DEVILLE C, QUAEGEBEUR J, OTTENKAMP J, SOURDILLE N, CHOUSSAT A, BROM G: Repair of tricuspid atresia in 100 patients. J Thorac Cardiovasc Surg 85:647–660, May 1983.

38. BULL C, DeLEVAL MR, STARK J, TAYLOR JFM, MacCARTNEY F: Use of a ventricular chamber in the Fontan repair. J Thorac Cardiovasc Surg 85:21–31, Jan 1983.

39. DeLeon SY, Idriss FS, Ilbawi MN, Muster AJ, Paul MH, Cole RB, Riggs TW, Berry TE: The role of the Glenn shunt in patients undergoing the Fontan operation. J Thorac Cardiovasc Surg 85:669–677, May 1983.

40. Shiina A, Seward JB, Tagika J, Hagler DJ, Danielson GK: Two dimensional echocardiographic-surgical correlation in Ebstein's anomaly: preoperative determination of patients requiring tricuspid valve plication versus replacement. Circulation 68:534–544, Sept 1983.

41. Duncan WJ, Ninomiya K, Cook DH, Rowe RD: Noninvasive diagnosis of neonatal aortic coarctation and associated anomalies using two-dimensional echocardiography. Am Heart J 106:63–69, July 1983.

42. Smallhorn JR, Huhta JC, Adams PA, Anderson RH, Wilkinson JO, Macartney J: Cross Sectional echocardiographic assessment of coarctation in the sick infant. Br Heart J 50:349–361, Oct 1983.

43. Glancy DL, Morrow AG, Simon AL, Roberts WC: Juxtaductal aortic coarctation: analysis of 84 patients studied hemodynamically, angiographically, and morphologically after age 1 year. Am J Cardiol 51:537–551, Feb 1983.

44. Sperling DR, Dorsey TJ, Rowen M, Gazzaniga AB: Percutaneous transluminal angioplasty of congenital coarctation of the aorta. Am J Cardiol 51:562–564, Feb 1983.

45. Lock JE, Bass JL, Amplatz K, Fuhrman BP, Castaneda-Zuniga W: Balloon angioplasty of coarctation. Circulation 68:109–116, July 1983.

46. Kan JS, White RI, Mitchell SE, Farmlatt EJ, Donahoo JS, Gardiner TJ: Treatment of restenosis of coarctation by percutaneous transluminal angioplasty. Circulation 68:1087–1094, Nov 1983.

47. Bergdahl L, Bjork VO, Jonasson R: Surgical correction of coarctation of the aorta. Influence of age on late results. J Thorac Cardiovasc Surg 85:532–536, Apr 1983.

48. Todd PJ, Dangerfield PH, Hamilton DI, Wilkinson JL: Late effects on the left upper limb of subclavian flap aortoplasty. J Thorac Cardiovasc Surg 85:678–681, May 1983.

49. Fripp RR, Whitman V, Werner JC, Nicholas GG, Waldhausen JA: Blood pressure response to exercise in children following the subclavian flap procedure for coarctation of the aorta. J Thorac Cardiovasc Surg 85:682–685, May 1983.

50. Waldman JD, Lamberti JJ, Goodman AH, Mathewson JW, Kirkpatrick SE, George L, Turner SW, Pappelbaum SJ: Coarctation in the first year of life. Patterns of postoperative effect. J Thorac Cardiovasc Surg 86:9–17, July 1983.

51. Stark J, Smallhorn J, Huhta J, DeLaval M, MacCartney FJ, Rees PG, Taylor JFN: Surgery for congenital heart defects diagnosed with cross-sectional echocardiography. Circulation 68 (suppl II):129–138, Sept 1983.

52. Warnes C, Somerville J: Double mitral valve orifice in atrial ventricular defects. Br Heart J 49:59–64, Jan 1983.

53. Vargas Barron J, Sahn DJ, Attie F, Valdes-Cruz LM, Grenadier E, Allen HD, Lima CO, Goldberg SJ: Two-dimensional echocardiographic study of right ventricular outflow and great artery anatomy in pulmonary atresia with ventricular septal defects and in truncus arteriosus. Am Heart J 105:281–286, Feb 1983.

54. Matina D, VanDoesburg NH, Fouron J-C, Guerin R, Davignon A: Subziphoid two dimensional echocardiographic diagnosis of doubled chambered right ventricle. Circulation 67:885–888, Apr 1983.

55. Smallhorn JF, Anderson RH, Macartay MJ: Morphological characterization of ventricular septal defects associated with coarctation of aorta by cross sectional echocardiography. Br Heart J 49:485–494, May 1983.

56. Lappen RS, Riggs TW, Lapin D, Paul MH, Muster AJ: Two-dimensional echocardiographic measurement of right pulmonary artery diameter in infants and children. J Am Coll Cardiol 2:121–126, July 1983.

57. Caldwell RL, Hurwitz RA, Girod DA, Weyman AE, Feigenbaum H: Two-dimensional echocardiographic differentiation of anomalous left coronary artery from congestive cardiomyopathy. Am Heart J 106:710–716, Oct 1983.

58. Riggs TW, Lapin GD, Paul MH, Muster AJ, Berry TE, Tagcic SE, Berdusis K: Measurement of

mitral valve orifice area in infants and children by 2-dimensional echocardiography. J Am Coll Cardiol 1:873–878, March 1983.

59. KING ME, BRAUN H, GOLDBLATT A, LIBERTHSON R, WEYMAN A: Inter ventricular septal configuration as a predictor of right ventricular systolic hypertension in children: a cross sectional echocardiographic study. Circulation 68:68–75, July 1983.

60. HIRAISHI S, BARGERON LM, ISABEL-JONES JB, EMMANOUILIDES GC, FRIEDMAN WF, JARMAKANI JM: Ventricular and pulmonary artery volumes in patients with absent pulmonary valve: factors affecting the natural course. Circulation 67:183–190, Jan 1983.

61. PETER CA, BOWYER K, JONES RH: Radionuclide analysis of right and left ventricular response to exercise in patients with atrial and ventricular septal defects. Am Heart J 105:428–435, March 1983.

62. LEVIN AR, GOLBERG HL, BORER JS, ROTHENBERG LN, NOLAN FA, ENGLE MA, COHEN B, SKELLY NT, CARTER J: Digital angiography in the pediatric patient. Circulation 68:374–384, Aug 1983.

63. TAKAHASA M, SCHIEBER RA, WISHNER SH, RITCHIE GW, FRANCIS PS: Selective coronary arteriography in infants and children. Circulation 68:1021–1028, Nov 1983.

64. ST. JOHN SUTTON M, MEYER RA: Left ventricular function in persistent pulmonary hypertension in the newborn: computer analysis of the echocardiogram. Br Heart J 50:540–549, Dec 1983.

65. WELLES FC, COGHILL S, CAPLEN HL, LINCOLN C: Duration of circulatory arrest does influence the psychological development of children after cardiac operation in early life. J Thorac Cardiovasc Surg 86:823–831, Dec 1983.

66. URRUTIA-S CO, FALASCHI G, OTT DA, COOLEY DA: Surgical management of 56 patients with congenital coronary artery fistulas. Ann Thorac Surg 35:300–307, March 1983.

67. OGLIETTI J, COOLEY D, IZQUIERDO JP, VENTEMIGLIA R, MUASHER I, HALLMAN GL, REUL GJ JR: Cor triatriatum: operative results in 25 patients. Ann Thorac Surg 35:415–420, Apr 1983.

68. PENKOSKE PA, CASTANEDA AR, FYLER DC, VAN PRAAGH R: Origin of pulmonary artery branch from ascending aorta. Primary surgical repair in infancy. J Thorac Cardiovasc Surg 85:537–545, Apr 1983.

69. MAZZUCCO A, RIZZOLI G, FRACASSO A, STELLIN G, VALFRE C, PELLEGRINO P, BORTOLOTTI U, GALLUCCI V: Experience with operation for total anomalous pulmonary venous connection in infancy. J Thorac Cardiovasc Surg 85:686–690, May 1983.

70. KRON IL, RHEUBAN KS, CARPENTER MS, NOLAN SP: Interrupted aortic arch. A conservative approach for the sick neonate. J Thorac Cardiovasc Surg 86:37–40, July 1983.

71. LUBER JM, CASTANEDA AR, LANG P, NORWOOD WI: Repair of double-outlet right ventricle: early and late results. Circulation 68 (suppl II):144–147, Sept 1983.

72. STEVENSON JG, KAWABORI I, BAILEY WW: Noninvasive evaluation of Blalock-Taussig shunts: determination of patency and differentiation from patent ductus arteriosus by Doppler echocardiography. Am Heart J 106:1121–1132, Nov 1983.

73. GUYTON RA, OWENS JE, WAUMETT JD, DOOLEY KJ, HATCHER CR JR, WILLIAMS WH: The Blalock-Taussig shunt. Low risk, effective palliation, and pulmonary artery growth. J Thorac Cardiovasc Surg 85:917–922, June 1983.

74. LODGE FA, LAMBERTI JJ, GOODMAN AH, KIRKPATRICK SE, GEORGE L, MATHEWSON JW, WALDMAN JD: Vascular consequences of subclavian artery transection for the treatment of congenital heart disease. J Thorac Cardiovasc Surg 86:18–23, July 1983.

75. MURAOKA R, YOKOTA M, AOSHIMA M, NOMOTO S, KYOKU I, KOBAYASHI A, NAKANO H, UEDA K, SAITO A: Extrathoracically adjustable pulmonary artery banding. J Thorac Cardiovasc Surg 86:582–586, Oct 1983.

76. PIEHLER JM, DANIELSON GK, PLUTH JR, ORSZULAK TA, PUGA FJ, SCHAFF HV, EDWARDS WD, SHUB C: Enlargement of the aortic root or anulus with autogenous pericardial patch during aortic valve replacement. Long-term follow-up. J Thorac Cardiovasc Surg 86:350–358, Sept 1983.

77. DI CARLO D, MARCELLETTI C, NIJVELD A, LUBBERS LJ, BECKER AE: The Fontan procedure in the absence of the interatrial septum. Failure of its principle? J Thorac Cardiovasc Surg 85:923–927, June 1983.

78. STEWART S, MANNING J, ALEXSON C, HARRIS P: The Hancock external valved conduit. A

dichotomy between late clinical results and late cardiac catheterization findings. J Thorac Cardiovasc Surg 86:562–569, Oct 1983.

79. DASKALOPOULOS DA, EDWARDS WD, DRISCOLL DJ, DANIELSON GK, PUGA FJ: Coronary artery compression with fatal myocardial ischemia. A rare complication of valved extracardiac conduits in children with congenital heart disease. J Thorac Cardiovasc Surg: 85:546–551, April 1983.

80. LANSING AM, ELBL F, SOLINGER RE, REES AH: Left atrial-left ventricular bypass for congenital mitral stenosis. Ann Thorac Surg 35:667–669, June 1983.

8

Chronic Congestive Heart Failure

PROGNOSIS

Although CHF is known to be highly fatal, to assess efficacy of therapeutic interventions better, a greater understanding of its course is required. Previous studies of survival are limited by heterogeneity of patient populations and diverse criteria for diagnosing CHF. Franciosa and associates[1] from Minneapolis, Minnesota, and Philadelphia, Pennsylvania, followed up 182 patients with chronic LV failure who were symptomatic despite therapy. The length of follow-up averaged 12 ± 10 (mean ± SD) months (range, 1–41). The cause of CHF was CAD in 95 patients and idiopathic dilated cardiomyopathy (IDC) in 87. A total of 88 deaths occurred, of which 40 (45%) were sudden; the incidence of sudden death was similar in patients with CAD and IDC. The overall mortality rate was 34% at 1 year, 59% at 2 years, and 76% at 3 years. The mortality rate in patients with CAD was 46 and 69% at 1 and 2 years, compared with 23 and 48% at 1 and 2 years in those with IDC (p < 0.01). Comparison of all survivors and nonsurvivors showed no difference in age or duration of symptoms at entry. Clinical class was significantly worse in nonsurvivors. Nonsurvivors had higher LV filling pressure (29 ± 7 -vs- 24 ± 9 mmHg) and systemic vascular resistance (25 ± 10 -vs- 21 ± 8 U) (both p < 0.01); they also had lower mean arterial pressure (87 ± 13 -vs- 94 ± 13 mmHg), cardiac index (2.0 ± 0.7 -vs- 2.5 ± 0.8 liters/min/M^2), and stroke work (35 ± 19 -vs- 56 ± 33 g · m) than did the survivors (all p < 0.001). However, only LV filling pressure was correlated with length of survival (4 = −0.31, p < 0.01). Thus, 3-year mortality is very high in patients with severe chronic LV failure. The prognosis is poorer in patients with CHF due to CAD and, as expected, in those with worse symptoms and hemodynamic abnormalities.

Polak and associates[2] from Boston, Massachusetts, determined the predictive value of radionuclide ventriculography in 34 patients with depressed LV EF (<40%) and clinically evident CHF secondary to atherosclerotic CAD. The RV EF and the extent of LV wall motion abnormalities were identified. Sixteen patients alive after a 2-year follow-up had a higher RV EF and less extensive LV dyskinesia. Mortality was greater among the 21 patients with depressed RV EF (71% -vs- 23%), and depressed RV function was associated with more severely compromised LV function. The patients with RV dysfunction also had a greater prevalence of chronic lung disease and previous AMI. Thus, multiple factors may contribute to a reduction in RV EF in these patients, but the documentation of imparied RV function is of prognostic importance.

Wilson and associates[3] from Philadelphia, Pennsylvania, evaluated 77 patients with functional class III or IV CHF to determine clinical features that provide insight into prognosis. These patients were followed prospectively for 12 ± 11 months. M-mode echo and 24-hour Holter monitoring data and hemodynamic evaluation were used to classify these patients clinically. Holter monitoring demonstrated a high incidence of VPC, which were paired in 62% of the patients, multiform in 71%, and 3 or more consecutive VPC in 51%. Survival was dramatically reduced in this patient group, being 52% at 1 year and 32% at 2 years. Mortality was highest during the initial 4 months, after which the average mortality was 20%. Cardiac mortality was due equally to sudden death and CHF. Cardiac mortality during the first 4 months was related to functional class and to the presence of ≥5 consecutive VPCs. No variable was related to cardiac mortality after 4 months. Multivariate analysis identified only functional class as an independent prognostic variable. Thus, these data suggest that severe CHF is associated with a high mortality from both sudden and nonsudden cardiac death and that cardiac mortality is related primarily to ventricular functional status.

CATECHOLAMINES

Patients with chronic CHF are known to have elevated plasma concentrations of norepinephrine (NE). Although this elevation of catecholamines in plasma may facilitate myocardial contractility, it may also be toxic to the myocardium in the long term. The alpha-2 adrenoreceptor located on noradrenergic nerve terminals regulates neuronal NE release by feedback inhibition. This receptor is also located on human blood platelets. Weiss and associates[4] from Ann Arbor, Michigan, determined the status of platelet alpha-2 adrenoreceptors in 16 patients with CHF (classes I and II in 7 and classes III and IV in 9) and in 26 normal volunteers. Specific high affinity binding of the alpha-2 agonist ^{3}H-clonidine and the alpha-2 antagonist ^{3}H-yohimbine was used to determine the number (B_{max}) of alpha-2 receptors and the dissociation constant (K_D) for the 2 ligands. In the control population, the B_{max}) (in fmol/mg protein) for ^{3}H-clonidine was 33 ± 2 and for ^{3}H-yohimbine was 165 ± 12. There was a 25% difference in the maximum number of specific binding sites for ^{3}H-clonidine in the classes III and IV group (B_{max} 24 ± 2; p < 0.05) and a 43% difference in the maximum number of specific binding sites for ^{3}H-yohimbine (B_{max} 94 ± 9; p < 0.005). There was a smaller but nonsignificant difference in the number of receptors on platelets from patients in classes I and II. The K_D was similar in all 3 groups. These differences correlated well with the increases in plasma NE levels between the normal group (273.8 ± 44.1 pg/ml) and the patients in classes III and IV (1333.5 ± 244.9, p < 0.0005). This study supports the hypothesis that increased levels of circulating NE in CHF lead to a decrease in platelet alpha-2 adrenoreceptors.

Central and regional circulatory responses to orthostasis in patients with CHF were evaluated by Goldsmith and colleagues[5] from Minneapolis, Minnesota, in 22 subjects by measuring hemodynamic variables and forearm and hepatic blood flow at rest and during 65% head-up tilt. The results obtained were compared with those in 9 normal individuals. Heart rate and mean arterial BP increased during tilt in normal subjects, but did not change in patients with CHF. Forearm blood flow decreased in normal subjects with head-up tilt, but did not change from a lower baseline value in patients. Hepatic blood flow did not change with head-up tilt in either group. Total systemic resistance increased in patients with CHF, indicating that resistance does increase in some vascular beds. Plasma NE also increased modestly in patients with head-up tilt, but these changes did not correlate with changes in hepatic or forearm vascular resistance. Thus, the data obtained in this study demonstrate that the overall hemodynamic response and regulation of regional blood flow and resistance in some vascular beds differs in patients with CHF compared with normal subjects. Specifically, there is a smaller change in heart rate, blood pressure, forearm blood flow, and hepatic vascular resistance in patients with CHF when exposed to upright tilt. The reasons for these differences in hemodynamic responses are not clear.

Goldsmith and associates[6] from Milwaukee, Wisconsin, measured plasma vasopressin by radioimmunoassay in 31 patients with advanced CHF. The hypothesis tested was that vasopressin might contribute to both the vasoconstriction and impaired water handling in patients with CHF. Basal vasopressin levels in the patients were compared with those obtained from 51 normal subjects of similar age. The data obtained demonstrate: 1) the mean vasopressin level in the patients with CHF was 9.5 ± 0.89 pg/ml compared with 4.7 ± 0.66 (p < 0.001) in normal subjects; 2) vasopressin levels did not correlate with any hemodynamic variable or with plasma NE values; and 3) acute hemodynamic changes induced by nitroprusside and inhibition of the renin-angiotensin system with captopril did not influence vasopressin levels. Thus, the data demonstrate that serum vasopressin levels are usually increased in patients with CHF, but this increase does not appear to be related to the severity of CHF nor may it be manipulated by changing hemodynamics with pharmacologic intervention.

MISCELLANEOUS TOPICS

Hepatojugular reflux

Ducas and associates[7] from Montreal, Canada, described observations designed to test the validity of the hepatojugular reflux as an indicator of actual or incipient CHF. The central venous pressure (CVP) could be predicted from the height of the jugular venous pulsations in 44 of 48 comparisons. In the remaining comparisons, discrepancies ranged from 5–7 mmHg. In patients with normal resting cardiac function, abdominal compression did not cause an increase in CVP of >2 mmHg (2.7 mm H_2O). In 16 of 19 patients with impaired function, CVP increased by ≥3 mmHg. The increase in CVP was estimated from neck veins to within 2 mmHg in all but 3 instances. The CVP stabilized by 10 seconds and did not change over the subsequent 60 seconds. Abdominal compression caused no consistent change in cardiac output. Changes in venous pressure could not be attributed to changes in esophageal pressure or to compression of the heart by elevation of the diaphragm. Observations were consistent with the hypothesis that an increase in right-sided cardiac filling pressures resulting from abdominal compression, carried out as described, reflects both the volume of blood in the abdominal veins and the ability of the ventricles to respond to increased venous return, and this constitutes a useful clinical test for detecting CHF. An increase of 3 cm in the height of neck vein distention is a reasonable upper limit of normal.

Echo usefulness

Echeverria and associates[8] from Miami, Florida, assessed the role of echo in the evaluation of 50 patients with both acute and chronic CHF. Thirty patients (60%) had an EF <50% (mean ± SD, 30 ± 9%), LV dilation (6.5 ± 0.7 cm), and normal wall thicknesses (1.0 ± 0.2 cm). The echo findings were predictable on clinical grounds in 18 (60%) of the 30 patients and worse than clinically expected in 12 patients (40%). Management changes after echo were indicated in 11 (37%) of 30 patients. The remaining 20 (40%) of the 50-patient cohort had EF above 50% (mean, 70 ± 9%; p < 0.01), and, as a group, were characterized by normal LV size (5.1 ± 0.8 cm, p < 0.01) and borderline wall thicknesses (1.1 ± 0.2 cm, p < 0.01). The largest subgroup of these 20 patients had hypertensive CAD (7 patients, 35%) associated with the CHF syndrome, presumably related to LV diastolic (compliance) dysfunction. The normal EF was unexpected clinically in 18 (90%) of these 20 patients. Recommended management after echo changed in all 18 patients. Since standard clinical findings (history, physical examination, and chest roentgenography) failed to separate patients with normal and abnormal EF, or those in need of changes in management, echo was a useful and, at times, essential part of the evaluation of these patients with CHF.

Effects of discontinuing maintenance digoxin

To evaluate the importance of oral maintenance digoxin therapy in chronic CHF, Gheorghiade and Beller[9] from Charlottesville, Virginia, studied prospectively on and off the drug in 24 patients in sinus rhythm on maintenance digoxin for documented CHF. The average duration of therapy was 39 months (range, 2–180). All 24 patients had documented CAD: 22 were in New York Heart Association functional class III and 2 were in class II. Twenty-one patients (88%) were receiving diuretic or vasodilator therapy or both before digoxin discontinuance. At 1 month off digoxin and with no increase in doses of other medications except minor increases in antianginal therapy in 2 patients, no difference was observed in the group as a whole in symptoms, resting heart rate, arterial BP, physical findings, weight, cardiothoracic ratio, radiographic signs of pulmonary congestion, RNA LV EF, duration of symptom-limited treadmill exercise (14 patients), or CHF score, compared with evaluation during maintenance digoxin therapy. Similar results were obtained in a subgroup of 9 patients with a resting LV EF <0.35 (0.27 ± 0.02; mean ± SEM). Six patients had a decrease and 5 patients an increase in LV EF of ≥0.05 units after cessation of digoxin. Off digoxin, the CHF score increased by only 1 point in 2 patients, but also decreased in 2 patients. Thus, in this study population comprised of patients with CAD with documented CHF, most of whom were receiving diuretics or vasodilators or both, digoxin withdrawal had no adverse clinical or hemodynamic effects.

TREATMENT

Amrinone

In a study of Siegel and associates[10] from New York City, 7 patients with severe CHF were treated with oral amrinone for a mean duration of 39 weeks (range, 16–72). During the first week of therapy, exercise capacity as assessed on a treadmill using the Naughton protocol increased substantially from 7.6 ± 4.2–12.1 ± 4.4 minutes (p < 0.01). At an early period of follow-up (8–12 weeks), a further significant increase in exercise capacity to 15 ± 5 minutes (p < 0.05) was demonstrated, whereas at a later follow-up exercise capacity had decreased to 11 ± 7 minutes (p < 0.05). This was still significantly greater than prior to amrinone therapy (p < 0.01). The LV EF was increased from 14 ± 4–19 ± 4% (p < 0.05) during the first week of therapy, but was not significantly different from control at the early and later periods of follow-up. The LV end-diastolic dimension index increased from control value of 43 ± 5–47 ± 7 mm/M^2 (p < 0.01) at the late period of follow-up. Thus, long-term amrinone therapy resulted in a substantial improvement in exercise capacity despite a slow but progressive decline in cardiac performance.

Amrinone is a new bipyridine derivative that increases cardiac output and reduces filling pressures in patients with CHF. These improvements have been attributed by some investigators to the drug's having a predominant positive inotropic action, and others have suggested, at least in CHF, that the drug acts as a vasodilator with little or no inotropic effect. Wilsmhurst and Webb-Peploe[11] from London, England, investigated the side effects of both intravenous and orally administered amrinone to patients with chronic CHF. Acute intravenous administration in 40 patients caused a significant reduction in mean BP, and this was severe enough to require correction by plasma infusion in 5 patients. Oral amrinone in 18 patients was accompanied by thrombocytopenia in 10, but no complications were associated with the low platelet counts. Other potentially serious adverse effects were: abdominal pain (2 patients), nausea and vomiting (3 patients), jaundice (1 patient), myositis (1 patient), pulmonary infiltrates (2 patients), and polyserositis (1 patient). Other side effects included splenomegaly, eosinophilia, fever, headache, reduced tear secretion, dry skin, and nail discoloration. These real and potential severe adverse reactions with amrinone need to be weighed carefully against its benefits in the treatment of chronic CHF.

Bromocriptine

The sympathetic nervous system and the renin-angiotensin system are activated in patients with CHF and can be contributing to excessive peripheral vasoconstriction and impaired myocardial performance. Bromocriptine, an orally active ergot alkaloid with dopaminergic receptor agonist action, is known to lower plasma norepinephrine in the human. The agent also may possess direct vasodilator activity through vascular dopaminergic receptors. In a study by Francis and associates[12] from Minneapolis, Minnesota, to assess the effects of bromocriptine on hemodynamic measurements, sympathetic nervous system activity, and the renin-angiotensin system in CHF patients, standard hemodynamic parameters and plasma norepinephrine and plasma renin activity were measured before and following a single oral dose of 2.5 mg of bromocriptine in 10 patients with chronic stable CHF. The following statistically significant (p < 0.01) peak responses were noted: plasma norepinephrine decreased from a mean ± SD of 581 ± 194–366 ± 181 pg/ml; mean heart rate declined from 87 ± 16–78 ± 17 beats/minute; mean BP was reduced from 87 ± 9–73 ± 9 mmHg; systemic vascular resistance decreased from 1,494 ± 361–1,249 ± 289 dynes · s · cm^{-5}; stroke volume index increased from 27 ± 7–33 ± 10 ml/beat/M^2; LV filling pressure decreased from 28 ± 8–21 ± 8 mmHg; and mean RA pressure fell from 10 ± 4–7 ± 4 mmHg. Plasma renin activity did not change significantly. All patients tolerated the drug well. Although the effects of bromocriptine on plasma norepinephrine may contribute to an improved hemodynamic state, the direct vasodilator effect via vascular dopaminergic receptor stimulation appears to be a more likely mechanism. It was concluded that bromocriptine improves the hemodynamic profile in CHF acutely and that long-term studies are appropriate for enhanced characterization of the role of this agent in chronic CHF therapy.

Captopril

To determine the relation between the early and late hemodynamic effects of captopril in patients with severe CHF, Packer and colleagues[13] from New York City performed serial right-sided heart catheterizations in 51 such patients who were treated with the drug for 2–8 weeks. Four hemodynamic patterns of response were observed. Nine patients had minimal responses initially (type I), 6 failed to improve during long-term treatment, but 3 showed delayed hemodynamic benefits. Twenty-eight patients had initial beneficial drug effects that were sustained after 48 hours and after 2–8 weeks (type II). In 7 patients, first doses of captopril produced marked beneficial responses, but these became rapidly attenuated after 48 hours; nevertheless, continued therapy for 2–8 weeks was accompanied by spontaneous restoration of the hemodynamic effects of first doses of the drug, that is, triphasic response (type III). In the remaining 7 patients, attenuation of initial response was not reversed by prolonged captopril therapy; hemodynamic variables after 2–8 weeks had returned to their pretreatment values, that is, drug tolerance (type IV). Plasma renin activity was lower in patients with minimal responses and was higher in patients with triphasic responses than in patients with types II and IV response patterns. Although first-dose effects of captopril are frequently sustained, the occurrence of delayed, attenuated, and triphasic responses indicates that a complex and variable relation may exist between the early and late hemodynamic effects of vasodilator drugs in patients with severe CHF.

Although many studies have shown acute hemodynamic improvement in patients with CHF treated with vasodilating drugs, long-term control studies with both hemodynamic and exercise capacity measurements are not available. Kramer and associates[14] from San Francisco, California, studied captopril in 16 ambulatory patients in New York Heart Association functional classes II–IV CHF who were clinically stable on digoxin and diuretics. The acute response to open-label captopril was quantified by blood pool scintigraphy, right-sided heart catheterization at rest and during exercise, and measurements of exercise capacity. Patients were then randomized to maintenance therapy with captopril or matching placebo and were restudied after 3 months. The 2 groups were similar in their clinical characteristics and pretreatment rest and exercise hemodynamic measurements. Both displayed similar acute beneficial responses to captopril at rest, with a mean reduction in LV filling pressure from 24–14 mmHg and increases in cardiac index from 2.1–2.5 liters/min/M^2 and stroke index from 25–34 ml/M^2. Directionally similar hemodynamic improvement was noted during exercise. After 3 months, these beneficial hemodynamic changes were sustained only in the patients randomized to captopril. Concomitantly, the captopril patients increased their exercise capacity as measured by the duration of bicycle exercise, maximal work load, and oxygen consumption. The placebo group showed either no change or a worsening over the 3 months compared with their pretreatment measurements. These findings demonstrate that captopril is an effective adjunctive agent for the treatment of CHF and that it produces long-term hemodynamic improvement together with an increase in exercise capacity.

Captopril -vs- nitroprusside

Packer and associates[15] from New York City compared the hemodynamic effects of oral captopril and intravenous nitroprusside in 15 patients with severe CHF. At doses of both drugs titrated so as to produce similar decreases in systemic vascular resistance in each patient, nitroprusside produced substantially greater increases in cardiac index ($+0.67$ -vs- $+0.31$ liters/min/M^2; $p < 0.01$) but smaller decreases in mean arterial pressure (-18 -vs- -11 mmHg; $p < 0.01$) than did captopril. This finding was due to a significant decrease in heart rate with captopril (-7 beats/min; $p < 0.01$), which was not seen with nitroprusside, since changes in stroke volume index with both drugs were similar. Nitroprusside produced a decrease in pulmonary arteriolar resistance quantitatively similar to the decrease in systemic vascular resistance, but the decrease in pulmonary arteriolar resistance with captopril was not significant. Despite similar decreases in systemic resistance, captopril produced a greater decrease in LV filling pressure (-10 -vs- -7 mmHg; $p < 0.01$) but a smaller decrease in mean right atrial pressure (-3.1 -vs- -5.3 mmHg; $p < 0.01$) than did nitroprusside. Thus, captopril has actions independent of its systemic vasodilator effects, which account for the quantitative differences observed in its hemodynamic responses compared with those of nitroprusside in patients with severe CHF. These differences support experimental evidence that angiotensin, in addition to its direct systemic arterial vasoconstrictor actions, exerts positive chronotropic effects and alters ventricular compliance but has minimal direct effects on the limb venous circulation and on the pulmonary vasculature.

Clonidine

Peripherally acting vasodilators are now commonly used in the management of CHF. Many classes of agents (adrenergic blockers, nonspecific vasodilators, and angiotensin-converting enzyme inhibitors) have been extensively examined over the past decade. Numerous studies have demonstrated that these agents augment stroke volume and cardiac output, primarily by reducing ventricular afterload. In contrast to the peripheral class of compounds, centrally acting vasodilators have received little attention in the setting of low output CHF. One typical centrally acting agent is clonidine. Clonidine is used predominantly in hypertensive patients, in whom it effectively reduces systemic BP, systemic vascular resistance, and heart rate. It induces its antihypertensive effect by attenuating sympathetic outflow by way of complex interaction with the central alpha-adrenergic system. Hermiller and associates[16] from Columbus, Ohio, postulated that clonidine might be an effective vasodilator because it reduces sympathetic activity, a major cause of the elevated ventricular afterload accompanying CHF. They studied 14 patients with moderately severe CHF by giving 0.2–0.4 mg doses of clonidine orally. The 0.2 mg dose significantly reduced mean systemic (15%) and mean PA (20%) pressure; the corresponding reductions in vascular resistance were not as great because of a diminished cardiac output. Pulmonary capillary wedge pressure decreased significantly (27%). Heart rate decreased 11% and stroke volume remained unchanged. At a higher dose (0.4 mg), clonidine augmented these reductions but increased stroke volume modestly (15%). Isovolumic-developed pressure/duration of isovolumic contraction and the duration of the preejection period were used as indexes of inotropy. After both doses, isovolumic-developed pressure/duration of isovolumic contraction decreased dramatically ($\geq$33%) and the preejection period increased substantially ($\geq$18%) (both $p < 0.05$). Compared with currently employed vasodilating agents, the centrally acting agent clonidine appears unique in that the drug-induced systemic and pulmonary arterial vasodilation are not accompanied by a commensurate improvement in ventricular systolic function. This lack of improvement appears to be a result of negative inotropic effects.

Dibutyryl cyclic AMP

To evaluate the hemodynamic effects of dibutyryl cyclic AMP (DBcAMP) in chronic CHF, Matsui and associates[17] from Ishikawa-ken, Japan, performed right-sided cardiac catheterization in 11 patients with CHF and investigated hemodynamic variables before and after infusion of various doses of DBcAMP at a rate of 0.025–0.2 mg/kg/minute (mean, 0.14 ± 0.077 SD). Total systemic vascular resistance index was reduced from 3,171 ±

1,158–1,880 ± 554 dynes/s/cm^{-5} · M^2 (mean ± SD) and PA end-diastolic pressure from 23 ± 13–20 ± 11 mmHg, and increased cardiac index from 2.24 ± 0.06–3.41 ± 1.02 liters/min/M^2. Mean arterial BP decreased from 91 ± 14–84 ± 13 mmHg, and heart rate increased from 91 ± 16–99 ± 13 beats/minute. The increase in cardiac index was accompanied by a proportional decrease in total systemic vascular resistance index in all but 1 patient. In 8 patients the decrease in pulmonary arterial end-diastolic pressure was accompanied by an increase or no change in the LV stroke work index. In 6 patients, DBcAMP was given in incremental doses of 0.05, 0.1, and 0.2 mg/kg/minute every 20 minutes, and 5 of 6 patients tolerated the full dose and showed dose-related hemodynamic changes for the incremental doses of DBcAMP. These data suggest that DBcAMP has powerful vasodilating effects on resistance vessels in patients with CHF; hence, it can be a useful vasodilating agent for treatment of CHF.

Dobutamine

Applefeld and associates[18] from Baltimore, Maryland, described the use of outpatient dobutamine infusions by small, portable infusion pump in 3 patients with intractable CHF. With this therapy, LV function improved and CHF resolved in each. Tolerance to dobutamine was obviated by giving infusions twice weekly. Except for 3 mild infections around the catheter exit site, there were no complications of this therapy in 58 cumulative patient weeks. The portable infusion pump that contains the dobutamine is connected to a chronic indwelling venous catheter inserted surgically into the external jugular vein and located proximal to the right atrium. The distal end of the catheter exited into the parasternal region.

Dobutamine -vs- hydralazine

Magorien and associates[19] from Columbus, Ohio, evaluated 10 patients with severe CHF (New York Heart Association functional classes III and IV) to determine the efficacy of a combination of a powerful inotropic intervention (dobutamine) and an oral vasodilator (hydralazine) in treatment. Dobutamine (5 µg/kg/min) and hydralazine (1 mg/kg) caused an identical increase in cardiac index and stroke volume index and both agents increased coronary blood flow while reducing coronary vascular resistance. Both forms of therapy caused a significant increase in myocardial oxygen consumption. Dobutamine had a balanced effect on the coronary circulation, producing a proportional increase in coronary blood flow and oxygen consumption, whereas hydralazine increased oxygen supply -vs- demand. Thus, dobutamine exerts a balanced effect on coronary circulation, whereas hydralazine causes a greater increase in coronary flow than myocardial oxygen demand in patients with nonischemic CHF.

Dopamine

Maskin and associates[20] from New York City studied hemodynamic and metabolic effects of dopamine at rest and during maximal exercise in 13 patients with severe chronic CHF. During exercise before the administration of dopamine, the stroke volume index increased from 17.1 ± 5.2 ml/M^2 at rest to 28.1 ± 10.9 ml/M² (p < 0.001) at exhaustion, whereas pulmonary capillary wedge (PCW) pressure increased from 23 ± 13–44 ± 12 mmHg (p < 0.001). The arteriovenous oxygen difference increased from 9 ± 3–12 ± 2 ml/100 ml (p < 0.001) and oxygen uptake increased from 4 ± 1–12 ± 3 ml/kg/minute (p < 0.001). At rest, dopamine increased the stroke volume index to 23 ± 8 ml/M² (p < 0.001) and reduced the PCW pressure to 21 ± 1 mmHg (p < 0.05). However, during maximal exercise, the stroke volume index and PCW pressure were not changed by dopamine: 28 ± 11 -vs- 29 ± 10 ml/M² (NS) and 44 ± 12 -vs- 43 ± 11 mmHg (NS), respectively. In contrast, the maximal heart rate achieved during exercise was significantly higher with dopamine, 140 ± 29 -vs- 136 ± 30 beats/minute (p < 0.05), which contributed to a slight augmentation in the maximal cardiac index, 3.8 ± 1.1 -vs- 3.6 ± 1.2 liters/min/M² (p < 0.05). Nonetheless, neither peak arteriovenous oxygen difference nor maximal oxygen uptake was significantly changed by dopamine. Thus, administration of dopamine to patients with severe chronic CHF appears to exert a slight chronotropic effect, but does not improve ventricular performance during maximal exercise.

Enalapril

DiCarlo and associates[21] from San Francisco, California, evaluated 15 patients with chronic CHF to determine the efficacy of a new oral angiotensin-converting enzyme inhibitor, enalapril. Initial hemodynamic effects were characterized by significant increase in cardiac index (2.1 ± 0.7–2.6 ± 0.7 liters/min/M²) and a decrease in PA wedge pressure (30 ± 6–24 ± 7 mmHg), RA pressure (14 ± 5–11 ± 4 mmHg), mean systemic arterial pressure (96 ± 16–80 ± 17 mmHg) and systemic vascular resistance (1,820 ± 480–1,200 ± 410 dynes · s · cm⁻⁵) without any significant change in heart rate, PA pressure, and pulmonary vascular resistance. During maintenance therapy, diuretic drugs had to be administered in increasing dosage because of systemic venous hypertension. Chronic therapy resulted in sustained hemodynamic improvement in 7 patients followed for 4 weeks. Plasma renin activity increased and plasma norepinephrine levels decreased after enalapril therapy. All patients had symptomatic improvement. However, significant hypotension developed in 5 patients at the initiation of therapy and this appeared to be the major side effect of this agent. These data suggest that enalapril has the potential to improve cardiac function and symptoms in patients with chronic CHF, but that hypotension and venous hypertension are important side effects of this agent.

Endralazine

Quyyumi and associates[22] from London, England, made invasive hemodynamic measurements in 10 supine patients with chronic refractory CHF from CAD or dilated cardiomyopathy before and after oral administration of a new arteriolar vasodilator, endralazine. In 9 patients, a 10 mg dose of endralazine produced maximal increases in cardiac and stroke volume indexes of 56 and 41%, respectively, with a 45% reduction in total systemic resistance. After a 5 mg dose of endralazine, cardiac index increased maximally by 38% and stroke volume index by 34%, with a 31% decrease in total systemic resistance. Mean arterial pressure decreased 11 ± 4 mmHg (mean ± SEM) with the 5 mg dose and 17 ± 5 mmHg after the 10 mg dose. There were no significant changes in the RA, PA, or PA wedge pressures. After administration of a single dose of endralazine, statistically significant hemodynamic changes were observed from 1–8 hours with peak responses at 3–4 hours. These observations suggest that endralazine has hemodynamic properties similar to those of its structural analog, hydralazine. However, endralazine metabolism is largely independent of the patients' acetylator status, and no cases of systemic lupus erythematosus have been reported after long-term oral administration. These findings suggest that endralazine may be an efficacious drug that is potentially safer than hydralazine in the treatment of chronic CHF.

Hydralazine

To determine whether the circulatory response to hydralazine in patients with CHF is influenced by initial hemodynamic status of LV chamber size, Wilson and associates[23] from Philadelphia, Pennsylvania, studied 28 patients with chronic LV dysfunction. Hemodynamic measurements and ECG LV end-diastolic dimension were correlated with the response to 20 mg of intravenous hydralazine and to a dose titrated in each patient to reduce systemic resistance by ≥20%. Hydralazine, 20 mg, decreased systemic resistance from 23 ± 8–18 ± 8 U (p < 0.01) and increased the cardiac index from 2.0 ± 0.5–2.5 ± 0.6 liters/min/M^2 (p < 0.01) and the stroke work index from 21 ± 11–24 ± 9 g · m/M^2 (p < 0.05). Titrating the dose to decrease systemic resistance by ≥20% increased the cardiac index further to 2.7 ± 0.6 liters/min/M^2 and the stroke work index to 32 ± 9 g · m/M^2. The change in systemic resistance produced by 20 mg of hydralazine correlated only with initial systemic resistance (r = 0.53), suggesting that vascular response to hydralazine is a direct function of initial vascular resistance. The percentage change in stroke work index produced by 20 mg of hydralazine correlated directly with indexes of LV preload-end-diastolic wall stress (r = 0.69) and pulmonary wedge pressure (4 = 0.43) and inversely with stroke work index (4 = −0.49), an index of ventricular work. Similar but less close correlations were observed when the dose of hydralazine was titrated. The hemodynamic response to hydralazine did not correlate with LV end-diastolic dimension or RA pressure. Thus, vascular response to moderate doses of hydralazine is related to initial systemic vascular resistance. The LV pump response is related to the level of initial LV pump dysfunction but not to LV chamber size or RA pressure.

The aerobic exercise capacity of patients with chronic CHF is frequently impaired because of inadequate oxygen transport to working skeletal muscle. To determine whether hydralazine improves oxygen transport to working muscle, Wilson and coinvestigators[24] from Philadelphia, Pennsylvania, examined the effect of intravenous hydralazine on blood flow measured by thermodilution and metabolism in the leg during maximal upright bicycle exercise in 10 patients with chronic CHF. Hydralazine increased maximal exercise cardiac output and decreased systemic oxygen extraction but did not alter oxygen uptake. Leg blood flow at maximal exercise increased 1.6–2.1 liters/minute. The proportion of cardiac output delivered to the leg remained unchanged. This increase in flow was associated with a decrease in oxygen extraction in the leg and no change in peak femoral venous lactate, suggesting that there is functional or anatomic shunting of the augmented limb flow rather than delivery to metabolizing muscle. These data suggest that hydralazine augments flow to the exercising limb in patients with CHF but that this augmented flow does not increase oxygen availability within the working muscle.

Imipramine

The ECG effects of the tricyclic antidepressants are well studied and are quinidine like. In patients with ventricular arrhythmias, several tricyclic antidepressants have been shown to exert substantial antiarrhythmic activity. In depressed patients free of heart disease, therapeutic doses will frequently lengthen the P-R, QRS, and Q-T intervals, but these effects are rarely, if ever, of clinical importance. In patients with preexisting BBB or in cases of overdose, the risk of high degree AV heart block increases substantially. The effects of tricyclic antidepressants on LV performance have not been extensively studied. To fill this void, Glassman and associates[25] from New York City assessed by RNA the effect of imipramine hydrochloride on LV performance in a group of depressed patients with preexisting chronic CHF. The EF was measured at rest by first-pass RNA before and after treatment with imipramine, and it was unchanged during treatment, but 7 of 15 patients had orthostatic hypotension of such severity that administration of the drug had to be discontinued. Plasma concentrations of the drug were essentially twice those usually seen. It is important to appreciate that although imipramine does not further impair resting LV performance, this does not mean it is without risk. Orthostatic hypotension must be watched for when using imipramine in depressed patients with impaired LV performance.

Isosorbide dinitrate

Leier and colleagues[26] from Columbus, Ohio, studied 30 patients with moderate to severe CHF in a double-blind, randomized, placebo-controlled trial to determine the immediate and long-term effects of isosorbide dinitrate on clinical status and on resting and exercise hemodynamics. Seventeen patients received placebo and 13, isosorbide dinitrate. First dose of isosorbide dinitrate (40 mg orally) decreased resting and exercise PA wedge pressure, PA and systemic arterial pressures, and pulmonic and systemic vascular resistances without augmenting exercise capacity. Compared with placebo, chronic therapy with isosorbide dinitrate (40 mg orally every 6 hours for 12 weeks) significantly improved clinical status and exercise capacity. Resting and exercise systemic BP and systemic vascular resistance returned to baseline values during chronic isosorbide dinitrate therapy, but pulmonary capillary wedge pressure, PA pressure, and pulmonary vascular resistance remained improved. In patients with CHF, 12 weeks of isosorbide dinitrate therapy improved resting and exercise hemodynamics, exercise capacity, and clinical status; tolerance developed to the systemic arterial vascular effects without attenuation of the venous and pulmonary vascular effects.

MDL 17043

A new agent for the treatment of CHF, MDL 17043, administered intravenously or orally exerts positive inotropic and vasodilator actions in experimental animal preparations. Uretsky and coworkers[27] from Cincinnati, Ohio, studied its acute hemodynamic effects in 15 patients with severe CHF by right heart catheterization. Intravenous MDL 17043 at 10 minutes increased cardiac index (3.4 -vs- 1.9 liters/min/M^2) narrowed arterial venous oxygen content (4.6 -vs- 7.8 vol%) increased heart rate (98 -vs- 89 beats/min) and decreased systemic arterial (67 -vs- 83 mmHg), PA wedge (12 -vs- 24 mmHg), and RA (6 -vs- 12 mmHg) mean pressures significantly. In 11 patients, hemodynamics were monitored hourly for 6 hours. Compared with baseline, the cardiac index and heart rate were higher and mean systemic arterial pressure was lower for 6 hours; PA wedge and RA mean pressures were significantly lower for 5 hours. No serious arrhythmias or side effects occurred. Thus, these data suggest that MDL 17043 may be useful for treating CHF.

Milrinone

Milrinone, a derivative of amrinone, has nearly 20 times the inotropic potency of the parent compound and does not cause fever or thrombocytopenia in normal volunteers or in animals sensitive to amrinone. In 20 patients with severe CHF, Baim and associates[28] from Boston, Massachusetts, administered milrinone intravenously and it caused significant decreases in LV end-diastolic pressure (from 27 ± 2–18 ± 2 mmHg), PA wedge pressure, RA pressure, systemic vascular resistance, and a slight reduction in mean systemic arterial pressure. Significant increases occurred in cardiac index (from 1.9 ± 0.1–2.9 ± 0.2 liters/min/M^2) and the peak positive first derivative of LV pressure, with a slight increase in heart rate. Hemodynamic improvement was sustained during a 24-hour continuous infusion. Nineteen of the 20 patients subsequently received oral milrinone (29 ± 2 mg/day) for up to 11 months (mean, 6 ± 1), with sustained improvement in symptoms of CHF. In 10 patients receiving long-term oral milrinone (≥6 months) radionuclide ventriculography showed continued responsiveness, with a 27% increase in LV EF after 7.5 mg of the drug. Four patients died after a mean of 4.8 months of therapy, and 3 patients with severe underlying CAD and angina pectoris required additional antianginal therapy. No patient had fever, thrombocytopenia, gastrointestinal intolerance, or aggravation of ventricular ectopy. Thus, milrinone shows promise for the long-term treatment of CHF.

Minoxidil -vs- hydralazine -vs- nitroprusside

Minoxidil is a potent oral vasodilator of potential value in patients with CHF, although preliminary studies show that it causes fluid retention. To test whether minoxidil acts primarily as an arterial vasodilator in CHF, Markham and associates[29] from Dallas, Texas, compared minoxidil with hydralazine and nitroprusside. To evaluate its chronic efficacy and mechanism of fluid retention, the effects of minoxidil (7 patients) were compared, in a double-blind manner, with those of hydralazine (8 patients) on central and regional hemodynamics and the renin-angiotensin-aldosterone and sympathetic nervous systems. There was no demonstrable difference in the central hemodynamic effects of minoxidil and hydralazine in the dosages used. After 6 hours both drugs increased cardiac index (minoxidil group, from 1.65 ± 0.29–2.26 ± 0.40 liters/min/M^2, $p < 0.0001$; hydralazine group, from 1.88 ± 0.61–2.34 ± 0.90 liters/min/M^2, $p < 0.0001$), decreased systemic vascular resistance, and increased heart rate without change in PA, PA wedge, or RA pressures. Nitroprusside effects differed from those of minoxidil and hydralazine with respect to heart rate ($p < 0.005$) and mean PA ($p < 0.007$) and RA ($p < 0.009$) pressures. Nitroprusside also decreased relative hepatomesenteric flow compared with the other 2 agents ($p < 0.005$). Neither renal blood flow, glomerular filtration rate, filtration fraction, nor urinary sodium excretion were significantly altered acutely by any of the 3 drugs. Minoxidil and hydralazine did not differ in their neurohumoral effects: both agents produced an increase in plasma norepinephrine concentration ($p < 0.003$) and plasma renin activity ($p < 0.04$), but no change in plasma epinephrine or aldosterone concentrations. After 1 week of double-blind therapy, fluid retention was a greater problem with minoxidil than with hydralazine. Thus, minoxidil behaves primarily as an arterial vasodilator in CHF, fluid retention is a severe adverse effect, and the greater degree of fluid retention with minoxidil than hydralazine is not attributable to differing acute effects on total renal blood flow or function, or to differing effects on the renin-angiotensin-aldosterone or sympathetic nervous systems.

Nitroglycerin

Olivari and associates[30] from Minneapolis, Minnesota, evaluated the hemodynamic and hormonal response to nitroglycerin administered transdermally in a gel-like matrix in 9 patients with severe CHF and in 9 normal subjects. In patients with CHF, nitroglycerin produced sustained hemodynamic effects that began 30 minutes after application and persisted for ≥ 6 hours. The hemodynamic alterations resulting from nitroglycerin, included a significant decrease in RV and LV filling pressures, a significant increase in stroke index, and a significant decrease in forearm and pulmonary vascular resistance. There was no change in heart rate and systemic arterial pressure or in plasma norepinephrine or renin activity. After 24 hours, pressures partially returned to control levels, but mean PA pressure was still significantly lower than during the control period. With removal of the nitroglycerin, the hemodynamic alterations returned toward control values and there was an increase above control values in PA and systemic arterial pressure and pulmonary, systemic, and forearm vascular resistances. Thus, transdermal absorption of nitroglycerin may favorably influence hemodynamics for at least 6 hours following the application of the material, but there is a vasoconstrictor effect that occurs following removal of the nitroglycerin.

Nifedipine

In an investigation carried out by Cantelli and associates[31] from Bologna, Italy, the acute hemodynamic effects of combining administration of digoxin (0.01 mg/kg intravenously) with nifedipine (10 mg sublingually) were compared with those of the drugs alone in 12 patients with chronic CHF due to CAD (7 patients) or dilated cardiomyopathy (IDC, 5 patients); 4 patients also had MR. Nifedipine significantly reduced systolic and diastolic BP, systemic vascular resistance (SVR) from 1,925 ± 400 (mean ± SD) to 1,333 ± 256 dyne · s · cm^{-5} after 30 minutes, and LV filling pressure from 19 ± 8–16 ± 4 mmHg. The cardiac index increased from 2.2 ± 0.5–2.8 ± 0.6 liters/min/M^2. Digoxin induced a significant reduction in LV filling pressure from 18 ± 8–14 ± 5 mmHg after 90 minutes and a slight increase in stroke volume index; no significant change in BP, cardiac index, and SVR was seen. The combination of digoxin and nifedipine produced a significant increase in cardiac index from control value of 2.2 ± 0.5–3.0 ± 0.4 liters/min/M^2, and a significant reduction in LV filling pressure from 18 ± 8–13 ± 5 mmHg, and in SVR. No significant difference was seen between the hemodynamic response to the 3 drug regimens in patients with CAD -vs- patients with IDC. Nifedipine produced a greater improvement in cardiac performance in patients with than without MR. Simultaneous administration of both drugs resulted in an augmentation of cardiac performance greater than that achieved with either agent alone. Thus, the combination produced a greater cardiac output increase and a greater LV filling pressure reduction, indicating a shift upward and to the left to a more improved LV function curve.

Elkayam and associates[32] from Los Angeles, California, evaluated the temporal hemodynamic effects of oral nifedipine after a single dose of 20–40 mg in 11 patients with severe chronic CHF (LV EF, 0.22 ± 0.7). Nifedipine significantly reduced systemic vascular resistance, from 1,850 ± 493–1,315 ± 398 dynes/s/cm^{-5} at 1 hour (20%), to 1,410 ± 246 at 3 hours, and to 1,523 ± 286 at 6 hours (p < 0.05). Cardiac index increased 21%, from 2.1 ± 0.5–2.5 ± 0.8 liters/min/M^2 at 1 hour, to 2.4 ± 0.5 liters/min/M^2 at 3 hours (p < 0.05), and to 2.2 ± 0.4 liters/min/M^2 at 6 hours. The group response of stroke volume to nifedipine was smaller. A peak increase of 17% was seen 3 hours after initiation of therapy (23 ± 7 -vs- 26 ± 6 ml/M^2). This difference did not reach statistical significance. Mean BP declined significantly, from 94 ± 20–80 ± 13 mmHg at 1 hour, to 83 ± 15 mmHg at 3 hours, and to 86 ± 17 mmHg at 6 hours (p < 0.05) and was associated with no significant change in heart rate. The marked decrease in BP resulted in a decrease in rate-pressure product from 12,272 ± 4,230–10,500 ± 2,074 mmHg/minute at 1 hour, to 10,374 ± 2,735 mmHg/minute at 3 hours, and to 11,047 ± 3,813 mmHg/minute at 6 hours (p < 0.05). The PA wedge pressure, RA pressure, pulmonary vascular resistance and LV stroke work index showed no significant change after oral nifedipine. This study therefore shows that oral nifedipine, when administered to patients with chronic severe CHF, markedly reduces systemic vascular resistance. However, this change is followed by no change in stroke work index and only a mild change in stroke volume and PA wedge pressure. These findings suggest that nifedipine has a limited effect on cardiac performance and raise doubt regarding the role of this drug as a vasodilating agent in the treatment of chronic CHF.

Nitroprusside

Yin and colleagues[33] from Baltimore, Maryland, studied the effects of nitroprusside on the hydraulic RV and LV vascular load in 7 patients with severe LV failure. At doses of 0.25–0.75 μg/kg/minute, stroke volume increased progressively from 40–49 ml and LV end-diastolic pressure decreased from 25–11 mmHg. Accompanying this improvement in LV performance were dose-related decreases in mean ventricular pressures, pulmonic and systemic resistances, and the lower frequency components of input impedance moduli. Characteristic impedance and both total and oscillatory external power were decreased in the pulmonic but not the aortic vasculature. In this class of patients, RV unloading is a striking and direct effect of nitroprusside and may account, in part, for improved LV performance through ventricular interdependence.

Activation of the sympathetic nervous system, manifested by an increase in heart rate and circulating plasma norepinephrine, can occur in normal subjects when they are given vasodilators. The extent to which this activation occurs in patients with CHF and whether this activation could account for the hemodynamic rebound sometimes observed following abrupt withdrawal of nitroprusside in such patients has been unclear. Francis and associates[34] from Minneapolis, Minnesota, studied the effects of nitroprusside on plasma norepinephrine in 38 patients with CHF to determine if acute vasodilator therapy activates this vasoconstrictor system during or following such treatment. Thirty-six patients also had plasma renin activity (PRA) measured and plasma arginine vasopressin was measured in 12 patients. Baseline supine plasma norepinephrine (714 ± 72 pg/ml, ±SEM), PRA (15 ± 2 ng/ml/h), and arginine vasopressin (10 ± 1 pg/ml) were increased at least 2-fold in the CHF patients. Nitroprusside (96 ± 11 μg/min) was infused for 64 minutes after achieving an optimal hemodynamic response: cardiac index increased (2.01 ± 0.08–2.67 ± 0.1 liters/min/M^2; p < 0.001), pulmonary artery wedge pressure decreased (25 ± 1–16 ± 1 mmHg; p < 0.001), mean arterial pressure decreased (83 ± 1–72 ± 1 mmHg; p < 0.001), and heart rate was unchanged. Plasma norepinephrine (632 ± 43 pg/ml), PRA (18 ± 3 ng/ml/h), and arginine vasopressin (11 ± 1 pg/ml) did not change significantly for the group during peak effect of the vasodilator. Nitroprusside was abruptly stopped and 36 ± 2 minutes later there was no significant change for the group in plasma norepinephrine (755 ± 72 pg/ml), PRA (18 ± 3 ng/ml/h), or arginine vasopressin (11 ± 1 pg/ml). There was no hemodynamic rebound for the group following nitroprusside withdrawal, although some individual patients did show a rebound increase in systemic vascular resistance. In these individuals there was no consistent relation between changes in plasma norepinephrine, renin activity, and arginine vasopressin and the observed increase in the systemic vascular resistance. It was concluded that short-term nitroprusside therapy for CHF does not consistently alter plasma norepinephrine, PRA, or plasma arginine vasopressin concentration. The rebound in systemic vascular resistance that may be observed in individual patients when nitroprusside is abruptly withdrawn does not appear to be modulated by activation of the sympathetic nervous system, the renin-angiotensin system, or arginine vasopressin.

On the basis of preload manipulations, an optimal LV filling pressure of 14–18 mmHg has been suggested for patients with LV failure. Since afterload reduction results in increased cardiac output in CHF, Franciosa and associates[35] from Philadelphia, Pennsylvania, tested the hypothesis that LV filling pressure could be reduced to normal by nitroprusside without compromising cardiac output in 15 patients with acutely decompensated chronic CHF from either CAD or idiopathic dilated cardiomyopathy. Cardiac index was measured after each 4–6 mmHg decrease in PA wedge pressure until the latter fell below 14 mmHg (group I, 9 patients) or until systolic arterial pressure reached 90 mmHg during nitroprusside infusion (group II, 6 patients). In group I, PA wedge pressure fell in significant decrements ($p < 0.001$) from 28 ± 4 (SD) to 24 ± 3, 17 ± 2, and 11 ± 2 mmHg during nitroprusside infusion. Cardiac index rose in significant increments ($p < 0.05$) from 2.5 ± 0.8–2.8 ± 0.6, 3.3 ± 0.7, and 3.7 ± 1.1 liter/min/M^2 with each increase in nitroprusside dosage. Mean arterial pressure fell during nitroprusside infusion from 97 ± 16–70 ± 8 mmHg ($p < 0.001$) without any change in heart rate. In group II, directionally identical changes in hemodynamics were observed during nitroprusside infusion; the highest cardiac index occurred at the lowest PA wedge pressure attained, and no side effects were observed despite the fall in systolic arterial pressure to 90 mmHg. Thus, reduction of LV filling pressure to within the normal range by nitroprusside infusion in patients with chronic LV failure can raise cardiac output beyond levels observed at LV filling pressure of 14–18 mmHg. Normalization of filling pressure may improve subendocardial coronary perfusion, and invasive monitoring of filling pressure during nitroprusside infusion may not be routinely required.

Prazosin

The beneficial effects of acute prazosin therapy in patients with CHF have been well documented, but its chronic efficacy over several months had not previously been evaluated in a placebo-controlled manner. Therefore Markham and associates[36] from Dallas, Texas, assessed by radionuclide ventriculography the effect of prazosin, 20 mg/day, on LV EF and end-systolic and end-diastolic volumes at rest and on peak upright bicycle exercise and also its effects on RV EF at rest, exercise time, and work load, and standard clinical variables in 23 patients with stable class III symptoms of CHF. The study consisted of a 6-month randomized, double-blind, controlled evaluation of prazosin -vs- placebo in patients receiving a stable dose of digitalis and diuretics for at least 1 month. At entry, the prazosin and placebo groups did not differ in any respect. Prazosin caused no demonstrable effect on clinical variables, such as status of symptoms, heart rate, mean arterial pressure, and cardiothoracic ratio when compared with placebo. Prazosin also caused no demonstrable effect compared with placebo on absolute or percent changes in radionuclide variables at rest or on peak exercise, exercise time, or exercise work load. In addition, prazosin had no consistent effect compared with placebo on plasma renin activity or plasma catecholamine levels. However, there was a slight but significant increase in weight ($p < 0.0001$) and in plasma renin activity in the upright position ($p < 0.002$) with time, as well as a tendency for the diuretic dose to increase with time in both groups. Thus, long-term prazosin therapy generally produces no demonstrable subjective or objective improvement in patients with stable, chronic class III CHF receiving digitalis and diuretic therapy.

Higginbotham and associates[37] from Durham, North Carolina, assessed the effects of oral prazosin (15–20 mg/day) on symptoms, exercise performance, and LV function in a 6-month, double-blind, placebo-controlled study of patients in New York Heart Association functional class III. The EF was measured at rest and during upright bicycle exercise by equilibrium radionuclide angiography; end-diastolic volume, stroke volume, and cardiac output were derived from corresponding count measurements. Although there was no statistically significant difference between clinical responses in the prazosin and placebo groups, qualitative differences suggested a clinical response to prazosin. Of the 9 patients who received prazosin, 5 improved to functional class II and 2 became asymptomatic; the 2 nonresponders deteriorated to functional class IV when prazosin was stopped. Four of 9 patients who received placebo improved to functional class II and 2 deteriorated to class IV. Exercise time tended to increase in the prazosin group (from 541 ± 204–630 ± 100 at 6 months) and decrease in the placebo group (from 539 ± 141–435 ± 148 at 6 months), but neither change was significant. Prazosin effected a sustained decrease in mean BP of approximately 10 mmHg at rest, and a quantitatively similar but insignificant decrease during exercise. Radionuclide EF increased and LV end-diastolic counts decreased significantly at rest and during exercise in the prazosin group, but not in the placebo group. Because changes in EF and end-diastolic counts were similar, stroke counts and count output were unchanged. Thus, long-term oral prazosin therapy caused sustained changes in BP and LV function in most patients in functional class III, but these changes were not uniformly translated into clinical improvement or increased exercise tolerance. Prazosin does not appear to increase cardiac output during exercise in patients with CHF.

Pirbuterol

In 20 patients with severe CHF, Pamelia and associates[38] from Charlottesville, Virginia, studied the effects of the beta-adrenergic agonist pirbuterol compared with placebo in both an acute double-blind randomized trial and after long-term treatment. Acutely, pirbuterol patients (n, 10) demonstrated a significant rise in cardiac index (2.2 ± 0.14–3.2 ± 0.32 liters/min/M^2), stroke index (26 ± 2.6–35 ± 2.9 ml/beat/M^2), stroke work index (22 ± 2.4–30 ± 2.7 g · m/M^2), and EF (22 ± 4–30 ± 5%). These hemodynamic variables did not significantly change in 10 placebo patients. After 3 weeks of pirbuterol therapy, 14 patients (70%) were symptomatically improved and were continued on the drug for another 3 weeks; 13 of 14 patients who were symptomatically improved underwent restudy. Compared with pretreatment baseline, there was continued improvement in cardiac index (2.5 ± 0.16–3.2 ± 0.24 liters/min/M^2), stroke index (30 ± 2.5–38 ± 2.9 ml/beat/M^2), stroke work index (26 ± 2.3–35 ± 3.1 g · m/M^2), and EF (24 ± 1–28 ± 4%). Patients who more frequently improved were those with nonischemic cardiomyopathy and those with higher initial EF. These results demonstrate the acute beneficial effects of oral pirbuterol -vs- placebo in a double-blind randomized trial. Improvement was maintained during long-term therapy in most CHF patients.

Prenalterol

Fitzpatrick and colleagues[39] from Christchurch, New Zealand, studied the hemodynamic, hormonal, and electrolyte effects of prenalterol, a synthetic selective beta-1 agonist, in 6 patients with New York Heart Association functional classes II and III heart failure. Prenalterol was infused incrementally at 60, 120, and 240 nmol/minute for each rate for 24 hours, producing steady-state plasma prenalterol levels of 52, 121, and 194 nmol/liter, respectively. Hemodynamic and hormonal measurements were performed before, during, and after prenalterol administration under conditions of constant body posture and a regulated intake of dietary sodium and potassium. Prenalterol induced a statistically significant increase in cardiac index from 2.6–3.1 liters/min/M^2 with parallel increases in stroke index. Forearm blood flow measurements increased from 2.9–4.1 ml/min/100 g, while calculated systemic vascular resistance fell, as did PA wedge pressure from 14–11 mmHg. The drug did not alter heart rate, arterial pressure, right-sided heart pressure, or the frequency of VPC. Prenalterol increased plasma renin activity from 2.9–6.6 nmol/liter/h, angiotensin II from 59–89 pmol/liter, urinary aldosterone excretion from 41–78 nmol/day, and plasma insulin from 11–20 mU/liter. Circulating catecholamines, cortisol, glucose, glucagon, or pancreatic polypeptide did not change. Dose response studies in 5 patients showed dose-dependent increments in hemodynamic variables, whereas hormonal changes plateaued at the second dose level. These investigators conclude that prenalterol infusion augments myocardial contractility, reduces systemic vascular resistance, and stimulates insulin release and the renin-angiotensin-aldosterone system.

Propylbutyldopamine

The cardiovascular actions of a dopamine analog, propylbutyldopamine (PBDA) were examined by Fennell and colleagues[40] from Chicago, Illinois, for the first time in conscious dogs, normal human volunteers, and patients with CHF. The PBDA lowered BP without reflex increases in heart rate, increased renal blood flow, and decreased renal vascular resistance in dogs previously instrumented to allow measurement of arterial pressure and regional vascular flows in the conscious, unrestrained state. Pretreatment of the dogs with S-sulpiride, an antagonist selective for the dopamine receptor located on noradrenergic neurons (DA$_2$), attenuated the reduction in arterial pressure but not the increase in renal blood flow produced by PBDA. The emetic potency of this dopamine analog was also examined in conscious dogs; the drug caused vomiting on 2 of 22 occasions. In contrast to its effects in conscious dogs, PBDA in nonemetic dosages failed to lower BP in 3 normal volunteers but slightly increased heart rate and doubled renal blood flow as measured by the changes in the clearance of p-aminohippurate. Pretreatment of the volunteers with metoclopramide, antagonized the increase in both heart rate and renal blood flow produced by PBDA. In 11 patients with CHF not due to valvular or congenital heart disease, intravenous infusion of PBDA resulted in dose-dependent reduction in mean arterial pressure, LV filling pressure, and pulmonary and systemic vascular resistances, and increases in cardiac index, without changes in either stroke work index or heart rate. The demonstration that PBDA decreases systemic vascular resistance and BP in patients with CHF and increases renal blood flow in dogs and normal volunteers introduces a new class of drugs with unique mechanisms of action and advantages for the treatment of such conditions as CHF and hypertension. The possibility that this drug acts through activation or peripheral DA_2 presynaptic and DA_1 postsynaptic dopamine receptors appears strong, and further studies with this and similar agonists should stimulate the study of DA_2 receptors in man.

Trimazosin

In a study by Ports and associates[41] from San Francisco, California, the hemodynamic effects of the oral vasodilator trimazosin were evaluated in patients with chronic CHF, initially over a 72-hour period (13 patients) and after 3 months of maintenance therapy (7 patients). During the initial evaluation, cardiac index and stroke work index increased an average of 24 and 37%, respectively, and PA wedge pressure decreased by 26%. These beneficial hemodynamic effects were maintained during supine bicycle exercise. After 3 months of maintenance therapy, cardiac index (+30%) and stroke work index (+38%) remained elevated, and PA wedge pressure was lower (+38%). Improved hemodynamics during exercise also were seen after maintenance therapy. Withdrawal of trimazosin was associated with deterioration in hemodynamics and LV function. Thus, trimazosin has the potential to cause sustained improvements in LV function, both at rest and during exercise, in patients with chronic CHF.

Verapamil

Because of its intrinsic negative inotropic effect, the administration of verapamil is believed to be contraindicated in the presence of CHF. Because CHF, however, is frequently associated with arrhythmias and angina pectoris and because verapamil possesses potent antiarrhythmic and antianginal properties, Ferlinz and Citron[42] from Long Beach and Irvine, California, studied 14 patients with CHF both hemodynamically and by cineangiography. These studies were performed in both a controlled state and during intravenous verapamil administration (0.1 mg/kg bolus, followed by 0.005 mg/kg/min infusion). Verapamil markedly lowered mean aortic pressure (95 ± 19–81 ± 12 mmHg; $p < 0.001$) and systemic vascular resistance (1,953 ± 873–1,417 ± 454 dynes/s/cm^{-5}; $p < 0.01$). Simultaneously, indexes of LV performance substantially improved: the EF increased from 29 ± 13–37 ± 17% ($p < 0.01$), and mean velocity of circumferential fiber shortening increased from 0.45 ± 0.18–0.64 ± 0.28 circ/s ($p < 0.001$). Cardiac index also increased (from 1.98 ± 0.49 liters/min/M^2 before verapamil to 2.24 ± 0.60 liters/min/M^2 after verapamil), although this improvement did not become statistically significant. No appreciable changes were noted in the heart rate, LV end-diastolic pressure, or mean PA or PA wedge pressure. Thus, the intrinsic negative inotropic activity of intravenous verapamil in therapeutic doses generally does not represent a serious drawback even in patients with CHF; its potent unloading vasodilatory properties more than compensate for any intrinsic decrease in LV contractility, and can thereby actually improve overall cardiac function.

WIN 47203

Maskin and coinvestigators[43] from New York City studied the hemodynamic and clinical effects of WIN 47203, a newly synthesized noncatecholamine, nonglycosidic inotropic agent, in 11 patients with severe CHF. Intravenous WIN 47203 increased cardiac index from 1.93–2.87 liters/min/M^2 and reduced PA wedge pressure from 27–16 mmHg. Mean systemic arterial pressure decreased from 75–72 mmHg and systemic vascular resistance from 1,591–1,071 dynes/s/cm^5; heart rate was unchanged. Oral WIN 47203 produced similar hemodynamic improvement. Hemodynamic monitoring of 6 consecutive doses did not demonstrate any evidence for attenuation of effectiveness. Chronic therapy with WIN 47203 produced substantial symptomatic improvement and increased maximal oxygen uptake at 1 week. Patients were further improved after 4 weeks of WIN 47203, and maximal oxygen uptake increased from 9–11.6 ml/kg/minute. No overt clinical or laboratory manifestations of toxicity were observed. Withdrawal of WIN 47203 in 2 patients in whom clinical benefit was not sustained resulted in clinical and hemodynamic deterioration, which was reversed by reinstitution of the drug. Therefore this study demonstrates the acute and sustained cardiotonic efficacy of WIN 47203 in man. If long-term administration remains well tolerated and without side effects, this drug appears to be very promising for treatment of chronic severe CHF.

Sinoway and associates[44] from New York City evaluated 7 patients with severe CHF treated with WIN 47203, an analog of amrinone, for an average of 7.4 weeks. Hemodynamic improvement occurred in all patients initially, with cardiac index increasing from 1.79 ± 0.39–2.30 ± 0.44 liters/min/M^2 and PA wedge pressure decreasing from 24.1 ± 6.7–16.1 ± 7.8 mmHg ($p < 0.05$). In 5 of the 7 patients, long-term therapy produced symptomatic improvement. Withdrawal of WIN 47203 resulted in hemodynamic deterioration in all patients. During long-term therapy, no major side effects or hematologic changes were observed. Thus, these data suggest that WIN 47203 can improve symptoms and hemodynamic abnormalities in some patients with severe CHF.

References

1. FRANCIOSA JA, WILEN M, ZIESCHE S, COHN JN: Survival in men with severe chronic left ventricular failure due to either coronary heart disease or idiopathic dilated cardiomyopathy. Am J Cardiol 51:831–836, March 1983.
2. POLAK JF, HOLMAN BL, WYNNE J, COLUCCI WS: Right ventricular ejection fraction: an indicator of increased mortality in patients with congestive heart failure associated with coronary artery disease. J Am Coll Cardiol 2:217–224, Aug 1983.
3. WILSON JR, SCHWARTZ JS, SUTTON MSJ, FERRARO N, HOROWITZ LN, REICHEK N, JOSEPHSON ME: Prognosis in severe heart failure: relation to hemodynamic measurements and ventricular ectopic activity. J Am Coll Cardiol 2:403–410, Sept 1983.
4. WEISS RJ, TOBES M, WERTZ CE, SMITH CB: Platelet alpha$_2$ adrenoreceptors in chronic congestive heart failure. Am J Cardiol 52:101–105, July 1983.
5. GOLDSMITH SR, FRANCIS GS, LEVINE TB, COHN JN: Regional blood flow response to orthostasis in patients with congestive heart failure. J Am Coll Cardiol 1:1391–1395, June 1983.
6. GOLDSMITH SR, FRANCIS GS, COWLEY AW, LEVINE TB, COHN JN: Increased plasma arginine vasopressin levels in patients with congestive heart failure. J Am Coll Cardiol 1:1385–1390, June 1983.
7. DUCAS J, MAGDER S, McGREGOR M: Validity of the hepatojugular reflux as a clinical test for congestive heart failure. Am J Cardiol 52:1299–1303, Dec 1983.

8. ECHEVERRIA HH, BILSKER MS, MYERSBURG RJ, KESSLER KM: Congestive heart failure: echocardiographic insights. Am J Med 75:750–755, Nov 1983.

9. GHEORGHIADE M, BELLER GA: Effects of discontinuing maintenance digoxin therapy in patients with ischemic heart disease and congestive heart failure in sinus rhythm. Am J Cardiol 51:1243–1250, May 1983.

10. SIEGEL LA, LEJEMTEL TH, STROM J, MASKIN C, FORMAN R, FRISHMAN W, WEXLER J, RIBNER H, SONNENBLICK EH: Improvement in exercise capacity despite cardiac deterioration: noninvasive assessment of long-term therapy with amrinone in severe heart failure. Am Heart J 106:1042–1047, Nov 1983.

11. WILSMHURST PT, WEBB-PEPLOE MM: Side effects of amrinone therapy. Br Heart J 49:447–451, May 1983.

12. FRANCIS GS, PARKS R, COHN JN: The effects of bromocriptine in patients with congestive heart failure. Am Heart J 106:100–106, July 1983.

13. PACKER M, MEDINA N, YUSHAK M, MELLER J: Hemodynamic patterns of response during long-term captopril therapy for severe chronic heart failure. Circulation 68:803–812, Oct 1983.

14. KRAMER BL, MASSIE BM, TOPIC N: Controlled trial of captopril in chronic heart failure: a rest and exercise hemodynamic study. Circulation 67:807–816, April 1983.

15. PACKER M, MELLER J, MEDINA N, YUSHAK M: Quantitative differences in the hemodynamic effects of captopril and nitroprusside in severe chronic heart failure. Am J Cardiol 51:183–188, Jan 1983.

16. HERMILLER JB, MAGORIEN RD, LEITHE ME, UNVERFERTH DV, LEIER CV: Clonidine in congestive heart failure: A vasodilator with negative inotropic effects. Am J Cardiol 51:791–795, March 1983.

17. MATSUI S, MURAKAMI E, TAKEKOSHI, EMOTO J, MATOBA M: Hemodynamic effects of dibutyryl cyclic AMP in congestive heart failure. Am J Cardiol 51:1364–1368, May 1983.

18. APPLEFELD MM, NEWMAN KA, GROVE WR, SUTTON FJ, ROFFMAN DS, REED WP, LINBERG SE: Intermittent, continuous outpatient dobutamine infusion in the management of congestive heart failure. Am J Cardiol 51:455–458, Feb 1983.

19. MAGORIEN RD, UNVERFERTH DV, BROWN GP, LEIER CV: Dobutamine and hydralazine: comparative influences of positive inotropy and vasodilation on coronary blood flow and myocardial energetics in nonischemic congestive heart failure. J Am Coll Cardiol 1:499–505, Feb 1983.

20. MASKIN CS, KUGLER J, SONNENBLICK EH, LEJEMTEL TH: Acute inotropic stimulation with dopamine in severe congestive heart failure: beneficial hemodynamic effect at rest but not during maximal exercise. Am J Cardiol 52:1028–1032, Nov 1983.

21. DICARLO L, CHATTERJEE K, PARMLEY WW, SWEDBERG K, ATHERTON B, CURRAN D, CUCCI M: Enalapril: a new angiotensin-converting enzyme inhibitor in chronic heart failure: acute and chronic hemodynamic evaluations. J Am Coll Cardiol 2:865–871, Nov 1983.

22. QUYYUMI AA, WAGSTAFF D, EVANS TR: Acute hemodynamic effects of endralazine: a new vasodilator for chronic refractory congestive heart failure. Am J Cardiol 51:1353–1357, May 1983.

23. WILSON JR, SUTTON MS, SCHWARTS JS, FERRARO N, REICHEK N: Determinants of circulatory response to intravenous hydralazine in congestive heart failure. Am J Cardiol 52:299–303, Aug 1983.

24. WILSON JR, MARTIN JL, FERRARO N, WEBER KT: Effect of hydralazine on perfusion and metabolism in the leg during upright bicycle exercise in patients with heart failure. Circulation 68:425–432, Aug 1983.

25. GLASSMAN AH, JOHNSON LL, GIARDINA EGV, WALSH T, ROOSE SP, COOPER TB, BIGGER T: The use of imipramine in depressed patients with congestive heart failure. JAMA 250:1997–2001, Oct 21, 1983.

26. LEIER CV, HUSS R, MAGORIEN RD, UNVERFERTH DV: Improved exercise capacity and differing arterial and venous tolerance during chronic isosorbide dinitrate therapy for congestive heart failure. Circulation 67:817–822, Apr 1983.

27. URETSKY BF, GENERALOVICH T, REDDY PS, SPANGENBERG RB, FOLLANSBEE WP: The acute hemodynamic effects of a new agent, MDL 17,043, in the treatment of congestive heart failure. Circulation 67:823–828, Apr 1983.

28. BAIM DS, McDOWELL AV, CHERNILES J, MONRAD ES, PARKER JA, EDELSON J, BRAUNWALD E, GROSSMAN W: Evaluation of a new bipyridine inotropic agent—milrinone—in patients with severe congestive heart failure. N Engl J Med 309:748–756, Sept 29, 1983.

29. MARKHAM RV, GILMORE A, PETTINGER WA, BRATER DC, CORBETT JR, FIRTH BG: Central and regional hemodynamic effects and neurohumoral consequences of minoxidil in severe congestive heart failure and comparison to hydralazine and nitroprusside. Am J Cardiol 52:774–781, Oct 1983.

30. OLIVARI MT, CARLYLE PF, LEVIN TB, COHN JN: Hemodynamic and hormonal response to transdermal nitroglycerin in normal subjects and in patients with congestive heart failure. J Am Coll Cardiol 2:872–878, Nov 1983.

31. CANTELLI I, PAVESI PC, PARCHI C, NACCARELLA F, BRACCHETTI D: Acute hemodynamic effects of combined therapy with digoxin and nifedipine in patients with chronic heart failure. Am Heart J 106:308–315, Aug 1983.

32. ELKAYAM U, WEBER L, TORKAN B, BERMAN D, RAHIMTOOLA SH: Acute hemodynamic effect of oral nifedipine in severe chronic congestive heart failure. Am J Cardiol 52:1041–1045, Nov 1983.

33. YIN FCP, GUZMAN PA, BRIN KP, MAUGHAN WL, BRINKER JA, TRAILL TA, WEISS JL, WEISFELDT ML: Effect of nitroprusside on hydraulic vascular loads on the right and left ventricle of patients with heart failure. Circulation 67:1330–1339, June 1983.

34. FRANCIS GS, OLIVARI MT, GOLDSMITH SR, LEVINE TB, PIERPONT G, COHN JN: The acute response of plasma norepinephrine, renin activity, and arginine vasopressin to short-term nitroprusside and nitroprusside withdrawal in patients with congestive heart failure. Am Heart J 106:1315–1320, Dec 1983.

35. FRANCIOSA JA, DUNKMAN WB, WILEN M, SILVERSTEIN SR: "Optimal" left ventricular filling pressure during nitroprusside infusion for congestive heart failure. Am J Med 74:457–464, March 1983.

36. MARKHAM RV, CORBETT JR, GILMORE A, PETTINGER WA, FIRTH BG: Efficacy of prazosin in the management of chronic congestive heart failure: a 6-month randomized, double-blind, placebo-controlled study. Am J Cardiol 51:1346–1352, Jan 1983.

37. HIGGINBOTHAM MB, MORRIS KG, BRAMLET DA, COLEMAN RE, COBB FR: Long-term ambulatory therapy with prazosin versus placebo for chronic heart failure: relation between clinical response and left ventricular function at rest and during exercise. Am J Cardiol 52:782–788, Oct 1983.

38. PAMELIA FX, GEORGHIADE M, BELLER GA, BISHOP HL, OLUKOTUN AY, TAYLOR CR, WATSON DD, GRUNWALD AM, SIROWATKA J, CARABELLOW BA: Acute and long-term hemodynamic effects of oral pirbuterol in patients with chronic severe congestive heart failure: randomized double-blind trial. Am Heart J 106:1369–1376, Dec 1984.

39. FITZPATRICK D, IKRAM H, NICHOLLS MG, ESPINER EA: Hemodynamic, hormonal and electrolyte responses to prenalterol infusion in heart failure. Circulation 67:613–619, March 1983.

40. FENNELL WH, TAYLOR AA, YOUNG JB, BRANDON TA, GINOS JZ, GOLDBERG LI, MITCHELL JR: Propylbutyldopamine: hemodynamic effects in conscious dogs, normal human volunteers and patients with heart failure. Circulation 67:829–836, Apr 1983.

41. PORTS TA, CHATTERJEE K, WILKINSON P, AVAKIAN D, PARMLEY WW: Trimazosin in chronic congestive heart failure: improved left ventricular function at rest and during exercise. Am Heart J 102:1036–1042, Nov 1983.

42. FERLINZ J, CITRON PD: Hemodynamic and myocardial performance characteristics after verapamil use in congestive heart failure. Am J Cardiol 51:1339–1345, May 1983.

43. MASKIN CS, SINOWAY L, CHADWICK B, SONNENBLICK EH, LeJEMTEL TH: Sustained hemodynamic and clinical effects of a new cardiotonic agent, WIN 47203, in patients with severe congestive heart failure. Circulation 67:1065–1070, May 1983.

44. SINOWAY LS, MASKIN CS, CHADWICK B, FORMAN R, SONNENBLICK EH, LeJEMTEL TH: Long-term therapy with a new cardiotonic agent, WIN 47203: drug-dependent improvement in cardiac performance and progression of the underlying disease. J Am Coll Cardiol 2:327–331, Aug 1983.

9

Miscellaneous Topics

PERICARDIAL HEART DISEASE

Subepicardial adipose tissue: frequency, confusion with pericardial effusion

Roberts and Roberts[1] from Bethesda, Maryland, described certain clinical and morphologic findings in 55 patients whose hearts at necropsy contained so much fat that they floated in water. The patients were 47–89 years old (mean, 67). Symptomatic CAD was present in 28 (51%) and valvular heart disease (MS) in 3 (5%). The heart at necropsy was enlarged (>350 g for women and >400 g for men) in 45 patients (82%). The mean heart weight for the 31 women was 470 g and for the 24 men, 515 g. In addition to the severe increase in fat in the AV sulci and over both ventricles, the amount of fat in the atrial septum was increased in all patients. In 14 patients (25%), the thickness of the atrial septum cephalad to the fossa ovale was ≥2 cm. Excessive fat in this location is called "lipomatous hypertrophy of the atrial septum." Of the 16 patients (29%) with fatal AMI, 7 (44%) had rupture of either the LV free wall or ventricular septum. The high frequency of cardiac rupture in these patients supports the contention that rupture during AMI is more common in the fatty than in the nonfatty heart.

An isolated anterior echo-free space is generally regarded as a false positive echo finding for pericardial effusion. Even when an anterior echo-free space is accompanied by a posterior echo-free space, the echo-free spaces have been occasionally reported to be falsely positive for pericardial effusion, principally in patients with cardiac neoplasms. The basis for these findings was not fully explained until Isner and associates[2] from Boston, Massachusetts, and Bethesda, Maryland, evaluated by computed tomographic imaging or necropsy 5 patients in whom there was either an anterior or a posterior echo-free space or both. This technique demonstrated that subepicardial adipose tissue is the echo imitator of pericardial effusion.

To obtain epidemiologic information on extra echo spaces immediately posterior to the LV free wall, Savage and associates[3] from Framingham and Boston, Massachusetts, and Bethesda, Maryland, evaluated 2,028 subjects in the original Framingham cohort study (mean age, 70 ± 7 years) and 3,624 of the offspring of the cohort (and their spouses) (mean age, 44 ± 10 years) with adequate echo. Extra echo spaces were detected in 370 (6.5%) of the 5,652 subjects. The prevalence ranged from <1% in subjects in the 20- to 30-year age decade to >15% for those in their 80s. Extra echo spaces tended to be more common in subjects who were older, female, obese, more hypertensive, and who had higher blood sugar levels and higher LDL cholesterol levels (measured 8 years earlier). The high prevalence of extra echo spaces and the independent association with age (cohort and offspring), obesity (cohort and male offspring), and ventricular septal hypertrophy (cohort and male offspring) is compatible with at least 2 hypotheses, among others, that should be tested: 1) subepicardial fat may often masquerade as pericardial fluid and thus producing a posterior extra echo space, especially in obese elderly subjects; 2) small posterior extra echo spaces often may be early markers of subclinical hypertensive heart disease.

Pericardial effusion

During CHF, unilateral pleural effusion tends to be right sided, and bilateral pleural effusions tend to show more fluid on the right. Weiss and Spodick[4] from Worcester, Massachusetts, tested their impression that the opposite was true for pericardial heart disease—i.e., that unilateral pleural effusions tended to be left-sided and bilateral effusions larger on the left—by reviewing 133 consecutively discharged patients with any pericardial heart disease. Among the 35 patients with pericardial heart disease and pleural effusion, the pleural effusion was predominantly right sided in only 3 patients and solely or predominantly left-sided in 25 (Table 9-1).

Chandraratna and associates[5] from Los Angeles, California, performed 2-D echo contrast studies in 16 patients with pericardial effusion. A 4-chamber view was obtained by positioning the transducer at the apex. The exploratory needle was visualized in 9 patients. Five milliliters of saline solution were injected through the exploring needle and a cloud of echoes indicated its position. Microbubbles were seen in all 16 patients. This technique enabled the operator to identify that the needle was inadvertently in the LV cavity in 2 patients and in the RV cavity in 1. Furthermore, in 2 patients, when fluid could not be aspirated, the contrast study confirmed that the needle was in the pericardial sac; in both cases, pericardial fluid could be aspirated with slight manipulation of the needle. In a patient with a stab wound a negative contrast effect indicated the probable site of laceration. Thus, 2-D contrast echo is useful in locating needle position, which facilitated pericardiocentesis.

A diagnosis of active pericardial bleeding traditionally has depended on an invasive documentation by needle aspiration, angiography, or direct

TABLE 9-1. *Sites of pleural effusion in 35 patients with pericarditis. Reproduced with permission from Weiss and Spodick.*[4]

GROUP	NO. IN GROUP	RUB	PLEURAL EFFUSION				
			LEFT ONLY	LEFT > RIGHT	LEFT = RIGHT	RIGHT > LEFT	RIGHT ONLY
			NUMBER OF PATIENTS				
A. Pericarditis (n, 21) Pericardial fluid							
A1. Definite	11	10*	8	1	2	0	0
A2. Not demonstrable	4	3	3	0	1	0	0
A3. Status unknown	6	6	4	2	0	0	0
B. Pericarditis with cardiac failure	5	5	1	0	2	2	0
C. Pericardial fluid; no definite inflammatory signs	6	0	3	1	1	0	1
D. Constrictive pericarditis	3	2	2	0	1	0	0
Totals	35	26	21	4	7	2	1

* One effusion proved to be inflammatory on pericardiocentesis.

inspection. Bateman and associates[6] from Los Angeles, California, performed blood pool scintigraphy in 2 patients just before and after the development of hemopericardium revealed unique images in which acute pericardial bleeding manifested itself by an additional blood chamber adjacent to the cardiac chambers. The authors believe that such distinctive images were highly specific for active bleeding into the pericardial sac.

The relation of right RA inversion, a previously undescribed cross-sectional echo sign, to presence of cardiac tamponade was investigated by Gillam and coworkers[7] from Boston, Massachusetts. These investigators studied 127 patients with moderate or large pericardial effusions. Cardiac tamponade was present in 19 and absent in 104. Four patients with equivocal tamponade were excluded from analysis. A RA inversion was present in all 19 patients with cardiac tamponade and 19 of 104 without cardiac tamponade (sensitivity 100%; specificity 82%). The degree of inversion as quantitated by the area-corrected curvature did not improve the ability to discriminate between patients with and without cardiac tamponade. However, consideration of the duration of inversion by the RA inversion time index (duration of inversion/cardiac cycle length) and an empirically derived cut-off of 0.34 did improve the specificity and predictive value (100%) without a significant loss of sensitivity (94%). These investigators concluded that RA inversion, particularly if prolonged, is a useful echo marker of cardiac tamponade that may be of particular diagnostic value when the clinical picture is unclear.

Effects of mediastinal irradiation for Hodgkin's disease

Gottdiener and associates[8] from Bethesda, Maryland, used noninvasive techniques to document a high frequency of cardiac abnormalities (diminished LV size, pericardial effusion, and decreased LV function and functional reserve) in 25 patients who had no cardiac disease before being treated for Hodgkin's disease 5–15 years (mean, 11) earlier. These patients had received mediastinal irradiation through a single anteroposterior port—a technique formerly used at some centers but no longer employed. The average age of the 25 patients at the time of cardiac evaluation was 39 years (range, 25–59); 16 were women and 9 were men. All but 1 patient had received ≤4,000 rads to the mediastinum over a 16-week interval. The other patient received >4,600 rads. Symptoms suggestive of CAD were present in 4 of the 25 patients. Twelve (48%) patients had ECG abnormalities, including LA abnormality (5 patients), decreased QRS voltage (3 patients), intraventricular conduction abnormality (1 patient), and nonspecific ST-T wave abnormalities (2 patients). By echo, LV end-diastolic dimension was decreased in 12 of 24 patients who could be evaluated. The thickness of the LV free wall was decreased in 5 of 23 patients and increased in 1. The thickness of the ventricular septum was decreased in 4 of 21 patients who could be evaluated. The LA dimensions were decreased in 4 patients and increased in 3. Mitral valve closure velocity was decreased in 7 of 18 patients and LV fractional shortening was decreased in 3 of 16 who could be evaluated. Pericardial effusion was present in 9 patients (36%). Thus, this study indicates that multiple cardiac abnormalities are common even in asymptomatic young persons 5–15 years after therapeutic anterior irradiation of the mediastinum for Hodgkin's disease.

Occult or overt but delayed cardiac disease after thoracic radiotherapy for Hodgkin's disease is common. Applefeld and Wiernik[9] from Baltimore, Maryland, performed detailed cardiac evaluations in 48 patients with Hodgkin's disease a mean of 97 months after radiotherapy. The study protocol included echo, gated RNA, and cardiac catheterization. Cardiac disease was found in 46 patients (96%) and included constrictive or occult constrictive pericarditis (24 patients), abnormal hemodynamic response to a fluid challenge (14 patients), CAD (6 patients), and LV dysfunction (2 patients). Most patients (53%) had normal echoes. Gated blood pool RNA was performed in 42 patients. Excluding patients with occlusive CAD, the LV EF at rest (mean, 59%) and during exercise (mean, 69%) was within normal limits. Two patients had CHF. Six patients had pericardiectomy for constrictive pericarditis and 3 patients had CABG for CAD. Thus 1) delayed cardiac disease after radiotherapy is common, 2) chronic pericardial disorders are the most frequent manifestations of this disease, and 3) the prognosis for patients who have radiation-induced cardiac disease is generally favorable.

Postpericardiotomy syndrome

The postpericardiotomy syndrome remains an ill-defined and perplexing entity. Bufalino and associates[10] from Maywood, Illinois, utilized gallium-67 citrate scanning to define the postpericardiotomy syndrome better in 16 patients who had recently undergone cardiac surgery and were complaining of chest pain and sweats. The diagnosis was based on clear evidence of pericardial inflammation (friction rub plus elevated erythrocyte sedimentation rate or elevated white blood cell count). These patients received gallium-67 (5 mCi) and 72 hours later scintigraphic imaging was performed in 3 projections. Gallium-67 uptake over the heart was seen in 7 patients. None had evidence of recent infarction. All 7 positive scans occurred in patients >2 weeks into recovery from surgery, and 5 patients were >4 weeks into recovery. The 9 patients with no significant gallium-67 uptake over the heart were each 8 days or less into recovery. These results suggest that "early" pericarditis may have a different pathophysiology than "late" pericarditis, and the early pericarditis was more traumatic than immunologic. The classic postpericardiotomy syndrome, which may occur quite late after surgery, probably does not occur until a latent period has elapsed during which an immune-inflammatory response has developed. It was concluded that gallium-67 imaging is a useful tool in the differential diagnosis of chest pain and fever that occur in patients ≥2 weeks after cardiac surgery.

Chronic constrictive pericarditis

Blake and associates[11] from Dublin, Ireland, reviewed the causes of chronic constrictive pericarditis treated by pericardiectomy during the past 25 years. Of their 32 patients, the etiology of the constriction was rheumatoid disease in 4, trauma in 2, sarcoidosis in 1, tuberculosis in 4 and undetermined in 21.

Distinguishing pericardial constriction from myocardial restriction

Janos and associates[12] from Cincinnati, Ohio, evaluated 3 patients with restrictive cardiomyopathy and 4 patients with restrictive pericarditis to determine whether digitized echo could allow identification of these 2 processes. The LV diastolic function was evaluated by computer analysis of digitized M-mode echoes and the data compared with those obtained in normal subjects. Distinguishing echo features of constrictive pericarditis and restrictive cardiomyopathy were: 1) the major LV filling period was 78 ± 9% of normal -vs- 128 ± 4%; 2) minimal LV dimension to peak filling interval was 50 ± 10 -vs- 110 ms; and 3) the maximal rate of LV posterior wall thinning was −4.9 -vs- −2.3 seconds. Thus, these data suggest that it may be possible to diagnose the 2 disease entities using this technique at the bedside.

PRIMARY PULMONARY HYPERTENSION

Seven women with primary pulmonary hypertension (PPH) underwent hemodynamic evaluation by Leier and coworkers[13] from Columbus, Ohio, at rest and during exercise, before and after the oral administration of captopril. Dose-response curves were generated for the 25, 50, and 100 mg doses. Captopril significantly reduced systemic BP and systemic vascular resistance; and these effects persisted at submaximal levels of exercise. Captopril did not alter PA pressure resistance, cardiac output, or stroke volume at rest or during exercise. Furthermore, exercise tolerance did not improve. Four patients received captopril for 12 weeks at doses of 75 and 100 mg every 8 hours. Resting and exercise hemodynamic evaluation was repeated at the end of the 12-week period. Except for a persistent reduction in mean systemic BP at rest, chronic captopril administration did not evoke hemodynamic changes. Measured exercise duration did not change during continuing captopril treatment, although 1 patient described mild subjective improvement in activity tolerance. In PPH, captopril exerts its major effect on systemic vasculature with little or no effect on the pulmonary circuit. As observed in this study, an occasional patient may experience some clinical improvement with captopril therapy, but most adult patients with severe PPH will not benefit from long-term administration.

To evaluate the potential value of nifedipine for PPH, Rubin and associates[14] from Dallas, Texas, made hemodynamic and scintigraphic measurements before and 15–30 minutes after nifedipine, 10–20 mg, given sublingually to 9 patients. Nifedipine treatment increased cardiac output (mean ± SD, 3.6 ± 1.7–5.3 ± 2.8 liters/min) and decreased mean aortic pressure (99 ± 19–85 ± 12 mmHg) and total pulmonary and total systemic resistances (1,605 ± 787–1,025 ± 540 dynes $\cdot$ s $\cdot$ cm^{-5} and 2,761 ± 1,557–1,591 ± 823 dynes $\cdot$ s $\cdot$ cm^{-5}, respectively). Heart rate and mean PA pressure did not change significantly. The RV end-diastolic volume decreased 10%, end-systolic volume decreased 15%, and RV EF increased 18% in 8 patients. After 4–14 months (mean, 7.3 ± 3.8) of treatment with nifedipine, 40–120 mg/day, in 6 patients, cardiac output increased (3.6 ± 2.0–5.0 ± 1.8 liters/min) and total pulmonary resistance decreased (1,572 ± 730–987 ± 586 dynes $\cdot$ s $\cdot$ cm^{-5}), whereas PA pressure remained unchanged (59 ± 23.2–55 ± 28.6 mmHg) compared with baseline values. Thus, nifedipine therapy may be useful in the chronic management of patients with PPH.

Rich and associates[15] from Chicago, Illinois, evaluated the effects of 3 types of vasoactive agents, hydralazine, nifedipine, and amrinone, in 7 patients with PPH. Hemodynamic values were measured before and after drug administration in every patient. All drugs increased cardiac output and reduced both systemic and pulmonary resistance in the patients studied. Only nifedipine significantly reduced PA pressure (6 ± 5 mmHg). In addition, it decreased pulmonary resistance to a greater degree than systemic resistance in 2 of the 7 patients, suggesting that nifedipine can cause selective pulmonary vasodilation in some patients. Hydralazine appeared to increase cardiac output and stroke volume by reducing systemic resistance. There was no evidence of direct pulmonary vasodilating effects; it decreased systemic resistance more than pulmonary resistance in every case. The increase in cardiac output from amrinone was secondary to a decrease in systemic arterial pressure with reflex tachycardia; stroke volume was unchanged. Amrinone had little pulmonary effect in all but 1 patient, in whom it substantially reduced PA pressure and pulmonary resistance. The mechanism of action of these 3 drugs in PPH differs. Nifedipine holds the most promise as an effective pulmonary vasodilator. A study of the effects of long-term administration of nifedipine in PPH is warranted.

SECONDARY PULMONARY HYPERTENSION

Thirty-eight patients admitted to the hospital with clinical and radiologic findings of PA hypertension and RV failure 2 months after ingestion of toxic rapeseed oil were evaluated by Garcia-Dorado and coworkers[16] from Madrid, Spain, and Montreal, Canada, utilizing invasive and noninvasive tests. Noninvasive evaluation demonstrated RV enlargement in 84% of the patients. Invasive evaluation in 11 patients demonstrated a mean PA pressure of 40 ± 9 mmHg, mean pulmonary vascular resistance of 0.45 ± 0.12, and mean RV end-diastolic pressure of 13 ± 4 mmHg. Pulmonary arterial hypertension was sustained after the acute administration of 100% oxygen and persisted in 6 patients restudied within 6 months. These data suggest that symptomatic PA hypertension and associated RV dysfunction may complicate toxic rapeseed oil ingestion and that these findings persist for at least several months.

CHRONIC OBSTRUCTIVE PULMONARY DISEASE

Brent and associates[17] from New Haven, Connecticut, studied 14 patients with chronic obstructive pulmonary disease (COPD), mild to moderate PA hypertension, and diminished RV EF with use of combined RNA-hemodynamic approach to assess and contrast the acute effects of 3 vasodilators on RV performance and central hemodynamic function. Nitroglycerin significantly decreased mean RA pressure, RV end-diastolic volume index, mean PA pressure, cardiac index, and arterial oxygen tension, but did not affect pulmonary vascular resistance index and increased RV EF. Nitroprusside had similar effects on mean RA pressure, RV end-diastolic volume index, mean PA pressure, cardiac index, and arterial oxygen tension, but also mildly decreased pulmonary vascular resistance index and did not alter RV EF. In contrast, hydralazine decreased pulmonary vascular resistance index and increased cardiac index and RV EF. The increase in EF correlated well with the decrease in pulmonary vascular resistance. These data suggest that in patients with mild to moderate secondary PA hypertension, acute administration of hydralazine results in a substantial improvement in RV performance by virtue of decreasing pulmonary vascular resistance. In contrast, nitroglycerin and nitroprusside demonstrate predominant effects that reduce preload, cardiac index, and arterial oxygen tension. Based on these data, afterload reduction with vasodilators, such as hydralazine, may be potentially useful in selected patients with pulmonary disease and secondary PA hypertension and appear preferable to agents that primarily reduce preload.

Mehrotra and associates[18] from Washington, D.C., evaluated 6 patients with angina pectoris and COPD with mild to moderate hypoxemia at rest. These 6 patients had reversible perfusion defects on stress and redistribution thallium imaging and 3 patients had positive ECG abnormalities with exercise. No patient had significant CAD on arteriography. It is presumed that cellular dysfunction secondary to hypoxemia was responsible for reducing the uptake of thallium-201 during stress.

Morrison and associates[19] in Tucson, Arizona, evaluated the influence of low flow oxygen and isosorbide dinitrate on rest and exercise biventricular EF in patients with COPD. Nine patients with stable, moderate to severe COPD, who had no prior history of CHF were evaluated during supine exercise with simultaneous hemodynamic and radionuclide ventriculographic monitoring. A second exercise evaluation was performed in 8 patients during low flow oxygen breathing and in 5 persons, a third exercise test was performed after they had received 10 mg of oral isosorbide. Oxygen administration decreased exercise PA pressure in all subjects and diminished total pulmonary vascular resistance in 5 of the 7 patients in whom it was measured. RV EF increased by ≥0.05 in subjects with a decrease in total pulmonary resistance. Isosorbide increased rest and exercise RV and LV EF with simultaneous decreases in PA pressure, total pulmonary resistance, BP, and arterial oxygen tension.

These data demonstrate that in patients with COPD, but without a history of CHF, RV systolic functional responses to low flow oxygen and isosorbide at rest and exercise is determined by changes in total pulmonary resistance.

EXERCISING AND EXERCISERS

Exercise capacity after bed rest

Hung and associates[20] from Stanford and Moffett Field, California, assessed the mechanisms responsible for the decrease in exercise capacity after bed rest in 12 apparently healthy men aged 50 ± 4 years who underwent equilibrium-gated blood pool scintigraphy during supine and upright multistage bicycle ergometry before and after 10 days of bed rest. After bed rest, echo measured supine resting LV end-diastolic volume decreased by 16% (p < 0.05). Peak oxygen uptake during supine effort after bed rest was diminished by 6% (p, NS), whereas peak oxygen uptake during upright effort declined by 15% (p < 0.05). After bed rest, increases in heart rate were also greater during exercise in the upright than in the supine position (p < 0.05). Values of LV EF increased normally during both supine and upright effort after bed rest and were higher than corresponding values before bed rest (p < 0.05). After bed rest, increased LV EF and heart rate largely compensated for the reduced cardiac volume during supine effort, but these mechanisms were insufficient to maintain oxygen transport capacity at levels during upright effort before bed rest. These results indicate that orthostatically induced cardiac underfilling, not physical deconditioning or LV dysfunction, is the major cause of reduced effort tolerance after 10 days of bed rest in normal middle-aged men.

Of 12 healthy men with a mean age of 50 years who had bed rest for 10 days, 6 were randomly assigned by DeBusk and associates[21] from Palo Alto, California, to perform individually prescribed physical exercise daily for 60 days after bed rest (exercise group) and 6 simply resumed their customary activities (control group). Exercise group subjects were significantly more active than control subjects during this interval. Two classic training effects observed in the 60 days after bed rest were significantly larger among exercise than among control group subjects; compared with values immediately after bed rest, heart rate at a constant submaximal workload declined by 36 beats/minute in the exercise group -vs- 16 beats/minute in the control group, and peak oxygen consumption increased by 4.8 -vs- 2.2 ml/kg/minute. Despite these differences in the cardiovascular response to exercise, peak oxygen consumption in both groups returned to before bed rest levels by 30 days after bed rest, and this was accompanied by significant and similar increases in resting LV end-diastolic and stroke volumes in both groups. Simple resumption of usual physical activities after bed rest was as effective as formal exercise conditioning in restoring functional capacity to before bed rest levels.

In elderly

In contrast to young persons, normal elderly persons who undergo symptom-limited dynamic exercise have a decrease in LV contractile performance characterized by a decrease in LV EF. To test the hypothesis that physical conditioning can be achieved in older persons and produces improvement in the exercise-induced decrease in LV EF observed during normal aging, Schocken and associates[22] from Durham, North Carolina, examined 24 normal elderly persons ≥ age 65 years (mean age, 72 years) before and after a 12-week program of physical training. The subjects had been screened for evidence of cardiovascular disease, including rest and exercise stress ECG. All subjects underwent rest and exercise upright sitting RNA before and after the training program. The subjects achieved cardiovascular training effects as measured by increased functional capacity and decreased double product at one-half the maximum work load attained at the initial stress test. A significant increase occurred after training in the cardiac index response to exercise ($p < 0.02$) and in the augmentation of the end-diastolic volume index produced by exercise ($p < 0.05$). The exercise-induced decrease in LV EF and increase in LV end-systolic volume index remained unaltered by training. In conclusion, although older persons can achieve overall training effects from a program of physical conditioning, the age-associated differences in LV contractile performance remained unchanged. The data suggest that deconditioning is not a significant contributor to the decline in LV contractile performance in the elderly.

Abnormal ST segment in young athletes

Treadmill stress ECG is employed widely to detect underlying cardiovascular disease in asymptomatic patients. To determine the frequency and significance of an abnormal ST segment response to exercise in young athletes with increased LV mass induced by physical conditioning, Spirito and associates[23] from Bethesda, Maryland, studied by M-mode echo and exercise ECG in 75 male isometrically trained athletes without evidence of heart disease (mean age, 21 years) and 48 nonathletic young normal subjects. Ventricular septal and LV free wall thicknesses and calculated LV mass was significantly greater in athletes than in control subjects. An abnormal ST segment response to exercise was present in 7 (9%) of the 75 athletes, all of whom had a LV mass >275 g and in 5 the LV mass was above the 95th percentile of that of the control subjects. An abnormal treadmill exercise test result also was present in 3 (6%) of 48 control subjects. Seven of the 10 subjects with abnormal exercise test results had RNA at rest and with exercise, each of which was normal. It was concluded that 1) abnormal exercise test results occur commonly in both athletes and nonathletes; 2) almost 10% of isometrically trained athletes have a "false positive" exercise ECG, suggesting that this test has major limitations in screening for underlying cardiovascular disease in athletes; and 3) in athletes, a relation was present between "physiologically" increased LV mass and false positive exercise test results.

Myocardial mechanics in athletic hearts

Sugishita and colleagues[24] from Tsukuba, Japan, measured parameters of myocardial mechanics at rest by means of echo in 31 competitive runners and 17 judo champions, which were compared with those in 25 normal control subjects and 15 patients with volume-overloaded (AR) and 13 with pressure overloaded (systemic hypertension [SH]) hearts, 14 patients with dilated cardiomyopathy (DC), and 11 patients with HC. In runners, the ratio of LV radius to wall thickness (R/Th) was maintained in the normal range, but fractional shortening (FS) was decreased slightly ($p < 0.01$). Patients with decompensated DC and AR had increased R/Th ($p < 0.001$) and decreased FS ($p < 0.001$). In judo champions, FS was maintained in the normal range, but R/Th was decreased ($p < 0.001$). In patients with SH, R/Th was decreased slightly ($p < 0.05$), but FS and peak systolic wall stress were maintained in the normal range. In patients with HC, FS was maintained in the normal range, but R/Th was decreased ($p < 0.001$). It was concluded that 1) hearts of runners (isotonic exercise) are cardiomechanically similar to those of patients with compensated AR or DC and have enhanced cardiac reserve, whereas 2) hearts of judo champions (isometric exercise) are similar to those of HC patients with inappropriately increased hypertrophy.

Skeletal muscle creatine kinase MB isoenzyme in marathon runners

Siegel and associates[25] from Boston, Massachusetts, measured serum creatine kinase (CK) MB isoenzyme activity in 108 trained marathon runners. The mean serum CK-MB was 98 ± 66 U/liter measured by quantitative electrophoretic technique (normal, <5 U/liter), or 8% of total CK activity. These levels in asymptomatic runners were comparable with peak serum values reported in patients during AMI. Elevated serum levels of CK-MB in runners can arise from skeletal muscle through exertional rhabdomyolysis, from silent injury to myocardium, or from a combined tissue source. To investigate this directly, skeletal muscle obtained by needle biopsy was analyzed for CK isoenzymes from 25 trained male marathon runners and 10 sedentary male subjects. The MB isoenzyme accounted for $9\% \pm 1\%$ (SD) of total CK activity per gram of total protein in the skeletal muscle of runners and $3\% \pm 1\%$ in control tissue, which was significant. Total CK activity was not statistically different between the 2 groups. Similar relative concentrations of CK-MB in skeletal muscle (9%) and serum after competition (8%) strongly suggest that elevated serum CK-MB activity in asymptomatic runners arises from a noncardiac or skeletal muscle source.

Cyclists

Noninvasive studies were performed by Fagard and coworkers[26] from Leuven, Belguim in 12 male bicyclists in the competitive season (CS) and in the resting season (RS) and in 12 matched control subjects to determine seasonal variations in cardiac structure and function in athletes and to compare the data with those of nonathletes. In athletes, peak oxygen uptake was 6% lower in the RS than the CS: the RS value was 40% higher than in nonathletes. The echos of athletes showed a higher LV total diameter at end diastole in the CS than in the RS; this difference was due to a greater septal and posterior wall thickness with unchanged internal diameter. On the ECG, R-wave voltages were larger in the CS in leads I, V_5, and V_6. Athletes had greater LV dimension and wall thickness than nonathletes, and their ratio of wall thickness to internal radius of the left ventricle was higher. Various echo and mechanocardiographic indexes of LV function were determined. During the RS, the athletes had a lower percent shortening and maximal velocity of

LV internal diameter, lower maximal and minimal velocities of the endocardium of the posterior wall, a longer preejection period, and a larger ratio of preejection period to LV ejection time. These findings are probably related to a greater LV end-systolic stress and index of myocardial afterload in the RS. The investigators conclude that cyclists in the CS, compared with nonathletes, have greater LV internal dimension and increased wall thickness, with similar LV function. During the RS, internal dimension does not change from the level in the CS, but wall thickness is somewhat reduced and LV function is slightly depressed, most likely because of a higher afterload in RS.

Sauna bathing

Ishikawa and associates[27] from Tokyo, Japan, studied 36 healthy men age 22–46 years (mean, 28) during and after a Finnish sauna with an air temperature of 80–90°C and 30–40% relative humidity. The amount of fluid lost during bathing, estimated from the decrease in body weight, ranged from 1,200–3,400 ml (mean, 2,100 ml). Measurements were carried out before and 1 hour after bathing. No intake of fluid or food was allowed until all investigations had been completed. The spatial QRS magnitude, and the magnitudes of the R and Q waves in lead Z and of the S wave in lead X, were significantly increased after sauna bathing. The internal LV dimensions in both diastole and systole tended to be smaller after sauna bathing, although a less pronounced change occurred in systole. The mean hematocrit increased from 44.4% before sauna bathing to 46.3% afterward. The internal LV dimensions by echo in systole and diastole were 44.3 and 30.4 mm before and 40.4 and 30.2 mm after sauna bathing. These findings indicate that a decrease in the intraventricular volume was accompanied by an increase in the body surface potential. In patients therefore who sweat profusely LV hypertrophy may be erroneously diagnosed on ECG.

DIGITAL SUBTRACTION VENTRICULOGRAPHY

Cardiac applications for digital subtraction angiography appear promising, but few correlative studies with contrast ventriculography have been done. Kronenberg and associates[28] from Nashville, Tennessee, evaluated LV volume, EF, and regional wall motion by digital subtraction angiography after intravenous injection of 40 ml of iodinated contrast medium and after LV injection of 5–10 ml of contrast medium. A film-based system of the authors' own design was used. Results were compared with those after direct LV injection of 40 ml of contrast medium. The ventriculograms after intravenous injection were of diagnostic quality in 9 of 12 studies, and there were close correlations between intravenous and direct injection studies for LV EF and for LV volume. Regional wall motion scores showed close correspondence in 83% of sectors. After small volume LV injections, the ventricular image was enhanced considerably by digital subtraction. Correlations between small and large volume ventriculograms were close for LV EF and for LV volume. There was close correspondence of wall motion scores in 87% of sectors. Thus, digital subtraction angiography improves the visibility of the LV after either intravenous or small volume direct LV injection. Digital images produce excellent estimates of LV volume and should have considerable usefulness for the study of cardiac performance and anatomy.

Norris and associates[29] from San Diego, California, used digital images of the LV obtained at 20 frames/s from continuous fluoroscopy after intravenous injection of contrast medium (digital intravenous ventriculography) to estimate LV volumes and EF with the use of several techniques for identifying the ventriculographic silhouette. The digital technique was compared with direct contrast left ventriculography in 26 patients undergoing diagnostic cardiac catheterization. End-diastolic (EDV) and end-systolic volumes (ESV) calculated from digital intravenous and direct left ventriculograms were obtained with use of a standard area-length formula. Both EDV and ESV determined from digital intravenous ventriculography (mask mode images) correlated closely with those obtained by direct left ventriculography. Combining the EDV and ESV to define the relation between the 2 techniques yielded an even closer correlation. There was also good correlation between the 2 techniques for measurement of EF. Measurements from direct left ventriculography were frequently invalidated by ventricular arrhythmias during the time of opacification of the LV; this was rarely the case for digital intravenous ventriculography. It is concluded that area-length estimates of LV volumes and EF can be accurately obtained from digital processing of fluoroscopic LV images after intravenous injection of contrast medium.

Tobis and associates[30] from Orange, California, calculated LV EF from 25 first-pass digital subtraction angiograms using a densitometric analysis. Digital subtraction angiograms were obtained in a computerized format; therefore they can be readily analyzed with computer software to measure the density of the iodine signal within the image. The video signals from the image intensifier were logarithmically amplified so that there was a linear correlation between the video signal intensity and the depth of the iodine contrast material represented by that video signal. The LV EF was also calculated by the area-length method from the same digital subtraction angiograms. There was close correlation between these 2 techniques. The videodensitometric EF technique is simple to perform, it correlates well with the standard area-length method, and it is not dependent on geometric assumptions of LV geometry.

Nissen and associates[31] from Lexington, Kentucky, compared the accuracy and reproducibility of measurements of LV EDV, ESV, EF, and regional wall motion obtained by digital subtraction ventriculography (DSV) with values of direct cineangiography in 40 patients, 21 of whom were ambulatory. The DSV was performed with a 1-second, 30 ml contrast injection, which yielded real-time fluoroimages composed of 512 × 512 pixels at 30 frames/second. Single-plane right anterior oblique LV volumes were calculated by area-length methods for both DSV and cineangiography. Wall motion was assessed as percent area shortening for 12 equal myocardial segments, with results classified as abnormal if greater than 2 SD below the mean of 20 normal values. The DSV technique exhibited close correlation with angiography for EDV, ESV, and EF. Intravenous DSV and direct cineangiography were concordant in classification of LV contractile pattern in 436 of 480 (91%) myocardial segments. Measurements of DSV obtained by 2 observers showed close correlations for EDV, ESV, and EF, and wall motion classification was in agreement in 434 of 480 (90%) LV segments. Artifacts induced by respiratory motion, persistence of contrast in the RV or left atrium, or low cardiac output may have contributed to the discrepancies observed. These data indicate that DSV is accurate in assessing LV volume and EF, correlates well with cineangiography, and exhibits good interobserver reproducibility.

PHARMACOLOGIC TOPICS

Pindolol

Frishman[32] from New York City reviewed pharmacologic features of pindolol and pointed out that pindolol differs from other beta-blocking drugs currently available in the USA because of its partial agonist activity.

Ethanol

Kupari[33] from Helsinki, Finland, examined the acute cardiac effect of ethanol (1 gm/kg orally within 60 minutes) in 22 healthy volunteers by M-mode echo and systolic time intervals for 3 hours after beginning ingestion. Each subject also took part in a control study in which the same volume of juice was substituted for ethanol. Heart rate increased by 15% and cardiac output by 17% during ethanol intake, but total peripheral resistance decreased by 15%. The LV end-diastolic diameter was shortened by 2% during the declining phase of blood ethanol concentration; stroke volume and circumferential wall stress were simultaneously decreased by 7 and 5%, respectively. No ethanol-related changes were noted in echo indices of LV function; neither were any sex differences observed in the cardiovascular changes after ethanol ingestion. Each of the systolic time intervals was significantly altered, even during the control experiment. The responses of each of these intervals to ethanol differed significantly from those in the control test as well. Notably, the preejection period/ejection time ratio rose after ethanol, this change, according to simultaneous echo data, resulting from reduced preload instead of impaired contractility, as maintained in previous investigations. It is concluded that alcohol in modest doses is capable of altering each of the extramyocaridal influences on LV function—heart rate, preload, and afterload—but does not impair myocardial performance, at least in normal subjects.

UNCATEGORIZABLE

Cardiovascular disease in persons ≥90 years of age

Although the average age at death has increased dramatically during this century, the maximum length of life has not changed. The percentage of individuals surviving for 90 years and beyond, however, is increasing. In 1980 about 1% of the USA population was ≥90 years old. Very few autopsies are performed in patients dying after age 90 years (frequency, about 4%) and therefore little attention has been focused on the clinical and morphologic frequencies in types of cardiovascular diseases observed in these very elderly

TABLE 9-2. *Morphologic cardiac observations in 40 necropsy patients aged 90–103 years.*

	PATIENTS	
	N	%
Coronary arterial disease		
Calcium	37	92
Luminal narrowing 76–100% in XSA by atherosclerotic plaques of ≥1 major coronary arteries	28	70
Acute myocardial infarction	10	25
Healed myocardial infarction	14	35
Aortic valve disease		
Calcium	22	55
Stenosis	2	5
Mitral anular disease		
Calcium	19	47
Cardiac amyloidosis (fatal)	4	10
Dilated cardiomyopathy	1	3
Obliterative pericardial disease		
Idiopathic	1	5
Iatrogenic	1	5

TABLE 9-3. *Electrocardiographic observations in 30 patients aged 90–103 years.*

ABNORMALITY	CLINICAL HEART DISEASE		TOTAL	
	PRESENT* (N, 8)	ABSENT (N, 22)	N	%
Atrial fibrillation	5	7	12	40
Abnormal QRS axis			12	40
Left (−30 to −90°)	4	6		
Right (+111 to +210°)	1	1		
Complete (QRS ≥0.12 second) BBB			12	40
Left	6	1		
Right	1	4		
Ventricular premature complexes	4	6	10	33
Atrial premature complexes	1	2	3	10
Heart Block			8	27
P-R interval >0.20 second	3	3		
Second degree	0	1		
Third degree (complete)	1[†]	0		
Q-wave abnormality without BBB			4	13
Q II, III, aV₁	0	1		
Q-S V₁–V₃	0	1		
Both	0	2		
Left ventricular hypertrophy without BBB (R in V₅ or V₆ + S in V₁ ≥35 mm)	1	0	1	3
Low voltage (QRS ≤15 mm in I + II + III)	0	1	1	3

* Coronary heart disease = 3; cardiac amyloidosis = 4; aortic valve stenosis = 1.
† Pacemaker inserted 6 years before death.

persons. To fill this void, Waller and Roberts[34] from Bethesda, Maryland, described clinical and necropsy observations in 40 patients (29 women) ≥90 years old. Most (21 patients [57%]) died during the 4 coldest months, and 12 (30%), during the 4 warmest months. At necropsy, 39 had ≥1 major cardiac abnormalities, the most frequent being calcific deposits in the major epicardial coronary arteries in 37 (92%) (Table 9-2). In 28 patients (70%), 1 or more of the 4 major arteries was narrowed 76–100% in cross-sectional area (XSA) by atherosclerotic plaques, an average of 1.9/4.0 per patient: the 12 patients with clinical events compatible with myocardial ischemia (angina pectoris or AMI) had an average of 2.2/4 and the other 28 patients had an average of 1.0/4.0. In 36 patients, a histologic section was examined from each 5 mm long segment from each of the 4 major coronary arteries: of the 1,789 segments, only 6 (<1%) were narrowed 96–100% in XSA by plaques; 147 (8%), 76–95%; 339 (19%), 51–75%; 930 (52%), 26–50%, and 367 (21%), 0–25%. The average amount of XSA narrowing for the 1,789 segments was about 42%. In 10 patients with clinical evidence of myocardial ischemia, the average amount of narrowing per segment was approximately 55%; in the 26 patients without clinical ischemia, the average was about 38%. Of the 40 patients, 18 (45%) had LV transmural foci of fibrosis or necrosis or both. Of 14 patients with transmural scars, only 1 had a clinical event compatible with AMI; of the 10 with AMI at necropsy, only 4 had typical clinical features of infarction. Calcific deposits were present in ≥1 aortic valve cusps in 22 patients (55%), causing AS in 2, and in the mitral anulus in 19 (47%), probably causing MS in 1. Amyloid deposits were present in the heart in at least 9 patients; they were grossly visible and caused fatal cardiac dysfunction in 4, and microscopically visible only in 5, causing no cardiac dysfunction. Eight patients (20%) had chronic CHF; 27 of 39 (69%) had either a history of systemic hypertension or BP >140/90 mmHg during their final year of life. Precordial murmurs were recorded in 25 (62%) patients, systolic only in 24 and both systolic and diastolic in 1. Data from ECGs were available in 30 patients: 12 (40%) had AF; 12 (40%), abnormal axis; 12, complete BBB; 1, criteria for LV hypertrophy (despite increased cardiac mass in 67%); and 1, low voltage (Table 9-3). All patients had fairly extensive atherosclerosis of the aorta, with aneurysmal formation in 5 with fatal rupture in 3. Five had strokes, which were fatal in 4. At least 5 had leg claudication. Two had massive pulmonary emboli superimposed on chronic obstructive pulmonary disease. Thus, cardiovascular disease was present at necropsy in 39 of the 40 patients, but frequently it was not diagnosed clinically.

Lipomatous hypertrophy of the atrial septum

Fyke and associates[35] from Rochester, Minnesota, identified 17 patients by retrospective analysis of 2-D echo as having features consistent with lipomatous hypertrophy of the atrial septum. The atrial septum viewed from the subcostal transducer position demonstrated a distinctive echo-dense globular thickening that did not involve the valve of the fossa ovalis. The tomographic image of the atrial septum had a dumbbell appearance and the mean thickness of the atrial septum was 21 mm. Seven patients had supraventricular arrhythmias. Thus, there is a distinctive echo alteration of the atrial septum that suggests the diagnosis of lipomatous hypertrophy.

Interpreting chest roentgenogram

In the training of cardiologists, considerable emphasis is placed on learning proper precordial examination and how to obtain and interpret ECGs, echoes, hemodynamics, and contrast and radionuclide angiograms. In contrast, relatively little emphasis is placed on learning how to interpret "routine" radiographs of the chest. Waters and associates[36] from Washington, D.C., and Bethesda, Maryland, described a simple technique to aid in the interpretation of the cardiac and aortic silhouette on the chest roentgenogram (Fig. 9-1). A 3 × 5 inch (7.6 ± 12.7 mm) card is cut so that it is square (3 × 3 inches) (7.6 × 7.6 mm). On the card, 4 equal-sized circles are drawn, as demonstrated in Fig. 9-1, upper left. After the structures are drawn on the card, the ends of a pipe-cleaning wick are placed through the aortic valve and descending aorta and secured by bending the wire on the back of the card. The wick then represents the ascending, transverse, and proximal descending thoracic aorta. The bottom of the card represents the anterior chest wall, the right edge, the right side of the chest, the top, the posterior wall, and the left edge, the left lateral wall of the chest. The card can now be viewed from the front (Fig. 9-1, upper left), left lateral position (Fig. 9-1, upper right), left anterior oblique (LAO) position (Fig. 9-1, lower left), and right anterior oblique (RAO) position (Fig. 9-1, lower right) simply by rotating the card. In the left lateral position the RV chamber is the most anterior and the LA chamber is the most posterior. The LV and RA chambers are midway in between. In the LAO position the RA and RV chambers are to the left and the LA and LV, to the right. This is the best view for seeing the ascending and descending thoracic aorta (Ao). In the RAO position right and left atria form the right lateral border and the right and left ventricles, the left lateral border. The ascending and descending thoracic aorta are superimposed.

Diagnosis of cardiac injury from blunt trauma by radionuclide angiography

Sutherland and associates[37] from London, Canada, prospectively evaluated 77 patients who had sustained multisystem trauma, including severe blunt chest trauma, to assess the frequency of associated traumatic myocardial injury. Traumatic injury to either the right or left ventricle was defined by the presence of discrete abnormalities of wall motion by ECG gated cardiac scintigraphy in patients without a clinical history of heart disease. Forty-two patients (55%) (group 1) had focal abnormalities of wall motion; 27 involved the right ventricle, 7 the left ventricle, 7 were biventricular, and 1 involved only the septum. Both the right and LV EFs were significantly (p < 0.01) lower (31 ± 11% and 47 ± 14%, respectively) than those in the 35 traumatized patients without wall motion abnormalities on scintigraphy (group 2) (49 ± 8% and 58 ± 11%, respectively). Repeat scintigraphic examination in 32 group 1 patients at a time remote from initial injury showed improvement or resolution of previously defined focal wall motion abnormalities in 27 patients (84%). The ECG and serum enzyme tests were insensitive indexes of traumatic myocardial injury when defined by the scintigraphic abnormalities. Thus, severe blunt chest trauma results in a higher frequency of traumatic myocardial injury than heretofore recognized, and frequently involves the anteriorly situated right ventricle.

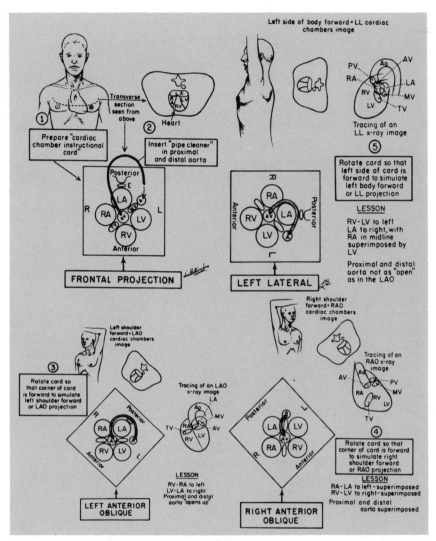

Fig. 9-1. Technique for interpreting the cardiac and aortic silhouette on the chest roentgenogram. Ao = aorta; AV = aortic valve; MV = mitral valve; PV = pulmonic valve; TV = tricuspid valve; A = descending thoracic aorta; E = esophagus; LAO = left anterior oblique; LL = left lateral; RAO = right anterior oblique.

Left atrial myxoma

Salcedo and associates[38] from Cleveland, Ohio, evaluated 25 patients with LA myxoma to determine echo features. All patients had M-mode echo and 14 had 2-D evaluations. The data obtained demonstrated that most patients with LA myxoma have a detectable "mass" of extraneous echoes in the left atrium. The only other consistent abnormality on M-mode study was a decreased EF slope of the mitral valve. The LA, RV, LV end-diastolic, and LV end-systolic dimensions were usually normal. Two-D echo identified the presence of a LA myxoma in all 14 patients studied by this technique, and it also provided additional information concerning size, shape, mobility, and site of insertion of the tumor. Thus, these data indicate that echo is a sensitive means for detecting and visualizing LA myxoma and that 2-D echo provides important information concerning size, shape, and site of insertion of the tumor.

Ultrasonic tissue characterization

Interactions between an ultrasonic signal and cardiac tissue have been used to characterize the histologic state of myocardium in vitro. To assess the utility of in vivo ultrasonic tissue characterization, Green and associates[39] from Stanford, California, applied stochastic analysis to the digitized echo signals from 15 patients with 2-D echoes suggesting intracardiac masses. Ten subjects with echoes suggesting mural thrombi underwent subsequent surgery or necropsy, which confirmed thrombi in 6 and revealed no thrombi (designated artifact) in 4. Five other patients had intracardiac tumors. The amplitudes within the digitized ultrasonic signals were displayed as histograms, which were described by a parameter k that represented the degree to which each histogram departed from a totally random probability density function. In 5 of 6 thrombi k = 0, but in all 4 artifacts, k > 0. The sixth thrombus had k = 0.5 due to the specular effect of the interface between the 2 lobes of the thrombus. All 5 tumors had k > 0. Ultrasonic tissue characterization using a stochastic analysis of backscatter can be performed in vivo and helps differentiate thrombus from artifact and tumor in the heart.

Intracardiac thrombi by computed tomography

Tomoda and associates[40] from Kanagawa, Japan, evaluated LA and LV thrombi by computed tomography (CT) in 56 patients. The patients were divided into group I, 28 patients with mitral valve disease, and group II, 28 patients with AMI. Two-D echo and CT were performed in all the patients studied. Cineangiocardiography was performed in all group I and in 13 group II patients. Open heart surgery or autopsy was performed in all group I and 4 group II patients. The sensitivity in detecting LA thrombus was 100% with CT, 70% with angiocardiography, and 60% with 2-D echo. The specificity in detecting LA thrombus was 91% with CT, 86% with 2-D echo, and 88% with angiocardiography. Thrombi located at the LA appendage were associated with great difficulties in detection by other methods, but were well delineated with CT. The LV thrombus was also visualized by CT with similar or greater accuracy than other diagnostic methods, although the sensitivity and specificity were not ascertained because surgery or autopsy was performed in only a few group II patients. Therefore, as far as the detection of intracardiac thrombus is concerned, CT has the advantage of offering uniform slices of the heart in an attempt to detect thrombi in unknown areas of cardiac chambers, including the LA appendage or LV apex, without being disturbed by the surrounding cardiac and noncardiac structures. Thus, CT has excellent accuracy in the detection of intracardia thrombus.

TABLE 9-4. *Comparison of the regular issues of 4 major USA cardiovascular journals for 1983.*

	AJC		CIRCU-LATION		JACC		AHJ	
Number pages (average/ month)	3250	(271)	2982	(249)	2679	(223)	2231	(186)
For articles (pages/ article)	3130	(4.9)	2793	(7.7)	2569	(7.6)	2096	(5.3)
For letters (number)	27	(53)	21	(19)	22	(18)	50	(43)
For abstracts (number)	0		0		0		0	
For society news	0		96		9		0	
For nonsociety news	0		0		0		0	
For books	2		0		3		9	
For indexes	79		58		52		52	
For information for authors	12		14		24		24	
For blank pages	0		0		0		0	
Number articles (average/ month)	643	(54)	362	(30)	337	(28)	392	(33)
Coronary heart disease	132	(20.5%)	92	(25.4%)	70	(20.8%)	87	(22.2%)
Arrhythmias & CD	74	(11.5%)	40	(11.0%)	40	(11.9%)	38	(9.7%)
Systemic hypertension	18	(2.9%)	10	(2.8%)	6	(1.8%)	9	(2.3%)
Congestive heart failure	22	(3.4%)	16	(4.4%)	15	(4.4%)	8	(2.0%)
Valvular heart disease	47	(7.3%)	16	(4.4%)	19	(5.6%)	14	(3.6%)
Cardiomyopathy	22	(3.4%)	10	(2.8%)	8	(2.4%)	10	(2.5%)
Pericardial heart disease	3	(0.5%)	1	(0.3%)	5	(1.5%)	1	(0.3%)
Congenital heart disease	79	(12.3%)	23	(6.3%)	21	(6.2%)	17	(4.3%)
Miscellaneous	36	(5.6%)	22	(6.1%)	13	(3.9%)	15	(3.8%)
Methods	29	(4.5%)	16	(4.4%)	34	(10.1%)	11	(2.8%)
Experimental Studies	52	(8.1%)	86	(23.8%)	48	(14.2%)	47	(12.0%)
Editorials & point of view	19	(2.9%)	6	(1.7%)	15	(4.4%)	24	(6.1%)
C-V pharmacology & therapy	5	(0.8%)	8	(2.2%)	7	(2.1%)	6	(1.5%)
Historical studies	10	(1.6%)	2	(0.5%)	5	(1.5%)	0	
Brief reports (case reports)	81	(12.6%)	13	(3.6%)	28	(8.3%)	105	(26.8%)
From-the-editor	14	(2.2%)	1	(0.3%)	3*	(0.9%)	0	
Number figures (per article)	2033	(3.2)	1759	(4.9)	1363	(4.0)	1204	(3.1)
Number of tables (per article)	1154	(1.8)	804	(2.2)	635	(1.9)	630	(1.6)
Number authors (per article)	3051	(4.7)	1895	(5.2)	1476	(4.4)	1775	(4.5)
Individual subscription (USA)	$52.00		$46.00		$50.00		$41.00	
Number subscribers	28,000		24,000		20,000		12,000	

Abbreviations: AJC = American Journal of Cardiology; AHJ = American Heart Journal; JACC = Journal of the American College of Cardiology; CD = conduction disturbances; CV = cardiovascular.
* Two were by guest editors.

Effect of verapamil on LV function

Verapamil has a negative inotropic action in isolated cardiac muscle. Its effects on LV function were tested by Vlietstra and associates[41] from Rochester, Minnesota, in 25 patients with suspected CAD. A double-blind, randomized, placebo-controlled study design was used. Verapamil (0.2

TABLE 9-5. *Comparison of the regular issues of 3 non–USA English language cardiovascular journals for 1983.*

	BHJ	EHJ[a]	IJC[b]
Number pages (avg/month)	1,257 (105)	995 (83)	1,244 (104)
For articles (pages/article)	1,171 (6.0)	872 (6.7)	1,063 (5.6)
For letters (number)	20 (12)	1 (2)	7 (3)
For abstracts (number)	24 (67)	0	0
For society news	2	60[c]	0
For non-society news	0	0	37
For books	0	23	2
For indexes	39	29[d]	49
For information for authors	0	10	18
For blank pages	1	0	68
Number articles (avg/month)	195 (16)	131 (11)	190 (16)
Coronary heart disease	43 (22.1%)	38 (29.0%)	18 (9.5%)
Arrhythmias & CD	10 (5.1%)	19 (14.5%)	6 (3.2%)
Systemic hypertension	3 (1.5%)	7 (5.3%)	0
Congestive heart failure	6 (3.1%)	3 (2.3%)	0
Valvular heart disease	20 (10.3%)	13 (9.9%)	1 (0.5%)
Cardiomyopathy	8 (4.1%)	2 (1.5%)	1 (0.5%)
Pericardial heart disease	1 (0.5%)	1 (0.8%)	0
Congenital heart disease	30 (15.4%)	8 (6.1%)	1 (0.5%)
Miscellaneous	19 (9.7%)	12 (9.2%)	7 (3.7%)
Methods	8 (4.1%)	4 (3.1%)	1 (0.5%)
Experimental studies	0	4 (3.1%)	5 (2.6%)
Editorials & Point of View	11 (5.6%)	1 (0.8%)	112 (59.0%)
CV pharmacology & therapy	4 (2.1%)	7 (5.3%)	2 (1.0%)
Historical studies	1 (0.5%)	0	6 (3.2%)
Brief reports (case reports)	31 (15.9%)	6 (4.6%)	27 (14.2%)
From-the-Editor	0	6 (4.5%)	3 (1.6%)
Number figures (per article)	668 (3.4)	365 (2.8)	234 (1.2)
Number tables (per article)	321 (1.6)	296 (2.3)	138 (0.7)
Number authors (per article)	753 (3.9)	575 (4.4)	442 (2.3)
Individual subscription (USA)	$109.00	$70.50	$35.00
Number subscribers	5,500	1,800	1,500

[a] At the time that this table was prepared, the December regular issue of the EHJ had not arrived. Thus, these numbers are based on compilations of 11 issues (January–November) plus the average numbers for 1 additional issue so that the totals are for 12 months or 12 issues.

[b] Ten rather than 12 issues of this Journal were published in 1983. These tabulations include numbers 3 and 4 of volume 2 (a single issue), numbers 5 and 6 of volume 2 (a single issue), all 4 numbers of volume 3 (April, May, June and July) and all 4 numbers of volume 4 (August, September, October and November/December).

[c] The quality of the paper used for these pages was inferior to that used for the other pages.

[d] This number is an estimate because the December 1983 issue had not been published when this table was prepared.

Abbreviations: BHJ—British Heart Journal; EHJ—European Heart Journal; IJC—International Journal of Cardiology; CD—conduction disturbance; CV—cardiovascular.

mg/kg over 10 minutes) significantly lowered mean arterial pressure (from 105–89 mmHg) while increasing the cardiac index (from 2.8–3.1 liters/min/M^2). No statistically significant effect was seen on heart rate, LV end-diastolic pressure or end-systolic volume index, EF, peak rates of systolic wall thickening or diastolic wall thinning, or percentage of hemiaxial shortening. However, there was a small increase in the LV end-diastolic volume index (from 94–102 ml/M^2). Important findings were a reduction in systemic vascular resistance (from 39–30 U · M^2), an increase in LV end-diastolic volume index consistent with a negative inotropic effect, and no evidence of improved regional wall dynamics in portions of the LV wall considered hypokinetic because of myocardial ischemia.

Comparison of 7 English language cardiology journals for 1983

Roberts[42] analyzed and compared 7 English language cardiology journals for the year 1983 in terms of numbers of pages, articles, types of articles, figures and tables published, and numbers of authors per article. The 7 journals included the 4 major USA cardiology journals—*American Journal of Cardiology* (AJC), *Circulation*, *Journal of the American College of Cardiology* (JACC), and *American Heart Journal* (AHJ)—and 3 non-USA journals—*British Heart Journal* (BHJ), *European Heart Journal* (EHJ), and *International Journal of Cardiology* (IJC) (Tables 9-4 and 9-5). Although *Circulation* published the most total pages (because of its huge abstract issue), the AJC published more total pages for articles, the most articles (in its regular issue, 44% more than *Circulation*, 48% more than JACC, 39% more than AHJ) and the AJC provided the most words per page (its maximal number being 20% higher than the maximal number in *Circulation*, 16% higher than in JACC, and 26% higher than in AHJ). Each of the 3 non-USA journals was much smaller in terms of pages and articles published than were any of the USA journals. In types of articles published, several differences among the 7 journals were apparent. Of the articles concerning experimental (nonhuman) studies *Circulation* had 24%, JACC had 14%, AHJ had 12%, AJC had 8%, and it was zero or nearly so in BHJ, EHJ, and IJC. Brief reports accounted for 27% of the 392 articles in AHJ and 13% of the 643 articles in AJC. Of the 190 articles in IJC, 112 (59%) were editorials and 14% were brief reports. Articles concerning systemic hypertension accounted for only 2% of the 2,250 articles published in the regular issues of all 7 journals. The 4 USA journals averaged 4.7 authors per article and the 3 non-USA journals, 3.4 authors per article.

References

1. Roberts WC, Roberts JD: The floating heart or the heart too fat to sink: analysis of 55 necropsy patients. Am J Cardiol 52:1286–1289, Dec 1983.
2. Isner JM, Carter BL, Roberts WC, Bankoff MS: Subepicardial adipose tissue producing echocardiographic appearance of pericardial effusion: Documentation by computed tomography and necropsy. Am J Cardiol 51:565–569, Feb 1983.
3. Savage DD, Garrison RJ, Brand F, Anderson SJ, Castelli WP, Kannel WB, Feinleib M:

Prevalence and correlates of posterior extra echocardiographic spaces in a free-living population based sample (the Framingham study). Am J Cardiol 51:1207–1212, Apr 1983.

4. WEISS JM, SPODICK DH: Association of left pleural effusion with pericardial disease. N Engl J Med 308:696–697, March 24, 1983.

5. CHANDRARATNA PA, REID CL, NIMALASURIYA A, KAWANISHI D, RAHIMTOOLA SH: Application of 2-dimensional contrast studies during pericardiocentesis. Am J Cardiol 52:1120–1122, Nov 1983.

6. BATEMAN TM, MASSUMI R, GRAY RJ, CHAUX A, DEROBERTIS MA, BROWN DE, MATLOFF JM, BERMAN DS: Noninvasive detection of active pericardial bleeding using cardiac blood pool scintigraphy. Am J Cardiol 51:329–331, Jan 1983.

7. GILLAM LD, GUYER DE, GIBSON TC, KING ME, MARSHALL JE, WEYNAM AE: Hydrodynamic compression of the right atrium: a new echocardiographic sign of cardiac tamponade. Circulation 68:294–301, Aug 1983.

8. GOTTDIENER JS, KATIN MJ, BORER JS, BACHARACH SL, GREEN MV: Late cardiac effects of therapeutic mediastinal irradiation: assessment by echocardiography and radionuclide angiography. N Engl J Med 308:569–572, March 10, 1983.

9. APPLEFELD MM, WIERNIK PH: Cardiac disease after radiation therapy for Hodgkin's disease: analysis of 48 patients. Am J Cardiol 51:1679–1681, June 1983.

10. BUFALINO VJ, ROBINSON JA, HENKIN R, O'CONNELL J, GUNNARY R: Gallium-67 scanning: a new diagnostic approach to the post-pericardiotomy syndrome. Am Heart J 106:1138–1143, Nov 1983.

11. BLAKE S, BONAR S, O'NEILL H, HANLY P, DRURY I, FLANAGAN M, GARRETT J: Aetiology of chronic constrictive pericarditis. Br Heart J 50:273–276, Sept 1983.

12. JANOS GG, ARJUNAN K, MEYER RA, ENGEL P, KAPLAN S: Differentiation of constrictive pericarditis and restrictive cardiomyopathy using digitized echocardiography. J Am Coll Cardiol 1:541–549, Feb 1983.

13. LEIER CV, BAMBACH D, NELSON S, HERMILLER JB, HUSS P, MAGORIEN RD, UNVERFERTH DV: Captopril in primary pulmonary hypertension. Circulation 67:155–161, Jan 1983.

14. RUBIN LJ, NICOD P, HILLIS D, FIRTH BG: Treatment of primary pulmonary hypertension with nifedipine. Ann Intern Med 99:433–438, Oct 1983.

15. RICH S, GANZ R, LEVY PS: Comparative actions of hydralazine, nifedipine and amrinone in primary pulmonary hypertension. Am J Cardiol 52:1104–1107, Nov 1983.

16. GARCIA-DORADO D, MILLER DD, GARCIA EJ, DELCAN JL, MAROTO E, CHAITMAN BR: An epidemic of pulmonary hypertension after toxic rapeseed oil ingestion in Spain. J Am Coll Cardiol 1:1216–1222, May 1983.

17. BRENT BN, BERGER HJ, MATTHAY RA, MAHLER D, PYTLIK L, ZARET BL: Contrasting acute effects of vasodilators (nitroglycerin, nitroprusside, and hydralazine) on right ventricular performance in patients with chronic obstructive pulmonary disease and pulmonary hypertension: a combined radionuclide-hemodynamic study. Am J Cardiol 51:1682–1688, June 1983.

18. MEHROTRA PP, WEAVER YJ, HIGGINBOTHAM EA: Myocardial perfusion defect on thallium-201 imaging in patients with chronic obstructive pulmonary disease. J Am Coll Cardiol 2:233–239, Aug 1983.

19. MORRISON D, CALDWELL J, LAKSHMINARYAN S, RITCHIE JL, KENNEDY JW: The acute effects of low flow oxygen and isosorbide dinitrate on left and right ventricular ejection fractions in chronic obstructive pulmonary disease. J Am Coll Cardiol 2:652–660, Oct 1983.

20. HUNG J, GOLDWATER D, CONVERTINO VA, McKILLOP JH, GORIS ML, DEBUSK RF: Mechanisms for decreased exercise capacity after bed rest in normal middle-aged men. Am J Cardiol 51:344–348, Jan 1983.

21. DEBUSK RF, CONVERTINO VA, HUNG J, GOLDWATER D: Exercise conditioning in middle-aged men after 10 days of bed rest. Circulation 68:245–250, Aug 1983.

22. SCHOCKEN DD, BLUMENTHAL JA, PORT S, HINDLE P, COLEMAN RE: Physical conditioning and left ventricular performance in the elderly: assessment by radionuclide angiocardiography. Am J Cardiol 52:359–364, Aug 1983.

23. Spirito P, Maron BJ, Bonow RO, Epstein SE: Prevalence and significance of an abnormal S-T segment response to exercise in a young athletic population. Am J Cardiol 51:1663–1666, June 1983.

24. Sugishita Y, Koseki S, Matsuda M, Yamaguchi T, Ito I: Myocardial mechanics of athletic hearts in comparison with diseased hearts. Am Heart J 105:273–280, Feb 1983.

25. Siegel AJ, Silverman LM, Evans WJ: Elevated skeletal muscle creatine kinase MB isoenzyme levels in marathon runners. JAMA 250:2835–2837, Nov 25, 1983.

26. Fagard R, Aubert A, Lysens R, Staessen J, Vanhees L, Amery A: Noninvasive assessment of seasonal variations in cardiac structure and function in cyclists. Circulation 67:896–901, Apr 1983.

27. Ishikawa K, Shirato C, Yanagisawa A: Electrocardiographic changes due to sauna bathing: influence of acute reduction in circulating blood volume on body surface potentials with special reference to the Brody effect. Br Heart J 50:469–475, Nov 1983.

28. Kronenberg MW, Price RR, Smith CW, Robertson RM, Perry JM, Pickens DR, Domanski MJ, Partain L, Friesinger GC: Evaluation of left ventricular performance using digital subtraction angiography. Am J Cardiol 51:837–842, March 1983.

29. Norris SL, Slutsky RA, Mancini J, Ashburn WL, Gregoratos G, Peterson KL, Higgins CB, Einsidler E, Dillon W: Comparison of digital intravenous ventriculography with direct left ventriculography for quantitation of left ventricular volumes and ejection fractions. Am J Cardiol 51:1399–1403, May 1983.

30. Tobis J, Nalcioglu O, Seibert A, Johnston WD, Henry WL: Measurement of left ventricular ejection fraction by videodensitometric analysis of digital subtraction angiograms. Am J Cardiol 52:871–875, Oct 1983.

31. Nissen SE, Booth D, Waters J, Fassas T, Demaria AN: Evaluation of left ventricular contractile pattern by intravenous digital subtraction ventriculography: comparison with cineangiography and assessment of interobserver variability. Am J Cardiol 52:1293–1298, Dec 1983.

32. Frishman WH: Pindolol: a new β-adrenoceptor antagonist with partial agonist activity. N Engl J Med 308:940–944, Apr 21, 1983.

33. Kupari: Acute cardiovascular effects of ethanol: a controlled non-invasive study. Br Heart J 49:174–182, Feb 1983.

34. Waller BF, Roberts WC: Cardiovascular disease in the very elderly: analysis of 40 necropsy patients aged 90 years or over. Am J Cardiol 51:403–421, Feb 1983.

35. Fyke FE, Tajik AJ, Edwards WD, Seward JB: Diagnosis of lipomatous hypertrophy of the atrial septum by two-dimensional echocardiography. J Am Coll Cardiol 1:1352–1357, May 1983.

36. Waters TJ, Rubin RE, Roberts WC: A simple method to interpret cardiac and aortic anatomy from chest radiographs. Am J Cardiol 52:644–645, Sept 1983.

37. Sutherland GR, Driedger AA, Holliday RL, Cheung HW, Sibbald WJ: Frequency of myocardial injury after blunt chest trauma as eveluted by radionuclide angiography. Am J Cardiol 52:1099–1103, Nov 1983.

38. Salcedo EE, Adams KV, Lever HM, Gill CC, Lombardo H: Echocardiographic findings in 25 patients with left atrial myxoma. J Am Coll Cardiol 1:1162–1166, Apr 1983.

39. Green SE, Joynt LF, Fitzgerald PJ, Rubenson DS, Popp RL: In vivo ultrasonic tissue characterization of human intracardiac masses. Am J Cardiol 51:231–236, Jan 1983.

40. Tomoda H, Hoshiai M, Furuya H, Kuribayash S, Ootaki M, Matsuyama S, Koide S, Kawada S, Shotsu A: Evaluation of intracardiac thrombus with computed tomography. Am J Cardiol 51:843–852, March 1983.

41. Vliestra RE, Farias MAC, Frye RL, Smith HC, Ritman E: Effect of verapamil on left ventricular function: a randomized, placebo-controlled study. Am J Cardiol 51:1213–1217, Apr 1983.

42. Roberts WC: Comparison of 7 English-language cardiology journals for 1983. Am J Cardiol 53:862–869, March 1, 1984.

Author Index

Ueda K, 388
Uhl GS, 163
Ulvenstam G, 162
Untereker WJ, 285
Unverferth BJ, 325
Unverferth DV, 325, 328,
402, 403, 406, 423
Urban PL, 145
Uretsky BF, 407
Uretz E, 185
Urrutia-S CO, 384
Ursell PC, 344
Uther JB, 123

Vaislic C, 93
Val PG, 90
Valantine H, 42
Valdellon B, 135
Valdes-Cruz LM, 355, 366,
377
Valfre C, 385
Valkenburg HA, 249
Valle M, 45, 76
Van de Carr S, 163
Van Den Brand M, 152
van der Wall EE, 146
van der Werf T, 305
Van Dyk D, 240
van Eenige MJ, 146
van Engelen CLJ, 146
van Hoogenhuijze E, 287
Van Praagh R, 385
Van Trigt P, 87
Vance WS, 44
Vandenbrand MJBM, 83
Vandermoten PP, 45
VanDoesburg NH, 361,
377
Vanhees L, 428
Vardan S, 237, 253, 258
Vargas Barron J, 377
Varghese PJ, 17
Varma VM, 3
Vartiainen E, 252
Vasiliedes AJ, 334
Vedin A, 159, 162
Ventemiglia R, 385
Ventura HO, 243, 256
Verdel G, 305
Verdouw PD, 142
Vered Z, 295
Verghese CP, 181, 203
Vessey MP, 37
Vetrovec GW, 96
Victor E, 343

Victor MF, 266
Viet TT, 269
Vignola PA, 12
Vilarem C, 221
Villar J, 253
Virmani R, 345
Visser CA, 295
Visser FC, 146
Vlay SC, 193
Vliestra RE, 15, 96, 145,
438
Vohringer HF, 154
Volpin N, 39
Von Der Lippe G, 125
Von Olshausen K, 147
Vukovich RA, 253
Vuylsteek, 41

Waagstein F, 159
Wackers FJ, 11, 43, 345
Wagner GS, 6, 85, 122,
123
Wagstaff D, 404
Waites TF, 77
Wakasugi T, 30
Waldenstrom A, 159
Waldenstrom J, 159
Waldhausen JA, 376
Waldman JD, 376, 387
Waldo AL, 190, 210
Waleffe A, 208
Walinsky P, 145
Walker WE, 150
Walker WS, 181
Wallace RB, 302
Waller BF, 99, 333, 338,
433
Waller JL, 96
Wallsh E, 96
Walsh CK, 211
Walsh T, 406
Walton JA, 146
Wappel MA, 293
Ward DE, 42, 286
Warner R, 237, 253, 258
Warner RA, 114, 224
Warnes CA, 305, 309, 377
Warnica JW, 158
Waspe LE, 200, 207
Wasserman AG, 3, 17
Watanabe A, 30
Waters DD, 44, 64, 66, 67
Waters J, 430
Waters TJ, 434
Watkins L, 208

Watson DD, 77, 412
Watson RDS, 256
Watson RM, 62
Watt DAL, 133
Watt EW, 77
Watt GCM, 243
Waugh RA, 6
Waumett JD, 387
Waxman A, 9
Waxman HL, 140, 186,
192, 194, 195, 200, 202,
209, 214
Wayne VS, 223
Weaver YJ, 425
Webb-Peploe MM, 399
Weber KT, 405
Weber L, 409
Weber MA, 246, 258
Weber P, 252
Wechsler AS, 87
Wedel H, 159, 162
Wegscheider K, 154
Wei JY, 116, 145, 157, 243
Weightman, 280
Weiler–Ravell D, 48, 60
Weiner DA, 19, 51, 52
Weinrich DJ, 2
Weins RD, 90
Weinstein IR, 307
Weinstein L, 288
Weintraub RM, 86
Weintraub WS, 8
Weisel RD, 90
Weisfeldt ML, 157, 409
Weiss JL, 157, 409
Weiss JM, 420
Weiss MB, 344
Weiss R, 146
Weiss RJ, 396
Weiss ST, 247
Weissman RH, 222
Wellens HJJ, 127, 140,
183, 194, 208
Welles FC, 384
Wellons HL, 77
Wells W, 355
Welson CS, 363
Wenger NK, 167
Werner JA, 193
Werner JC, 376
Wertz CE, 396
Westerman GR, 362
Wexler J, 399
Wexler LF, 15
Weyman A, 381
Weyman AE, 380

Subject Index